PSYCHOPATHOLOGY

PSYCHOPATHOLOGY

Lee Willerman
University of Texas at Austin

David B. Cohen
University of Texas at Austin

McGRAW-HILL PUBLISHING COMPANY

New York St. Louis San Francisco Auckland Bogotá Caracas
Hamburg Lisbon London Madrid Mexico Milan Montreal New Delhi
Oklahoma City Paris San Juan São Paulo Singapore Sydney Tokyo Toronto

This book was set in Times Roman by the College Composition Unit in cooperation with Waldman Graphics, Inc.
The editors were James D. Anker and David Dunham;
the production supervisor was Leroy A. Young.
The cover was designed by Tony Paccione.
R. R. Donnelley & Sons Company was printer and binder.

PSYCHOPATHOLOGY

2 3 4 5 6 7 8 9 0 **DOH DOH**   9 4 3 2 1 0

ISBN 0-07-070311-6

Library of Congress Cataloging-in-Publication Data

Willerman, Lee, (date).
    Psychopathology / Lee Willerman, David B. Cohen.
        p.   cm.—(McGraw-Hill series in psychology)
    Includes bibliographical references.
    ISBN 0-07-070311-6
    1. Psychology, Pathological.   2. Biological psychiatry.
I. Cohen, David B., (date).   II. Title.   III. Series.
RC454.W535   1990
616.89—dc20   89-12793

ABOUT
THE AUTHORS

After obtaining his Ph.D. in clinical psychology from Wayne State University in 1967, Lee Willerman was a research psychologist at the National Institute of Neurological Diseases and Stroke until 1970. From 1970 to 71 he was an NIH Postdoctoral Fellow in the Department of Human Genetics at the University of Michigan Medical School. In 1971 he moved to the University of Texas at Austin, where he is now the Sarah M. and Charles E. Seay Regents Professor in Clinical Psychology and Director of the Clinical Psychology Training Program. He has authored many articles in scientific journals and has written *The Psychology of Individual and Group Differences* (1979) and coedited *Readings about Individual and Group Differences* (1979). His research interests are in the biological bases and behavior genetics of intelligence, personality, and psychopathology.

David B. Cohen, a native Brooklynite, received his B.A. degree in 1963 from Columbia College before moving to Ann Arbor as a doctoral student in the graduate program in clinical psychology at the University of Michigan. In 1969 he moved to the University of Texas at Austin to become a member of the clinical psychology program where he is now Professor of Psychology. His major research interests include the psychology of dreaming, personality, and abnormal behavior. His research on the recall, content, and function of dreams resulted in numerous articles, book chapters, and a book, *Sleep and Dreaming: Origins, Nature, and Functions (1979)*. His interests in personality and abnormal behavior are directed in particular to questions about the biological mechanisms and risk factors in psychopathology and their implications for the classification of psychiatric disorders.

To Benné and Leslie

CONTENTS

PREFACE

All textbooks on abnormal behavior typically combine two general aspects of behavior disorders: the *psychopathological* aspect of causes and mechanisms revealed by theory and research, and the *clinical* aspect of assessment and treatment. Although this book is no exception, its title, *Psychopathology,* suggests a major focus on the causes and mechanisms of abnormal behavior. In keeping with current theory and research in psychopathology, we give special emphasis to genetics, neurology, and neuropsychology when warranted by the evidence, but try to couch the material at a level accessible to students with little or no background in these fields.

The psychopathological emphasis depends on the particular question being asked, however. Causes differ among disorders so that the accent for some disorders such as schizophrenia and manic-depression will be on biological causation, whereas for others psychological and social factors will be of greater relevance.

Despite limited knowledge about the causes of abnormal behavior, we are inherently optimistic. We believe that many yet unresolved questions will eventually yield answers through scientific research. The real challenge, as we see it, is to ask the right questions about abnormality, questions that narrow down the possibilities and zero in on the essence of each disorder.

Compared to other texts, our book has somewhat more technical description and analysis of environmental, genetic, and biological mechanisms. The section on facets of psychopathology (Chapters 5-8) may be particularly challenging because it introduces concepts and vocabulary that may be unfamiliar to many readers. Nevertheless, we believe that an effort to understand these chapters will pay off in deeper knowledge about the specific disorders discussed in more detail later, in the third section of the book. It is our greatest hope that some readers will be sufficiently motivated by the material to embark on careers in psychopathology. There is much yet to be discovered, and it will take the efforts of many insightful investigators to advance the field significantly.

ACKNOWLEDGMENTS

A book like this depends on the work of many people. In particular we want to thank Professors Irving Gottesman, University of Virginia; Brian Kolb, University of Lethbridge; and S. J. Rachman, University of British Columbia, who critically read an early draft of the entire manuscript; their incisive and penetrating analyses were of inestimable value to shaping the eventual form and substance of the work. We want to give special acknowledgment to colleagues—in particular, to Erin Bigler, Jan Bruell, Arnold Buss, Steve Finn, Edna Foa, Joe Horn, John Loehlin, Gerry Metalsky, Sue Mineka, Tim Schallert, and Michael Telch—for their enthusiastic encouragement and generous help. We also wish to thank the many other reviewers whose comments on the manuscript were very helpful in its development: Stanley Berent, University of Michigan; Paul H. Blaney, University of Miami; Clifford L. Fawl, Nebraska Wesleyan University; Russell Leaf, Rutgers University; Boyd S. Richards, University of New Brunswick; Dennis P. Saccuzzo, San Diego State University; Dennison Smith, Oberlin College; Herman A. Walters, University of Montana; and David G. Weight, Brigham Young University. We are most grateful to Cheryl Kupper for her gentle but forceful guidance for improving the organization, logic, and clarity of the exposition. Finally, we want to thank Patty Ardies, Cheri Lourcey, Cathy Papke, Marie Stephens, and especially Sonia Prideaux, whose typing, photocopying, and other administrative efforts were carried out with uncommon faithfulness, cheerfulness, and forbearance.

Lee Willerman

David B. Cohen

PSYCHOPATHOLOGY

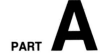

GENERAL INTRODUCTION

Concepts of Psychopathology

OUTLINE

In 1969 Charles Manson, a charismatic leader of an obscure cult, was found guilty, along with several of his followers, of brutally torturing and murdering a pregnant movie starlet and two of her houseguests. Manson believed that these murders would create a race war from which he would emerge a leader. The trial captured much publicity partly because the murderers seemed so bizarre: they held strange ideas, were unrepentant, and worshipped Manson.

Manson was the child of a neglectful, unwed, alcoholic mother, herself convicted of armed robbery when the boy was 5. At age 12 Manson had been placed in a home for boys because his mother could not find foster care. At 13 he began a life of crime that led to more than twenty years in various institutions, some quite brutal. On the day of his last release before the murders, he pleaded unsuccessfully to remain behind bars because he could not "adjust to the outside world." Manson had resisted formal schooling and could barely read and write, although his IQ was in the average range. A caseworker earlier had reported that he was "aggressively antisocial" and "definitely in need of some psychiatric" treatment. After his last arrest Manson said:

> ...I haven't decided yet what I am or who I am. I was given a name in a cell with a name and a number....I never went to school, so I never growed up in the respect to learn, to read and write too good. So I stayed in that jail and I have stayed stupid. I have ate out of your garbage cans to stay out of jail....I have done my best to get along in your world and now you want to kill me....Ha! I'm already dead, have been dead all my life. I've lived in your tomb that you built. I did seven years for a $37.50 check. I did 12 years because I didn't have any parents....When you were out riding your bicycle, I was sitting in your cell looking out the window (Wooden, 1980, p. 54)

The Manson case is clearly extreme by most standards of behavioral abnormality. Few people, whether disturbed or not, are capable of being so charismatic, and people with mental disorders, even those who are primarily antisocial, rarely become murderers. Manson's behavior is especially interesting because it raises many basic questions about abnormality: How does it arise, what maintains it, how can it be treated, and could it have been prevented?

In Manson's case there are many adverse factors that could have caused or contributed to his chronic behavioral peculiarities. We would like to know, for example, whether Manson's bizarre antisocial behavior was caused by his mother's neglect, what abuse he experienced in institutions, and/or an whether there was inherited abnormality.

Unfortunately, it is usually difficult to disentangle and evaluate all potential explanations for the behavior of any single person, let alone someone as unusual as Manson. Manson's history is unique and it is unlikely that other people with similar experiences would have committed grisly murders or attracted worshipful followers.

Only by examining groups of roughly similar cases can the various possible explanations be evaluated. We are on firmer scientific ground when we ask "How can we explain people like Manson?" than when we ask "Why did Manson turn out the way he did?" By comparing a group of cases of people similar to Manson with a group that did not turn out that way, we might be able to determine whether the frequency of parental neglect, parental criminality, and/or child abuse is elevated in the target group.

An even more powerful approach is to use adopted children. In the case of adoptees, the biological parents contribute only their genes, but the adoptive parents provide the rearing environment. The distinctive contributions of the biological parents and adoptive parents thus permit the independent evaluation of genes and environment to outcomes of interest. For example, suppose someone argued that inherited factors played a role in Manson's antisocial behavior, pointing to the fact that Manson's mother was a convicted criminal. This hypothesis could be tested by seeing whether criminality in a biological parent increases the risk for criminality even in children who are adopted early in life into nurturant environments. If the children do not become criminal, then a social explanation would seem more likely than a genetic one.

Although these and many other questions about the mechanisms of abnormal behavior lack definitive answers, our understanding increases with each year's new discoveries. We have an abiding conviction that future discoveries will help clarify not only the causes and treatment, but also ways to prevent abnormality. However, we will need to define some basic concepts of abnormality before tackling more difficult questions about its origins.

CONCEPT OF ABNORMALITY

Whether abnormal behaviors are identical in all societies is a question that has not been resolved. *Relativists* argue that symptoms of a disorder vary across cultures and that its causes vary from culture to culture. *Absolutists* argue that Western criteria for abnormality truly carve nature at its joints, that is, a specific disorder is caused by the same biological factors in every culture (Butcher & Bemis, 1984). Cross-cultural studies of schizophrenia tend to sustain the absolutist view for that disorder, although the specific content of a person's problems differs across cultures—an Asian schizophrenic may claim to be Confucius rather than Jesus. The present authors suspect that for abnormalities in which physiological factors figure strongly, the absolutist position will be supported. For other abnormalities the relativist position may turn out to be more useful both for understanding causes and for finding appropriate treatments.

Different Perspectives

Abnormality is defined somewhat differently by society, affected individuals, and mental health professionals—clinical psychologists and psychiatrists. We will take a look at how these perspectives differ as well as what their commonalities are.

Society focuses on the inability to be a responsible adult or to achieve certain expected milestones such as learning how to feed oneself if a child. Since expectations vary from culture to culture, the same set of expectations cannot be applied universally as criteria for abnormality in all societies.

The personal perspective is represented by self-reported symptoms of suffering such as anxiety, depression, or inability to cope. Some people seek help because of distress while others with similar degrees of distress suffer silently. Some disturbed people have so little insight that they cannot report accurately about their behavior and feelings, and may even deny any problems. Thus, like the societal perspective, the personal perspective alone is a fallible index of abnormality.

Mental health experts try to use objective criteria to encourage agreement at least amongst themselves about the presence or absence of abnormality. Experts examine the person, using interviews and psychological or neurological tests of various kinds, often in a standardized format, so that the results can be compared to findings obtained from other patients or from people in the general population. Using these methods, it is possible to determine how well a person performs compared with the average in the population. Generally, the more extreme the departure from the population average, the more likely it is that the person will be judged deviant.

Deviance alone is not a sufficient criterion for labeling someone as abnormal. Extremely high intelligence is as deviant as mental retardation in the sense that both are fairly rare departures from the average, yet only retardation is regarded as abnormal. The label of "abnormality" requires the presence of maladaptation in addition to deviation. "Maladaptation" is an inference about behavior that suggests sabotaged well-being and/or a diminished capacity to cope.

The expert initially gathers information about abnormality primarily by assessing thinking, emotion, overt behavior, and interpersonal relationships (Kaplan & Sadock, 1985), usually obtained from interviews and tests about the following:

Consciousness Is the person oriented to time and place?

Emotion Is the person's affective expression appropriate and properly regulated?

Thinking Do the person's ideas have goal direction and are they reasonably congruent with reality?

Perception Does the person see things that aren't there (hallucinate)?

Memory Is information properly stored and retrieved from memory?

Intelligence Can the person solve intellectual problems at a level expected for his or her age?

Interpersonal relationships Does the person display the capacity to maintain a proper give-and-take in relationships with significant others?

Inadequacies in one or more of these functions may be sufficient to label the person as abnormal since poor performance is almost always maladaptive as well as deviant.

There are no hard-and-fast rules for distinguishing between normal and abnormal behavior. For example, where do we draw the line between sadness and depression, fear and panic, self-assertion and aggressiveness, or below-average intellectual functioning and mental retardation? Typically, the expert uses implicit or explicit statistical criteria regarding the rarity and severity of the maladaptation; the rarer and more maladaptive the behavior relative to social norms, the more likely it is to be judged abnormal.

We do not want to leave the impression that disagreements between societal, personal, and professional perspectives are inevitable. Such disagreements tend to occur when symptoms are mild rather than severe. Thus, a person who believes that his ideas are being monitored or hears voices giving a running commentary on his thoughts will be labeled abnormal from any perspective. On the other hand, a cult member who believes in snake worship but otherwise is in contact with reality, functions adequately at home and at work, and feels good about himself might be labeled abnormal only by society because of his unconventional belief.

Mental Health

Behavioral abnormality can be understood better by distinguishing it from its conceptual counterpart, mental health, which, like abnormality, also can be described from three perspectives. Each of these perspectives on mental health can be debated too, because assessing normality requires judgments about the absence of abnormality.

Consider the comprehensive approach to mental health proposed by Strupp, Hadley, and Gomes-Schwartz (1977). Its three-component perspective incorporates (1) the society's view of appropriate roles and responsibilities, such as being an attentive pupil, a productive worker, or a good parent, (2) the person's subjective sense of well-being, and (3) an expert's evaluation of the person's ability to cope with stress and maintain a healthy balance between selfish impulses and demands of family and society (Table 1.1).

Discrepancies among the components of this model of mental health often characterize specific types of abnormality. For example, there are people with no subjective complaints whom society and mental health professionals believe to be disturbed. This pattern of inconsistency is common for antisocial individuals such as Manson who tend to deny having personal problems.

Psychopathology

This book focuses on the underlying causes of abnormal behavior, and therefore its title is *Psychopathology,* a term derived from the Greek words for *psyche* (mind) and *pathos* (suffering). Abnormality often derives from genetic and neurophysiological aberrations as well as abnormal psychological processes and mistaken beliefs. The psychopathological approach attempts to go beneath the surface to provide answers—sometimes admittedly speculative answers—to fundamental questions about how and why abnormality arises.

TABLE 1.1 PRIMARY PERSPECTIVES ON MENTAL HEALTH

Source	Standards/values	"Measures"
Society (behavior)	Orderly world in which individuals assume responsibility for their assigned social roles (e.g., parent, breadwinner), conform to prevailing mores, and meet situational requirements	Extent to which individual fulfills society's expectations and measures up to prevailing standards
Individual (well-being)	Happiness; gratification of needs	Subjective perceptions of self-esteem, acceptance, and well-being
Mental health professional (psychological structure)	Sound personality structure characterized by autonomy, reality orientation, ability to cope with stress, and self-actualization	Clinical judgment aided by behavioral observations and psychological tests of variables such as self-concept, sense of identity, freedom from debilitating conflict, unified outlook on life, resistance to stress, self-regulation, ability to cope with reality, absence of mental and behavioral symptoms, and adequacy in love, work, play, and interpersonal relations

Source: Modified from H. H. Strupp, S. W. Hadley, and B. Gomes-Schwartz, *Psychotherapy for Better or Worse.* New York: Jason Aronson, 1977, p. 100.

Two Languages for Psychopathology Psychopathological explanations rely on two different but related languages. Neurophysiological language describes brain mechanisms involving neurons, their interconnections, and neural metabolism. Psychological language refers to psychological mechanisms such as perception, learning, motivation, and self-concept. Each language reflects a different aspect of behavior—a brain and a mind aspect. Unfortunately, the rules for translating one language into the other are often unknown. For example, a well-adjusted and intelligent person was in an accident that damaged the front part of his brain. Although his IQ score remained high, he became unreliable, irritable, and impulsive. The neurological damage could easily be seen on an X-ray, but the precise means by which the brain damage was translated into these undesirable behaviors is still mysterious.

But sometimes the two languages complement one another like two sides of a coin—for example, in Alzheimer's disease, a degenerative disease of the brain. In the language of psychology, Alzheimer's disease produces impaired memory, diminished intelligence, and disorientation. In the language of neurophysiology, it is associated with deterioration of a memory center in the brain (Hymen et al., 1984). The memory center defect prevents the retrieval of information and it is therefore not surprising that the affected person has reduced intelligence and becomes disoriented. Such established correlations between neural and psychological abnormalities help illuminate the relationship between biological and psychological functions.

Symptoms of Abnormal Behavior   Symptoms of psychopathology are indications that something is wrong with a person. Generally, symptoms are of two types. One type involves observable or quantifiable abnormalities such as abnormal brain waves or behavioral indications that the person cannot cope effectively; these can be measured *objectively*. The other type includes complaints reported by the affected person such as fearful preoccupations, confusion about reality, and demoralization about the inability to cope; these clearly are *subjective*. Correlations between objective and subjective symptoms vary considerably. For some of the abnormalities to be discussed the correlation between subjective and objective abnormalities is fairly high, but there are many exceptions. Thus, it is not unusual to see a person with many subjective symptoms who displays few objective abnormalities. For example, some depressed people have many doubts and complain about themselves and their capacity to function, yet lack objective signs of abnormality such as disrupted sleep patterns, memory failures, and deteriorating job performance.

No single symptom—difficulty recalling new information, depressive feelings, or severe headaches—however disturbing to the patient or those around him, can tell us what is really wrong. That is best revealed by discovering a distinctive cluster of symptoms, or a *syndrome* (*syn*: together; *drome*: run) that, through a sort of triangulation, increases the likelihood that a core problem can be identified. For example, the symptom triad of headache, fever, and aching joints is more likely to indicate an influenza syndrome than any one of the symptoms alone. Likewise, a refusal to maintain normal body weight accompanied by an intense fear of becoming fat and a belief that one is overweight despite being emaciated is likely to indicate anorexia nervosa rather than a normal attempt to diet or an intestinal malabsorption disorder.

Coping with Psychopathology   It was the founder of psychoanalysis, Sigmund Freud, who first pointed out that behavioral symptoms themselves can be compromise formations. By *compromise formations* Freud meant that a symptom was a product of an underlying problem combined with the effort to cope with or defend against that problem—for example, a person plagued by self-doubt nevertheless acts as if extremely confident. Sometimes behavior reflects the normal or healthy side of personality coping with the abnormal side, as when a claustrophobic person confronts his fear by taking an elevator. However, coping can be as abnormal as the abnormality it is directed against—for example, when a patient truly blinded by brain damage denies blindness and claims to see (Critchley, 1979).

Consider the symptoms in each of the following cases:

1 A brain-damaged patient with impaired memory for recent events follows the same ritual day after day, demanding that her shoes be put on her in a fixed order.

2 A braggart, severely criticized by his boss for incompetence, becomes depressed and attempts suicide.

In the first example, memory failure is directly traceable to the brain injury, but the bizarre ritual for putting on shoes represents an attempt to avoid surprises that perplex and cause intolerable anxiety. By becoming a creature of habit, this person avoids surprise, but at the cost of exhausting the people around her. In the second case, the patient's braggadocio is probably a defense against deeper feelings of inadequacy, but criticism demolishes the cover-up and precipitates a severe depression.

These examples reveal that overt behavior may be a product of hidden problems. A penetrating analysis of behavior thus requires knowledge about aspects of people other than their most conspicuous behavioral peculiarities.

Epidemiology

One of the most important questions about abnormal behaviors is their frequencies in the general population, and epidemiology refers to the methods by which these frequencies are determined. It is surprisingly difficult to obtain reliable information on rates of abnormality, yet such estimates are often necessary for intelligently planning health care facilities, providing clues to how or why abnormalities arise, and experimenting with ways to reduce their frequency. For example, in 1855 John Snow traced the rates of cholera in different London neighborhoods, and discovered that a high percentage of people with cholera lived near a specific water well. He inferred that the well was contaminated, and by removing the pump handle, he ended the epidemic. More recently, epidemiologists have indicated that the transmission of acquired immune deficiency syndrome (AIDS) is greatly increased by multiple sexual partners and the practice of anal intercourse (Winkelstein et al., 1987).

The true frequency of mental disorders has been difficult to determine for at least three reasons: study-to-study variation in diagnostic criteria for specific disorders, lack of centralized records for all cases, and little or no information on the number of mentally ill in the general population who have been missed. Estimates of the proportion of disturbed people who have sought treatment for a mental disorder vary from study to study and vary with the severity of the disorder; the average estimate is that only 25 percent of the mentally disordered population ever seeks treatment (Link & Dohrenwend, 1982a; Shapiro et al., 1984).

Thus, to obtain true frequencies of disorders in the population, one must survey people in their homes rather than rely on the number of people who go to mental health facilities. The survey used in Figure 1.1 did this by going directly to people's homes and extensively interviewing a representative sample of more than 9000 adults in three cities, excluding those residing in hospitals, nursing homes, or prisons or on the street. The purpose of each interview was to determine whether that person had had any of the disorders in question in the past month.

The most striking numbers in this figure are the high rates of major depression, alcoholism, phobias, and mild cognitive impairment. Cognitive impairment is not a formal diagnosis, but is used to estimate the proportion of people who might have mental debilities such as Alzheimer's dementia. It is determined from a series of questions tapping fairly simple aspects of intellectual functioning—for example, testing memory by asking who the president of the United States is.

One conclusion from these data is that there is much misery and debilitation in the general population. Yet why do so few affected people ever seek treatment? Many experts believe that demoralization rather than behavioral abnormality per se is the major motive for seeking professional help. *Demoralization*

FIGURE 1.1   One-month prevalence rates of disorder per 100 community residents.

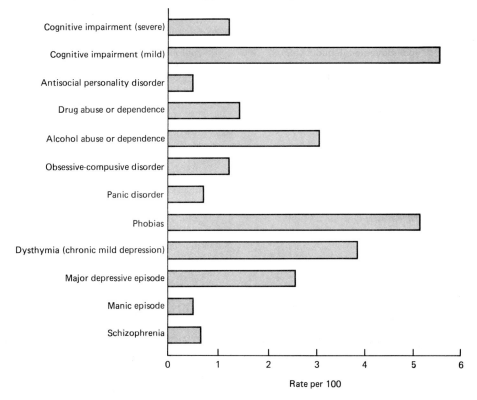

Rate per 100

refers to a constellation of factors like low self-esteem, a sense of helplessness, and a pessimistic outlook (Frank, 1973; Link & Dohrenwend, 1982b). Having a mental disorder in the absence of demoralization usually means that the affected person will not voluntarily seek help. Often it is the relatives who urge these persons to seek treatment.

The economic, like the personal, costs of mental disorders are enormous. Conservative estimates for 1980 alone suggested that mental disorders cost American society $20 billion in direct expenses for hospitals, doctors, and medication. If we also factor in the loss in work productivity, the figure exceeds $100 billion (Vischi, 1984). For schizophrenia alone, costs of treatment and the loss in productivity resulting from the fact that schizophrenics often cannot work are now estimated to be $48 billion per year (Holden, 1987). The expense of long-term care either at home or in nursing facilities for the dementing brain diseases like Alzheimer's dementia is now $40 billion per year for those over age 64, and will probably increase as a greater proportion of the population enters old age.

These costs to society provide an additional incentive to improve treatment. One recent innovation, the introduction of lithium for alleviating the severe mood swings in manic-depressive disorders, provides a clear example of the economic benefits possible. In the ten years that followed the 1969 introduction of lithium carbonate in the United States, shortened hospital stays and reduced likelihood that manic-depressive illness would recur saved nearly $3 billion in the direct costs of treatment.

While everybody agrees that the personal, family, and economic costs of mental disorders are staggering, experts do not necessarily agree about how mental disturbances arise or how they should be treated. The next section focuses on four major perspectives on the cause and treatment of psychopathology.

MODELS OF PSYCHOPATHOLOGY

There is more than one way to think about the origins and mechanisms of abnormal behavior, but generally we concentrate on environmental, biological, and psychological factors. This diversity has important consequences on how research is conducted and what questions are asked.

Each model of psychopathology is actually a loose set of propositions to explain some, but typically not all, aspects of abnormality. Using a single model to explain abnormal behavior is like trying to describe a cylinder from only one of the shadows it casts. With light shining from one end, the cylinder casts a circular shadow; with light shining from the side, it casts a rectangular shadow. Any inference about the nature of the hidden cylinder that is drawn from either shadow alone can only be partially correct. Clearly, the cylindrical nature of the object is more than its circular or rectangular aspect, or even the sum of the two. In short, no single model of abnormal behavior captures the essence of all forms of psychopathology.

All of the models to be described contribute to our understanding of abnormal behavior because all psychological phenomena have environmental, psychological, and physiological aspects. However, one model may be especially important for explaining a particular facet of a disorder—for example, its origins (or etiology), mechanisms, course, or treatment. The relative usefulness of a model will therefore depend on the specific disorder, the questions being asked about it, and the available research evidence.

We now consider the four major etiological models of abnormality—the behavioral, cognitive, psychodynamic, and physiological (or disease) models. Our discussion will also underscore their significant differences in focus and impact.

Behavioral Model

According to the behavioral model, abnormality is caused by unfortunate arrangements of environmental events that, through the normal mechanisms of learning, have become transformed into abnormal behavior. For example, suppose a person contracts food poisoning after dining in a restaurant. From then on, the person may refuse to eat any of the same foods or go to any other restaurants; even the prospect of eating these foods produces anxiety and upsets his stomach. To explain his avoidance, the behavioral model would focus on the objective observations of causal connections between environment and behavior rather than on speculations about abnormalities of brain or mind. Behaviorists regard abnormal programming as the major source of abnormal behavior, not faulty wiring in the brain. To correct abnormality, behaviorists seek to identify those environmental factors that elicit or maintain undesirable reactions and then manipulate them to produce the learning of more desirable responses.

Principles   The behavioral model involves two basic learning mechanisms to explain how environmental events result in abnormal behavior: *classical conditioning* and *instrumental conditioning*. For both the classical and instrumental conditioning approaches, the basic idea is that both normal and abnormal behavior are shaped by external events. The classical conditioning model focuses on unconditioned stimuli in the environment that elicit specific reactions called unconditioned responses. They are called unconditioned because the stimulus-response connections are wired into the organism like reflexes rather than programmed by prior learning.

For example, the unconditioned stimulus of cold produces a shivering response, food produces salivation, and physical injury produces pain. Learning occurs when a new and otherwise neutral stimulus is paired with an unconditioned stimulus. After one or more exposures to this pairing, the neutral stimulus comes to elicit the response even in the absence of the unconditioned stimulus. The new stimulus then becomes a conditioned stimulus and its associated reaction is called a conditioned (or learned) response.

Ivan Pavlov (1927), the Russian physiologist who initially formulated classical conditioning theory, placed a drop of lemon juice (the unconditioned stimulus) on a dog's tongue, which promptly elicited salivation (the unconditioned response). After a tone (the neutral, or to-be-conditioned stimulus) was repeatedly paired with the lemon juice, the tone itself could elicit salivation (the conditioned response). After repeatedly presenting the tone in the absence of the lemon juice reinforcer, however, the salivation in response to the tone eventually disappeared, a phenomenon called extinction. Many psychologists believe that classical conditioning mechanisms can explain the acquisition of some abnormal behaviors. For example, a height phobia could arise from a prior traumatic experience involving height.

The instrumental form of conditioning theory, formulated largely by B. F. Skinner (1938), works on the principle that behavior is controlled by its consequences. Thus, for example, rewarded behaviors are more likely to increase, and punished behaviors are more likely to decrease in frequency over time.

Skinner distinguishes between positive and negative reinforcement. *Positive reinforcers* are stimuli such as food or approval, which increase the probability that a given response will be repeated. *Negative reinforcers* are aversive stimuli whose removal—for example, turning off an electric shock after a certain response—increases the probability of that response recurring. Negative reinforcement is thus different from *punishment* because punishment is a noxious stimulus that is applied rather than removed after a particular response is made. An individual who makes a response that turns off a shock is receiving negative reinforcement; an individual who makes a response that turns on the shock is receiving punishment.

Let's see how a specific behavioral problem might be treated depending on whether classical or instrumental conditioning is used. A pedophile, a person sexually attracted to children, might receive a classical conditioning therapy that repeatedly pairs pictures of children with an intense shock. Over repeated trials, the pictures would become classically conditioned stimuli for fear rather than sexual arousal, the ultimate goal being to reduce the pedophile's sexual arousal in the presence of real children. An instrumental conditioning approach to the same problem might focus on repeatedly rewarding the patient for initiating and maintaining positive social interactions with potential sex partners of appropriate age.

By focusing on objective external events to explain behavior, the behavioral model avoids complex and ambiguous hidden psychological causes, particularly those featured in Freud's psychodynamic model discussed below. Moreover, since the causal external events and the resulting abnormal behaviors are observable, presumed causal connections between them can be tested and verified. A proponent of the instrumental conditioning model will say, for example, that the chronic whining of a child was maintained because parents positively reinforced the behavior by giving in to the child's complaints and that this hypothesis can be tested by having the parents change their behavior toward the child.

Criticisms   The success of therapies using principles of conditioning to correct abnormal behavior is not enough proof that the abnormal behavior arose initially from earlier unfortunate reinforcements (Marks, 1987). The behavioral model also cannot reconcile the observation that many abnormalities run in families even when the family members are not reared together, implying the importance of genetic factors in the genesis of psychopathology. For example, adopted-away children of schizophrenic biological parents reared in normal adoptive homes have the same elevated risk of developing schizophrenia as do children of schizophrenics reared by those parents, suggesting the importance of genetic factors in the disorder.

Moreover, critics argue that by focusing exclusively on the objectively verifiable consequences of external events, the behavioral model often seems to downplay the importance of thinking, and thus to underestimate the richness, unpredictability, and causal implications of unconscious and subjective experience. Obviously, psychologically important external events must be interpreted by a perceiver, and differences in interpretation lead to differences in the meanings derived from the same external event (see Chapters 5 and 6). Mechanisms for perceiving, processing, and retrieving information about the environment are built into the organism, and defects in the "mental machinery" of brain function can occur for genetic or other biological reasons that alter the way information is normally understood or remembered (see Chapters 7 and 8).

In sum, in its emphasis on environment and conditioning, the behavioral model provides an antidote to unverifiable theorizing about the brain or mental pathology, but often by minimizing or ignoring evidence that the physiological and subjective aspects of mental life have causal significance.

To some extent, the classical conditioning aspect of the behavioral model is being modified in ways that bring it closer to cognitive psychology (Rescorla, 1988). In essence, the new view emphasizes the information that one stimulus—e.g., the conditioned stimulus (CS)—provides about another—e.g., the unconditioned stimulus (UCS)—beyond the mere temporal contiguity of the CS and UCS. In other words, conditioning is now seen as the learning of *relations* among external events. Advances in the theory underlying Pavlovian conditioning are too complex to describe here, but the advances acknowledge internal representations of external events, leaving open the possibility that aberrations in these representations can lead to abnormal behavior.

Cognitive Model

Principles   The cognitive model gives special causal weight to the mental processes of perceiving, knowing, believing, and recalling that are not included in the behavioral model. The cognitive model proposes that unhappiness and distress arise from negative thoughts. While acknowledging the role of reinforcement and extinction in influencing behavior, it emphasizes that a perceiver gives meaning to events, and it is these meanings that shape behavior. When the imposed meaning is irrational or self-defeating, the consequent behavior is often maladaptive.

The major difference between the cognitive and behavioral models can be illustrated by a simple example. Suppose two people are denied a job for the exact same reason. One person interprets the denial as a personal criticism, prompting feelings of worthlessness and depression, whereas the other person interprets the denial only as the prospective employer's loss. In both cases, the objective events are identical, but the interpretations and the subsequent feelings aroused are different. Behaviorists would argue that knowledge about their prior reinforcement histories would have explained why these two people reacted differently to the denial of the job. The behaviorist would regard the depressive thoughts and feelings merely as conditioned responses with no causal significance for future behavior. The cognitivist, on the other hand, would argue that the thoughts themselves cause the depressive feelings and shape future behavior.

The cognitive view advocates the idea that humans use fantasy and forethought and can acquire information about the world in the absence of reinforcement that is controlled by external agents. They can also learn by reading and listening, and even by observing consequences to others without themselves having to be directly reinforced, in a process called *observational* or *vicarious learning*. One experimental demonstration of observational learning showed, for example, that a young monkey can learn a snake phobia merely by observing an adult monkey react fearfully to a snake (Mineka et al., 1984).

According to the cognitive model, among the most important mental processes that influence behavior are *appraisals* and *attributions*. Appraisals are often unwarranted evaluations about future behavior that predict, for example, that "I am going to fail." Attributions are explanations for a past event that say, for example, "I failed because I'm incompetent." Negative appraisals and attributions often elicit disruptive emotions that make it less likely that the most desired consequences will occur. For example, assuming that a date will be a personal disaster may result in excessive anxiety on the date, causing competence to deteriorate and creating a negative outcome.

Albert Ellis is the founder of *rational-emotive therapy,* a form of therapy based on a cognitive model. Ellis believes that much human misery stems from hidden, often unverbalized irrational beliefs which he calls *musts* (Ellis, 1987). These include beliefs that one must be loved by everyone, that one must be supremely competent in all endeavors, and that one's worth is quite justifiably judged only by the quality of one's deeds (Bandura, 1986). People with such beliefs erroneously exaggerate the consequences of not living up to their lofty standards, which can lead to negative attributions of worthlessness. Ellis attempts through verbal persuasion, disputation, and counterexample to poke holes in the patient's "musts" and replace them with a more rational perspective. The idea driving this approach is that thoughts are the prime movers of behavior and that changing thoughts will change behavior.

Another brand of cognitive therapy, identified with the work of Aaron T. Beck, overlaps considerably with the approach of Ellis. Beck also uses rational analysis to expose faulty thinking habits (Hollon & Beck, 1986). Where the two approaches differ most is in Beck's use of Socratic methods rather than disputation to help the person discover the error of his ways and in the systematic use of homework assignments. Beck may ask a male patient, for example, to ask out several women so that the patient can learn that it is not catastrophic to be refused a date. Hence, Beck's approach is really a *cognitive-behavioral* therapy because it explicitly relies on feedback, that is, reinforcement for changing cognitions and behavior.

If a patient can be forced to confront something that is inappropriately feared, positive reinforcement from the confrontation can reduce fearful cognitions. In other words, the cognitive-behavioral approach emphasizes a reciprocal relationship between cognitions and behavioral outcomes, and either one can drive the other. An interesting example of this reciprocity comes from a study of social recovery after a heart attack. Patients often worry that sexual arousal might be lethal even if the physician tells them that sexual arousal is not dangerous. If these patients are encouraged to observe their elevated heart rates during strenuous performance on a treadmill, however, they acquire increased confidence about their capacity to resume normal sexual activities (Taylor et al., 1985).

Let us see how a cognitive therapist would treat agoraphobia, a disorder characterized by a fear of being in public places (*agora* is the Greek word for market). Research indicates that most agoraphobics have a history of panic attacks, terrifying feelings of being unable to breathe, dying, or going insane. The cognitive therapist may observe that the agoraphobic patient has panic attacks at home as well as in public. The fear of going out is really a worry that a panic attack in public would be embarrassing and that would be catastrophic. To dispel this worry, a therapist might take the patient to the supermarket and pretend to have a panic attack while standing in line. The simulation might be very realistic, the therapist yelling and falling to the floor as if in a faint. The agoraphobic would see that customers and staff are solicitous and learn that although it is not good to have a panic attack in public, it is certainly not catastrophic (Telch, 1988). Thus, the agoraphobic observes that even if a panic attack cannot be prevented, it need not restrict one's life because of the exaggerated fear of embarrassing consequences.

Criticisms   Biologically oriented critics argue that the purely cognitive model does not explain how faulty thinking habits develop and also that it ignores evidence of genetic and other biological factors in behavior. Behaviorally oriented critics of the purely cognitive model argue that cognitions are shaped by reinforcements in the same way that other forms of behavior are shaped and therefore are not independent of the laws of learning. In their view, maladaptive cognitions arise because of unfortunate prior learning experiences and not spontaneously. Critics also argue that purely cognitive approaches to treatment such as rational analyses and disputation are ineffective unless systematic reinforcement procedures are used to eliminate undesired behaviors or to increase desired behaviors (Beidel & Turner, 1986).

Psychodynamic Model

Principles   Like the cognitive model, the psychodynamic model deals with faulty cognitions, especially those that arise from *intrapsychic conflict*—the constant inner tension among the selfish, realistic, and moral tendencies of the personality.

In the course of becoming socialized, *every* individual must reconcile selfish impulses and other needs with an external reality. The emerging components of personality—what Sigmund Freud called the id, ego, and superego—are the characters in this drama of reluctant reconciliation. The *id*—the blindly selfish part of personality—is devoted to the unbridled satisfaction of instinctive pleasures. The *ego*—the expedient part of personality—serves the id by learning how to achieve id satisfaction without eliciting physical punishment. Eventually, an emerging component of the ego, the *superego,* acquires the ability to appreciate moral aspects of the social environment and to make the ego experience guilty feelings. This superego aspect of personality prompts the ego to avoid moral violations and consequent guilt while searching out opportunities for id satisfaction.

Conflict is assumed to be *developmental*, that is, rooted in early life when a child's selfish pleasure-striving clashes with the social reality provided by the parents. These infantile conflicts may produce anxiety and be forced out of awareness; that is, they may become *unconscious*. Defense mechanisms such as repression develop to block impulses and to prevent them and the inner conflicts they create from erupting into consciousness. Nevertheless, unconscious memories remain active, continually striving for expression. According to psychoanalytic theory, one way they find conscious expression is by being *symbolically* disguised before entering consciousness, as in a dream. The disguise expresses the impulse in a way that does not further provoke the defense mechanism of repression.

The ego mobilizes mechanisms of defense as the means of coping with anxiety and guilt aroused by conflict-ridden id impulses close to reaching behavioral expression and/or consciousness. Defenses are often mobilized at the cost of distorting reality, heightening inner conflict, and sapping energy. According to the psychodynamic model, overused or failing mechanisms of defense are responsible for the emergence of symptoms.

Let us again use agoraphobia to see how a psychodynamically oriented therapist might treat the behavior as expressing a defense against an unconscious anxiety-provoking impulse. A patient may have sexual desires that are kept out of consciousness by repression when seeing strangers on the street, for example. Deeper analysis may reveal intense guilt about sexuality and perhaps early childhood memories of being frightened by expressions of sexual feelings. The agoraphobia is thus interpreted to be a defense against consciously acknowledging sexual feelings stirred by opportunities irrationally perceived to exist in the street. The consequence is a symbolic transformation of the sexual anxiety to a fear of being outside. The goal of the therapist would be to make the patient's sexual feelings and fears conscious so that they can then be reexamined from a more mature perspective.

It is important to keep in mind that the psychodynamic view argues that defenses are present in everyone as a consequence of socialization and therefore that defenses are not necessarily bad. Defenses that are exaggerated and rigidly applied and distort reality to a significant degree are judged to be maladaptive. But the line between normal and abnormal defenses can be difficult to define. Surprisingly, defenses of normal people can result in distorted, overly favorable self-appraisals that may make them even less in touch with social reality than those who are abnormal (Lewinsohn et al., 1980). For example, mildly depressed people often see themselves in a negative light, yet in comparison to normal controls, their self-perceptions are in fact closer to the perceptions that other people have of them. In his characterization of a severely depressed person Freud noticed this "depressive realism" and remarked that:

> When in his exacerbation of self-criticism he describes himself as petty, egoistic, dishonest, lacking in independence, one whose sole aim has been to hide the weaknesses of his own nature, for all we know it may be that he has come very near to self-knowledge; we can only wonder why a man must become ill before he can discover truth of this kind (Freud, p. 156, 1917/1959).

A moderately inflated ego that is slightly out of touch with social reality thus may actually be a healthy sign.

In the classic psychodynamic model just described, ego defenses are the sometimes pathological mechanisms for resolving *conflict* between selfish impulses (id) and moral sentiments (superego). In short, the ego is a strong but embattled component of personality, threatened from within by the equally strong and demanding components of id and superego. In recent revisions of the model —especially the newer theories that focus on a person's relationship to his own personality (self theory) and to significant others (object relations theory)—defensive behavior is viewed as an attempt to deal with ego *deficits*; these are reflected in feelings of emptiness and unreality, an uncertain sense of self, and a consequent inability to develop truly affectionate and trusting relationships. Defense against such ego weakness is reflected in compliant, combative, or avoidant relationships, pervasive suspiciousness and hostility, and the sense that one's behavior is artificial or "unreal."

In sum, the psychodynamic model deals with the socialization of human nature as played out in mental life. Classic conflict theory addresses the problem of how self-control evolves out of selfish pleasure-striving. Revisions of the theory deal with the problem of how a sense of self evolves out of dependency needs. While classical and modern aspects of the psychodynamic model deal with different, but equally fundamental, problems, both assume that the child is vulnerable, and that the frustration and gratification of needs by caretakers largely determine whether psychological development will be normal or abnormal.

Criticisms   The psychodynamic model proposes that psychological experiences are often transformed by unconscious cognitive mechanisms into sometimes unrecognizable forms. By acknowledging the richness of a mental life that imperfectly reflects external reality, the model can account for seemingly irrational behavior.

Nevertheless, it has been subject to harsh criticisms, at least in scientific circles, for at least two good reasons, which we detail further in Chapter 6. First, many of the assumptions are either scientifically untestable or, when tested, found to be unsupportable. For example, the role of early childhood experience in indelibly shaping adult personality is inconsistent with the research evidence suggesting a less powerful role for these early experiences. Second, scientifically more defensible explanations involving biology, conditioning, and cognition often seem to fit the facts about abnormality better. For example, increasing knowledge of genetics and brain function, although still far from complete, better characterizes some forms of psychopathology as neuropsychological diseases.

Physiological Model

Thus far the models described can be regarded as psychological, meaning that the causes of abnormal behavior are believed to be rooted in psychological experiences. The physiological, or disease, model proposes that much abnormal behavior arises from faulty physiological processes or diseases.

Principles   The physiological model assumes that abnormal thinking and behavior result from physiological abnormalities. In actuality, there are three major disease concepts and it is not always clear which of the three is being invoked. Sometimes a disease refers to the direct pathological actions of an environmental agent such as a virus invading the brain. A disease can also refer to an inherited abnormality; an example is the disease *phenylketonuria*, caused by an abnormal pair of genes that prevents the metabolism of an amino acid essential to proper brain development. This type of genetic defect, unless treated with a special diet, leaves the person with faulty neural wiring.

Finally, a disease can be inferred when a person reacts adversely to an environmental agent that is not generally deleterious. The clearest example of this kind is an allergy arising from an environmental ''allergen'' that is harmless to most people, but produces an adverse immunological reaction in genetically susceptible people. In contrast to phenylketonuria, which represents a genetic defect that will invariably produce a disease in any natural environment, allergy indicates a genetic abnormality that need never occur in a favorable environment. Thus the distinction between a defect producing a disease such as phenylketonuria and the allergic type of defect is really about the degree to which chance environmental factors contribute to the eventual manifestation of a disease in a genetically vulnerable person.

When an inborn vulnerability requires a special environmental agent to produce a full-fledged disorder, as in the allergy example, we speak of a *diathesis-stress* interaction. A diathesis refers to any inborn predisposition that eventuates in a disease, but only in the presence of certain environmental stresses. It is often argued that schizophrenia, a disorder associated with aberrant thinking processes, is a mental disease that behaves in accordance with a diathesis-stress model with its genetic component requiring a stress to produce disorganized behavior (Meehl, 1962).

It is difficult *not* to adopt a disease perspective for disorders characterized by the following: (1) a heritable component—for example, manic-depressive disorder, schizophrenia, antisocial personality, and the many genetic forms of mental retardation; (2) a higher incidence of pregnancy complications or physical anomalies detectable at birth suggesting that something went awry in embryological development—for example, infantile autism, some types of learning disabilities, and hyperactivity; and (3) evidence that hormonal dysregulation and drugs such as amphetamine and cocaine can produce symptoms of mental disorder—for example, anxiety, depression, delusion, and hallucination. That certain brain abnormalities and drugs can mimic symptoms seen in some mental disorders suggests, but does not prove, that analogous neural or chemical abnormalities may sometimes underlie behavioral dysfunctions for which a biological basis cannot yet be demonstrated.

For some conditions such as phobias, the behavioral, cognitive, or psychodynamic models often seem more useful than the physiological model for conceptualizing causes and treatments. Laboratory studies of learning, for example, indicate that phobic avoidance and addictive behaviors can be caused and treated by environmental manipulations, although biological factors also may be influential.

Nevertheless, even if abnormalities such as phobias or anxiety disorders are thought of as largely psychological disorders, it doesn't necessarily follow that they are beyond the physiological approach. For example, agoraphobia is often preceded by a panic attack, and both have a tendency to run in families, suggesting a disease with a possible genetic basis. The panic attacks might be treated by administering a drug such as imipramine that can reduce their frequency. By diminishing the frequency of panic attacks, perhaps the patient would gain the courage to venture outdoors and the agoraphobia would disappear as the person learns that the panic attacks will no longer occur. Antipanic drugs need not be used alone. In fact, behavioral, cognitive, and drug therapies often are used together for panic attacks and agoraphobia. Drugs are administered to reduce the frequency of panic attacks and the behavioral and cognitive therapies help the person learn that the consequences of having a panic attack are exaggerated, and thus need not be intensely feared.

Stress and Vulnerability   The physiological model of psychopathology recognizes that psychological stresses frequently have a role in precipitating disease. Generally, stress upsets the mechanisms for preserving the stability of physiology, cognition, and personality. Normally when we are exposed to heat stress, we sweat to maintain a constant body temperature; when we are stressed by boredom, we seek out stimulation. The preservation of stability around an internal physiological norm is called *homeostasis* (Cannon, 1939). Stressors—anything that potentially can disrupt stability—produce disease only when they sabotage the mechanisms that maintain the internal status quo. They can do this alone if the stresses are extreme, or if they are operating on a vulnerable organism, even when the stresses are relatively minor.

Labeling a stressor as a *pathogenic,* or a disease-causing, agent often oversimplifies the case: pathology, or disease, may be as much a matter of the situation within the organism—the degree of vulnerability or resiliency—as of what it is in the environment that attacks the organism from without (see Chapter 5). In other words, vulnerability can be as important as environmental stressors in producing disease.

Depending on the particular disease and the perspective of the investigator, a stressor or a homeostatic failure may be emphasized. For example, schizophrenics may deteriorate following a relatively common anxiety-provoking stressor such as looking for a job. To focus on the stressor as the cause overlooks the schizophrenic's vulnerability and ignores the fact that such stresses are an inherent part of living that most of us successfully cope with regularly. Returning the schizophrenic to a relatively normal life may require a reduction in vulnerability to such unexceptional stressors, rather than simply avoiding them entirely.

One illustrative study of the interplay of stress and vulnerability was prompted by an earlier observation that although 20 percent of all children have a positive throat culture for streptococcus, only about 1 percent have a sore throat and fever indicating a strep infection (Meyer & Haggerty, 1962; Haggerty, 1980). Does stress increase vulnerability to infection? To help researchers answer this question, parents of 100 children in sixteen families kept diaries about "upsetting" stressful events and illnesses in their children for one year while throat cultures in the children were taken biweekly. As Figure 1.2 indicates, except for the two weeks immediately preceding an infection, a fairly consistent average of approximately four upsetting events occurred every two weeks to each child. But during the two weeks immediately preceding an infection in a specific child, sixteen stressful events occurred. Apparently, multiple stressful events can exhaust coping resources, making some individuals more susceptible to infection.

Infections often followed stressful events, but some infections were *not* preceded by excessive stress. Thus external stress cannot explain all instances of infection; other resiliencies or vulnerabilities must also be considered, not to mention the presence of the offending germ. Clearly, pathogens and other stressors are common facts of life, yet most individuals do not deteriorate in

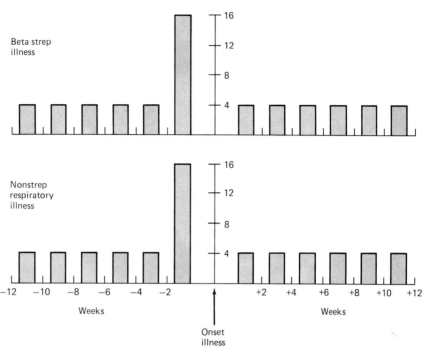

Figure 1.2   Respiratory infections in families in relation to acute life stress (100 children). Vertical axis shows number of stressful life events recorded in each two-week period, before and after respiratory infections. Note marked increase in stressful events in two weeks preceding streptococcal and other respiratory illness in the infected children. (From R. J. Haggerty (1980) *Developmental Medicine and Child Neurology*, 22, 391–400, p. 392.)

their presence. It seems likely that psychological stressors operate analogously to physiological stressors. Psychological or social stress can exhaust compensatory mechanisms, particularly if the stresses are chronic or the coping mechanisms are ineffective.

A recent study of significant life events preceding the onset of first episodes of mania, a mood disorder characterized by extreme elation, shows how stresses can precipitate a mental disorder. Two-thirds of first-admission manic patients had suffered a major emotional upheaval in the month just prior to onset of the disorder, in contrast to only 8 percent of a control group of surgical patients (Ambelas, 1987). These events were predominantly births and deaths over which the patient had little influence. We also know that mania is often an expression of an underlying manic-depressive disorder, a condition with a heritable component. These data therefore suggest a diathesis-stress model in which emotional stresses can precipitate a manic disorder in a genetically predisposed person.

What personality qualities could make individuals less vulnerable to the effects of social stress? One quality may be "hardiness," a personality constellation characterized by commitment to work, a sense of personal control, and the belief that stress is a challenge rather than a threat (Kobasa & Puccetti, 1983). Otherwise undesirable factors like selfishness and unreflectiveness may be adaptive under some circumstances because they lead to a shallowness in interpersonal relations that diminishes the potential adverse impact of psychological stressors such as loss of a loved one (Hinkle, 1974). Thus even undesirable qualities of personality sometimes may be beneficial.

Criticisms Critics of the physiological model and its application say that it ignores the question of how physiological abnormalities produce psychological symptoms. Perhaps more importantly, it often hypothesizes the existence of physiological abnormalities even when they cannot be objectively demonstrated. This may have negative consequences when drugs or other physical interventions produce serious and irreversible side effects.

Thomas Szasz (1970), the most vociferous critic of the disease model, focuses specifically on the mental disease concept and the harmful consequences of the *medical* treatment of behaviorally deviant people who display no signs of physical disease. The term disease, he says, should refer only to *tangible* bodily dysfunction established by objective assessment. Therefore, if a brain disease causes abnormal behavior, it should be called a neurological disease, not a mental disease, because the ''mind'' is an abstraction, and abstractions cannot be diseased. Here is how Szasz puts it:

> Disease means bodily disease. *Gould's Medical Dictionary* defines disease as a disturbance of the function or structure of an organ or a part of the body. The mind (whatever it is) is not an organ or a part of the body. Hence, it cannot be diseased in the same sense as the body can. When we speak of mental illness, then, we speak metaphorically. To say that a person's mind is sick is like saying that the economy is sick or that a joke is sick. When metaphor is mistaken for reality and then used for social purposes, then we have the makings of myth. I hold that the concepts of mental health and mental illness are mythological concepts, used strategically to advance some social interests and to retard others, much as national and religious myths have been used in the past (Szasz, as quoted in Miller et al., 1976, pp. 9–10).

According to Szasz, most so-called mental illnesses are merely deviant behaviors. Viewing them *as though* they were the products of a disease promotes a medical approach to essentially nonmedical problems of living. Finally, the disease model tends to explain offensive behavior by shifting the onus from the patient's personal responsibility to a hypothetical disease process. To Szasz this implies that the person can be freed of culpability, an outcome that he regards as undesirable because it minimizes the person's own motives and values in producing or maintaining the deviant behavior.

Critics of the physiological model also say that even if a drug is effective for treating a mental disorder, it does not imply that a physiological abnormality was at the root of the original problem (any more than an effective behavioral treatment implies that a psychological abnormality was the cause of a behavioral problem). Tension headaches arising from psychological stresses can be relieved by aspirin, yet no one claims that an aspirin deficiency was the cause of the headache or that the best long-term treatment warrants the use of drugs.

Hardly any researchers believe that all mental disorders are best viewed solely as physiological abnormalities. For some disorders, the physiological perspective may indeed be the most promising, but for others, psychological perspectives may be better. This is an empirical question and not one to be decided on the basis of philosophy or ideology, however. Thus, to some of his adversaries in the physiological camp, Szasz often seems to be tilting at windmills.

PLAN OF THIS BOOK

Our intention is to provide a grounding in the theories and data of psychopathology. We have sifted through thousands of ideas and empirical observations, many of which are conflicting or at least difficult to reconcile, and have come up with our own selection of what is significant. Other psychologists may see things somewhat differently, so this book cannot be regarded as a completely unslanted appraisal of the status of psychopathology. A book of this sort is, in reality, a progress report, and until the final answers are known, different people will identify different themes as being the most significant and most promising for future investigation.

Researchers are on the threshold of making important discoveries in psychopathology. Indeed, with the emergence of technologies that permit closer examination of individual cells, better imaging of brain structure and function, and more powerful methods of genetic and behavioral assessment, future explanations of abnormal behavior will no doubt be more penetrating at all levels of analysis.

The next three chapters in the book cover the history, classification, and assessment of psychopathology. The following four chapters on "facets" of psychopathology constitute the heart of the book because they offer expanded discussion of the models and their wider implications. Some of what is currently believed about the specific causes of psychopathology may turn out to be off the mark, but these methodologically and theoretically oriented "facet" chapters do not depend heavily on the day-to-day accumulation of new knowledge. They represent broad perspectives that can usually accommodate new data within existing models. On the other hand, each of the following 13 "content" chapters on specific disorders may be altered by the publication of a single important paper that radically changes our views. The final chapter in the book offers a summary of the effects of treatment for various behavioral abnormalities. Not surprisingly, some abnormalities are relatively easily treated while others remain resistant to current approaches.

SUMMARY

Abnormality, like normality, is difficult to define. The society, the person, and the professional may disagree about the definition. In this book abnormality refers to behavioral deviations judged to be maladaptive. Psychopathology refers to the underlying biological and psychological dysfunctions hypothesized to explain the abnormalities. Moreover, theories of physiological and psychological causation employ different languages, which sometimes makes translation from one language to the other difficult. Consequently, theorists of different perspectives often seem to talk past each other, though they are dealing with different aspects of the same underlying problem.

Models of psychopathology tend to be behavioral, cognitive, psychodynamic, or physiological. The behavioral model emphasizes deviant and maladaptive learning caused by adverse environmental factors in otherwise normal individuals. The cognitive model highlights the personal meanings of various events, while the psychodynamic model emphasizes intrapsychic conflicts, that is, conflicts among the selfish, realistic, and moral aspects of personality. The physiological model emphasizes brain and genetic abnormalities in the genesis of mental disorders. Unfortunately, singleminded theories of psychopathology are confounded by evidence that disorders usually have multiple causes involving both physiology and experience.

Historical Roots

OUTLINE

An historical approach provides us with a special appreciation of both the evolution and persistence of ideas going back to antiquity. In the apparent timelessness and universality of certain problems and solutions, we come to appreciate our indebtedness to the intellectual and humanitarian forerunners of contemporary psychopathology.

In this chapter, we trace the evolution of theories and treatments of psychopathology, and of the institutional management of the severest behavior disorders. We see how earlier views on the organic, supernatural, and psychological sources of abnormality gave way while influencing the development of more modern, scientifically based theories. Finally, we focus on the complex problem of institutionalization, its social roots, its humane and inhumane aspects, and changes toward increased personal freedom, effective treatment, and legal protection.

PERSPECTIVES ON PSYCHOPATHOLOGY

Efforts to reduce the complexities of abnormal behavior to a few common denominators typically invoke the following basic criteria: psychological dysfunction, social disapproval, and personal unhappiness. From these criteria, a few basic types of abnormality—cognitive disorganization, emotional dysfunction, and antisocial behavior—are universally recognized throughout history and across cultures (Al-Issa, 1982; Draguns, 1982; Linton, 1956).

Ancient medical writings describe specific examples of dementia (confusion, loss of memory, and other cognitive disabilities), psychosis (disorganized and/or bizarre thinking), mental retardation, depression, mania, paranoia, anxiety, and hysteria (neurologically inexplicable bodily complaints). Moreover, behavior disorders appear in Greek mythology (the epilepsy of Hercules), biblical stories (the manic-depression of King Saul), and Renaissance literature (the paranoia of Othello).

Three broad views of abnormal behavior have competed throughout history. The *organic* view emphasizes the influence of brain dysfunctions determined by hereditary and environmental factors. The *supernatural* view is composed of metaphysical speculation about soul sickness and possession by evil spirits. The *psychological* view focuses on the frustrations, conflicts, and irrationalities of mental life. Table 2.1 presents a sampling of historical ideas, to which we now turn.

Organic View

Hippocratic Humoral Notions   An early champion of the organic view was the Greek physician Hippocrates (460–370 B.C.E.). He assumed that the brain is the origin of all psychological functions, and that an abnormal brain is the cause of abnormal behavior. "If you cut open the head, you will find the brain humid, full of sweat and smelling badly. And in this way you may see that it is not a god which injures the body, but disease."

Hippocrates developed a primitive but influential and historically durable physiological theory of temperament that could be applied to abnormal behavior. According to this theory, the brain, and therefore mental life, is influenced by four basic fluids, or *humors,* that circulate in the body: yellow bile, blood, phlegm, and black bile. An excess of yellow bile accounts for "choleric" temper, or extreme irritability. An excess of blood explains cheerfulness, optimism, and changeability. Too much phlegm accounts for sluggishness, dull-

TABLE 2.1   HISTORICAL ROOTS OF MENTAL ILLNESS CONCEPTS

Viewpoint	Historical period		
	Ancient	Medieval-Renaissance	Premodern
Organic	Humoral theory (Hippocrates; Galen) emphasizes physiology and natural causes	Humoral theory complicated by astrological and demonological views (Arnauld of Villanova) Brain pathology causes madness (Bartholomaeus) Environmental factors (e.g., poisons, diet) can cause brain pathology (Paracelsus)	"Magnetic" abnormalities of body and brain cause physical and mental illness (Mesmer) Electrochemical nature of the brain (Galvani) Location of psychological functions (Broca) Advent of bacterial, traumatic, and hereditary models of mental illness (Greisinger; Kraepelin)
Supernatural	Gods create abnormalities for revenge or revelation (Plato)	Some forms of abnormal behavior represent evil (sin and possession) rather than illness (Sprenger; Kraemer)	Decline of spiritual view with the advent of modern science
Psychological	Inner conflict and defects of judgment disorganize mental life (Cicero)	Little or no psychological theory documented for Middle Ages Speculation during Renaissance and Enlightenment periods about inner conflict (Paracelsus; Weyer) and about psychosomatics (Stahl)	Rediscovery of inner conflict in psychological theories (Braid; Charcot; Freud) Elaboration of learning mechanisms in behaviorism (Pavlov)

ness, and apathy, while excessive black bile causes a pessimistic outlook and deep depression. (Indeed, our term melancholy originates in *melaina chole,* the Greek phrase for black bile.)

The Hippocratic theory of humors was further developed by Galen (130–200 C.E.), the greatest physician of Roman times (Kroll, 1973). Galen theorized that the humors influenced the body, the brain, and therefore behavior because of their unique qualities: heat, cold, moisture, and dryness. Each humor presumably embodied a pair of these qualities: warm and moist (blood), warm and dry (yellow bile), cold and dry (black bile), and cold and moist (phlegm). Galen assumed that mental illness can arise from an imbalance as well as an excess of these qualities. Thus, for example, melancholia reflected excess cold and dryness carried by black bile. Modern scientific work on brain chemistry and hormones—in severe depression, for example—gives new life to the ancient notion of bodily humors.

The influence of Hippocrates and Galen continued well into the European Middle Ages. Prior to 1200 C.E., physicians emphasized natural causes, including humoral imbalance, and they often prescribed medical treatment (Kroll, 1973; Schoeneman, 1977). Different types of psychopathology were recognized: *Vesani* caused by poisons or unhealthy diet, *Insani* by bad heredity, *Lunatici* by lunar influence, and *Melancholici* by unbalanced temperament. Supernatural factors were invoked more often later in the Middle Ages; for example, a devil-influenced type of abnormality (*Obsessi*) was recognized. Nevertheless, despite a rise in supernatural speculation (described below), a medical model still predominated; the mentally ill were typically viewed as suffering from *physical* illness that could be treated by doctors (Neugebauer, 1978).

Brain Mechanisms and Behavior Speculation about the relationship between mental life and the brain continued in Europe throughout the Middle Ages, the Renaissance (fifteenth to seventeenth centuries), and the Enlightenment (eighteenth century). For example, the widely used thirteenth-century reference work, *Encyclopedia of Bartholomaeus,* written by a Franciscan monk, offered a theory (Kroll, 1973): madness is caused by defects near the lateral ventricles, fluid-filled cavities near the center of the brain (see Chapter 8, p. 203). Interestingly, contemporary research suggests a relationship between lateral ventricle abnormalities and some types of schizophrenia (see Chapter 12).

Theories about abnormal brain mechanisms became less speculative only during the nineteenth century with the coming of new scientific findings such as the electrical nature of neural conductivity, first discovered by Galvani in 1791. Some seventy years after Galvani's discoveries, Paul Broca (1824–1880) autopsied the brain of a man hospitalized for thirty years for a severe speech deficit. On the basis of the autopsy, Broca reported that the speech center of the human brain is located in the frontal lobe of the left cerebral hemisphere, a region now called Broca's area after its discoverer. The year 1861 thus marks the first scientific confirmation of a long-held idea that specific psychological functions are located in specific parts of the brain. Broca's work was thus a landmark in the historical evolution of the organic view and a cornerstone of modern neuroscience.

The pioneer nineteenth-century neuropsychologist Jean Pierre Falret (1794–1870) expressed the strong conviction that an understanding of abnormal behavior requires the scientific study of brain anatomy and function. Falret believed that every case of severe mental disorder expresses a corresponding brain lesion. Many of Falret's influential contemporaries including the German psychiatrist Wilhelm Griesinger (1817–1868) embraced this rather uncompromisingly organic viewpoint. Modern neuroscientific research is providing increasing evidence that, indeed, brain abnormalities distinguish not only psychopathology from normalcy, but also specific disorders from one another (John, Prichep, & Easton, 1988).

General Paresis and Neuropathology Not until the nineteenth century did the convergence of physics, biochemistry, anatomy, and physiology provide the groundwork for a truly scientific organic (disease) model of abnormal behavior. This development is best exemplified by the discovery of a causal connection between a specific disease agent, the syphilis bacterium (*Spirochaeta pallida*), and the brain disorder, *general paresis,* a progressive deterioration of perceptual, cognitive, and memory functions and a corresponding impairment of motor capacity that progresses from weakness to paralysis.

In 1897, Richard Krafft-Ebing observed that paretic patients innoculated with material from syphilitic sores failed to develop the rashes and other symptoms of syphilis; this immunity to infection indicated that the patients had earlier contracted the disease. Subsequent developments included the discovery of the syphilitic spirochete by two German researchers, Schaudinn and Hoffmann (in 1905), identification of syphilitic infection in postmortem studies of the brain by Noguchi and Moore (in 1913), and the introduction in 1943 of penicillin as a treatment (see Figure 2.1). These and other discoveries constituted additional milestones in the historical development of the organic model.

Perhaps more than anyone else, the German psychiatrist and experimental psychopathologist Emil Kraepelin (1856–1926) should be considered the founder of the modern organic model of psychopathology. Kraepelin used the techniques of Wundt's new experimental psychology (see below) to study the psychological dysfunctions and drug-responsiveness of psychiatric patients. Kraepelin's most lasting contribution, however, was his textbook, *Clinical Psychiatry,* which described a system for classifying the varieties of psychopathology into discrete disorders, each with a distinctive biological basis and clinical course. The best-known example of Kraepelin's system was his divi-

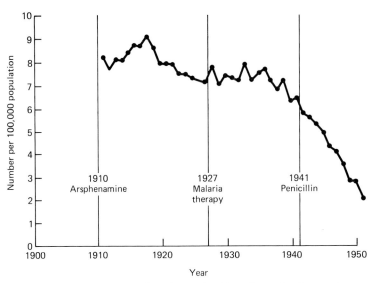

FIGURE 2.1 First admissions to New York State hospitals with a diagnosis of general paresis, 1911 to 1951. (From New York State Department of Mental Hygiene annual report, 1951.)

sion of manic-depressive and schizophrenic disorders into separate disease categories (see Chapter 11).

Genetic Mechanisms The organic model of psychopathology recognizes that abnormal behavior can arise from genetic as well as traumatic and infectious causes. Vague notions about the heritability of behavioral traits have a long history (McClearn & DeFries, 1973). Hippocrates' organic view included a biological influence passed down through the generations of a family—what might be called a hereditary factor. During the medieval and Renaissance period, a hereditary type of psychopathology (*Insani*) was distinguished. However, the exact nature of genetic mechanisms was entirely unknown prior to the nineteenth century. All this changed dramatically with the work of Charles Darwin and Gregor Mendel.

Darwin's (1859, 1871) theories of evolution through natural and sexual selection (see Chapters 7 and 20) hypothesized that many physical and behavioral traits first arose by chance, but evolved because they served some adaptive purpose. Organisms possessing the trait were more likely to survive in the struggle for life, and, if the trait had any genetic component at all, its selective advantage could be passed to the next generation. These offspring would, in turn, have a greater chance of survival, and so on. The idea of a hereditary basis to behavioral traits was soon applied to psychopathological traits, as we will see.

Darwin's ideas about the specific physiological mechanisms of heredity were vague and incorrectly formulated. It was the botanist Gregor Mendel who showed in 1865 the statistical foundations for the manner in which traits are transmitted (see Chapter 7). The implications of his theory were that familial dissimilarities as well as resemblances could arise from common hereditary principles which he called dominance, recessiveness, and segregation. His theory could explain how a disease could be present in a child of two normal parents (who we now know are each carriers of a recessive abnormal gene)—for example, *phenylketonuria,* an enzyme defect that causes brain deterioration and mental retardation unless treated early in life.

Nowadays, a great deal more is known about specific genetic mechanisms including genetically based dissimilarities between parents and children. We will have more to say about Darwin and Mendel in Chapter 7. Suffice it to say that advances in behavior-genetic research have figured profoundly in the advancement of the organic view, including the idea that certain forms of psychopathology—panic or depression, for example—are heritable exaggerations of genetically selected survival mechanisms.

Somatotherapies   Throughout history, therapeutic efforts with severely disturbed patients were based on the assumption of organic disease. The early twentieth century saw the introduction of new and powerful biological treatments, or somatotherapies (*soma*: body), including induced convulsion, psychosurgery, and drugs.

By the 1930s, psychiatrists had noted that a psychotic condition might be less severe following a convulsion. In 1934, the Portuguese neurosurgeon Ladislas von Meduna suggested that there might be some sort of biological antagonism between psychosis and seizures, the neurological "storms" underlying behavioral convulsions. Meduna used the convulsant drug metrazol to test his idea that seizure tends to inhibit psychosis. In 1938, the Italian neuropsychiatrists Ugo Cerletti and Lucio Bini introduced an alternative version, the electrically induced seizure treatment we now call electroconvulsive therapy, or ECT. Modified forms of this therapy are especially effective for treating the severe depression of patients who, often psychotic and/or suicidal, are unresponsive to other treatments. Procedures, controversies, and evaluation of ECT are discussed in Chapters 13 and 22.

Isolated efforts to treat disorganized behavior by *psychosurgery* had been carried out in Switzerland and Russia since the beginning of the twentieth century. Psychosurgery refers to the alteration of behavior by deliberate lesions made in selected parts of the brain. In 1936, Antonio de Egas Moniz introduced new procedures for calming highly agitated, depressed, or dangerous patients. An early version of Moniz's *frontal lobotomy* technique, for which he was awarded the Nobel prize, involved passing a wire loop through a hollow needle that had been inserted into the brain, typically the anterior part. The compressed wire loop was pushed through the needle until, emerging at the other end, it expanded; the expanded loop was then rotated to produce circular cuts in the tissue (see Figure 2.2).

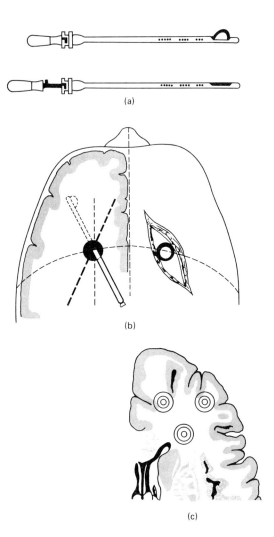

FIGURE 2.2   The "core" lobotomy procedure of Egas Moniz and Almeida Lima. (a) The leucotome. (b) The leucotome was inserted at different angles through a burr hole in the skull. When the leucotome was believed to be in place the cutting wire was extruded and the instrument rotated. (c) Sketch of a horizontal slice (parallel to the top of the head) through the brain illustrating three "cores" of destroyed nerve fibers in the frontal lobe. (From Valenstein, E. S., 1973, p. 278. *Brain Control: A Critical Examination of Brain Stimulation and Psychosurgery.* Reprinted with permission from John Wiley & Sons, Publisher)

The more than 50,000 psychosurgical procedures carried out in the 1940s and 1950s were guided by brain-behavior theories that were primitive at best. Scientific, therapeutic, and ethical questions have always surrounded psychosurgical treatment which is occasionally used today in highly selected and otherwise unresponsive cases (Culliton, 1976; Valenstein, 1973, 1980).

Perhaps the greatest somatotherapeutic advance came in the 1950s and 1960s with the introduction of potent drugs for treating psychopathology. To appreciate just how widespread the use of therapeutic drugs is, consider one statistic: in 1977, Americans consumed more than 8000 tons of the antianxiety drug Valium (Paul & Skolnick, 1981). Many of these drugs were initially developed by researchers interested in nonpsychiatric agents such as antihistamines and antihypertensives. The discovery of their relevance to psychiatric disorders was thus sometimes a matter of luck.

A discussion of drug therapy is given in Chapter 22. It is enough to say here that the effectiveness of drugs has been critical in promoting the organic viewpoint and, in particular, neuropsychological models of abnormal behaviors. For example, there is increasing evidence that psychosis, depression, and anxiety can be provoked or blocked by certain drugs whose structure and locus of action in the brain are becoming increasingly understood.

Supernatural View

Like the organic view, the supernatural view has a long history. Metaphysical speculation on the causes of abnormal behavior is evident in ancient Greek literature, but probably has even earlier origins.

Natural and Supernatural Causes   In his dialogues, Plato (428–348 B.C.E.) distinguished two causes of madness: natural causes related to physiology and environment, and supernatural causes from gods like Apollo, Eros, and Dionysus. Unlike the natural type, divine madness was insightful and prophetic, a vehicle by which the gods communicated to humans, therefore requiring interpretation rather than therapy. (Divine madness was, however, sometimes sinister—for example, the madness that the Furies, portrayed in Greek drama, induced in transgressors of social and religious convention.) The distinction between natural and supernatural causes of abnormal behavior persisted through the Middle Ages to the modern era.

Ancient notions about a supernatural basis of abnormal behavior evolved during the Middle Ages both in Christian theology and folk tradition. A mixture of ideas involving humors, demons, and astrological "facts" characterized some of the more complex and fanciful speculations. For example, some metaphysicians argued that devilish spirits called *incubi* were especially likely to take possession of a person with an excess of warm humors (Zilboorg & Henry, 1941, p. 137).

Nevertheless, even churchmen considered most instances of abnormal behavior to be the result of natural rather than spiritual causes. Psychopathology was therefore typically treated at home or in local churches with folk remedies and prayerful attention (Alldridge, 1979; Kroll, 1973). Some cases, however, were believed to reflect the influence of spirits (incubi, succubi, sylvani) or malevolent humans practicing witchcraft. A person so transformed was considered both mad and evil. The most vigorous, systematic, and terrifying institutional response to such behavior was the Inquisition of the Roman Catholic Church.

Until the eleventh century, the Church had tended to downplay if not censure ideas about witchcraft and demonic possession. Thereafter, for complex economic and political reasons, it began to use these ideas to reinforce and expand its power (Spanos, 1978). In 1233, the Church Inquisition, a kind of medieval secret police, was initially founded by Pope Gregory IX to combat heresy and encourage repentance. During the European Renaissance period, especially during the sixteenth century, it heightened its efforts against witchcraft and demonic possession. Although establishment of the Inquisition was primarily a political reaction against the threat of heresy, it also represented an intellectual commitment to a supernatural view of some types of abnormal behavior.

Witches' Hammer   One of the best-known and most malevolent products of this historical period was the *Malleus Maleficarum*, or Witches' Hammer. *Malleus,* which became the official handbook of the Inquisition, was written toward the end of the fifteenth century by two German Dominican brothers, Johann Sprenger and Heinrich Kraemer, and approved by Pope Innocent VIII in his papal edict of 1484.

Malleus suggested ways to detect evil supernatural influences caused by witchcraft, and to punish witches while attempting to save victims by requiring fasting, prayer, and exorcism. Even the notorious *Malleus* recognized natural forms of abnormal behavior, but it is remembered primarily for the ghastly excesses it promoted in the name of supernatural causes. Whether accused by Inquisitional or by local authorities, witches were intimidated psychologically and physically in order to coerce repentance; when this failed, the accused might be beaten, broken on the rack, or, rather infrequently, burned at the stake.

Some of the mostly female victims of politicoreligious fervor and sadistic impulse were probably suffering from diagnosable mental abnormalities; for example, some had hallucinations, delusions, and emotional turmoil suggesting psychotic disorder while others displayed evidence of medically inexplicable abnormalities of sensation, movement, and consciousness suggesting hysterical disorder. Nevertheless, most were probably just nonconformists, social nuisances, or the victims of neighbors with vivid imaginations or personal grudges (Spanos, 1978).

Even after the declining influence of the Inquisition, witch hunts and witchcraft trials continued unabated in both Catholic and Protestant countries through the seventeenth century; they became progressively less frequent only in the eighteenth century during the Age of Reason with its new scientific discoveries of physical and physiological causality. Yet even during the eighteenth century, some women were decapitated for witchcraft, the last case occurring in 1782 in Switzerland.

The last major incident occurring in North America involved a witchcraft scare in colonial Salem at the end of the seventeenth century. A group of eight girls began showing signs of "distemper," including bizarre speech and convulsive fits. The girls began accusing people of witchcraft. Hundreds were indicted and imprisoned though few were ever brought to trial and almost no one was killed. One interesting speculation is that the apparently psychotic and hysterical symptoms of the so-called victims of witchery were actually signs of a temporary organic mental disorder caused by ergot poisoning from a virulent parasitic fungus that had contaminated the grain products consumed by the inhabitants of one section of the town (Caporael, 1976). Unfortunately, there is simply no way to be sure if this speculation has any validity.

Any tendency to be too judgmental about the seemingly frequent barbarisms of past cultures should be weighted against both the barbarisms of the modern era and an appreciation of how difficult it is, despite all our advances, to make reliable distinctions and rational decisions regarding illness, evil, and just plain idiosyncracy.

Psychological View

The psychological view, reflecting both philosophical and scientific traditions, focuses on conscious experience, mental mechanisms, and social environmental causes. Like so many themes in Western culture, speculations about the psychological basis of abnormal behavior are rooted in ancient Greek and Roman thought.

Greek Tradition   Plato theorized about two kinds of psychopathology. One of these, related to our modern concept of neurosis, involves *conflicts* among personal traits—for example, desire versus inhibition. Another, related to our concepts of psychosis and dementia, involve *defects* of reason, especially poor insight or faulty self-knowledge. The Roman orator/philosopher Cicero (106–43 B.C.E.) similarly emphasized the influence of imbalances among reason (intellect), instinct (appetites), and passions (temper) in causing abnormal behavior. He argued that there are four tempers: discomfort, fear, pleasure, and violent desire (*libido*), the last-named most likely to disorganize behavior. Almost 2000 years later, the libido concept would dramatically reemerge in Sigmund Freud's psychodynamic model (see Chapter 6).

Postmedieval Notions about Conflict and Repression   Purely psychological theories of abnormal behavior during the Middle Ages are hard to find. More typically, mixtures of Greco-Roman psychology and medieval notions of supernatural influence prevailed. Paracelsus (1493–1541), the Swiss physician, mystic, and iconoclast, was the first to argue that repressed needs and thoughts could cause mental disorder, another idea that was to emerge centuries later in psychodynamic models of the modern era.

Johann Weyer (1515–1588) (Figure 2.3), a humanitarian and physician, spoke out forcefully against the "silly and often godless absurdities" of *Malleus Maleficarum* and the atrocities of the Inquisition. Although he still believed in supernatural causes of abnormal behavior, Weyer thought that the pathological effect of such influence was more likely if a person were predisposed by natural factors including diet, personality, and social condition. In short, Weyer actually formulated an early version of what we now call the *diathesis-stress* hypothesis, which holds that a constitutional weakness (diathesis) may interact with stresses of external origin to produce an increased risk for developing mental disorder.

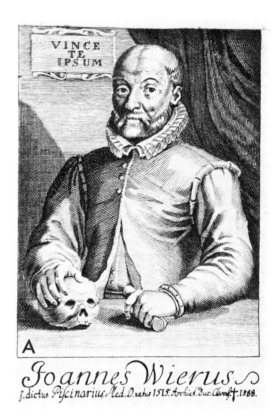

FIGURE 2.3   Johann Weyer (1515–1588).

Weyer recommended studying patients' dreams and fantasies for evidence of inner conflicts. He argued that psychological investigation could reveal natural explanations for so-called miraculous phenomena. For example, by careful and controlled observation, Weyer was able to establish conclusively that secret feedings rather than miraculous powers explained the apparent ability of a young maid, Barbara Kremers, to go without food indefinitely. The Kremers case shows that Weyer was indeed far ahead of his time in arguing for careful observation guided by scientific objectivity.

Weyer's efforts to distinguish between the reality of fantasy and the fantasy of demonology represents an historical bridge between ancient and modern psychological theories about the role of impulse, emotion, conflict, and repression in explaining abnormal behavior (see Chapter 6).

From Mesmerism to Hypnosis   The gradual evolution of premodern psychological theories takes a somewhat bizarre detour through the pseudoscientific theories of Franz Mesmer (Darnton, 1968; Fuller, 1982). Mesmer (1734–1815) believed that all things in the universe, and indeed the universe itself, is filled with an invisible magnetic fluid; disorganized magnetic fluids in the human body could therefore explain abnormal behavior. Mesmer believed that by gaining control over these fluids, he could heal the physically and mentally ill.

In practice, *mesmerism* was an elaborate and theatrical hocus-pocus involving a troughlike oaken apparatus called a *baquet* (see Figure 2.4). Filled with water and iron filings, the baquet had iron rods, supposedly magnetized by Mesmer, sticking out on all sides. By touching, stroking, and sheer charismatic "presence," Mesmer elicited crying, convulsions, and other hysterical crises in those who gathered around the baquet.

In late-eighteenth-century Paris, Mesmer's was the best act in town. The scientific presumptions, therapeutic promise, occult quality, and just plain razzle-dazzle of mesmerism accounted for its incredibly widespread appeal. This was an era in transition between the Enlightenment and romanticism when many fascinating new ideas about mysterious invisible factors such as gravity, magnetism, and electricity were very much in the air, so to speak.

However, as an explanation of human behavior, animal magnetism could not survive scientific test, and Mesmer's notions lost considerable steam when Louis XVI convened a Royal Commission that included scientists like Lavoisier and Benjamin Franklin to investigate them. Published in 1784, the commission's report made clear that "magnetism" without suggestion produced nothing, whereas suggestion without magnetism produced all the "magnetic" phenomena.

FIGURE 2.4   Mesmer and patients around the baquet. (Courtesy The Mansell Collection)

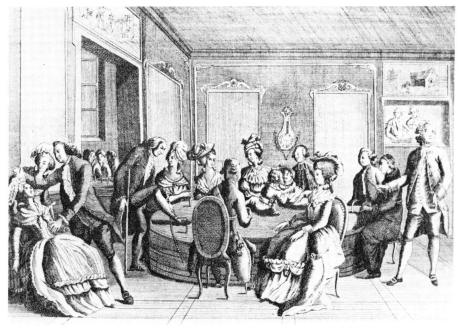

While Mesmer faded from the scene, his ideas flourished throughout Europe, in large part because of the influence of the Marquis de Puysegeur (1751–1825). An artillery officer and aristocrat, de Puysegeur used "magnetic" techniques to treat the illnesses of people living on his estate (Ellenberger, 1970). He was able to induce "perfect crises," altered states of consciousness associated with mental clarity, hyperresponsiveness to the "magnetizer," and subsequent amnesia for the experience. This state came to be known as artificial somnambulism. It soon became apparent that neither baquet nor other props were necessary to induce artificial somnambulism or to produce cures; the main ingredient was the will of the "magnetizer" and the belief and desire of the patient.

The highly influential ideas and practices of de Puysegeur and others spread to England. There, James Braid (1795–1860), a surgeon renowned for his successful treatments of clubfoot, developed a physiological-psychological theory of artificial somnambulism which he renamed "neuro-hypnosis," partly to distinguish his research from the discredited views of the mesmerists. Braid thought of neuro-hypnosis as a kind of "nervous sleep" involving visual fixation, narrowed attention, impressionability, and imagination whose combined effects exhaust the brain, thereby sending the mind "out of gear" and into an altered state of intense concentration (Kravis, 1988).

Two aspects of the hypnotic state investigated by Braid would prove to have special importance to the evolving field of psychopathology. The use of hypnosis to induce bodily changes such as flushing, fainting, or paralysis provided a basis for theorizing about psychosomatic and hysterical symptoms, theorizing that was sometimes rather controversial (see below). The use of hypnosis to induce "double consciousness"—a state of heightened responsiveness and lucid experiences, the memories of which are completely lost (amnesia) upon "awakening"—provided a basis for theorizing about dissociative disorders—in particular, multiple personality. Braid's research on both the psychosomatic and dissociative aspects of hypnosis are forerunners of two contemporary models of psychopathology and psychological therapy: the psychodynamic model, which focuses on unconscious, conflict-ridden, idiosyncratic ideation, and the cognitive model, which focuses on attitudes, expectations, and learning (Kravis, 1988).

The same medical and scientific communities that had rejected Mesmer and his followers cast a more favorable eye on Braid's experiment-based psychophysiological theories and therapeutic methods. By the late nineteenth century, Braidism had become highly influential in Europe and the United States, and hypnotism was increasingly used both as a therapeutic procedure and as a research vehicle for exploring the mental mechanisms of psychopathology.

Controversies arose about the significance of *hypnotizability,* a readiness to be hypnotized or to enter the hypnotic state spontaneously. The controversy about hypnotizability was based partly on its connection to *hysterical* symptoms such as neurologically inexplicable blindness or paralysis. The Paris school of psychiatry headed by Jean Martin Charcot (1825–1893) and Pierre Janet (1859–1947) argued that hypnotizability is symptomatic of a neuropathological disposition, something like hyperactivity or morbid sensitivity. In contrast, the Nancy school of Ambrose-Auguste Liebeault (1823–1904) and Hippolyte-Marie Bernheim (1837–1919) argued that hypnotic suggestibility is a normal human tendency, something like sociability or curiosity. It is interesting that the leaders of these competing schools based their arguments in part on differing interpretations of Braid's work. Even today, the debate continues as to whether hypnotizability represents a pathological disposition or simply a talent for mimicry (see Chapters 16 and 17.)

From Hypnosis to Psychoanalysis Despite theoretical differences, the research of both the Paris and Nancy schools reinforced the psychological perspective of unconscious mental processes that influence behavior. The most ambitious expression of this view was the psychoanalytic theory of neurosis developed by Sigmund Freud (1856–1939) (Figure 2.5), a brilliant physician with extensive neurophysiological training and an abiding interest in questions about brain and mind.

Freud was deeply impressed by the hypnosis-hysteria connection. From the work of the Paris school he developed the idea that neurotic behavior is a symptom of unconscious conflict about expressing forbidden desires. For example, several interviews under hypnosis might reveal that a case of hysterical blindness or paralysis expressed a pathological avoidance of sexual or aggressive ideas about which the person was deeply conflicted. From the work of the Nancy school, Freud developed the idea that a psychological theory of conflict could be applied to normal as well as to neurotic behavior, and that techniques other than hypnosis could be used to analyze behaviors, promote insight, and thereby achieve therapeutic changes (see Chapter 6).

Experience with neurotic patients led Freud to dispense with hypnosis. Instead, the patient was encouraged to reveal unconscious motivation through *free association*, that is, a process by which ideas and fantasies are expressed without regard for their content or logic. Associations freed from the constraints of logic or propriety would constitute the raw material for interpreting behavior and enhancing insight into otherwise obscure mental mechanisms that accounted for symptomatology. Reviving conflict-ridden memories would have therapeutic value by inducing an emotional release (catharsis) or by facilitating rational self-control.

Psychoanalysis and Behaviorism The historical evolution from mesmerism to hypnosis to psychoanalysis represented progress in the scientific understanding of at least some types of abnormal behavior. By the early twentieth century, behaviorism was competing successfully with psychoanalysis for influence over the scientific community. The behaviorist approach to abnormal behavior (see Chapters 1, 5, and 15) is a modern by-product of experimental research on conditioned reflexes that had been pioneered by the great Russian neurophysiologist Ivan Pavlov (1849–1936).

Behaviorists rejected the basic psychoanalytic idea that symptoms are symbolic expressions of unconscious, conflict-ridden, erotic, or aggressive preoccupations originating in early childhood. Instead, they attempted to document experimentally how even animals who enjoy no symbolic abilities would nevertheless develop neurotic behaviors if exposed to noxious environments. If neurotic behavior could be produced experimentally in animals, then, they argued, murky psychoanalytic concepts about morbid mental mechanisms could be dispensed with as so much excess theoretical baggage. Not only that, but the scientifically testable principles of behaviorism could be applied to the therapeutic elimination of abnormal behavior through new learning.

In the psychoanalytic view, the human capacity for symbolic and imaginative thought makes tenuous any connection between behavior and its external causes. It therefore follows that a theory and therapy for *human* neuroses requires the analysis of personal meanings as much as (or more than) the reconstruction of objective event–behavior relationships (Taylor, 1984). In contrast, the behavioral view underscores the direct and discoverable influences of spe-

FIGURE 2.5 Sigmund Freud (1856–1939).

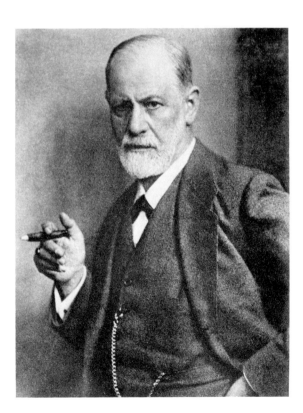

cific external stimuli over behavior. It therefore follows that theory, research, and therapy should be devoted to making those environment-behavior connections more explicit and controllable. Major differences between the environmental approach of behaviorism and the intrapsychic focus of psychoanalysis are given in Table 2.2.

Over the years, developments in psychoanalysis and behaviorism have tended to blur some of their differences. The psychoanalytic model has evolved perceptibly toward behaviorist views—for example, in exposing some of its concepts to *scientific test,* increasing its attention to basic motives (for security, affiliation, and competence) other than the one (libido) emphasized by Freud, and, perhaps most importantly, by increasing its attention to current environmental influences on behavior. The behaviorist tradition has also evolved, in some ways even more perceptibly in its cognitive-behavioral model, toward the psychoanalytic view by increasingly considering the role of *conflict* and symbolic *cognitive* processes that can make the connection between external events and abnormal behavior somewhat less direct (see Chapter 5).

Nevertheless, changes in these psychological models are minor compared to basic differences that remain, especially in the psychoanalytic emphasis on

TABLE 2.2   MAJOR DIFFERENCES BETWEEN BEHAVIORAL AND PSYCHOANALYTIC PSYCHOLOGIES

Dimension	Behavioral psychology	Psychoanalytic psychology
Method	*Laboratory* study typcially of normal animals or humans subject to frustrations caused by pain, conflict, uncertainty, or unpredictability	*Clinical* study, typically of psychiatric patients, using hypnosis, free association, and fantasy interpretation
Mechanisms	Conditioning and observational *learning* common to animals and humans	*Symbolic process* and repression unique to human mental life
Environment-behavior relationship	*Straightforward:* normal learning mechanisms yield abnormal behavior from abnormal environments	*Ambiguous:* repression and immature symbolic processes introduce an inventive element that distorts the environment-behavior relationship
Frustrated motives	*Any* basic motivation: safety, food, predictability, controllability	Special focus on *sexual* and aggressive motivation
Special predispositions	None emphasized	Two hypothesized: (1) *Developmental* (universal vulnerability): fantasy (prelogical thinking) dominates early childhood experience (2) *Psychopathological* (unique vulnerability): sensitization from adverse early experiences
Attitude toward "human nature"	Indifferent or optimistic	Pessimistic

early experience, infantile sexuality, unconscious mental life, and symbolic interpretation, as opposed to the behaviorist emphasis on conditioned reactions, conscious thought processes, and relatively predictable environment-behavior connections.

Experimental Psychopathology Toward the end of the nineteenth century, the psychological approach was developing experimental techniques to be used in the study of abnormal behavior. In 1879, Wilhelm Wundt (1832–1920) established in Leipzig, Germany the first laboratory devoted exclusively to the experimental analysis of conscious experience, emotions, and mental mechanisms (Boring, 1950). The scientific discipline of psychology dates its origin from the 1879 establishment of Wundt's laboratory. New techniques were developed for this research, including the scaling of subjective experience, the measurement of reaction time, and, during the early part of the twentieth century, the electronic monitoring of brain waves, heart rate, and other psychophysiological aspects of behavior. The new experimental techniques would soon be applied to the abnormalities of perception, thinking, and memory characteristic of different disorders.

An example of these developments is the work of Carl Gustav Jung (1875–1961) and his students, who combined their interest in psychoanalytic theory and their training in experimental methods to develop a psychophysiological approach to thought processes. They used a newly developed technique of measuring the electrical conductivity of the skin—the galvanic skin response, or GSR—to study the responses of subjects while taking a word-association test. Research on GSR patterns associated with idiosyncratic word associations led to theorizing about largely unconscious preoccupations or "complexes" that motivate individual behavior and that could at least partially explain the origins of mental illness.

The twentieth century has witnessed an explosive growth in experimental research on environmental causes of abnormal behavior—for example, animal research carried out during the first half of the twentieth century by Pavlov (1927/1960), Maier (1949), and Masserman (1950/1966). This research showed how "neurotic" reactions—excessive emotionality, inhibition, and avoidance behavior—can come under the control of even innocuous stimuli such as lights or tones that have been systematically associated with noxious experiences that are uncontrollable or unpredictable. The effect of this laboratory work was to confer increasing scientific respectability to age-old notions about conflict, frustration, and demoralization, and to reinforce cognitive-behavioral and psychodynamic theories about the social learning of psychopathology (see Chapters 5 and 6).

We have concluded our discussion of the historical evolution of organic, spiritual, and psychological perspectives on the nature of abnormal behavior. In the next section we provide a brief history of the treatment of severe behavioral disorders in mental institutions.

MENTAL INSTITUTIONS

The institutional approach to the social management of severe abnormality has a long history going back to ancient notions of sanctuary. We begin with a description of early asylums. We then describe both the humanitarian and inhumane aspects of mental institutions, and the reform movements that improved the lot of institutionalized patients. Modern society continues to grapple with questions of how to balance the needs for institutional treatment and protection of personal rights.

Asylums

Early History The concept of asylum, or therapeutic sanctuary for the physically and mentally ill, reached an early high point in ancient Greece. During the sixth century B.C.E., a sanctuary was erected at Epidauros in the name of Aesculapius, the god of healing. Patients were treated with baths, diet, remedies, exercise, instruction, and emotional support. Fasting, prayers, and rituals were also used, sometimes in combination with hypnotic and hallucinogenic drugs. Less fortunate patients might be treated with bloodletting, flogging, or weird concoctions such as sheep dung mixed with wine. The goal of all these ministrations was the promotion of insight and inspiration if not simple conformity to social norms.

Throughout the ancient period, special asylums existed for the mentally ill, usually as part of some religious or charitable organization. During the early Middle Ages, most of the asylums were either almshouses or monasteries where monks provided prayer and comfort to the mentally ill alongside the poor, the aged, or physically ill people who had no families to support them. Over the years, the asylum function was increasingly taken over by laymen working under the auspices of the state or for private profit. By the fifteenth century, secular asylums—often modified cloisters or monasteries—were springing up throughout Europe.

Renaissance Period Spain and England led the way in building asylums exclusively for the mentally ill. The first of these was founded in 1409 in Valencia, Spain. The most famous asylum of this period, however, was St. Mary of Bethlehem in London. Originally a monastery, it became an asylum for the mentally ill in 1377. In 1547, King Henry VIII, who seized and closed all the monasteries after his break with the Roman Catholic Church, gave the institution to the city of London. Despite the humanitarian intentions of its founders, conditions in the asylum deteriorated to an appalling state over the years. The moon-mad "lunatics" of Bethlehem, or Bedlam as it came to be known, were daily put on display for a small fee to amuse the population, and the Bedlam asylum became one of the great tourist attractions of the time (Figure 2.6).

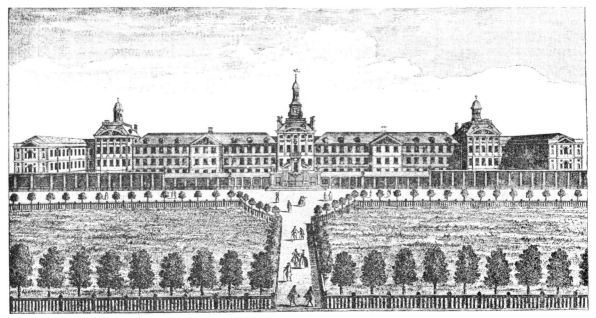

FIGURE 2.6   Bethlehem Hospital ("Bedlam") circa the seventeenth century.

By the seventeenth century, the housing of mental patients was big business. Private homes were converted into madhouses for patients who could pay. Two kinds of abuse were all too typical of these residences: the traditional neglect, mistreatment, and exploitation, and the more sinister abuse of wrongful incarceration. In the absence of protective laws, seemingly normal individuals could be locked away for months or years on slender pretext. A husband could have his wife put away for speaking her mind or acting independently, or to get at her money. A businessman, fallen on hard times and unable to pay his bills, might be institutionalized by the authorities at the behest of his creditors. The asylum thus came to serve as a penal institution as well as a psychiatric one (see Peterson, 1982, for example). Despite some attempts at legal reform over the years, adequate protection against wrongful incarceration had to wait until the mid-twentieth century.

Humanitarian Reformers 1700s–1900s

The mentally ill were not without their champions. At the end of the eighteenth century, a major reform movement began to take shape. Five of its most important figures were Edward Tyson, Philippe Pinel, and William Tuke, and, later, Dorothea Dix and Clifford Beers in America.

The least celebrated of the major humanitarian reformers was Edward Tyson (1651–1708), a prosperous English physician and renowned anatomist who proved by dissection that the porpoise is actually a mammal and not a fish. His later anatomical work established the striking resemblance of apes and humans, a connection explained some 150 years later when Darwin published his work on natural selection and evolution. After his election to the Royal College of Physicians, Tyson was put in charge of the by-then notorious Bethlehem hospital where he initiated major humanitarian reforms: improved nursing care, better clothing, and an innovative program for the follow-up of discharged patients (see Boorstein, 1983, for details).

Perhaps the most celebrated reformer was the French physician Philippe Pinel (1745–1826). A modest man of great erudition and humane motives, Pinel earned his claim to fame with his vigorous adoption of certain reforms begun earlier by a remarkable yet virtually unknown man named Jean-Baptiste Pussin (whose interesting story is described by Weiner, 1979).

Pussin, a tanner by trade, had been a patient in Paris in the Bicêtre hospital for men, where he received treatment for scrofula, a tubercular condition of the lymph glands in the neck. After recovering, he gained employment at the hospital, eventually becoming superintendent of the ward for "incurable" mental patients. In this capacity, Pussin instituted firm but humanitarian treatment, including freeing patients from shackles and encouraging meaningful work for them. He did all he could to provide nutritious food, bright open spaces, and kind attention in place of meager rations, dark cells, chains, bloodletting, and other "therapeutic" horrors.

Pinel, enjoying a fine reputation, was appointed in 1793 by the authorities of the French Revolution to work at the Bicêtre hospital. There, despite his higher status, Pinel adopted and expanded upon Pussin's pioneering reforms. Two years later, Pinel was transferred to the other great hospital of Paris, la Salpêtrière for women patients (where 100 years later Freud was to get the better part of his clinical training in hypnosis). Eventually, Pinel's efforts to get his mentor transferred to la Salpêtrière was successful, and in 1802, the two men were reunited to continue their collaboration. Together, they fought to free all but the most intractable inmates, and to provide a gentler and more understanding form of care (Figure 2.7).

The themes of these changes, collectively known as "moral treatment," were simple enough. Psychopathology was to be considered a natural illness rather than sinfulness, depravity, or criminality. Jailers were to become healers, and inmates were no longer to be thought of as wild beasts. In a way, moral treatment represented a return to the classic sanctuary model of ancient Greece, but without the religious overtones.

In England, the Quaker tea and coffee merchant William Tuke became so incensed at the wretched treatment of the mentally ill, he took up the cause of reform. On his own initiative, Tuke used private funds to establish in 1796 the York retreat for the care and study of abnormal behavior. His efforts to provide sanctuary and a healthful environment for patients were based on the humanitarian model of Pussin and Pinel. Tuke's son, grandson, and great-

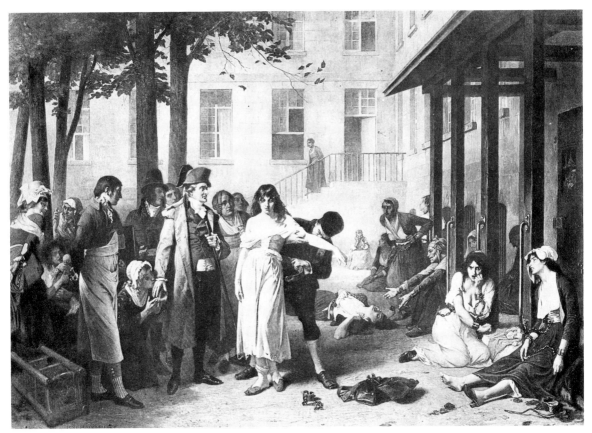

FIGURE 2.7   Pinel ordering the unshackling of patients at the Salpetrière, from a painting by Fleury. (The Bettman Archive)

grandson continued the tradition of moral treatment right up to the twentieth century.

While Pussin, Pinel, and others labored in revolutionary France and Tuke took up the cause in England, Benjamin Rush (1745–1813) promoted the concept of moral treatment in the United States from his position at the Pennsylvania Hospital. Though a minor figure in the pantheon of reformers, this signer of the Declaration of Independence is considered the "father of American psychiatry." Rush also gets credit for initiating the modern penal system. Only 200 years ago, convicted criminals typically were flogged, maimed, or publicly humiliated in the stocks. Rush, in a paper read in 1787 to a group of Quakers at Benjamin Franklin's home, suggested an alternative form of punishment: solitary confinement and hard work plus Bible study for penitence. The upshot was a new penitentiary movement, first in Pennsylvania and later throughout the United States.

Dorothea Lynde Dix (1802–1887) (Figure 2.8), an ex-school teacher forced by tuberculosis into early retirement, devoted her remaining years to an indefatigable campaign for the reform of prisons and asylums, first in the United States and later in Canada and Europe. She wrote to Congress about the

> ...more than 9000 idiots, epileptics and insane in the United States, destitute of appropriate care and protection...bound with galling chains, bowed beneath fetters and heavy iron balls attached to drag-chains, lacerated with ropes, scourged with rods and terrified beneath storms of execration and cruel blows; now subject to jibes and scorn and torturing tricks; now abandoned to the most outrageous violations (quoted in Zilboorg & Henry, 1941, pp. 583–584).

Dix traveled throughout the country, lobbying politicians, bureaucrats, and rich businessmen. Through her amazingly successful efforts, she raised millions of dollars toward the founding of thirty-two mental hospitals. But as good intentions sometimes have unfortunate consequences, Dix's unyielding fervor and authoritarian manner promoted changes that actually undercut her humanitarian goals.

As the many new hospitals filled up, treatment values changed and therapy became less effective. According to Bockoven (1963), "the inundation of mental hospitals with long-standing chronic cases ruined moral [i.e., humane]

FIGURE 2.8   Dorothea Lynde Dix by S. B. Waugh. (Courtesy New Jersey State Hospital)

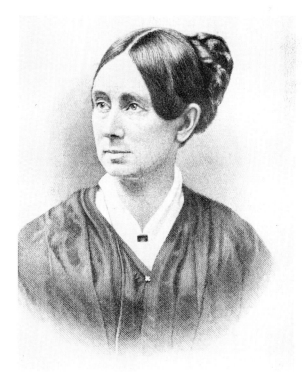

treatment. Neither the chronic cases transferred to the hospitals from jails, almshouses, cellars and attics nor the new cases of recently acquired insanity could benefit from the art and therapeutic know-how which had been learned by moral therapists since the time of Pinel and Tuke''(p. 38). Thus, the thrust of psychiatric treatment shifted from the earlier moral model of Pussin, Pinel, and Tuke to a medical or custodial model. The optimism, enthusiasm, and spirit of experimentation that had characterized work with the mentally ill and had been carried out largely by individual initiative were overwhelmed by a new emphasis on diagnosis, custodial care, and increased attention to bureaucratic and legalistic matters.

The final figure in our pantheon of reformers is Clifford Beers (1876–1943) (Figure 2.9). A Yale graduate and aspiring businessman, Beers published an account of his own mental breakdown and subsequent institutionalization in a classic autobiography that gave an inspirational push to the mental hygiene

FIGURE 2.9   Clifford W. Beers. (Bettman Archive)

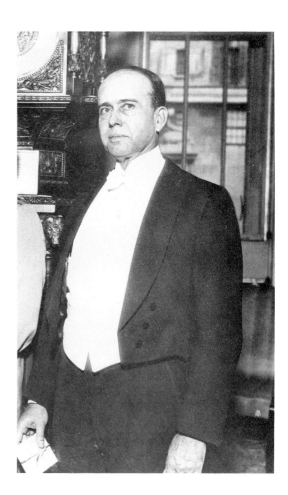

movement in the United States. In *A Mind That Found Itself* (1908), Beers documents his suicidal depression over fears of becoming epileptic, his deepening isolation and withdrawal, his paranoid psychosis, and his manic grandiosity.

Fortunately, Beers recovered sufficiently to write about his psychosis and the appalling treatment of inmates at the private sanitarium to which he was sent by well-meaning relatives. Like the madhouses of the seventeenth and eighteenth centuries, private sanitariums available to the Beers family were run for profit, often at the expense of genuine treatment. Here, the strait-jacket, physical abuse, and other forms of mistreatment were the rule.

Beers' book served as the literary inspiration for a new movement to reform hospital treatment and educate the public on ways to prevent mental illness. His efforts were based on his fervent belief that "so-called madmen are too often man-made, and that he who is potentially mad may keep a saving grip on his own reason if he is fortunate enough to receive that kindly and intelligent treatment to which one on the brink of mental chaos is entitled" (Beers, 1907/ 1981, p. 190).

With the support of prominent psychiatrists and psychologists like Adolph Meyer and William James, Beers worked tirelessly to establish the *mental hygiene movement* designed to promote mental health and a greater understanding of mental illness. In 1908, he founded the Connecticut Society for Mental Hygiene, and a year later, the National Committee for Mental Hygiene. These and numerous other organizations soon grew in influence, attracting philanthropic support, political backing, and international attention. They provided information, funded research, and promoted legislation in the interests of mental health.

Custodial Hospitals 1900–1950s

Despite the often heroic efforts of people like Dix and Beers, and despite a new optimism about even severe disorders spurred by behaviorism and psychoanalysis, the lot of the average institutionalized mental patient in mid-century Europe and America was unenviable. In fact, considering the frequently humane standards of late-nineteenth-century mental hospitals (see Maher & Maher, 1979), subsequent developments might be considered regressive.

By mid-century, the number of psychiatric patients in the United States was growing twelve times faster than the general population. By 1944, more than half a million patients were housed in mental hospitals, which had grown in size from the 200 to 500 patients typical of nineteenth-century asylums to well over a thousand. By 1950, some of the larger hospitals reached gargantuan proportions, the biggest being the Pilgrim State Hospital in New York with a capacity of 10,000.

It is difficult to know exactly what it was like for the average patient because only the more abusive conditions tended to catch the attention of the press and public. Patients were usually treated as custodial wards of the state whether they were or not. At best, they received mediocre food, little intellectual stimulation or emotional support, and even less medical or psychiatric treatment. At worst, they were subjected to some age-old mistreatments: isolation, beatings, and the misuse of straitjackets, wet packs, and sedation.

The war effort of the early 1940s diverted funds otherwise slated for these places, thus subjecting the typical mental patient to even further "economies." The custodial functions carried out by poorly trained personnel largely substituted for meaningful therapeutic treatment. Conformity, dependency, passivity, and even withdrawal into fantasy were considered "good" behavior. The worst of the abuses were dramatically documented by Mary Jane Ward in an autobiographical novel. *The Snake Pit* provides a disturbing and moving picture of patients treated like criminals, retardates, or animals subjected to caprice, indifference, or brutality.

Deinstitutionalization 1960s–1980s

Since the early 1960s certain positive changes, some profound and some superficial, have occurred in hospital care. Many of the more brutal aspects of custodial care have gone by the board. Food and physical amenities have improved, and professional treatment is more solicitous and more often genuinely therapeutic. More patients have access to drugs, behavior modification programs, individual or group psychotherapy, and vocational training.

Between 1961 and 1972 alone, the number of hospitalized patients dropped from 527,000 to 276,000 (see Figure 2.10). There are two reasons for this deinstitutionalization, both reflecting an increasing concern for patients' rights. First, state and local authorities adopted stricter criteria for hospitalization, sometimes requiring evidence only of danger to self or others; in other words, bizarre behavior in itself was often no longer considered a legitimate criterion. Second, increasing efforts were made to keep hospital stays as brief as possible; many newly admitted inpatients were discharged after seventy-five days.

Unfortunately, some of the effects of this deinstitutionalization, a modern expression of the reform movement, have been superficial if not negative. Many elderly patients simply went from mental hospitals to nursing homes. Younger patients, discharged back to families, halfway houses, or residence hotels, have become a burden to themselves and others, disrupting family life, straining social service agencies, and often winding up on the street or back in the hospital. Consider the following two examples.

> Until [this 42-year-old man] became psychotic he was enrolled in an Ivy League college. He was hospitalized briefly in a state institution, where he was given antipsychotic medication, but when we saw him, he was receiving no treatment. For a while after his discharge his mother cared for him; eventually, however, she became too depressed to continue. Frightened and too confused to care for himself, he now wanders the streets by day, muttering incoherently and responding to voices he

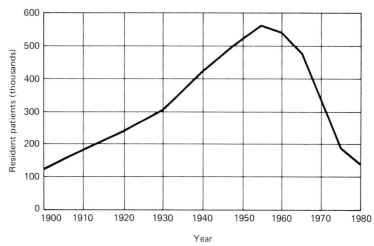

FIGURE 2.10   Deinstitutionalization of the mentally ill since the late 1950s has reduced the inpatient population at state and county mental hospitals. Because alternative residences and treatment programs have not been provided in many communities, many former patients, as well as some younger disturbed people who were never hospitalized, may now be homeless. (From "The Homeless Problem" by E. Bassuk. Copyright 1984 by Scientific American, Inc. All rights reserved.)

alone hears. At night he goes to a shelter where the staff are too busy feeding and clothing people to devote themselves to individual problems.

The court psychiatrist diagnosed [this 18-year-old man] as schizophrenic, and he was hospitalized in an institution for the criminally insane for the next 16 years. Since being discharged more than two years ago, he has lived both in shelters and on the streets; not long before we saw him he had been arrested for trespassing in a cemetery, where he was living in a tomb he had hollowed out. He says he receives messages from spirits who speak to him through spiders (Bassuk, 1984, p. 43).

Exploitation and degradation of former patients is often as great or greater under this new system, and there are many cases of unwanted and unmanageable pregnancies that would not have occurred in the hospital setting (Arnhoff, 1975). In addition, stiffer admission requirements bar many people from getting help who might benefit from brief hospitalization (Bassuk, 1984). These developments, in part, reflect important changes in the legal status of persons subject to hospitalization.

PSYCHOPATHOLOGY AND THE LAW

The 1960s and 1970s saw the proliferation of civil and criminal laws aimed at protecting the rights and promoting the welfare of mental patients. Where no crime has been committed, civil law permits *voluntary* commitment for those individuals who seek asylum. This can be done either on an informal basis, with the person free to leave at any time, or more often, in a more formal manner that requires a physician's certification of need and a psychiatric review during confinement. Under extraordinary circumstances, hospital officials may attempt to change the patient's voluntary status to involuntary, hopefully while recognizing legal safeguards that include concurrence of examiners, formal petition to the courts, a judicial hearing, and even a trial by jury when requested.

Institutionalization

Involuntary Commitment Civil law also permits *involuntary* commitment of dangerous, disorganized, or incompetent individuals. The term involuntary commitment refers *both* to people who resist confinement and to those who are so confused or incompetent that willingness or resistance is not an issue. Involuntary commitment thus reflects two functions of government: the police function that protects society against dangerous people, and the guardian, or *parens patriae,* function that protects persons who are frankly suicidal or otherwise incapable of taking care of themselves—for example, the severely mentally retarded.

The legal system has codified how the right of the public to protection should be balanced against the right of the individual to liberty (Miller et al., 1976, pp. 5–6). Under new legal protections gained since the early 1970s, involuntary admission to a mental hospital for reasons other than imminent danger to self or others has become increasingly difficult. Bizarre or offensive behavior no longer constitutes a compelling criterion for hospitalization in many instances.

The civil rights of presumptively dangerous individuals subject to involuntary commitment procedures have been enhanced by many laws—for example, acknowledging the right to examination by more than one clinician, the right to a judicial hearing, and, in some cases, the right to a trial by jury with full legal representation. The objective of psychiatric evaluation and judicial review is to establish an imminent danger to the person or to others, a major problem given the difficulty of predicting the future and the uncertainty of psychiatric assessment.

During the 1970s, legal rights to facilitate release of involuntary patients were codified. The most celebrated case was the suit against a Florida state hospital superintendent brought by Kenneth Donaldson (Figure 2.11), involuntarily committed by a father who thought his son was delusional. Donaldson was confined for almost fifteen years without meaningful treatment. Donaldson argued that he was repeatedly denied ground privileges, reliable access to a psychiatrist, and even occupational therapy. Further, he argued that he was neither mentally ill nor dangerous, and that he had repeatedly requested release to responsible persons willing to provide care, guidance, and job opportunities.

The court was impressed by the evidence that Donaldson was neither dangerous nor incompetent, that he was capable of living outside the hospital, and that the hospital officials had failed to respond to his right to be released, or to be treated and then released; Donaldson's perpetual confinement despite re-

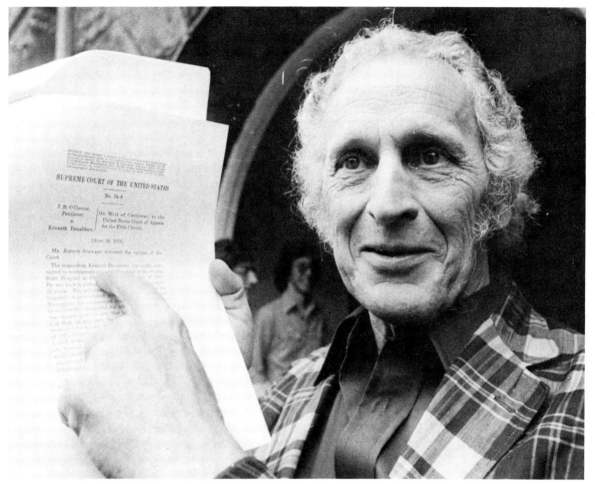

FIGURE 2.11   Kenneth Donalson after winning his case at the Supreme Court. (Wide World Photos)

peated attempts to prove his competence and harmlessness was deemed by the court to have been an unconstitutional misuse of authority.

Right to Treatment   Involuntary civil commitment would seem to confer the right to treatment including not only the obvious such as medication or psychotherapy, but also rooms with sufficient space, light, and toilet facilities, plus decent food, clean clothes, and opportunities for exercise. However, the courts have required only decent living conditions and some attempt at rehabilitation, if not a cure. In short, the right to "treatment" means the right to *some* treatment, not ideal treatment.

It should go without saying that the right to some treatment includes the right to be free from physical, psychological, or chemical abuse. And this raises an interesting question about a patient's right to *refuse* treatment. For example, if a suicidal individual can be committed involuntarily, may that individual be coerced to accept antidepressive medication or electroconvulsive therapy, seemingly drastic treatments that nevertheless have proven to be effective for normalizing behavior or speeding release in many cases? To help resolve such questions, guidelines have been established that are especially strict for drastic treatments that include psychosurgery, electroconvulsive shock, medication, or aversive conditioning.

Criminal Nonresponsibility

Individuals may occasionally be relieved of personal responsibility for illegal behavior. The development of legal guidelines to delineate such instances represents society's attempt to grapple with certain vital distinctions: evil versus illness, and guilt versus innocence. These distinctions go back to the ancient Hebrews and the Greco-Roman period when law and tradition protected children, psychotics, and the mentally retarded from the full application of punitive law.

A defendant accused of an illegal act is subject to laws designed to establish criminal responsibility and determine punishment or treatment. Under the law, criminal responsibility is based on criminal intent, literally "guilty mind" or *mens rea,* a combination of willful malevolence and comprehension of wrongdoing. In contrast, criminal *non*responsibility involves two broad categories: immaturity and insanity (see Figure 2.12). The immaturity concept is relatively simple, but the insanity concept is complex.

The term *immaturity* applies both to minors and to severely mentally retarded adults—in other words, people who, because of their chronological or "mental" age, are presumed to be unable to appreciate the nature of an illegal act such as shooting someone. Establishing that an individual is not guilty of a crime by reason of immaturity is relatively straightforward because age and IQ are easy to determine.

The legal term *insanity* identifies those *rare* cases of irresistible impulse or mental disorganization that can absolve a person from criminal responsibility. Establishing that a person is not guilty by reason of insanity is difficult because

FIGURE 2.12 Categories of criminal nonresponsibility.

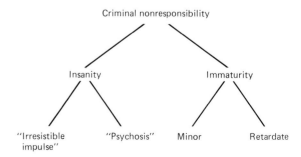

insanity criteria are not clear-cut. Such a determination also depends on highly questionable inferences about the mental state of a defendant *at the time of the act,* not at the time of the trial. Also, insanity and commitment are two different though related issues. If no longer insane, a person judged not guilty by reason of insanity may be discharged by the courts. However, if still insane or otherwise incompetent, such a person may be committed to a mental hospital for further treatment. We now turn to some important milestones in the historical development of the insanity concept.

Insanity Criteria 1840s–1980s

Irresistible Impulse   The decision in a criminal case tried in an Ohio court in 1834 established the so-called irresistible impulse criterion for determining insanity. The court ruled that in some cases a pathological impulse could drive an otherwise competent person to commit an illegal act despite that person's comprehension of right and wrong. To establish irresistible impulse, the defense would have to convince the court that during the act, the person could not have resisted the impulse even if a policeman were in the immediate vicinity. For example, insanity could be argued in a case in which a brain defect caused a seizurelike "fit" of murderous rage that overwhelmed an otherwise normal person in Jekyll-and-Hyde fashion; such a person might have no recollection of the criminal act carried out in the pathologically altered state of mind.

Critics of the irresistible impulse criterion argue that it is next-to-impossible to distinguish between an irresistible impulse (mental disease) and an impulse not resisted (culpable self-indulgence). Nowadays, the irresistible impulse argument is used less frequently and less successfully. Nevertheless, when the crime is determined to stem from seizurelike disorganization, a defendant is likely to be exonerated.

M'Naghten Rule   In 1843, a Scotsman named Daniel M'Naghten was acquitted of killing Edward Drummond, secretary to Sir Robert Peel, the Tory prime minister of England. M'Naghten was driven by the delusion that the Tories were tormenting and endangering him. After nine physicians testified that M'Naghten was "insane," the court ruled that he was not guilty by reason of insanity, and placed him in a lunatic asylum for the remainder of his life.

Displeased by the verdict, Queen Victoria set up a commission of fifteen common-law judges to study the case. Their subsequent deliberations produced what is called the M'Naghten rule.

> ...to establish a defense on the ground of insanity, it must be clearly proved that at the time of the committing of the act, the party accused with labouring under such a defect of reason, from disease of the mind, as not to know the nature and quality of the act he was doing; or if he did know it, that he did not know that he was doing what was wrong.

The rule includes two criteria, at least one of which must be met. First, there must be confusion as to the nature of the act—squeezing someone's neck be-

FIGURE 2.13 Daniel M'Naghten.

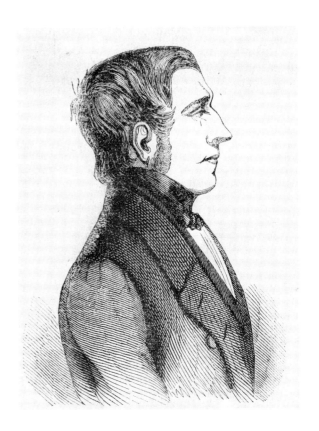

lieving it to be a lemon, or the person must be unable to appreciate the wrongfulness of the act—acting in self-defense in the delusional belief that one is being physically attacked at the time of the act (Slovenko, 1980).

The rule forces the court to take the perspective of the defendent and ask, specifically, if the defendant would be justified, under *existing law,* in committing the act if his beliefs, at the time of the act, were actually true. Ironically, M'Naghten himself would probably have been judged guilty as charged under the M'Naghten rule because (1) he did have criminal intent (*mens rea*), (2) he did know what he was doing, and (3) he would have been guilty under the law even if the Tories had actually been plotting to kill him (Slovenko, 1980).

Durham Product Rule In 1869, a New Hampshire court established that a finding of mental illness could preclude guilt for a crime. On the basis of this precedent, in *Durham vs. the United States,* Judge David Bazelon of the Court of Appeals for the District of Columbia formulated the Durham rule in 1954:

An accused is not criminally responsible if his unlawful act was the product of a mental disease or defect (Durham v. United States, 214 F.2d 862 [D.C.Cir. 1954]).

Originally designed to encourage maximum use of psychiatric testimony, the Durham rule was discarded in 1972 because of the difficulties posed by conflicting testimony and the ambiguity of terms like "product" and "mental illness." In its place, the American Law Institute adopted another rule, which appears to be a mixture of irresistible impulse, M'Naghten, and Durham criteria.

American Law Institute Rule   The American Law Institute (ALI) rule, first introduced in 1962 and later (1972) adopted by the D. C. Appeals Court, provides that

> (1) A person is not responsible for criminal conduct if at the time of such conduct as a result of mental disease or defect he lacks substantial capacity either to appreciate the criminality (wrongfulness) of his conduct or to conform his conduct to the requirement of the law; (2) As used in the Article, the terms "mental disease or defect" do not include an abnormality manifested only by repeated criminal or otherwise anti-social conduct (United States v. Brawner, 471 F 2d 969 [D.C. Dir. 1972]).

The ALI rule contains elements of several earlier rulings: Durham in the "mental disease or defect" criterion; M'Naghten in the "appreciation of criminality" (wrongfulness) criterion; and irresistible impulse in the "conformity of conduct" criterion. The ALI rule liberalized the standards for establishing insanity. For example, although under a strict interpretation of a M'Naghten-type rule, Daniel M'Naghten would probably have been convicted, under the more liberal ALI rule, he probably would have been acquitted by reason of insanity. Psychiatric testimony carried less weight under the ALI rule than under Durham because the latter is advisory rather than definitive, rarely delivering conclusive evidence regarding the mental state of the accused during the criminal act.

The ALI rule included two standards for determining insanity: a cognitive standard (inability to appreciate wrongfulness of an act) and a volitional standard (inability to conform conduct to requirements of law). The volitional standard has been removed by an act of Congress. The Insanity Reform Act of 1984 now requires only that the cognitive standard be used to determine insanity at the time of the act. (For an excellent critical discussion of this change, see Rogers, 1987.)

Ambiguities and controversies have always surrounded the various definitions and distinctions we have discussed in this and the preceding chapter: insanity versus criminal responsibility (*mens rea*); personal rights and responsibilities versus *parens patriae* and police powers of government; normality and mental health versus abnormality and psychopathology. Clearly, absolute answers continue to elude age-old questions about how to define and where to draw the line, and this will be apparent in the next chapter, which deals with the classification of abnormal behavior into distinct disorders.

SUMMARY

Throughout history, three major views of abnormal behavior have prevailed. The organic view holds that the causes of abnormal behavior lie in corresponding brain abnormalities. Notions about bodily fluids, or humors, gradually gave way to increasing knowledge of brain mechanisms, neurological diseases, and genetic causation; organic treatments also evolved from the diets and potions of ancient times to the pharmacological, electrical, and psychosurgical treatments of more recent times. The supernatural view that demonic forces cause some forms of abnormal behavior, though not taken seriously by modern scientists, did have extraordinary influence during certain historical periods. A prominent example occurred in Europe from the fifteenth to the seventeenth centuries during the Renaissance period when religious institutions, struggling to expand political power and to promote spiritual influence, spawned preoccupation with abnormal behavior. As a result, both sane and insane alike were caught up in witch hunts that occurred off and on up until the eighteenth century. In the psychological view, mental mechanisms described by ancient philosophers as tensions between passion and reason, and by modern psychologists as cognitive mechanisms and conditioned reactions, are believed to account for abnormal behavior.

The historical evolution of institutionalized treatment began with the priestly and secular asylums of ancient and modern times. With the rise of nation states and private enterprise, financial and administrative needs competed with humanitarian concerns, and the lot of the patient deteriorated. Attempts by humanitarian reformers to encourage the humane treatment of patients confined to mental hospitals met with mixed success, with initial reforms often being lost over the years. Even in modern times, the persistence of "snake pits" with ragged, ignored, or abused inmates reflected seemingly inevitable tensions between economic forces and philanthropic influences in societies still uncertain about the causes of severe abnormal behavior.

The modern reform movement in mental health has included a new emphasis on patient rights regarding hospitalization and treatment. The need to balance individual rights and social obligations is reflected in the evolution of criteria, including irresistible impulse, defective reason, mental illness, and inability to comprehend the nature of personal actions, for distinguishing between insanity and moral responsibility.

CHAPTER 3

Classification of Clinical Disorders

OUTLINE

Classification is the systematic arrangement of things—people, events, whatever—according to similarities and differences. A classification system says what goes with what—for example, the periodic table arranges chemical elements into distinct "families" on the basis of atomic structures. Classification systems also exist for organizing abnormal behavior into distinct disorders and groups of disorders. This chapter discusses psychiatric classification and then describes many of the disorders represented in one particular classification system, the *DSM-III-R*.

We should first be clear about the difference between the classification of disorders and the classification of individuals. A classification of *disorders* reflects our assumptions about the nature and arrangement of abnormal behavior in the general population—for example, our assumption that thought disorders (psychoses) and anxiety disorders (neuroses) are fundamentally different types of psychopathology. A classification of *individuals,* on the other hand, represents a match between an individual pattern of behavior—a pattern of delusions, hallucinations, and social withdrawal, for example—and behavioral criteria associated with a diagnostic category—in this example, the schizophrenia category. In other words, when we classify, or diagnose, a person, we "place" that person in the classification system. This chapter will focus mainly on the classification of disorders, while the next chapter will focus on the classification of persons (diagnosis.)

CLASSIFICATION OF DISORDERS

Our thinking and communication benefit from reducing complex experience to simpler, more manageable concepts. Young children soon learn to reduce a multitude of experiences with animals by using categories such as "dog" or "horse," and dimensions like "size" and "friendliness." Likewise, psychopathologists reduce the complexities of abnormal behavior by using categories such as schizophrenia or phobia, and dimensions such as anxiety level or degree of stress. The categorical approach dominates most systems currently used to classify abnormal behavior into distinct disorders.

Categorical Approach to Classification

Categories A category is defined by a set of criteria that formally identify the essential features of something—person, animal, or event. The more the observed features of something match the formal criteria for the category, the more likely it is that it will be classified as a member of the category. Thus, animals with orange feathers, two long legs, and an angled beak are likely to be included in the category of flamingo; in the same way, socially withdrawn people with abnormal thinking patterns are likely to be included in the category of schizophrenic disorder.

Assignment to a category tends to be an all-or-nothing affair—an animal either is or is not a flamingo; a person either is or is not a schizophrenic. Things within a category also tend to be seen as if they were alike but different from objects in other categories. This means that variations within a category are either ignored or minimized. Thus, the differences between types of schizophrenia are considered less important than the differences between any one type of schizophrenia and some other disorder like phobia (see Figure 3.1).

Approaches to Categorization There are different ways of approaching categorical classification. In one approach, each category is associated with criteria *all of which* are considered essential to the category's definition. Thus, if a category is defined by criteria a, b, c, d, e, and f, the only permissible exemplar would be a syndrome composed of *all* the definitive symptoms a through f. This approach to categorization is called *classical* because it represents the earliest view of how to classify things. (It is also called *monothetic,* referring to the unique theme, or inflexible idea, about what a category really means.) The effect of using a classical system to diagnose a disorder will be twofold: conparatively few persons will meet the criteria of any one category,

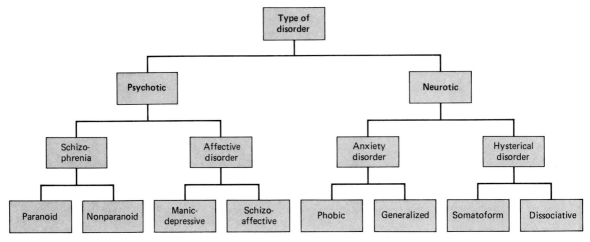

FIGURE 3.1 Hierarchical arrangement of a select group of categorically defined disorders. Specific examples (e.g., nonparanoid and paranoid) of a more general category (schizophrenia) are considered "closer" to each other than to the specific examples of other categories.

but those who do will show a high degree of behavioral similarity (Widiger & Frances, 1985).

In a different approach, each category is associated with criteria *only some* of which are necessary. An exemplar might be composed of symptoms a, c, d, and e, or b, c, e, and f, or some other permissible combination of, say, four out of six. In such a system, alternative exemplars, or *prototypes,* of a category can vary considerably. For example, some prototypes of schizophrenic disorder might display a more eccentric and delusional pattern while others might display a more withdrawn and apathetic pattern. This approach to categorization—which is common to the classification of psychopathology—is called *prototypal* because of the alternative exemplars (prototypes) that it permits. (The approach is also called *polythetic,* referring to permissible variations on a "theme," or flexible idea, about what a category really means.)

A mixed approach with both classical (monothetic) and prototypal (polythetic) aspects is often used. In these cases, some criteria—say a *and* b—are both considered definitive and necessary, and neither can substitute for the other; this is the classical aspect. Other criteria—say c, d, e, and f—may also be definitive but not all are necessary. Any combination of at least two out of the four may do, for example, so that any one may substitute for another; this is the prototypal aspect.

A prototypal approach, with its broadly and flexibly defined categories, has two advantages over a purely classical approach. First, it requires fewer categories to classify the great variety of behavioral variation, and this means greater simplicity. Second, it tends to be more reliable when used to diagnose persons because clinicians do not have to agree on every criterion to arrive at the same diagnosis.

Behavioral Discontinuity and Categorical Classification A categorical approach to classification rests on an assumption that discontinuities exist between behavioral phenomena (Blashfield, 1984). To appreciate what discontinuity means, look at Figure 3.2. The figure shows two different frequency distributions of individuals along a dimension. The dimension might be height, intelligence, extraversion, anxiety level, or severity of thought disorder.

The bell-shaped distribution shown in the top of the figure (a) is *unimodal*; it has a single peak indicating that most cases cluster in one region along the dimension. The distribution at the bottom of the figure (b) is *bimodal*; it has two peaks, indicating that most cases cluster in either of two regions of the dimension, with relatively few cases in between. Bimodality suggests some underlying discontinuity justifying the use of a categorical distinction. If "classification is the art of carving nature at the joints, it should indeed imply that there is a joint there [a region with few cases], that one is not sawing through bone" (Kendell, 1975, p. 65).

FIGURE 3.2 Two types of frequency distribution. (a) A *unimodal* (single-peaked) frequency distribution suggesting an underlying continuity. The justification for dividing this dimension at some cut-off point (vertical line) is less evident than in the case of the bimodal distribution. (b) A *bimodal* (two-peaked) frequency distribution suggesting an underlying discontinuity. The justification for dividing the dimension into two distinct regions (categories) is clearly evident.

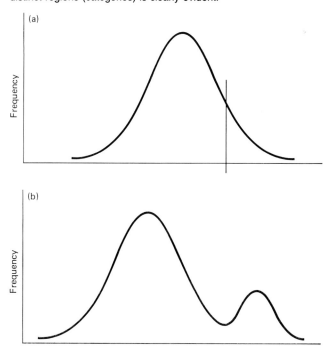

To the extent that patterns of behavior shade into one another without clear-cut boundaries, we may be "sawing through bone" when we use a cutoff point (the vertical line cutting the bell-shaped distribution in Figure 3.2, top) to divide dimensions. If most dimensions underlying abnormal behavior are continuously distributed, then, critics argue, serious questions can be raised about the use of a categorical approach for classifying psychopathology (Eysenck, 1986). Nevertheless, the categorical approach continues to yield useful information on the causes, course, and outcomes of discrete disorders.

Classification in the Context of Psychopathological Theory and Research

A classification system for abnormal behavior usually reflects both social conventions and scientific theory (Blashfield, 1984, 1986). But more, it provides a common language and conventional procedures to update knowledge and test theories. This link between theory and classification means that both evolve together on the basis of research and clinical experience. In short, a classification system is part of a larger scientific enterprise concerned with explaining behavior and testing those explanations (Skinner, 1981). To appreciate how this enterprise applies to abnormal behavior, we will discuss the interrelationship among theory, research, and classification as portrayed in Figure 3.3.

Theory   A theory is a formal representation of ideas about something. A theory of abnormal behavior usually specifies the symptoms, causes, and treatment of disorders (Figure 3.3, top). A theory may be rather modest, indicating merely the way that abnormalities are behaviorally organized and segregated from each other in time and place. On the other hand, a theory may be rather ambitious, specifying different physiological and/or mental mechanisms that explain the development, course, and treatment-responsiveness of different types of behavioral disorder.

A classification system like *DSM-III-R* (Figure 3.3, middle) translates theoretical ideas into the concrete terminology of behavioral definitions and conventional procedures for diagnosing specific instances of a disorder. In short, by representing theoretical ideas *operationally*—that is, in concrete and usable form—the classification system makes it possible to test those ideas in the light of research and clinical practice.

Validity   Such testing yields evidence of two kinds of validity for a disorder (Figure 3.3, bottom). *Internal validity* refers to evidence that a disorder is a coherent pattern of behaviors as theory says. *External validity* refers to evidence that associations exist between a disorder and other phenomena as predicted by the theory. Let us take a closer look at internal and external validity.

We said that a category is internally valid if its defining features cohere, or predict one another, as specified by theory. For example, the internal validity of schizophrenia rests on evidence that its major features—including disorganized and bizarre thinking and social withdrawal—co-occur more often than

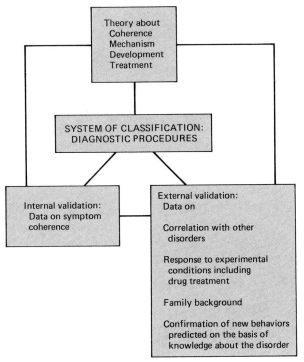

FIGURE 3.3   Interrelationship among theory, validation, and the classification system with its diagnostic procedures. (Adapted from Skinner, 1981.)

expected by chance. An internally valid category can be tested for external validity, the meaningful connections between a category and other phenomena predicted by theory. For example, consider the hypothesis that disorder X is determined by physiological mechanism m. Note that m is not yet part of the defining features of the category. It is an external phenomenon whose connection to disorder X, if established, would enhance our understanding of X. External validity for disorder X would be enhanced by evidence that it responds favorably to drugs that suppress m, but responds unfavorably to drugs that activate m.

Now that we have discussed the basic question of reliability and validity of categories, we can proceed to a description of a widely used system for classifying abnormal behavior.

DSM-III-R SYSTEM OF CLASSIFICATION

The third edition of the *Diagnostic and Statistical Manual of Mental Disorders,* or *DSM-III,* was published in 1980 by the American Psychiatric Association, and its revised form, the *DSM-III-R,* was published in 1987. *DSM-III* and *DSM-III-R* evolved out of earlier, less successful efforts (see Millon, 1986).

The Evolution of *DSM-III-R*

DSM-I, published in 1952, replaced a little used psychiatric section of the sixth edition of the *International Classification of Diseases* (*ICD-6*), published by the World Health Organization. *DSM-I* proved unsatisfactory for several reasons, including imprecise or ambiguous criteria; two clinicians working independently with *DSM-I* too often arrived at different diagnoses. *DSM-II* was published in 1968, sixteen years after the initial publication of its predecessor. The number of diagnostic categories was enlarged by 50 percent, proliferating with somewhat ambiguous terms like neurosis, psychosis, and condition. Despite the improvements over *DSM-I, DSM-II* immediately drew criticisms similar to those aimed at its forerunner. A radically new *DSM* appeared twelve years later in 1980.

The developers of *DSM-III* provided more detailed and explicit behavioral criteria for the new categories, and distinguished between *essential* (necessary) and *associated* criteria that were often, but not necessarily, observed. In addition to category-defining criteria, *DSM-III* provided *exclusionary* criteria to help define what a category is *not*. The result of these and other innovations was increased diagnostic reliability (discussed in Chapter 4).

The developers of *DSM-III* were also concerned about the usefulness of the system. To make it attractive even to nonmedically trained clinicians—such people are often antagonistic to the medical model, which suggests that psychiatrists must have primary if not exclusive responsibility for treating "mental illness"—the committee omitted any suggestion that psychopathology is a subset of medicine. Thus, the term disorder rather than disease was adopted, even for syndromes caused by observable brain abnormalities ("organic mental disorders"). Also, with rare exceptions, *DSM-III* categories were defined primarily or exclusively in terms of certain behavioral criteria; factors such as drug responsiveness, physiological abnormalities, and psychopathology in first-degree relatives were omitted as criteria. In short, to encourage widespread usage and to minimize professional antagonism, the *DSM-III* was aimed toward better diagnostic reliability and away from controversial theoretical terms.

The revision of *DSM-III,* or *DSM-III-R,* represents a refinement of, more than a departure from, *DSM-III. DSM-III-R* retains the essential form and rationale of the earlier document, including its categorical system of classification and a theoretical descriptive approach to abnormal behavior. Significant changes include (a) major modifications of the criteria of certain categories (especially those relating to childhood abnormalities), (b) modification of the hierarchical relationship of some categories (for example, some instances of agoraphobia are now classified as a subcategory of panic disorder), and (c) modification of the scales for rating both psychosocial stressors and overall behavioral functioning (as described in Chapter 4). All of these changes were made to clarify the categorical concepts, enhance their diagnostic reliability, and accommodate new information gained from clinical and empirical work with *DSM-III*.

DSM-III introduced, and *DSM-III-R* retains, a "multiaxial" format for classifying abnormal behavior. This multiaxial format is composed of five essential "axes." Axes I and II refer to two types of disorders (described in the next section). Axes III to V refer to other factors associated with disorders: Axis III to the medical conditions that contribute to an Axis I or II disorder or its management, Axis IV to stressful external situations that influence the disorder, and Axis V to potential strengths or weaknesses displayed by the individual both currently and during the past year. Because Axes III to V are supplementary rather than essential aspects of a formal diagnosis of the disorder, they are left for the next chapter, where assessment in general (including formal diagnosis) is discussed.

Symptom and Personality Disorders

DSM-III and *DSM-III-R* distinguish between two kinds of psychopathology: *symptom disorders* (Axis I) and *personality disorders* (Axis II). This is rooted in the old distinction of disease—a medical problem of illness that a person *has* versus personality or character, a social problem of conduct that reflects what a person *is* (Fenichel, 1945; Reich, 1933/1949). In its modern guise, the distinction, though still somewhat murky, can be boiled down to the following two ideas. Compared to the traitlike symptoms of personality disorders (Axis II), the symptom disorders of Axis I typically represent a shift from relatively normal to disturbed functioning, and are more often experienced as afflictions imposed from outside rather than normal ways of being oneself. See Table 3.1.

SYMPTOM DISORDERS (AXIS I)

We believe it desirable to get a clear idea early in the book about the range and variety of psychopathologies, and at the same time, to have an opportunity to

TABLE 3.1 SYMPTOMS VS. TRAITS

Dimensions	Symptom (Axis I)	Trait (Axis II)
Objective		
Origins	Varies	Childhood
Onset	Acute	Gradual
Time course	Episodic	Persistent
Subjective		
Personal experience	Ego-alien	Ego-syntonic
Motivation for treatment	Urgent	Little
Resistance to treatment	Less	Much

learn some important vocabulary. With these goals in mind, we describe only the basic features of a selected sample of some *DSM-III-R* categories, starting with symptom disorders classified on Axis I.

Disorders Usually First Evident in Infancy, Childhood, or Adolescence

This group includes many categories: (a) disorders of attention sometimes called hyperactivity; (b) conduct disorders; (c) eating disorders involving self-induced starvation (anorexia) and gorging (bulimia); (d) anxiety disorders including school phobia and excessive dependency; (e) disorders of gender identity involving acting and feeling like a person of the opposite sex; and (f) a mix of other disorders including stuttering, sleepwalking, and bedwetting. (Mental retardation and autistic disorder, formerly classified by *DSM-III* with these Axis I disorders, are now classified by *DSM-III-R* on Axis II.) Here, we will give a brief illustration of a disorder involving hyperactivity, leaving to Chapters 20 and 21 a fuller discussion of childhood disorders.

Attention-Deficit Hyperactivity Disorder

[Jerry's] activity was characterized by a high speed coupled with an erratic quality. He rarely stood still: when he was not running, jumping, or climbing he jiggled up and down in place much as a boxer does while waiting for his opponent's next move. He lacked fine motor skill and some of his gross motor behavior was characterized by clumsiness and awkwardness.... When he went to the toy corner he would throw all the toys off the shelves until he found the one he wanted. If another child had the toy he wanted, he took it by force, then, when an adult intervened, he had a tantrum. He had a short attention span and was unable to sit in a group and listen to a short story (Ross & Ross, 1976, p. 34).

Organic Mental Disorders

Organic mental disorders can be classified on the basis of their known or suspected neuropathological mechanisms. Further, these disorders can be described in terms of their major psychological patterns, three of which are delirium, dementia, and amnesia.

Delirium is typically a reversible disorder marked by clouding of consciousness, that is, a disorganized mix of thinking and dreaming, and agitation or withdrawal. *Dementia* is often a nonreversible progressive deterioration leading to a vegetative condition. Its early stages include forgetfulness and loss of long-term memories, disorganized thinking and the inability to think abstractly, the inability to handle novel situations, impaired judgment, impulsivity, and apathy. Prior personality traits such as rigidity or suspiciousness may become exaggerated. *Amnesia* includes impairments of memory both for information obtained since the onset of the disorder (*anterograde* amnesia), and often for experiences that occurred before onset of the disorder (*retrograde* amnesia).

Organic brain disorders have numerous causes or *etiologies*. These include heredity, pathological aging, poisons, drugs (for example, organic complications of alcoholism), bacteria or viruses, and physical trauma—in particular, head injury.

Psychoactive Substance Use Disorders

This category includes disorders resulting from the effects of excessive and persistent use of mind-altering agents like alcohol, barbiturates, heroin, cocaine, amphetamines, and psychedelics. These agents cause behavioral deterioration along with substance dependence, but often without obvious neurological damage as in the organic mental disorders. For example, the abuse of alcohol can produce a chronic dependency on alcohol with antisocial behavior (substance *use* disorder) or a chronic amnesia or acute delirium (substance-*induced* disorder) or both.

Schizophrenic Disorders

This category includes dysfunctions primarily of thinking, but also of affect (feelings and emotional expression), motivation, and movement. Thinking is *psychotic,*—that is, fragmented, delusional, and hallucinatory. (Psychosis is described fully in Chapter 10.) Affective life is often dominated by apathy. Other features include withdrawal, disinterest, and idiosyncratic gestures. However, in schizophrenia, there are typically no gross deficits of perception, memory, or comprehension as in the organic mental disorders.

Different types of schizophrenia can be distinguished. For example, the *disorganized* (formerly hebephrenic) type is marked by incoherent and bizarre thinking and peculiar mannerisms.

Disorganized Schizophrenic Disorder

Emilio is a 40-year-old man who looks ten years younger. He is brought to the hospital, his twelfth hospitalization, by his mother because she is afraid of him. He is dressed in a ragged overcoat, bedroom slippers, and a baseball cap and wears several medals around his neck. His affect ranges from anger at his mother—"She feeds me shit...what comes out of other people's rectums"—to a giggling, obsequious seductiveness toward the interviewer. His speech and manner have a childlike quality, and he walks with a mincing step and exaggerated hip movements. His mother reports that he stopped taking his medication about a month ago and has since begun to hear voices and to look and act more bizarrely. When asked what he has been doing, he says "eating wires and lighting fires." His spontaneous speech is often incoherent and marked by frequent rhyming and clang associations [i.e., strings of inappropriate rhymes, e.g., "I went to the store, roar, bore, more."] (Spitzer et al., 1981, p. 51).

Another type of schizophrenia, the *paranoid* type, is marked by bizarre persecutory delusions. A good example comes from a patient who wanted to reject his Christian name (Leon) because it was a "dupe" name.

Paranoid Schizophrenic Disorder

Sir, it so happens that my birth certificate says that I am Dr. *Domino Dominorum et Rex Resarum, Simplis Christianus Pueris Mentalis Doktor.*...It also states on my birth certificate that I am the incarnation of Jesus Christ of Nazareth, and I also salute, and I want to add this. I *do* salute the manliness in Jesus Christ also, because the vine is Jesus and the rock is Christ, pertaining to the penis and testicles; and it so happens that I was railroaded into this place because of prejudice and jealousy and duping that started before I was born, and that is the main issue why I am here. I want to be myself. I do not consent to their misuse of the frequency of my life [by] those unsound individuals who practice electronic imposition and duping. I am working for my redemption...(Rokeach, 1964, pp. 5–6).

Delusional Disorders

This category includes disorders that feature very pronounced delusions, typically about being persecuted (paranoid delusions), but without evidence that the delusions are merely the by-products of an organic, schizophrenic, or manic-depressive disorder. Suspiciousness, seclusiveness, resentment, jealousy, anger, and sometimes even violence characterize paranoia, the most familiar type of delusional disorder. It is a psychotic disorder, but without the fragmented and bizarre abnormalities of the schizophrenic (including the paranoid schizophrenic) disorder.

Paranoid Disorder

On graduating from college, the patient was gradually promoted in an accounting firm until a minor mistake was discovered in the accounts and he was blamed. He, in turn, blamed his chief, and an antagonistic relationship gradually developed between them. Although the mistake in the account was soon rectified, the patient continued to complain to higher authorities, including his congressman and the President. He was eventually fired from his job. He believed that his boss was solely responsible for his inability to find another position, and he became agitated. On hospitalization, his thinking was appropriate except for the delusion that his boss was conspiring against him....After discharge the patient was able to find a job as an accountant in another firm and on follow-up was doing well except for the continued belief that his former boss was attempting to persecute him. He continues to write letters to his congressman, complaining about his former boss, but he is not psychotic in any other way (Walker & Brodie, 1980, p. 1292).

Psychotic Disorders Not Elsewhere Classified

This category includes psychotic behavior that is either of relatively short duration (days or weeks more than months or years), and clearly associated with events that create marked psychosocial stress, or mixed with dramatic shifts in mood and emotional agitation (often called schizoaffective disorder).

Schizoaffective Disorder

Louis...would sit...in a stooped manner, quietly bemoaning the fate of God, to whom he claimed he spoke the night before, and who had told him that because of his and God's sins, life for everyone would soon be even more "hellish" than living in a state hospital. Every several weeks, and rather unpredictably, Louis would suddenly be buoyed up, begin clapping his hands, and loudly sing to a cheerfully melodic refrain, a song with pleasant neologistic words (e.g., goody dum dum, happimush), but one that was otherwise totally incomprehensible. Following these brief euphoric episodes, Louis would succumb to his more usual depressive agitation, moaning incoherently about the wretched state of man's sinfulness, the coming of doomsday, the "tastelessness" of the weather, his "dramink" of hundreds of little girls and so on (Millon, 1969, p. 356).

Manic and Depressive Disorders

These abnormalities—called affective disorders in *DSM-III* and mood disorders in *DSM-III-R*—refer to gross deviations along the happy-sad dimension of affective life. (A discussion of the affect concept is given in Chapter 13.)

In *bipolar* (manic-depressive) disorder, the patient displays the symptoms of both the manic and depressive poles of mood. Manic behavior includes euphoric or excited thought, speech, and movement, inflated self-esteem, boundless energy, irrepressible activity, grandiosity, and poor judgment. It may even include psychotic thinking. Consider this example of a manic disorder.

Manic Disorder

[The patient] is in poor contact with reality. "I can do anything you can do, better," he is *certain,* recognizing neither the outer difficulties nor his own inner limitations. "I shall fly to Rome, talk with the Pope, initiate changes in our beliefs about the Holy Virgin," one of Janet's patients announced while she was still confined to the Salpetrière. She added, as she tried to show how light she had become, walking about the ward on tiptoes as if she were about to take off in winged flight, "Don't put me on your scales. They are not to be relied upon. I *know* I am getting light enough to fly." In his airborne certitude the manic has no need for authorities, advice, the newspapers: he is clairvoyant, powerful (Cole, 1970, p. 545).

The depressive component of the bipolar disorder includes sadness, hopelessness, *a*nergy (lack of energy), loss of self-esteem, delusional self-deprecation, apathy, loss of the appetites for food, sex, sleep, information, and social communion, abnormalities of vegetative function involving hormones and sleep patterns, and enhanced risk for suicide.

The *unipolar* disorder (called major depressive disorder in *DSM-III-R*) involves only one pole of the bipolar continuum, typically only the depressive pole. The following passage illustrates the agitated form of unipolar depression with its anxious, complaining, sometimes histrionic qualities.

Unipolar Depressive Disorder

Constance began to grow less withdrawn and more aware of her surroundings. As she re-established contact with the hospital environment, her quiet grief gave way to restless agitation, and in place of brooding there were outspoken self-accusations and insistent demands that she be punished.... Now Constance denounced herself venomously as a person steeped in sin, a liar, a hypocrite and a cheat.... She confessed publicly an affair she had had with a man many years earlier. She demanded repeatedly, angrily, tormentingly, that she be brought to trial for her terrible crimes, that she be imprisoned for life, that she be beaten and thrown naked into the street. She continually harped on the refrain, "Get it over with!" meaning, "Bring me to trial and punishment!" (From Norman Cameron, *Personality Development and Psychopathology: A Dynamic Approach*, p. 529. Copyright © 1963 by Houghton Mifflin Company. Used with permission).

The *cyclothymic* disorder is a mild version of bipolar disorder. It includes inexplicable shifts between mildly manic and mildly depressive mood. *Dysthymic* disorder is a mild version of unipolar depression.

A conventional distinction should be made explicit before describing four additional categories. This is the distinction between *neurotic* and *psychotic* conditions. We have described organic, schizophrenic, paranoid, and affective disorders, which are always or sometimes associated with psychotic behavior—bizarre and disorganized thinking, delusions, hallucinations, and the like (see Chapter 10). The term neurosis is often used to characterize a different type of disorder. Neurotic conditions are aberrant, but the anxiety, inhibitions, and avoidance behaviors typical of these disorders are less bizarre and there is no loss of contact with reality. For example, the phobic knows that his consuming fear of heights is "crazy"; he therefore has no concern when a loved one climbs stairs or moves toward an open window. Table 3.2 gives some com-

TABLE 3.2   NEUROSIS VS. PSYCHOSIS

Category	Neurosis	Psychosis
Emotion	Anxious Insecure	Apathetic Vulnerable
Object relations	Inhibited/avoidant Disappointed Annoyed Guilt-ridden	Detached Alienated Paranoid Indifferent
Cognition	Phobic Obsessive Driven Imaginative Self-conscious	Delusional Autistic Fragmented Bizarre/idiosyncratic Without insight
Social impression	Childish Annoying Irresponsible Defensive	Sick/defective Scary Insane Disorganized

parative features of neurosis and psychosis, and Chapter 10 provides a thorough discussion of the differences.

Major categories of neurotic disorders include anxiety disorders, somatoform disorders, dissociative disorders, and the psychosexual dysfunctions. Some of these will now be described, starting with the anxiety disorders.

Anxiety Disorders

Anxiety disorders include phobias, nonphobic panic, obsessions, compulsions, and posttraumatic stress. There are three kinds of phobic disorder: (a) simple phobia, the irrational fear of "harmful" objects or animals, (b) social phobia, the irrational fear of social scrutiny—for example, of eating or speaking in public, and (c) agoraphobia, the avoidance of open or novel places and situations where panic attacks or other catastrophic experiences are anticipated. Panic disorder can occur with or without agoraphobia. In panic disorder, the person experiences inexplicable and unpredictable anxiety so extreme there may be a fear of dying or going crazy. For example, panic may well up while driving a car, or while sitting in a restaurant. The anxiety attack may be strong enough to drive the person to seek "safety" at home.

Obsessive-compulsive disorder involves ruminative preoccupations and irresistible compulsions. The following extract describes obsessive-compulsive behavior. Note how the phobiclike anxiety about a number is elaborated by morbid preoccupations and superstituous, rituallike avoidance behaviors.

Obsessive-Compulsive Disorder

The patient was a 49-year-old man whose main symptom was an obsession with the number 13. If he heard the word he felt a "shock" and experienced a subsequent period of acute anxiety. His everyday life was a continuous effort to avoid any reference to 13, so much so that his activities were seriously handicapped. In some way or another, it seems as if everyone was always saying 13 to him. If they met him in the morning they would say, "Oh, good morning," or later in the day it would be "Good afternoon" (13 letters in each). He stayed in bed on the thirteenth day of each month, skipped the thirteenth tread in a stairway, and found it necessary to count letters and phrases, his steps, and streets, to avoid the number 13...(Ross, 1937, pp. 219–221).

The final subcategory of anxiety disorder—posttraumatic stress disorder—includes two components: a traumatic or life-threatening stressor—a rape or a close encounter with death, for example—that triggers the reaction, and the anxiety reaction itself—nervousness, withdrawal, depression, obsession, irritability, insomnia, recurrent nightmares, memory disturbances, and flashbacks. This is an example of some prominent features of posttraumatic stress disorder.

Posttraumatic Stress Disorder

The patient was a 26-year-old married Vietnam veteran who was recently laid off from a job he had held for 3 years. He was admitted to the hospital for severe symptoms of anxiety, which began after he was laid off at work and found himself at home watching reports of the fall of South Vietnam on television.... At home with time on his hands and watching the fall of South Vietnam on television, he began to experience unwanted intrusive recollections of...the guerrilla he had killed and the death of his friend. He found himself ruminating about all the people who were killed or injured and wondering what the purpose of it all had been. He began to experience nightmares, during which he relived the moments when he himself was almost injured (Andreasen, 1980, p. 1521).

Somatoform Disorders

Disorders in this category feature multiple physical symptoms that appear to have psychological rather than physical causes. In other words, the bodily disturbances appear to express general tension or unconscious conflict. We will describe just two of the somatoform disorders: somatization and conversion.

The essential feature of *somatization* disorder is a long and complicated medical record of pseudomedical complaints in many of the following areas: (a) sensorimotor (muscular weakness, for example), (b) gastrointestinal (abdominal pain), (c) female reproductive (painful menstruation), (d) psychosexual (sexual indifference), and (e) cardiopulmonary (breathlessness or dizziness). Complications often include anxiety, depression, and threats of suicide, as well as various kinds of antisocial behavior. The patient repeatedly seeks medical help from various physicians who, recognizing an essentially psychological problem, refer the patient to a psychiatrist or psychologist. *Conversion* disorder seems to be a bodily representation of an unconscious idea—for example, an unfulfilled desire. The somatic "communication" may include paralysis, fainting, seizure, blindness, deafness, anaesthesia, aphonia (muteness), incoordination, paresthesia (tingling sensations), vomiting, or even pseudocyesis (false pregnancy complete with swollen belly, cramps, and sensations of fetal movement). Consider the following example of conversion disorder in a man pressured by his family to have a second operation for back pain.

Conversion Disorder

After the operation, he became totally bedridden and incapacitated—not because of pain but because of an extensive weakness of his entire spinal and neck musculature that prevented him from walking or even sitting. The weakness was clearly a conversion symptom. Investigation under amobarbital sodium (Amytal Sodium) narcosis uncovered the fact that the patient had been utterly opposed to further surgery and had deeply resented his family's pressure, to which he had finally felt he must submit. He described all this under narcosis, he began to express bitter anger at his family. Speaking of at last agreeing to the operation he said: "So I finally decided, if

I had to cut my throat, I *would* cut my throat—and here I am; the family needed a lesson." When fully conscious both before and after the amobarbital interview, the patient consciously felt and exhibited no anger whatsoever toward those who had forced him into surgery. His anger had been expressed by the physical symptom of muscular weakness, which, without his being aware of its meaning or the feelings it expressed, gave him the means for revenge against his family (Nemiah, 1980c, p. 1532).

Dissociative Disorders

This category includes (a) psychogenic amnesia, (b) psychogenic fugue, and (c) multiple personality. All these disorders involve a loss or splitting of consciousness that suggests a dissociation of different components of personality; although none of the "parts" of the personality is psychotic, the "whole" is lost. It is important to understand that the splitting of consciousness and personality in dissociative disorder and the fragmentation of cognition and affect in schizophrenia are psychologically different phenomena. In other words, dissociative disorder should not be confused with schizophrenia which involves different psychopathology and etiology, and which runs in different families.

In *psychogenic amnesia,* loss of memory is *motivated* in that the person seems to gain something by not being able to remember a painful experience; thus the term psychogenic or mentally caused as opposed to neurologically caused. Some cruel or immoral act may be completely forgotten—for example, a sexual encounter or the beating of a child. The person is conscious of the amnesia, but not of its content. The hallmarks of psychogenic amnesia are its selectivity, convenience, and reversibility.

In *psychogenic fugue,* the patient experiences massive amnesia for roles, relationships, and even chunks of personal history, and typically travels to a different location, assuming a new identity and a new way of life. If a sudden "awakening" should occur later, there is complete amnesia for the new life. The "awakened" person is confused by inexplicable surroundings and circumstances, and by a sense of lost life.

Dissociative disorder is most dramatically expressed in *multiple personality.* In this disorder, two or more personalities compete for control over the body. Each personality seems to represent a set of ideas and motives, temperament, and talents. One personality may be apologetic, awkward, and sickly while another may be impish, inventive, and healthy. Health, posture, gait, bearing, and handwriting often are unique to each. The original personality is usually amnesic for most or all of the others, experiencing "lost time" upon awakening.

Alternating personalities emerge and disappear suddenly, either spontaneously or in response to hypnotic suggestion. The "dominant" personality may come to realize that other behavior is going on during a lapse of consciousness because of certain obvious changes noticed upon "awakening": knitting may be unraveled, clothes and hairstyle changed, and even setting altered. An emergent personality may visit someone whom the "dominant" personality does not know, and then recede into unconsciousness, leaving a suddenly "awakened" other personality to figure out what has happened.

Sexual Disorders

This category includes, among other disorders, gender identity disorders and aberrant sexual preoccupations, or paraphilia—for example, fetishism, exhibitionism, and voyeurism.

In most people, gender *identity*—that is, one's sense of being male or female—is congruent with one's sexual anatomy. Those who experience an incongruity between gender identity and sexual anatomy would be regarded as having a gender identity disorder. The most striking form of gender identity disorder is *transsexuality,* manifested most typically by a strong desire for a change in anatomical sex so that it corresponds with gender identity. Transsexuality is not transvestism, a gender *role* disorder wherein a man with a masculine gender identity nevertheless often dresses like a woman. To make the distinction between transsexuality and transvestism clear, a male transsexual believes that he is a woman trapped in a man's body, whereas a male transvestite enjoys dressing in the clothes of a woman but feels that he is a man.

Factitious Disorders

Factitious disorder involves the feigning of psychiatric or medical illness. A patient with a factitious disorder may claim amnesia, act confused, or give approximate answers like "forty-seven" to questions like "What is four times twelve?" The patient may also simulate physical symptoms—for example, by mixing blood in the urine. (The term Munchausen syndrome is used for a chronic and incapacitating factitious disorder that involves many physical symptoms and multiple hospitalizations—see Goodwin, 1988.) Factitious behavior has three basic qualities: it is artificial—impressing people as false or unnatural; it is voluntary—willingly carried out in a deliberate though typically compulsive manner; and it is irrational—the behavior appears bizarrely self-destructive and the motivation is incomprehensible. When a self-serving motive is evident—to avoid the draft, for example—and when the illness-seeking behavior lacks a compulsive quality, the diagnosis is malingering.

A factitious disorder is indicated by the weight of the patient's medical file, the amount of scarring on the patient's body from countless exploratory operations, and the dramatic quality of the patient's self-presentation. For example, on six different occasions, a nurse swallowed a fork that had to be retrieved by operation. She finally died of a "relentless factitious disorder" (Enoch & Trethowan, 1979). Another patient had a record of 105 hospitalizations and arrests during a sixteen-year period (cited in Sussman & Hyler, 1980). Some patients display what appears to be a factitious disorder by proxy, the abuse of a child's body with chemical poisons to enable the pursuit of medical attention (Goodwin, 1988).

Impulse Disorders

This category includes behaviors such as pathological gambling, stealing (kleptomania), firesetting (pyromania), and explosive outbursts of aggression (dyscontrol) which cannot be explained by the presence of other disorders. The hallmark of these disorders is failure to resist impulses despite threats of physical harm or social humiliation. All of these problems involve increasing tension in the patient prior to taking the impulsive action, and tension reduction afterward. The two examples that follow illustrate impulse disorder.

Kleptomania

A wealthy and beautiful 34-year-old woman...experienced the urge to walk into one of the more elegant department stores in the city and steal an article of clothing. Over the course of the previous three or four years she had stolen several blouses, a couple of sweaters, and a skirt. Since her husband's income alone was over $150,000 a year and her investments worth many times that, she recognized the "absurdity" of her acts. She also indicated that what she stole was rarely very expensive and sometimes not even enough to her liking for her to wear. She would become aware of the desire to steal something several days before she actually did it. The thoughts would increasingly occupy her mind until, on impulse, she walked into the store, plucked an item off the rack, and stuffed it into a bag she happened to be carrying or under her coat. Once out the door she felt a sense of relaxation and satisfaction; but at home she experienced anxiety and guilt when she realized what she had done (Spitzer, Skodol, Gibbon, & Williams, 1981, p. 80).

Pathological Gambling

A 48-year-old male attorney...had been arrested for taking funds from his firm, which he stated he had fully intended to return after he had a "big win" at gambling. He appeared deeply humiliated and remorseful about his behavior, although he had a previous history of near-arrests for defrauding his company of funds....He had gambled on horse racing for many years. He had been losing heavily recently, had resorted to illegal borrowing, and was now being pressured for payment. He stated that he embezzled the money to pay off these illegal debts because the threats of the "loan sharks" were frightening him so that he could not concentrate or sleep.... During the interview the patient was tense and restless, at times having to stand up and pace. He said he was having a flare-up of a duodenal ulcer. He was somewhat tearful throughout the interview, and said that although he realized his problems stemmed from his gambling, he still had a strong urge to gamble (Spitzer et al., 1981, p. 75).

Psychological Factors Affecting Physical Condition

This "psychosomatic" category recognizes the physiological dimension of psychopathology. Psychological factors, possibly complicated by psychosocial stressors, can cause or aggravate physical disease such as neurodermatitis, migraine, arthritis, ulcer, angina, asthma, and colitis. Psychological factors can include the death of a loved one, the seemingly unending demands of a spouse or employer, or excessive dependence on someone who is perceived to be unreliable.

PERSONALITY DISORDERS (AXIS II)

The personality disorders of Axis II involve chronic and treatment-resistant pathological traits and defective interpersonal patterns (see Table 3.1) marked by emotional instability, poor work history, underachievement, unsatisfying marriages, and friendlessness. Also common are Axis I symptoms including affective, psychopathic (antisocial), organic, and addictive kinds (see Drake & Vaillant, 1985).

Eleven Personality Disorders

Table 3.3 lists eleven Axis II categories. A diagnosed personality disorder rarely displays all the defining features of a *DSM* category; in fact, *DSM-III-R* requires that only four to six criteria be met out of seven to ten (depending on the category). In addition, a personality disorder is rarely found in isolation; there will often be other traits that collectively satisfy the criteria of additional Axis II categories.

Paranoid Personality Disorder   The hallmarks of paranoid personality disorder include pervasive mistrust, vigilance, secretiveness, blame avoidance, hypersensitivity, and exaggerated and unforgiving reactions to "provocation." Such individuals are often unable to show affection, and feelings of inferiority or depression may be masked by ambitiousness and grandiosity.

Schizoid Personality Disorder   The schizoid person is aloof, detached, and humorless all suggesting "dark, hollow-eyed nothing—affective anemia...the cold breath of an arctic soullessness" (quoted in Millon, 1981, p. 277). Schizoids live a solitary, though not necessarily reclusive, life. They are prone to absentmindedness and daydreaming, yet are surprisingly deficient in the capacity for reflection. Because the schizoid disorder need not include peculiarity of thought or eccentricity of speech, it must be distinguished from schizotypal personality disorder.

TABLE 3.3   PERSONALITY DISORDERS

Disorder	Salient traits
Paranoid	Suspicious; hypervigilant; secretive
Schizoid	Social; detached
Schizotypal	Eccentric, schizophrenic; hypersensitive/apathetic
Histrionic	Theatrical; egocentric; labile; exhibitionistic
Narcissistic	Egotistical; insensitive
Antisocial (psychopathic)	Rule-breaking; aggressive; callous; impulsive
Borderline (unstable)	Chaotic; emotional; reckless; unpredictable
Avoidant	Withdrawn; timid; hypersensitive, hyperself-conscious
Dependent	Submissive; docile; ineffectual
Compulsive	Hidebound; perfectionistic; controlled; obstinate
Passive-aggressive	Negativistic; contrary; dysphoric

Schizotypal Personality Disorder   This category is diagnosed when a significant number of the following qualities occur: magical thinking (the belief that one's thoughts are being broadcast to others, for example); ideas of reference (delusional belief in the personal significance of trivial events); social isolation; vague hallucinations (sensing the presence of a dead mother, for example); odd, digressive, or idiosyncratic forms of communication without frank thought disorder, and affective abnormalities such as interpersonal remoteness or suspiciousness; and hypersensitivity regarding interpersonal contact. Because this pattern is mildly schizophrenic, and because it may evolve into or out of a more clearly psychotic form, it is sometimes called ambulatory, borderline, latent, larval, or residual schizophrenia (see Chapter 10).

> Clinicians have come to speak of ambulatory schizophrenia, an illness that has some of the components of the more serious disorder, yet is not incapacitating and does not require hospitalization. A well-to-do family can maintain a brother or a daughter in an artificial environment (even hiring paid companions to provide a kind of imitation of life); ensconced in a room of his own, the schizoid self can loaf, dream, engage in a kind of "work" (on the occult, on some grand design for politics, or sexuality, or some electronic gadget) that never comes to anything....Some of these near-schizophrenics are found among the perennial students who haunt the universities but never take a degree, the artists who move in and out of ateliers but never hang a picture, the cultists who are the first to be drawn to new religions, new drugs, new therapies. So closely do these persons simulate the true innovators, who are the lifeblood of any growing society, that they test our own discriminative powers. We have to examine their fantasies and probe for the negative signs in their behavior before we can separate the authentic from the near-schizophrenic. Some of these near-schizophrenics compose the band of narcotics addicts, drifters, dipsomaniacs, criminals, and deviates who clog the courts and keep alive the question: "Are these men and women sick, or just weak, or do they have essentially simple character problems; are they undisciplined selves whose families have failed to socialize them?" (Cole, 1970, pp. 619–629).

Histrionic Personality Disorder   Histrionic personality disorder is a mixture of theatricality, egocentricity, dependency, and dysphoric affect. The histrionic person indulges in shallow, unstable, and short-lived enthusiasms. A friendship "commences with idolatry and ends in bitterness...succeeded by detachment, isolation, depression and paranoid-like trends" (Easser & Lesser, 1965, pp. 399–400), a pattern that suggests superficiality and fickleness. The histrionic personality typically combines erotic seductiveness and sexual inhibition. Such incongruous tendencies are further complicated by swings between ardor and despair or, as Kretschmer put it, "a mixture of the droll and tragic." The histrionic condition, in which no behavior is what it seems for long, represents a mingling of theatricality, "little girl" immaturity, dependency, and emotional instability, all in extreme measures.

> They are fickle, emotionally labile, irresponsible, shallow, love-intoxicated, giddy and shortsighted....Seductive, manipulative, exploitive, and sexually provocative, they think emotionally and illogically. Easy prey to flattery and compliments...they are possessive, grasping, demanding, romantic...when frustrated or disappointed,

they become reproachful, tearful, abusive and vindictive....Rejection sensitivity is perhaps their outstanding clinical feature (D. Klein, 1972, p. 237).

Narcissistic Personality Disorder   The hallmark of this disorder is an excessive and grandiose sense of self-importance. Behavior and fantasy focus on achievements or victories that call attention to and magnify the value of the self to the exclusion of others. Like the histrionic personality, the narcissistic personality uses others for attention and admiration but never meaningfully reciprocates. Unlike the histrionic personality, the narcissistic personality is relatively independent of others and capable of sustaining positive self-regard while alone. However, when in the company of others, the narcissistic personality displays an unrealistic sense of "entitlement," presuming rights to goods and favors by taking advantage of others who may be deeply envied and therefore resented.

Antisocial Personality Disorder   From early childhood, antisocial people are known for incorrigible lying, stealing, running away, truancy, vandalism, and drug abuse. These behaviors are characterized by irresponsibility, unpredictability, blame avoidance, aggressiveness, and lack of guilt or remorse—qualities that make it difficult to sustain relationships or performance at anything undertaken. Children may be abandoned, contracts broken, obligations ignored, feelings disregarded, plans changed, truths distorted. The aggressiveness that can accompany this egocentricity make this kind of human detachment particularly dangerous and destructive.

Borderline Personality Disorder   Major features of borderline personality disorder suggest profound emotional and interpersonal instability—for example, impulsiveness or unpredictability where gambling, sex, or drugs are concerned. Chaotic and unstable interpersonal relationships are characterized by idealization, manipulation, rejection, and detachment. Other manifestations of this disorder include frantic efforts to defend against real or imagined threats of being abandoned; unpredictable or uncontrollable anger; chronic disturbance of identity; instability of mood such as frequent or uncontrollable shifts between enthusiasm and depression; impulsive and reckless outbursts including suicidal behavior; and chronic feelings of unworthiness, emptiness, or purposelessness.

Avoidant Personality Disorder   Unlike the schizoid, the avoidant person cultivates detachment out of a fear of rejection; rather than schizoid indifference, the patient's longing for involvement is mixed with exquisite sensitivity to rejection. Fundamental characteristics of this disorder include wish for social communion, hypersensitivity to social evaluation, and social avoidance. Timidity, introversion, and hyperconsciousness of self may also be noted.

Dependent Personality Disorder   This disorder is marked by a passive-submissive orientation with the goal of achieving emotional and intellectual support. The person avoids personal responsibility while seeking out nurturant others. Thus, needs are subordinated and a negative self-image is developed ("I am so stupid!"). Psychological and even physical abuse may be tolerated in the interest of maintaining the dependency relationship, and this may perpetuate a naive and pollyannaish tendency to deny unfortunate experience. The overall picture is one of dependency, docility, and ineffectuality.

Obsessive-Compulsive Personality Disorder   The essential features of compulsive personality disorder include preoccupation with detail, trivialities, order, schedules, and lists; emotional reserve as seen in the cultivating of interpersonal relations that are formal and judgmental rather than affectionate; hidebound and pleasureless devotion to work; conformity and predictability; and indecisiveness with rumination and avoidance of decisions. With regard to the latter feature, Reich (1949) notes the incongruity between indecision, doubt, and distrust on the one hand, and the appearance of reserve and self-possession on the other. In his introductory remarks to a paper on the disorder, Freud described the compulsive personality as follows.

> The persons whom I am about to describe are remarkable for a regular combination of the three following peculiarities: they are exceptionally *orderly, parsimonious,* and *obstinate*. Each of these words really covers a small group or series of traits which are related to one another. "Orderly" comprises both bodily cleanliness and reliability and conscientiousness in the performance of petty duties: the opposite of it would be "untidy" and "negligent." "Parsimony" may be exaggerated up to the point of avarice; and obstinacy may amount to defiance, with which irascibility and vindictiveness may easily be associated (Freud, 1908/1959, pp. 45–46).

Passive-Aggressive Personality Disorder   The dominant characteristic of this condition is resistance to demands for performance expressed in hostile negativism, untoward criticism, procrastination, intentional inefficiency, and "forgetfulness." The effect on others is irritating, and the result on others is interpersonal conflict and occupational difficulties. Millon (1981) suggests that people with this disorder are frequently high-strung, moody, faultfinding, and disillusioned, with contrary and changing attitudes and feelings toward others.

Personality Disorders as Categories

Symptom Overlap among Axis II Categories   Personality disorders rarely exist singly and in pure form, and indeed, diagnoses of more than one personality disorder per patient are common (Skodol, Rosnick, Kellman et al., 1988). Multiple diagnoses can occur because the person actually has more than one type of psychopathology, but also because the criteria of different categories are often so similar—for example, the "irritability and aggressiveness" criteria of the antisocial and the "irritability" and "inappropriate, intense anger" criteria of the borderline disorders (American Psychiatric Association, 1987). When outpatients were rated using a four-point scale of diagnosability for each of the eleven categories on Axis II, four groups of co-occurring personality disorders emerged: (1) an "odd-eccentric" group, including the paranoid, schizoid, and schizotypal disorders; (2) an "anxious/fearful" group, including the avoidant, dependent, and passive-aggressive disorders; (3) a "dramatic/erratic" group, including the antisocial and borderline disorders; and (4) a "group" defined by compulsive disorder (Kass et al., 1985).

Traits from Axis II categories are dimensional, going from mild to severe, and are intercorrelated—that is, they predict one another. The two facts raise questions about the "either-or" categorical approach of *DSM*, especially in the area of personality disorder.

Symptom Nonoverlap within Axis II Categories   You will recall that not every criterion of an Axis II category need be satisfied to identify a specific personality disorder—for example, any four of eight criteria for histrionic personality disorder. This means that people with the same diagnosis may display different patterns of behavior. It is assumed that these within-category differences are merely variations on a common theme and not of critical significance.

Nevertheless, questions about this assumption have been raised. Stone (1988) points out, for example, that "the *DSM-III-R* system, requiring only five of eight items, allows 93 combinations; any two cases need only overlap on two items. A borderline patient with identity disturbance, labile affect, impulsivity, rage and self-damaging acts might have little in common (etiologically, dynamically, or prognostically) with another exhibiting emptiness, rejection sensitivity, disturbed relationships, identity disturbances, and labile affect" (p. 3). In short, symptom overlap among categories and the lack of overlap within categories raise serious questions about the validity and usefulness of those categories. These and other questions about *DSM-III* and *DSM-III-R* classification system are now taken up.

CRITICAL REACTIONS TO *DSM-III* AND *DSM-III-R* CLASSIFICATION

DSM-III was greeted with praise for its clarity, comprehensiveness, and reliability yet with criticism for its alleged shallowness and inconsistency. Schacht and Nathan described a prepublication draft of the *DSM-III* as "a symphony written by a committee—the notes are all there, but the way they are put together reflects the mediocrity inherent in such a process rather than integrated purpose or understanding" (1977, p. 1017). We summarize a few of the general points raised initially against *DSM-III*, criticisms which, for the most part, are applicable to *DSM-III-R*.

Clinicians with strong theoretical convictions saw *DSM-III* as a fragmented collection of categories with little coherence or consistency. For example, clinicians with strong psychoanalytic commitments criticized *DSM-III* for retreating from theoretical insights about the defense mechanisms of personality (Vaillant, 1984) and about the common underlying psychopathology of disorders expressed by different behaviors (Nemiah, 1980c).

Clinicians with a strong biological orientation faulted *DSM-III* for at least two reasons. First, the decision to exclude as diagnostically relevant any information about disorders in first-degree relatives—done to accommodate widespread antipathy toward the "medical model" and genetic etiology—was, according to some critics, not legitimate from a scientific point of view. Second, Axis I of *DSM-III* left out certain organic conditions that would seem to be just as relevant to psychopathology as other organic disorders that are represented there. For example, the omission of temporal lobe epilepsy (discussed in Chapter 9) is odd given its interesting psychopathological features and also its value as a biobehavioral model of psychopathology. Likewise and equally inexplicable, other organic deficits like aphasia (deficit of language), agnosia (deficit of object recognition), and apraxia (deficit of action) are omitted, as are movement disorders such as Parkinsonism that are relevant to theorizing about physiological mechanisms of psychosis (Pincus & Tucker, 1985).

Clinicians with a strong developmental orientation faulted *DSM-III* for conveying a cross-sectional view of psychopathology—that is, a view of behavior as static rather than as evolving in time (Vaillant, 1984). *DSM-III* sometimes represented the developmental stages of a single disorder as separate categories—for example, hyperactivity (Axis I) and antisocial personality disorder (Axis II)—even though the former is often an early phase in the development of the latter. Likewise, schizotypal personality (Axis II) may disintegrate into schizophrenia (Axis I).

Clinicians with a strong statistical orientation faulted *DSM-III* for its categorical emphasis on "yes-no" decisions regarding the presence of disorder (Blashfield, 1984; Finn, 1982; Kendell, 1975). These investigators pointed out that people too frequently could not easily be classified within *DSM-III* categories; in other words, the basic categorical assumption failed real-world tests. For example, conditions such as the Axis II personality disorders are defined categorically yet appear to be extreme examples of qualities that vary *continuously* from the normal to the pathological (Frances, 1982). Given the evidence of continuity, critics suggest replacing categorical "yes-no" decisions with estimates of the *degree* to which a person displays the features of a disorder. Such estimates could represent (a) the *severity* of disorder, (b) the *probability* that a person has the disorder, (c) the *liability* to developing the full syndrome at some later date, or (d) a combination of these. (To be fair, it should be noted that the framers of *DSM-III-R* have acknowledged that, despite their belief in the utility of discrete categories, no assumption is implied about actual continuity or discontinuity of psychopathological conditions.)

Certain revisions of *DSM-III* illustrate how theory, new data, and diagnostic fashion have evolved together in *DSM-III-R*. For example, agoraphobia, a separate category from panic disorder in *DSM-III,* is now a subcategory of panic disorder in *DSM-III-R*; this change reflects growing evidence that although many patients with panic never develop agoraphobia, almost all agoraphobias arise from the panic experience (see Chapter 15).

Nevertheless, most of the revisions of *DSM-III* are relatively minor; its basic rationale and categorical approach remaining largely intact. Therefore, the major criticisms of *DSM-III* mentioned above still largely apply to *DSM-III-R*. No doubt, criticisms from the psychoanalytic, biological, developmental, and statistical camps will continue to spark controversy and pressure for change.

The current *DSM* system will most assuredly continue to evolve, and much of the material discussed in subsequent chapters will provide clues about the evolutionary direction of *DSM-IV* and beyond (see Millon & Klerman, 1986).

SUMMARY

Classification is fundamental to human thought; by classifying, we reduce complex experiences to manageable *categories* and *dimensions*. A category is a concept that expresses a unique set of qualities. By comparing the qualities of something to the qualities of the category, decisions to include it or exclude it in the category can be made—for example, a person either is or is not schizophrenic, depending on the match between that person's behavior and the defining behavioral criteria of the schizophrenia category. A dimension is a scaled characteristic that can vary continuously from little to much; that is, a person is or is not schizophrenic *to a certain degree*. A classification system reflects theory about the relative importance of behavioral features, underlying mechanisms, and developmental origins in deciding what goes with what. Thus, a classification system is both a concrete *model* of a theory about behavior and a useful vehicle for *testing* that theory.

The bulk of the chapter describes the structure and content of the classification system of the revised third edition of the *Diagnostic and Statistical Manual of Mental Disorders* (*DSM-III-R*) published by the American Psychiatric Association. The *DSM-III-R*, like its immediate predecessor, *DSM-III*, does two separate but related things. First, it represents the categorical approach to *classifying* psychopathology into distinct disorders: the symptom disorders of Axis I and the personality disorders of Axis II. Second, it provides behaviorial criteria for *diagnosing* specific instances of such disorders.

The many critical reactions to *DSM-III* and *DSM-III-R* make clear how difficult it is for any single comprehensive classification system to satisfy the many theoretical and practical requirements of the scientific and therapeutic communities. Nevertheless, flawed though it may be, the *DSM-III/-III-R* system has been widely adopted, and, along with its forerunners, is the basis of virtually all the research findings discussed throughout the book.

Assessment of Psychopathology

In the last chapter on the classification of psychopathology, we discussed abnormal behavior in terms of general categories of disorder. In this chapter, we focus on how the abnormal behavior of an individual can be described and diagnosed as an instance of one or more of those categories.

Psychological assessment involves the evaluation of symptoms, needs and defenses, personality strengths and weaknesses, attitudes and expectations, and interpersonal (including family) problems. Assessment includes making decisions about the need for additional evaluation—for example, a medical examination to assess the possibility that a physical illness is contributing to the problem. It also involves decisions about the best type of therapeutic intervention.

TECHNIQUES OF ASSESSMENT

A clinician charged with the responsibility of assessing abnormal behavior can use interviews and tests along with standard criteria and guidelines such as those of *DSM-III-R*. In addition, subjective factors play a role; clinicians often rely on personal experience and what we may call "educated intuition" to evaluate information.

The three psychological approaches to assessment that we have selected are (a) *behavioral,* which emphasizes specific environment-behavior relationships, (b) *psychodynamic,* which describes mental conflicts and symbolic meanings, and (c) *diagnostic,* which centers around the formal diagnosis of a specific disorder according to standard criteria, in particular, those of *DSM-III-R.* A clinician is, of course, free to use more than one approach.

Clinical assessment, whether behavioral, psychodynamic, or diagnostic, typically includes an interview. Therefore a general description of interviewing will be useful before proceeding to a more focused discussion of each of the three approaches.

Interviewing

An interviewer uses direct observation of, and information reported by, the individual; often these are supplemented by information obtained from relatives and others. The objective is to describe in summary form the basic features of abnormal behavior, the factors that cause and maintain them, and how they might best be treated.

Techniques   To facilitate information gathering, the clinician must establish rapport. An opening line such as "I gather from what you said over the phone that..." conveys the impression of competence and caring. It also gives the patient an opportunity to amend what was said earlier in the event that the initial communication was distorted. For each area to be probed—childhood experience, family conflicts, and educational achievement, for example—the interviewee is guided from generalities to specifics. The interviewer might begin with a general question like "Can you tell me about growing up in your family?" Then, in response to the interviewee's answer, a more focused question can be asked like "What were your reactions to your parents' arguments over financial matters?"

The interviewer has to be flexible. With someone who is defensive or particularly sensitive, for example, the interviewer may rely on indirect questions like "Can you tell me more about that?" rather than direct questions like "Did your mother actually throw you out or did you feel like you were being thrown out?" The interviewer may also temporarily defer questions about some painful area, returning to it when the interviewee appears ready. Interviewing "requires great sensitivity, tact, and skill to help the patient maintain a sense of dignity while exposing embarrassing or humiliating experiences" (MacKinnon, 1980, p. 896).

Some clinicians have noted that in some ways an interview can be like a therapy session—promoting insight, comfort, and, sometimes, even lasting positive changes (Malan, Heath, Bacal, & Balfour, 1975). The interviewee may get an opportunity to appreciate his situation, perhaps for the first time. "And what a relief it is to him to discover that his true meaning is anything but what he at first says, and that he is at long last uncovering some conventional self-deception that he has been pulling on himself for years" (Sullivan, 1954, p. 21).

The therapeutic aspect of an interview may be evident even with severely troubled people who might otherwise resist insights into their problems. For example,

> given a bright, intuitive [borderline or psychotic] patient, a compassionate but blunt confrontation, especially if laced with humor, will, in just a few words, bring the ironies of the patient's conflicting and split-off views of the world into his full view. This may provoke tears of recognition and at the same time a profound appreciation toward the interviewer for having *understood* correctly the patient's dilemma. The patient often drops his "crazy facade" and begins to talk in a down-to-earth fashion (Stone, 1980, pp. 289–299).

Objectives   The interviewer usually attempts to get as much relevant information as possible about the person's feelings, behaviors, situations, and family history. The following kinds of questions are usually addressed.

First, what are the *central features* of the problem? Is the individual acting irrationally against others, withdrawing, or tending to self-blame? Do the symptoms suggest abnormalities mainly of thinking, emotions, or action? How is the problem expressed in dreams, fantasies, attitudes, and values? Does the problem reflect personality instability and susceptibility to stress? What are the possible latent strengths of personality—intelligence, for example, or sensitivity, or resourcefulness—that are either masked or derailed by the symptoms?

Second, what are the *consequences* of the problem for the patient and for others? For instance, do the symptoms elicit sympathy or encouragement, thereby making them more resistant to change, or do they elicit resentment or retaliation from others, thereby increasing the person's social isolation? How does the problem affect the patient's educational, vocational, and other kinds of performance? These questions are germane to characterizing the problem, formulating therapeutic strategies, and predicting outcome.

Third, what are *immediate causes* of the patient's problem? What situations intensify or minimize the problem? Does evidence indicate that some underlying medical condition contributes to the problem?

Fourth, what are the likely *historical causes* (etiology) of the problem? Does it run in the family? Might long-standing social or biological factors explain the situation and indicate appropriate intervention?

Fifth, what is the *prognosis*—that is, the likely outcome—with and without intervention? Would other strengths and weaknesses of the person influence outcome? For example, antisocial behavior in someone of limited intelligence is unlikely to respond favorably to a psychoanalytic-type therapy that requires insight about sometimes subtle and complex meanings over a protracted period of time.

Behavioral Assessment

A clinician utilizing a behavioral approach to assessment will gather information about stimuli that control important aspects of the behavioral problem, the patient's responses to these stimuli, and the conditions that reinforce the relevant responses. The stimulus side of the assessment of phobic anxiety, for example, might involve detailed descriptions of the phobic object and other environmental factors that elicit the anxiety; it might involve the construction of a scale of the specific situations associated with mild, moderate, and severe anxiety for the individual. Responses to the anxiety can be scaled to yield a quantitative description of unpleasant feelings, apprehensive thoughts, and avoidance behaviors; for example, the emotional component can be measured in terms of amount of trembling, sweating, tension, coughing, or choking. In assessing reinforcement, the clinician would identify the conditions that sustain the phobic avoidance behavior—for example, secondary gain from attention and sympathy. Detailed description is important not only for defining problems but also for evaluating any improvements achieved by therapy (see Chapter 22).

Interviewing permits assessment of social behavior problems arising from family situations (Table 4.1), and of specific stimulus-response-reinforcement connections—for example, those involved in anxiety disorder (Table 4.2). The interviewer may also use questionnaires or ask the patient to role-play in order to make direct observations. The patient may also be asked to use a checklist

TABLE 4.1   ASSESSMENT OF FAMILY BEHAVIOR

Problem areas	Observations
Development level	Long-standing overprotection by parents has left George dependent on adults for support and guidance.
Roles	George's prematurity placed him in the "sickly role." Mrs. Adams relates to her family by the "martyr role." Mr. Adams plays the role of the "family dummy" by assuming a facade of not knowing what the family needs.
Generation boundary lines	In the Franklin family, Mr. & Mrs. Franklin function as children, whereas the 9-year-old daughter Diane seems to hold the power of decision-making.
Family hierarchy	Every time Mr. Thompson attempts to discipline Joe, Mrs. Thompson steps in and undercuts his efforts. She then relegates her husband to the level of Joe's sibling.
Special communications and family secrets and myths	Part of the family's problems involve Mr. and Mrs. Wilson's unspoken agreement not to discuss Nancy's illness and not to label feelings about this issue. George seems to know he is adopted, but when he inquires about this, his parents switch the subject.
Multigeneration problems	Mrs. Rogers denigrates her daughter-in-law's child-rearing techniques. She communicates her disagreement directly to her son and tries to draw him into an alliance against his wife; additionally, she indirectly communicates this to her grandchild, Amy. Amy will ignore her mother's discipline and guidance by telling her mother she doesn't have to obey her because "Granny knows best and Daddy says so too."
Special stimuli and response patterns	Apparently when Mrs. Green starts to weaken in her limits, her youngest son, Robert, becomes more aggressive.
Significant Individual issues in the child or adolescent	Fred, who was a temperamentally difficult child, apparently frustrated Mrs. Nesbitt, who was herself striving to please her own parents. Nancy's learning disability problem, which was poorly understood by her parents, led to nightly homework battles, which lowered her self-esteem.
Significant individual pathology in the parent	Adolph's low self-esteem seems to have been shaped by the consistent criticism of his father, a diagnosed paranoid schizophrenic.

Source: Manosevitz, M., and Stedman, J. M. Some thoughts on training the novice family therapist in the art of family assessment. *Family Therapy,* 1981, *13,* 67–76.

TABLE 4.2 DESCRIPTION OF PATIENT'S MAIN COMPLAINT (ANXIETY DISORDER)

External cues

Specifically elicit information about objects or situations that provoke high anxiety or discomfort—e.g., supermarket, social contacts, bridges, urine, locking a door.

Internal cues

1. Inquire about *thoughts, images,* or *impulses* that provoke anxiety or shame or disgust—e.g., images of rats, numbers, impulses to stab one's child.

2. Inquire about *bodily sensations* that disturb the patient—e.g., tachycardia, blushing, depersonalization.

Imagined consequences of external and internal cues

1. Elicit fears about possible harm that can be caused by the *external object or situation*—e.g., snakes can bite, rejection during social interactions, falling from a high place, disease from touching a contaminated object, burglary if a door is not properly locked.

2. Elicit fears about harm caused by *internal cues*—either from (a) thoughts, images, or impulses, (b) bodily sensations, or (c) the long-term experience of high anxiety. For example,

(1) God will punish me. I may actually stab my child.

(2) I'll have a heart attack, people will think less of me if they see me blush, I'll go crazy or lose control and shame myself in public.

Strength of belief system

Assess the degree to which the patient believes that the feared consequences may occur. What is the objective probability that confrontation with feared cues will actually result in psychological or physical harm? (Strong belief systems are found to interfere with satisfactory progress in behavioral treatment.)

Source: Adapted from Steketee & Foa, 1985.

during a week of self-monitoring in order to obtain more objective and systematic information not otherwise available.

Behavioral assessment can include objective test situations set up in or outside the office. For example, rather than responding to a rating scale or a set of hypothetical questions, a snake phobic might be induced to approach a real snake while the clinician assesses the intensity of the reaction. Similar real-life tests can be used at a later date to evaluate long-term treatment effectiveness.

Psychodynamic Assessment

Objectives and Tools Many clinicians believe that psychodynamic assessment is the key to understanding infantile, destructive, and irrational behavior. According to this view, while shifting external conditions promote behavioral change (Mischel, 1973), enduring psychodynamic patterns promote maladaptive behavioral inflexibility (Wachtel, 1973). Also according to this view, personality involves subjectively biased ways of perceiving the world, and it is these subjective, highly motivated meanings that organize and direct behavior (Klein, G. S., 1976, p. 26). Normally, these hidden meanings compete with external situations for control over behavior. When purely personal meanings predominate, behavior may appear egocentric, bizarre, or inflexible.

For example, unresolved infantile conflicts with parents may explain repeated and self-destructive difficulties with authority figures in general.

Psychodynamic assessment of personality may be done with projective tests designed to elicit hidden tendencies and personal meanings. The tests are based on the "projective hypothesis" that under relaxed conditions, needs, fears, and defenses will be expressed ("projected") in the subjective interpretations of ambiguous stimuli. Projective tests thus utilize ambiguous stimuli to which a wide range of acceptable responses are possible (see Figure 4.1). While responses can be scored for objective accuracy—for example, perceiving a toad in a batlike ink blot represents a significant departure from the norm—responses are also evaluated for their variety, imaginativeness, and personal significance. Both the objective and subjective aspects of responding to projective stimuli tell us something about the person's unique way of construing experience.

To the extent that projective tests utilize stimuli with many "acceptable" responses, they can be distinguished from objective tests which constrain the range of acceptable responses. In objective tests of ability, for example, a response to a question such as "What is the circumference of the Earth?" can be scored as *right or wrong*. Objective tests of personality include items such as "I like my mother," "I do not like thunderstorms," "My thoughts are controlled by others"—answers to which can be scored either *true or false* or *agree or disagree*.

Projective tests permit the clinician to assess how an individual balances the dual demands of external reality—what the card really looks like—and subjective reality—what the person feels about the card. People are especially challenged by the ambiguous and enigmatic quality of projective test stimuli (Piotrowski, 1982).

Thematic Apperception Test   The Thematic Apperception Test (TAT), developed by Henry Murray (1943), consists of a set of pictures, each of which represents some relatively ambiguous situation (see Figure 4.1, top). For example, two people may be embracing or they may be struggling; a person in silhouette at an open window may be reflecting on life, planning his future, or contemplating suicide. The respondent is asked to make up a story to each of the cards, elaborating on the people, situations, background, and outcome of the perceived events. The patient's own needs and preoccupations will presumably be projected as thematic patterns—for example, themes of rejection or hostility toward members of the opposite sex.

Card 1 of the TAT, shown in Figure 4.1 (top), typically brings out indications of achievement motivation and attitudes toward authority. Typically, a respondent makes up a story in which a boy is described either as reflecting on his future as a violinist, or as wishing he could be playing ball outside with the other kids, or something to that effect.

Here is one response to Card 1.

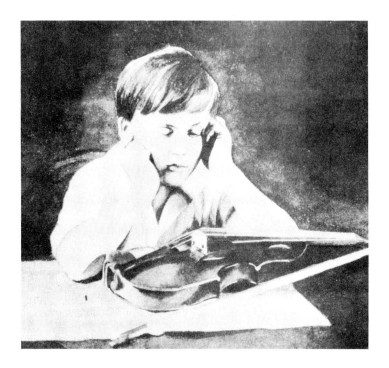

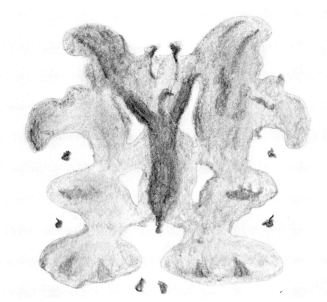

FIGURE 4.1   Stimulus cards like those used in the two most popular projective tests. The Thematic Apperception Test (top) and the Rorschach (bottom). (TAT card reprinted by permission of the publishers from *Thematic Apperception Test* by Henry A. Murray, Cambridge, Mass.: Harvard University Press. Copyright 1943 by the President and Fellows of Harvard College;1971 by Henry A. Murray.)

> That's a little boy sitting by his violin. It looks to me like he's kind of drowsy. He's been practicing or playing. It looks to me like he has kind of dozed off to sleep. It looks like the exercises have been kind of hard.

Schafer (1948, p. 135) interprets this response to reflect the person's tendency to withdraw passively from certain anxiety-arousing situations, perhaps especially those involving demands for high levels of personal achievement.

But consider this response:

> Grandpa's been a violinist for a long time. Billy admires this violin; what a great instrument. Billy will grow up to be a great pianist. (Examiner asks: "What is he thinking?") Oh what a pretty violin this is, excuse me, what a pretty piece of wood this is. Grandpa calls it a violin but I call it a bow...a modified bow and arrow set.

What can we make of this extraordinary "story"? Giving names to the figures in a card is highly unconventional. The inventive but mocking attitude reduces the testing situation to a game, perhaps expressing a unique way of defending against hostile impulses toward authority. Furthermore, two insidious features are evident: an arbitrary and peculiar transformation of Billy from ardent violinist to pianist, and an equally peculiar drift from the idea of violin bow (a conventional perception) to bow and arrow (a highly idiosyncratic association). This cognitive drift, or "slippage," suggests the possibility of some kind of thought disorder.

Rorschach Test   The Rorschach test is composed of ten ink blots including five with vivid color (see Figure 4.1, bottom). Because ink blots are more ambiguous than TAT pictures, the question "What might this be?" pushes the subject's intellectual and emotional resources somewhat harder. For example, a mothlike blot is typically recognized as a "moth" or a "bat." Atypically, it may be seen as a "bloodthirsty and menacing presence." Aberrant responses suggest that the personal significance of the card has interfered with accurate perception, and this in turn suggests some degree of cognitive impairment.

Piotrowski (1982) gives a particularly good example of the use of Rorschach testing to bring out an otherwise unsuspected liability to psychopathology. He describes a young woman of extraordinarily fine qualities—intelligent, competent, creative, hardworking, pleasant—yet lacking direction or sense of purpose, the early signs of a potential problem. Card III of the Rorschach typically elicits a response like "Two African women facing each other and carrying a cooking pot." Her response was:

> Two African fertility gods. First they looked like females, but now they're males. Male fertility gods. Stomachs are attached to their wrists. I don't know why, but they are very strange.

Piotrowski points out that her ability to recognize the peculiarity of her response indicates her remaining capacity for insight despite the growing presence of a schizophrenic disorder. This diagnostic impression was supported by subsequent developments in her behavior: intellectual deterioration, leaving school for a routine and low-paying job, and living a marginal existence. All these were significant losses considering the high plane of her former achievements.

Certain questions about a person's responses to the ink blots are of particular interest to the clinician. Does the person use the whole blot—indicating an ability to integrate details—or does the person focus on tiny areas—suggesting obsessive concern about detail? Is there a healthy balance of conventional and idiosyncratic perceptions? Is there a tendency to see "movement" in objectively static stimuli—suggesting both intelligence and imagination? Is there an overreaction to the colored parts of the blot—suggesting impulsivity—or to the shaded parts—suggesting anxiety and depression? What does the diversity of responses reveal about knowledge, interests, or pathological preoccupations?

To get the flavor of a psychodynamically oriented report based on projective test responses, consider the following example from the assessment of an obsessive-compulsive patient:

> The patient appears to be striving toward good rapport and objective attachments and does have the capacities for these; however, obsessional doubting and caution probably stand in the way of lasting, intense gratifications. He is aware of this inability to experience real enjoyment and feels lonely and depressed. A further hindrance appears to be the presence of strong, pent-up aggressions which he has inadequate means of expressing, and which he characteristically tends to rationalize, project, or deny through passive compliance. They are likely to be expressed mainly in aggressive fantasies and irritability. Rationalizing and isolation appear to be his chief defenses against all strong feelings. Anxiety is intense and the tolerance threshold is only fair. He appears to feel that he is too passive and there are indications of intense passive needs: the general impression is that by way of intellectual self-sufficiency he rigorously attempts to combat any admission of passivity that he can recognize, but, at the same time, he is very alert to nuances of interpersonal relationships and automatically assumes a passive, compliant role. In this setting of acute conflict over passive needs and intense anxiety, an addictive trend is likely to be present. Sexual adjustment appears to be poor and it is suggested that a strong latent feminine identification is present. Some sexual preoccupation is likely (Schafer, 1948, p. 119).

Evaluation of Projective Tests   Confidence in projective tests as "psychological X rays" has declined over the years. The main reason is that with some exceptions (Exner, 1986), diagnoses based on projective techniques tend to have poor reliability—particularly frequent disagreement between clinicians—and also poor validity—frequent discordance with real-world facts (Masling, 1960; Megargee, 1966; Maloney & Ward, 1976). Projective tests also show little *incremental* validity, that is, they do not increase validity when added to other procedures—a good interview, for example.

Nevertheless, projective tests may sometimes be useful—for example, when the results of nonprojective tests disagree or when testing young children, especially preschoolers, with whom nonprojective tests cannot easily be used. Moreover, projective tests may sometimes facilitate interviewing by building rapport and increasing the willingness of a client to reveal sensitive information (Butcher & Finn, 1983), helping bring out unique patterns of meaning and psychodynamics (Holt, 1960; Maloney & Ward, 1976), and facilitating therapeutic insights in patients with little insight into their problems (Bellak, 1954).

The mystique of projectives as the vehicle of choice for unearthing subterranean truths probably plays a major role in maintaining their credibility despite the evidence of their limited validity. The mystique is undoubtedly sustained by occasional noteworthy examples of diagnostic achievements by experts. Clearly, "much of what the expert achieves is a matter of art, the exercise of intuition and craft in a way that is difficult to verbalize..." (Holt, 1960, p. 25). Therefore, "viewed from this perspective, the problem of validity becomes first one of establishing the upper limits of what can be done by the most gifted diagnosticians, and then of finding out how they do it. Little research of these kinds has been done" (Holt, 1960, p. 33).

Formal Diagnostic Assessment

Achieving a formal diagnosis usually rests on information about signs and symptoms, personality strengths and weaknesses, possible medical conditions, and situational stresses—in short, the multiaxial considerations introduced by the *DSM-III*. The formal diagnostic approach makes use of certain types of assessment, three of which—structured interviewing, objective tests, and the use of *DSM-III-R* criteria—we describe next.

Structured Interviewing To achieve a formal diagnosis, a clinician often uses relatively informal interviewing procedures like those discussed early in the chapter. In recent years, structured interview procedures have been developed. In a structured interview, questions and their sequence are predetermined in a standard way. For example, the Present State Examination, or PSE (Wing, Cooper, & Sartorius, 1974), includes a standard set of questions that is administered according to certain rules. Some of the questions are obligatory, while others are used only as needed to clarify an apparently significant aspect of dysfunction revealed in the course of the examination. Suppose that a patient were asked the obligatory question, "Can you think quite clearly or is there any interference with your thoughts?" The patient's answer may require further, more specific inquiry: "Are thoughts put in your head that you know are not your own?" Obligatory and clarifying questions cover twenty areas of psychological functioning involving mood, thinking, motivation, perception, insight, and movement.

Information gathered with the PSE can be entered into a computer and transformed by a fixed set of rules into a diagnosis. Answers to the 500 PSE questions (raw data) are reduced to 140 symptoms (neologisms, muteness, guilt, and so on), and these can be reduced to thirty-five clusters of symptoms (visual hallucination, self-neglect, tension, and so on), and even further to broader "descriptive categories" (for example, psychotic, manic, schizophrenic).

Research is only just beginning to test the widespread assumption that, compared to unstructured interviews, structured interviews yield diagnoses that are more reliable and valid (Maier, Philipp, & Buller, 1988). A good example is the Personality Disorder Examination (PDE). The PDE organizes Axis II criteria into general areas of psychological functioning such as cognitive, interpersonal, and emotional. The interviewer introduces each area in a rather informal, open-ended way, and then asks a set of specific questions in fixed order. Initial tests of the PDE have yielded much higher interrater agreement for personality disorders than previously obtained by less structured assessments (Widiger & Frances, 1987).

Objective Tests of Personality The formal diagnostic process may benefit from the use of objective tests of personality. Made up of a fixed set of items typically of the "true/false" type, objective tests include *test norms,* expected or normal values against which deviant individual responses can be measured. One of the best known objective tests of psychopathology is the Minnesota Multiphasic Personality Inventory, or MMPI (Hathaway & McKinley, 1943). Items originally selected from older tests or made up by clinicians to represent significant features of psychopathology included questions about feelings, attitudes, beliefs, and cognitive style. During the development of the test, an item was retained only if it discriminated patients with a particular disorder from nonpatient controls—if it was endorsed by 30 percent of psychopaths but only by 5 percent of controls, for example.

Table 4.3 gives items that resemble real items on each of eight scales measuring abnormal personality and on three validity scales. Validity scales assess test-taking response patterns which, if prominent, call the results into question: (a) *lying* to make a favorable impression (endorsing many items such as "I have never hurt anyone's feelings" which are unlikely to be true of a normal person); (b) *carelessness,* eccentricity, or even faking pathology (endorsing items such as "Everything seems dark," which, taken on their own, are rare responses and which, collectively, do not constitute any known syndrome); and (c) *defensiveness* (endorsing items such as "Despite everything, I am better off than most people"), which suggests an unconscious retreat from objective self-evaluation into pollyannaish denial.

The utility of tests can be judged partly on the basis of external validity, that is, by agreement between the test results and "external criteria" that exist either at the same time (concurrent validity) or at some later time (predictive validity) (Cronbach, 1970). For example, the MMPI has modest concurrent validity; diagnoses made by computer analysis of MMPI responses are about as accurate as the diagnoses of skilled clinicians. At least some of the individual MMPI scales have modest *predictive* validity; for example, over 50 percent of ninth-grade boys with elevated scores on the Psychopathic deviancy and Hypomania scales later became delinquent, whereas none of the boys with in-

TABLE 4.3   ANALOGUE ITEMS FOR MMPI SCALES USED TO ASSESS PSYCHOPATHOLOGY

Scale	Sample item	High-score indication
Lie	I never engage in loose talk about other people.	Naive or calculated attempt to claim excessive virtue or appear "saintly"; overly scrupulous personal habits
Frequency	It is hard for me to tell one color from another.	Attempt to appear abnormal (also detects true abnormality)
Defensiveness	I am highly regarded by all my peers.	Attempt to appear healthy by denying even socially acceptable shortcomings
Hypochondriasis	New medicines hardly even work.	Excessive bodily concern and chronic dissatisfaction
Depression	My life is largely a series of disappointments.	Sad, troubled, hopeless
Hysteria	My limbs are sometimes very weak.	Multiple bodily complaints; poor insight; suggestible
Psychopathic deviation	I don't obey directions.	Antisocial; superficial relationships; impulsive
Paranoia	People are always trying to find out about me.	Suspiciousness and jealousy
Psychasthenia	I have never been very popular with my classmates.	Anxiety, doubt, rigidity
Schizophrenia	Sometimes I think my bones are getting soft.	Bizarre thinking and seclusive behavior
Hypomania	Taking action is better than contemplation.	Outgoing and impulsive

troverted and feminine interest patterns became delinquent (Hathaway & Monachesi, 1963).

Objective Tests of Organic Dysfunction   Neurological and neuropsychological tests provide the basis for the formal diagnosis of organic disorders. Neurological tests can provide direct information about brain pathology and indirect evidence about the metabolic organization of the central nervous system. X-ray pictures of the brain can determine if there is tissue loss or tumor growth. Pictures of the rate of metabolic activity in different parts of the brain may reveal neurological malfunctions that explain behavioral abnormalities.

Neuropsychological tests are designed to locate abnormalities of brain function through the use of behavioral tasks. For example, if maximal tapping speed of the right hand is much slower than that of the left, there is reason to suspect an abnormality of the areas of the left side of the brain responsible for skilled movements. If a person has trouble drawing a line connecting symbols from 1 to A to 2 to B and so on, an abnormality of the frontal part of the brain is suspected. In short, inferences about the location of brain dysfunction often can be made from behavioral patterns elicited by neuropsychological tests.

Because neurological and neuropsychological tests are so intimately tied up with brain-behavior relationships, we will defer further description until Chapter 8, where they are examined in more detail.

Objective Tests of Intelligence   Intelligence test items tap the capacity to make good judgments, think rationally, and manipulate information at an abstract level. The best estimates of intelligence and its impairments are derived from standardized tests. The terms "standardized" refers both to test norms against which individual performance is assessed and to fixed procedures and test items for gathering data (Cronbach, 1970). Figure 4.2 gives examples of the types of items included in IQ tests.

IQ scores are important and valuable because they are *reliable* over time—meaning that individuals tend to obtain similar scores on repeated testings—and because they have *external validity*—IQ estimates predicting performance on other tests and predicting performance in real-life situations that make demands on intellectual capacity (Willerman, 1979). Also, intelligence interacts with psychopathology—sometimes suppressing it, sometimes magnifying it, and always influencing the unique way that it is expressed. Therefore, clinicians assess intelligence to achieve a better understanding of a disorder and its long-term outlook.

DSM-III-R **Procedures**   One of the most frequent approaches to formal diagnostic assessment rests on the use of an interview to identify behavioral symptoms that satisfy the criteria of the recently revised *DSM-III*, or the *DSM-III-R*. Recall that *DSM-III-R* retains the prototypal format of *DSM-III* (see Chapter 3, pp. 63–64). This means that it provides polythetic criteria: both inclusional criteria that signify a particular disorder and exclusional criteria that tend to rule it out (Boyd et al., 1984). Both inclusional and exclusional criteria are defined in concrete behavioral terms rather than in the abstract terminology of some theory. For example, a phobia is diagnosed on the basis of the type, frequency, and intensity of anxious behaviors rather than from inferences about the presence of a hypothetical intrapsychic conflict.

DSM-III-R includes two general rules about making a formal diagnosis. Precedence is given first to *organic* factors because these can produce the symptoms of other disorders (see Chapter 9). For example, if the evidence warrants it, Organic Anxiety Disorder preempts Panic Disorder (American Psychiatric Association, 1987, p. xxv). Second, precedence is given to *pervasiveness,* with the more pervasive disorder—the one involving many psychological functions—preempting the less pervasive disorder; however, this rule applies only if the symptoms of the more pervasive disorder typically include the symptoms of the less pervasive disorder. Thus, schizophrenia preempts dysthymic disorder when the symptoms of both co-occur because dysthymia (mild chronic depression) is frequently an associated feature of schizophrenia. Nevertheless,

VERBAL IQ TEST ITEMS

(a) Information

1. Who wrote *Animal Farm*?

2. Where is Iceland?

3. At what temperature does water freeze?

4. What is oncology?

(b) Comprehension

1. Why should we obey no-smoking rules posted in public areas?

2. Why are legal contracts necessary?

3. Why do we sweat when we are hot?

4. What does this saying mean: "Two heads are better than one".

(c) Arithmetic

1. How many 22¢ stamps can you buy for a dollar?

2. How many hours will it take a motorist to travel 330 miles if he is going 55 miles an hour?

3. A man bought a TV set on sale for 15% off the regular retail price of $300. How much did he pay?

4. Eight men can finish a job in six days. How many men will be needed to finish the job in two days?

PERFORMANCE IQ TEST ITEMS

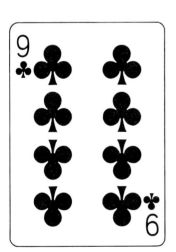

(a) Picture completion

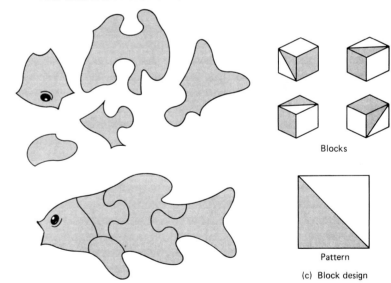

(b) Object assembly

Blocks

Pattern

(c) Block design

FIGURE 4.2   A sample of items analogous to those used in the *Wechsler Adult Intelligence Scale*. Top: Verbal test items. These include tests of (a) information, (b) comprehension, and (c) arithmetic. Bottom: Performance test items. These include (a) Picture Completion: recognize the missing part; (b) Object Assembly: rearrange the pieces to form a familiar object; (c) Block Design: blocks, with some sides all red, some all white, and some half red and half white, are to be arranged to reproduce a model design.

even with the organicity and pervasiveness rules, multiple diagnoses can still be made—for example, Depressive Disorder and Panic Disorder, or Borderline Personality Disorder and Alcohol Abuse (see Table 4.6).

Once a formal diagnosis of an Axis I and/or II disorder is made, three other kinds of information are sought to provide a fuller understanding of the disorder. These constitute three additional "axes" or dimensions of behavioral assessment. Recall that Axis III refers to possible physical disorder that may cause or exacerbate Axis I or II disorders or affect their clinical management (Hall et al., 1978). For example, diabetes mellitus would be indicated on Axis III for a patient whose psychiatric condition may be caused or aggravated by the disease. Axis III represents the idea that medical diseases often co-exist with and aggravate psychiatric disorders, and that a medical disease may pathologize the behavior even of an otherwise neurologically and psychologically normal person (see Hall, 1980a). One study (Koranyi, 1979) found that 46 percent of a sample of psychiatric patients had a co-existing medical disorder that caused the psychiatric condition in 18 percent of the cases and aggravated it in an additional 51 percent of the cases.

Axis IV refers to "psychosocial stressors" that may cause or aggravate an Axis I or II disorder—loss of loved one, family conflict, job-related difficulties, legal or financial problems, and so on. Axis IV is now defined by a scale of psychosocial stressors, both *acute* (less than six months) and *chronic*. This scale and examples of stressors at each level are shown in Table 4.4.

Axis V identifies the highest level of adaptive function achieved by the patient both currently and during the past twelve months. Evaluation along Axis V, using the Global Assessment of Functioning Scale (Table 4.5), indicates potential strengths in psychological, social, and occupational functioning that may be of practical significance in treatment and prognosis. Examples of formal diagnoses using the five axes of *DSM-III-R* are shown in Table 4.6.

DIAGNOSTIC RELIABILITY

Scientific progress in psychopathology requires that abnormal behavior be reliably identified. There are two kinds of diagnostic reliability. The *test-retest* type refers to agreement between the first and subsequent diagnoses made by the same diagnostician using the identical method. The *interrater* type refers to agreement between two independent raters evaluating the same set of behaviors at the same time. The ability to achieve reliable diagnoses in research and clinical settings has been a major consideration in evaluating and revising *DSM* classification systems (Grove, 1987).

There are many reasons that high reliability may not be achieved (Tsuang et al., 1987). Patients may actually change with time—for example, the disorder itself may be evolving or else the patient has different disorders at each time. In addition, two clinicians may acquire different information about the patient, perhaps because the patient tells a different story to each. Finally, unreliability may arise from certain inadequacies of the diagnostic system, in particular

TABLE 4.4   AXIS IV (*DSM-III-R*)

| Code | Term | Examples of stressors | |
		Acute events	Enduring circumstances
		Severity of psychological stressors scale: adults	
1	None	No acute events that may be relevant to the disorder	No enduring circumstances that may be relevant to the disorder
2	Mild	Broke up with boyfriend or girlfriend; started or graduated from school; child left home	Family arguments; job dissatisfaction; residence in high-crime neighborhood
3	Moderate	Marriage; marital separation; loss of job; retirement; miscarriage	Marital discord; serious financial problems; trouble with boss; being a single parent
4	Severe	Divorce; birth of first child	Unemployment; poverty
5	Extreme	Death of spouse; serious physical illness diagnosed; victim of rape	Serious chronic illness in self or child; ongoing physical or sexual abuse
6	Catastrophic	Death of child; suicide of spouse; devastating natural disaster	Captivity as hostage; concentration cap experience
0	Inadequate information, or no change in condition		
		Severity of psychological stressors scale: children and adolescents	
1	None	No acute events that may be relevant to the disorder	No enduring circumstances that may be relevant to the disorder
2	Mild	Broke up with boyfriend or girlfriend; change of school	Overcrowded living quarters; family arguments
3	Moderate	Expelled from school; birth of sibling	Chronic disabling illness in parent; chronic parental discord
4	Severe	Divorce of parents; unwanted pregnancy; arrest	Harsh or rejecting parents; chronic life-threatening illness in parent; multiple foster home placements
5	Extreme	Sexual or physical abuse; death of a parent	Recurrent sexual or physical abuse
6	Catastrophic	Death of both parents	Chronic life-threatening illness
0	Inadequate information, or no change in condition		

Source: Reprinted with permission from the *Diagnostic and Statistical Manual of Mental Disorders.* Third Edition Revised, p. 11. Copyright © 1987 American Psychiatric Association.

when diagnostic criteria are insufficiently detailed, overly abstract, or common to other categories (see Table 4.7) (Ward, Beck, Mendelson et al., 1962).

High, or even perfect, interrater reliability does not necessarily indicate external validity (accuracy); for example, two raters may agree on a diagnosis of schizophrenia though the patient may, in fact, be a manic-depressive. On the

TABLE 4.5 AXIS V (*DSM-III-R*)

Global Assessment of Functioning Scale (GAF Scale)

Consider psychological, social, and occupational functioning on a hypothetical continuum of mental health–illness. Do not include impairment in functioning due to physical (or environmental) limitations.*

Code	
90 | 81	Absent or minimal symptoms (e.g., mild anxiety before an exam), good functioning in all areas, interested and involved in a wide range of activities, socially effective, generally satisfied with life, no more than everyday problems or concerns (e.g., an occasional argument with family members).
80 | 71	If symptoms are present, they are transient and expectable reactions to psychosocial stressors (e.g., difficulty concentrating after family argument); no more than slight impairment in social, occupational, or school functioning (e.g., temporarily falling behind in school work).
70 | 61	Some mild symptoms (e.g., depressed mood and mild insomnia) or some difficulty in social, occupational, or school functioning (e.g., occasional truancy, or theft within the household), but generally functioning pretty well, has some meaningful interpersonal relationships.
60 | 51	Moderate symptoms (e.g., flat affect and circumstantial speech, occasional panic attacks) or moderate difficulty in social, occupational, or school functioning (e.g., few friends, conflicts with co-workers).
50 | 41	Serious symptoms (e.g., suicidal ideation, severe obsessional rituals, frequent shoplifting) or any serious impairment in social, occupational, or school functioning (e.g., no friends, unable to keep a job).
40 | 31	Some impairment in reality testing or communication (e.g., speech is at times illogical, obscure, or irrelevant) or major impairment in several areas, such as work or school, family relations, judgment, thinking, or mood (e.g., depressed man avoids friends, neglects family, and is unable to work; child frequently beats up younger children, is defiant at home, and is failing at school).
30 | 21	Behavior is considerably influenced by delusions or hallucinations or serious impairment in communication or judgment (e.g., sometimes incoherent, acts grossly inappropriately, suicidal preoccupation) or inability to function in almost all areas (e.g., stays in bed all day; no job, home, or friends).
20 | 11	Some danger of hurting self or others (e.g., suicide attempts without clear expectation of death; frequently violent, manic excitement) or occasionally fails to maintain minimal personal hygiene (e.g., smears feces) or gross impairment in communication (e.g., largely incoherent or mute).
10 | 1	Persistent danger of severely hurting self or others (e.g., recurrent violence) or persistent inability to maintain minimal personal hygiene or serious suicidal act with clear expectation of death.

*Use intermediate codes when appropriate, e.g., 45, 68, 72.
Source: Reprinted with permission from the *Diagnostic and Statistical Manual of Mental Disorders.* Third Edition Revised, p. 12. Copyright © 1987 American Psychiatric Association.

TABLE 4.6 EXAMPLES OF DIAGNOSTIC SUMMARIES RECORDED ACCORDING TO *DSM-III-R* FORMAT*

Example 1

Axis I:	296.23	Major Depression, Single Episode, Severe without Psychotic Features
	303.90	Alcohol Dependence
Axis II:	301.60	Dependent Personality Disorder (Provisional, rule out Borderline Personality Disorder)
Axis III:	Alcoholic cirrhosis of liver	
Axis IV:	Psychosocial stressors: anticipated retirement and change in residence, with loss of contact with friends Severity: 4—Moderate (Predominantly enduring circumstances)	
Axis V:	Current GAF: 44 Highest GAF past year: 55	

Example 2

Axis I:	295.94	Schizophrenia, Undifferentiated Type, Chronic with Acute Exacerbation
	V40.00	Borderline Intellectual Functioning (Provisional)
Axis II:	V71.09	No diagnosis on Axis II
Axis III:	Late effects of viral encephalitis	
Axis IV:	Psychosocial stressors: death of mother Severity: 6—Extreme (acute event)	
Axis V:	Current GAF: 28 Highest GAF past year: 40	

*Note that each diagnostic category of the *DSM-III-R* classification system is assigned a unique code number. A V code (in Example 2) refers to a condition not attributable to a mental disorder that is the focus of attention or treatment.

Source: Reprinted with permission from the *Diagnostic and Statistical Manual of Mental Disorders.* Third Edition, Revised, p. 21. Copyright © 1987 American Psychiatric Association.

other hand, lower interrater reliability need not indicate poor validity; for example, clinicians formulate diagnoses on the basis of questions about hallucinations, obsessional thoughts, or dysphoric feelings rather than on measures of the patient's height or head circumference; they do this even though asking questions about symptoms—a pertinent procedure—is far less reliable than the largely irrelevant physical measurements (see Meehl, 1986).

However, no matter how pertinent, if the procedures are so unreliable as to approach chance (random) agreement, they will be without validity because it will be unclear what, if anything, is "out there" to be explained. Which raises a fundamental point, namely, that to assess the reliability of a diagnostic procedure, we must determine to what extent observed agreement is better than chance agreement.

Reliability versus Chance

The idea of meaningful reliability can be appreciated by an example suggested by Spitzer and Fleiss (1974). Raters A and B *independently* assessed 100 peo-

TABLE 4.7 FACTORS AFFECTING DIAGNOSTIC AGREEMENT

Factor	Examples
Examiner	Training in observation and interviewing. Willingness to make diagnosis when uncertain. Assumptions about base rates for disorders. Sensitivity to nonexplicit information. Effect of examiners on patients.
Patient	Clarity and truthfulness of information given. Variability of symptom picture. Effect of patients on examiners.
Classification system	Quality of description and criteria. Breadth or generality of criteria.
Disorders	Base rates (rarity). Heterogeneity of symptom expression: different disorders may have common symptomatology.

ple for the presence or absence of "neurosis." Each of the 100 is seen, one at a time, by each of the two raters. Thus, across all 100, each rater generates a series of "yes" and "no" diagnoses. The basic question is this: To what extent does the set of "yes/no decisions of one rater agree, or overlap, with the set of "yes/no decisions of the other?

Table 4.8 shows the actual frequencies of "neurosis" or "other" used by each rater. Rater A discovered ten "neurotics" out of the 100 individuals rated, that is, rater A's *diagnostic rate* is 10 percent. Rater B discovered twelve "neurotics" out of the 100; that is, rater B's diagnostic rate is 12 percent.

Of the ten people labeled neurotic by rater A, rater B also called eight of them neurotic; likewise, of the twelve people labeled neurotic by rater B, rater A called eight of them neurotic. Thus, in eight out of the 100 cases, both raters agreed on the presence of neurosis. This agreement is shown in the top-left cell of Table 4.8. Note also that the bottom-right cell of the table shows that in 86 out of 100 cases, both raters agreed on the *absence* of neurosis. How good is

TABLE 4.8 HYPOTHETICAL FREQUENCIES OF DIAGNOSIS

	Rater B		
Rater A	"Neurosis"	"Other"	Diagnostic rate for rater A
"Neurosis"	8	2	10
"Other"	4	86	90
Diagnostic Rate for Rater B	12	88	100

Source: Adapted from Spitzer & Fleiss, 1974.

the overall 94 percent agreement of eight in 100 (neurosis) plus 86 in 100 (other)?

What looks like excellent overall agreement (94 percent) may look different when evaluated against chance agreement. How do we estimate the chance component of agreement? Consider the following ridiculous but instructive example: Suppose that each rater, being completely ignorant about clinical behavior, decided to assign the label "neurosis" *randomly* to 10 percent of the 100 cases. What would the expected chance agreement for "neurosis" be between two such raters? The answer is 10 percent of 10 percent, or 1 percent, because there is a 10 percent chance of one rater calling "neurotic" any of the ten "neurotics" chosen at random by the other rater. Thus, chance agreement is found by *multiplying the diagnostic rate of one rater by that of the other.*

What, then, would the expected agreement for "neurosis" be if rater A and rater B of Table 4.8 had assigned the label "neurosis" *at random* according to each rater's base rate (.10 for A, and .12 for B). The answer is .10 (rater A) × .12 (rater B) = .012. Therefore, the observed agreement on "neurosis" (.08, or 8/100) is 6.7 times better than the .012 expected by chance. Likewise, the .86, or 86/100, agreement for "other" is a little better than the .79 expected by chance (.90 for rater A × .88 for rater B).

The Kappa Statistic

A good estimate of reliability should have the chance part subtracted out. An important estimate of nonchance agreement is the kappa statistic (Cohen, J. A., 1960). *Kappa* (κ) is *observed* nonchance agreement (illustrated in the previous section) relative to possible nonchance agreement (explained shortly). To appreciate what κ really means, let's calculate kappa from the numbers in Table 4.8.

Recall that *observed nonchance* agreement is simply observed agreement minus chance agreement. Thus, the observed agreement proportion (Po) is 8/100 (for "neurosis") plus 86/100 (for "other"), that is, 94/100, or .94. We have already figured out chance agreement (Pc) as .012 (for "neurosis") plus .79 (for "other"). So our observed *non*chance agreement (Po − Pc) is .94 − .80 = .14. How good is this compared to *possible nonchance* agreement, that is, the highest possible agreement where only chance and no other factor spoils perfect agreement?

Perfect agreement is simply 100 in 100 = 1.00. Again, chance agreement (Pc) overall is .80. Thus, possible nonchance agreement is 1.00 minus .80, or .20. Now we can calculate kappa, the observed nonchance agreement relative to possible nonchance agreement:

$$\kappa = \frac{\text{observed nonchance}}{\text{possible nonchance}} = \frac{Po - Pc}{1.00 - Pc} = \frac{.94 - .80}{1.00 - .80} = \frac{.14}{.20} = .70$$

The .70 kappa can be interpreted to mean that 70 percent of the *nonchance* yes/no variability in A's ratings overlaps with B's, or vice versa. More simply, observed agreement is 70 percent of best possible agreement after chance agreement is factored out. Most studies now estimate interrater reliability in terms of kappa (see Table 4.9).

A difference between kappas is useful for evaluating changes in diagnostic procedures. For example, kappas of *DSM-III* categories (American Psychiatric Association, 1980, Appendix F) are generally higher than kappas of comparable *DSM-II* categories, which is a major reason for considering *DSM-III* to be a better system than *DSM-II*.

DIAGNOSTIC ACCURACY AND PREDICTIVE VALUE

The overall accuracy of a diagnostic procedure—an interview or a test—depends on the concordance between the diagnoses it yields and reality. Overall accuracy can be analyzed in terms of (1) *sensitivity,* the ability to detect *real* disorder, and (2) *specificity,* or ability to label *non*disorder correctly. For example, a test that detects 80 percent of the neurotics and 90 percent of the nonneurotics in a sample has greater overall accuracy (greater sensitivity and specificity) than a test that detects only 40 percent of neurotics and 70 percent of the nonneurotics in a sample.

We say that a diagnostic procedure has *predictive value* to the extent that it displays both high sensitivity and high specificity. Therefore, even a highly sensitive test may have low predictive value if such a test correctly identifies many true cases of disorder at the cost of falsely diagnosing many cases as "disorder" where no disorder actually exists. False diagnoses are called false positives, where the term positive, like in medicine, means disorder or disease. Diagnostic assessment can have low predictive value even if it detects all cases of actual disorder (perfect sensitivity) if it also generates many false positives (low specificity). To understand how the predictive value of assessment depends on both its sensitivity and its specificity, let us examine some numerical examples.

Imagine a sample of 100 patients diagnostically evaluated with a test of phobia. Table 4.10 shows that ten of these patients are actually phobic (base rate = 10/100 = .10). Nevertheless, the test has "identified" 20 phobics. How

TABLE 4.9 KAPPA COEFFICIENTS OF AGREEMENT FOR AXES I, II, IV, AND V OF *DSM-III*

Axis	Phase one* (Ns = 308–359)	Phase two† (Ns = 293–331)
I (Overall)	.88	.72
II (Overall)	.56	.64
IV	.60	.66
V	.75	.80

*Phase One assessment was done with an early draft of *DSM-III* criteria.
†Phase Two assessment was done with revised criteria.
Source: Adapted from American Psychiatric Association, 1980, Appendix F.

TABLE 4.10   ELEMENTS OF A HYPOTHETICAL TEST RESULT

Diagnostic vs. real-world distinctions		
Diagnostic distinctions		**Real-world distinctions**
"Phobia"	**"Not phobia"**	
8 True positives	2 False negatives	10 Actual phobics
12 False positives	78 True negatives	90 Actual nonphobics
20 (Subjects with test scores above criterion)	80 (Subjects with test scores below criterion)	100 Total

Evaluation of test		
Goal of assessment	**Accuracy**	**Predictive value**
Detect disorder	*Sensitivity:* 8/10 = .80	8/20 = .40
Identify nondisorder	*Specificity:* 78/90 = .87	

good is this test? The answer depends on the goal of assessment. If the goal is the detection of both disorder and nondisorder, then overall accuracy *and* predictive value are given by true positives (correct diagnosis of disorder) plus true negatives (correct diagnosis of nondisorder), 8 + 78 = 86, or 86 percent. However, if the goal of assessment is the detection of either disorder *or* nondisorder, then accurate detection and predictive value differ. Now let us consider accuracy versus predictive value when the goal is the detection of disorder (the usual goal of diagnostic assessment).

Detecting Disorder

Sensitivity   Recall that sensitivity is *the proportion of individuals whose disorder is correctly detected by the test.* In the example given in Table 4.10, eight of ten actual phobics are detected, so sensitivity is eight in ten, or .80. Note that a perfectly sensitive test would detect all phobics and there would be *no false negatives,* that is, no failures to detect disorder.

Predictive Value   Recall that predictive value is *the proportion of diagnoses that are correct.* What is the predictive value of using this test to diagnose phobia? In the example, eight of twenty people diagnosed as phobic are actual phobics, the rest being false positives (erroneously diagnosing nondisorder as disorder). Thus, this test of .80 sensitivity has a predictive value of only .40; that is, only 40 percent of the phobia diagnoses will be correct. In other words, the test correctly identifies a high percentage of true phobics, but at the cost of making many *false positives*. The practical utility of such a test depends on whether that cost is acceptable.

In the next section, we show why a test with high overall accuracy may, in certain applications, have virturally *no predictive value*. This happens when such an apparently "good" test is used to diagnose a rare disorder, that is, a disorder with a very low base rate.

Low-Base-Rate Problem

Suppose we have a test for predicting suicide. Suppose further that the test has incredibly high overall accuracy: a sensitivity of 1.00 and a specificity of .99. How confident would you be about the validity of diagnoses made with such a test? The problem is that the base rate of suicide is extremely small, only .0001 per year. Table 4.11 makes clear that this incredibly accurate test has low predictive value because, despite accurately detecting all the potential suicides, only 1 percent of the suicide diagnoses made on the basis of the test are true positives; the rest (99 percent of them) are false positives!

If the goal of assessment is to diagnose suicide potential regardless of the cost in false positives, clearly you might want to use this test; with its 100 percent sensitivity, all potential suicides are detected and there are no false negatives. However, the problem of identifying suicidal individuals is still not resolved; how do you separate out from the sample of 1010 diagnosed suicidals

TABLE 4.11 PREDICTING A LOW-BASE-RATE DISORDER (SUICIDE)

A. Predicted vs. real-world events

Predicted (diagnosed) events		Real-world events
"Suicide"	"Nonsuicide"	
10	0	10
True positive (TP)	False negative (FN)	Suicides
1,010	98,990	100,000
False positive (FP)	True negative (TN)	Nonsuicides
1,010	98,990	100,000

B. Diagnostic concepts

Sensitivity: detected suicides:	$\dfrac{T}{TP+FN}$	$= \dfrac{10}{10} = 1.00$
Specificity: detected nonsuicides:	$\dfrac{TN}{TN + FP}$	$= \dfrac{98,990}{99,990} = .99$
Predictive value for suicide: Actual suicide relative to predicted suicides:	$\dfrac{TP}{TP + FN}$	$= \dfrac{10}{1,010} = .01$
Overall accuracy: true suicides and nonsuicides:	$\dfrac{TP + TN}{100,000}$	$= \dfrac{99,000}{100,000} = .99$

the ten true positives from the 1000 false positives? The fact is, if our goal is merely overall accuracy, *not* using the test would be better; overall accuracy would be 99.9 percent because, if everyone is assumed to be "nonsuicidal," an error would occur in only ten of 100,000 cases, a level of accuracy ten times greater than the 99.0 percent overall accuracy using the test!

The low-base-rate problem means that the rarer the disorder, the greater the likelihood of making false positive diagnoses even when using a sensitive test. We can compensate for low base rate by using more stringent criteria and thus fewer diagnoses, but at the cost of making more false negatives (failing to detect disorder). In short, adequate prediction of rare events like suicide is always hazardous and typically impossible (Murphy, 1984).

FALLIBILITIES AND CONTROVERSIES

Missing Real Disorders

What Is a Miss?   Clearly, hits are better than misses (false positives and false negatives). Is one type of miss worse than another? Again, it depends on what is important. With suicide prediction, is it more important to avoid false negatives (missing a true suicide) or avoid false positives (erroneously labeling someone suicidal)? What about predicting homicide or schizophrenia? To illustrate the problem of misses, consider two different goals, selection versus intervention.

If selection is the goal of assessment, false positives are worse than false negatives. For example, a researcher cares less about the schizophrenics he fails to identify (false negatives) than erroneously labeling as schizophrenic people who are not truly schizophrenic (false positives) whom he selects for study. Our hypothetical researcher could use a strict set of criteria to help limit false positives at the expense of false negatives. Table 4.12 shows how shifting from a liberal requirement of four symptoms to a stricter requirement of eight symptoms reduces false positives from 40 to 5 percent, even though false negatives increase from 20 to 60 percent. This procedure ensures that a purer sample of schizophrenics will be selected, but at the cost of missing more true schizophrenics.

If clinical intervention is the goal of assessment, both types of misses are troublesome. A false negative would go untreated. A false positive, on the

TABLE 4.12   EFFECT OF USING STRICT OR LIBERAL SELECTION CRITERIA

Criteria: number of valid schizophrenic signs required	Percentage of real schizophrenics selected	Percentage of nonschizophrenics selected	Ratio of real to false schizophrenics: purity of sample
4	80	40	2:1
8	40	5	8:1

other hand, might suffer significant consequences of psychiatric labeling. We will now consider two interesting problems in assessment from the framework of misses: undiagnosed medical conditions presenting as "functional" psychiatric disorder (false negatives), and psychiatric labeling of normals (false positives).

Missing Physical Disease Failure to detect pathology, whether physical or psychological, can have serious consequences. Cancer and bipolar depression are two pathologies which, if undetected, can be lethal. With the advent of *DSM-III,* nonmedical clinicians became even more concerned with the importance of diagnosing medical conditions. The codification of this requirement in Axis III reflects evidence that many medical conditions can manifest as symptoms of functional neurotic, psychopathic (antisocial), and psychotic disorders (Hall et al., 1978). But how many medical conditions go undetected during psychiatric assessment?

It is estimated that from 5 to 45 percent of psychiatric patients (depending on health, social, and economic factors) suffer from medical conditions that either cause or aggravate psychiatric disorder (Hall, 1980a). Koranyi (1979) has provided evidence that medical and mental health professionals can be insensitive to medical conditions that influence psychopathology. He found that *undetected* physical disease, which was later discovered through medical examination, could be classified into three categories: (a) causal: diseases that are entirely responsible for the psychiatric symptoms; (b) aggravating: diseases that augment an existing psychiatric condition; and (c) coexisting: diseases with relatively little implication for psychiatric symptomatology.

Figure 4.3 shows that 43 percent of this sample of 2090 psychiatric outpatients (911 men; 1179 women) were suffering from a major medical disease. Of these 902 patients, 417, or 46 percent, were undiagnosed by the referring source.

The Social Psychology of Psychiatric Labeling

Recall that the diagnosis of a disorder where no disorder exists is called a false positive error. A noteworthy report by Rosenhan (1973) described a study involving the hospitalization of eight "pseudopatients": normal people who had agreed to simulate psychopathology in order to gain admission to a mental hospital. The pseudopatients presented themselves at the hospital complaining of hearing voices saying "empty," "hollow," and "thud." Other than falsifying this symptom and information regarding their vocation and employment, they truthfully reported personal information about their life histories, family relationships, and current experience.

Each pseudopatient gained admission, and some repeated the performance at more than one hospital, resulting in a total of twelve admissions. Each received a diagnosis of psychosis (in eleven cases, schizophrenic, in one case, manic-depressive). The pseudopatients remained in the hospital with little

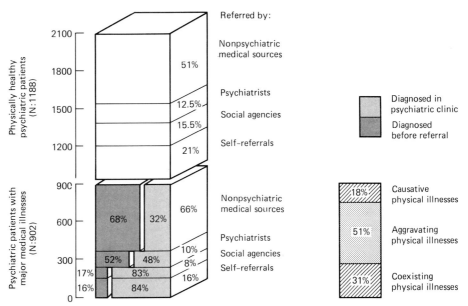

FIGURE 4.3 Rates of diagnosed and undiagnosed major medical illness in a sample of psychiatric clinic patients (Koranyi, 1979, p. 416). The figure shows that psychiatrists accounted for 10 percent of the 902 referrals who turned out to have serious physical disease. Yet diagnosticians failed to detect the disease in 43 percent of their medically ill cases. Nonmedical sources of referral such as social workers did far worse, failing to detect disease in 83 percent of their medically ill cases. (Koranyi, 1979. Archives of General Psychiatry, 1979, *36*, 414–419. Copyright 1979, American Medical Association)

treatment beyond the standard dispensation of various pills—almost 2100, of which only two were actually swallowed. Pseudopatients remained for an average of nineteen days before being discharged, typically with the diagnostic phrase "in remission."

On the face of it, Rosenhan's paper constitutes an indictment of psychiatric hospitals in general, and the diagnostic assessment available there in particular. However, critical evaluation (Millon, 1975; Spitzer, 1975) suggests that this report had its most important effect in sharpening discussion of difficult and legitimate problems in the assessment and treatment of psychopathology, rather than in indicting hospital procedures.

Faking Craziness Clearly, psychiatric symptoms can be faked just as medical symptoms can be faked. The fact that clinicians can be fooled does not, in itself, constitute an indictment of either psychological or medical assessment. That an occasional person can successfully feign psychotic symptoms raises the following questions: How often do normal people receive psychiatric diagnoses (false positives), and how often do disturbed people fail to get diagnosed (false negatives)?

The Rosenhan study does not tell us that. Given that an almost invisibly small number of normal people fake craziness, if a person shows enough concern about hallucinations to seek help at a mental hospital, that person probably does have schizophrenia or some other serious mental disorder. Furthermore, since bizarre cognitive symptoms can discriminate psychosis, a logical clinician, faced with a complaint of hallucination with no evidence of organic disease, *should* diagnose psychosis (Davis, 1976).

Detecting Normalcy According to Rosenhan's paper, the normalcy of the pseudopatient was obvious to real patients on the ward, suggesting that diagnostic biases can prevent clinicians from recognizing true normalcy. However, the fact that the average pseudopatient was discharged in only nineteen days without being given a prescription for antipsychotic medication seems inconsistent with the charge. But let us take a look from a different angle. Rosenhan does not report how many pseudopatients were discovered, only that some pseudopatients were discovered. Also, Rosenhan does not tell us how many *real* patients are typically thought to be "normal" by their fellow patients. Does this happen?

Consider the case of Clifford Beers, who was hospitalized for disorganized, paranoid, and suicidal behavior and who later wrote a landmark book on the subject (Chapter 2, pp. 50–51). One day a fellow patient declared "Why you are kept here I cannot understand. Apparently you are as sane as anyone. You have never made any but sensible remarks to me" (Beers, 1907/1981). Clearly, over a short hospitalization, a psychotic person may give the false impression of mental health. So even if *all* of Rosenhan's pseudopatients had been judged normal by other patients, the significance of such a finding would be ambiguous without the relevant comparison group of pseudonormals, or false negatives.

Criticisms of Psychiatric Labeling The Rosenhan (1973) paper raises some important questions about three characteristics of psychiatric labels: their stickiness, their generality, and their stigmatizing effects. With regard to stickiness, Rosenhan argues that the discharge diagnosis "schizophrenia in remission" shows how a label can stay with a person despite every sign that the person's behavior is normal. However, a diagnostic label often refers to a disorder that a person has regardless of fluctuations in behavior, and schizophrenia is a very good example of such a disorder. The evidence strongly suggests that schizophrenia can be a lifelong *vulnerability* whose behavioral expression may wax or wane, sometimes rather unpredictably (Astrachan, Brauer, Harrow, & Schwartz, 1974). In short, a label ought to stick with a person—at least with a person's psychiatric record—if, rather than merely summarizing behavior, it signifies an enduring condition that increases the risk for abnormal behavior.

When hallucinatory and other psychotic features of a schizophrenic condition subside, the disorder is typically described as "improved" rather than "in remission," that is, symptom-free (Spitzer, 1975). Therefore, it is noteworthy that in eleven of the twelve cases a pseudopatient was discharged with the diagnostic description of "schizophrenia in remission," suggesting that at the time of discharge, the clinician's decision was indeed guided by the pseudopatient's nonpsychotic behavior.

Labels have been criticized as generalizations, and generalizations, it is said, deflect attention from the unique qualities of individuals. In fact, attention to commonalities and attention to uniqueness need not conflict. Classifying a person as male or female, introverted or extraverted, neurotic or psychotic in no way implies the absence of unique qualities. No two people, including genetically identical twins, are exactly alike. But all people have certain things in common. Two people may be placed in the same category if they are each diabetic or schizophrenic despite the unique way each expresses the disorder symptomatically. Labels may be used by bad clinicians or ignorant laymen to avoid clear thinking and humane responsibility, but this does not invalidate the legitimate scientific investigation of commonalities.

Another argument is that labeling stigmatizes individuals—that such people are rejected, despised, and presumed to be incompetent (Mosher, 1978). On the other hand, Weiner (1982, pp. 46–48) suggests that although labeled individuals may be rated less attractive or desirable, the treatment they get from others depends more on how they behave than on what their condition is called. This seems especially true in the light of the growing understanding and tolerance of deviant behavior in contemporary America. The inclusion of Axis V (highest level of adaptive functioning in the past year) in *DSM-III-R* represents the desire not to stigmatize a person but rather to indicate, wherever possible, the strengths and capacities that should moderate the diagnosis and prognosis of abnormal behavior (Millon, 1986).

In sum, labels may in fact be sticky generalizations that can stigmatize. But stickiness *is* appropriate in the case of chronic disorders or persistent vulnerabilities, regardless of behavior. Generalizability *is* appropriate when commonality rather than uniqueness is the focus of attention. The fact that labels may be invalid or that labeling may be abusive should not obscure the legitimate scientific and humanitarian aspects of the diagnostic enterprise. As Spitzer says, psychiatric diagnosis exists

> to enable mental health professionals to (a) communicate with each other about the subject matter of their concern, (b) comprehend the pathological processes involved in psychiatric illness, and (c) control psychiatric disorders. Control consists of the ability to predict outcome, prevent the disorder from developing, and treat it once it has developed. Any serious discussion of the validity of psychiatric diagnosis, or suggestions for alternative systems of classifying psychological disturbance, must address itself to these purposes of psychiatric diagnosis (1975, p. 449).

Though diagnoses may sometimes seem inadequate for explaining the causes and workings of mental disorders, they nevertheless often yield information of value in predicting the likely course of illness—for example, an early recovery, chronicity, or recurrent episodes. Furthermore, for many mental disorders, diagnosis is useful in suggesting the best available treatment (Spitzer, 1975, p. 449).

SUMMARY

Psychiatric assessment consists of identifying abnormalities, making diagnoses, and evaluating outcomes and treatment strategies. Most assessment includes interviewing, the techniques and goals of which are determined by the interviewer's theoretical orientation. Behavioral assessment focuses on specific abnormal behaviors occurring in specific situations. Psychodynamic assessment focuses on inner conflict, symbolic meanings, and the presumed infantile origins of behavior. This type of assessment is often based on projective tests (Rorschach, TAT) composed of ambiguous stimuli. When the goal of assessment is diagnosis, the accent is on the underlying disorder as defined conventionally by classification systems like *DSM-III-R*. Diagnosing a disorder sometimes requires supplementing interviewing with objective tests like the MMPI whose items have answers that do not depend on clinical interpretation.

Three fundamental questions—of reliability, validity, and predictive value—can be asked about any assessment procedure. The reliability question is basically about *agreement*: Can two raters, operating independently with the same procedures, arrive at the same diagnostic formulation from the same set of behavioral data? The validity question is basically about *accuracy*: Can a diagnostic procedure yield a formulation that agrees with objective psychopathology? The predictive value question is about the *utility* of a diagnostic procedure: Specifically, what proportion of all the diagnoses made are valid? This is an important question because a procedure that detects most, or even all, actual disorders may be used at the cost of labeling too many people abnormal. The reliability and validity of psychiatric diagnosis must be weighted against their social implications, that is, the personal and interpersonal consequences of being labeled abnormal. The controversial questions about the value and costs of psychiatric labeling continue to be debated while efforts to improve the classification systems that guide diagnostic decisions proceed apace.

THEORETICAL FACETS

Ecopathological Facet

OUTLINE

RESILIENCY AND VULNERABILITY
  Resiliency
  Vulnerability
  The Ecopathology-Psychopathology Correlation
THE PROBLEM OF UNPREDICTABILITY
SUMMARY

It is one thing to describe abnormal behavior. It is quite another to explain how abnormal behavior arises and why it occurs in some people but not in others. An obvious place to look for explanations is in the environment. Therefore, in this chapter, we take a critical look at two closely related assumptions that have often been made about the environment and its connection to abnormal behavior. The first assumption is that strong correlations, or correspondences, exist between environmental and behavioral characteristics. The second assumption is that such correlations reflect the causal influence of the environment or, more specifically, that adverse environments typically produce abnormal behavior, while benign environments typically produce normal behavior.

We will use the term *ecopathology* for adverse environments, and also for the theoretical perspective that describes the different ways that adverse environments can become connected to psychopathology. We will see that ecopathology-psychopathology correlations are often rather modest, and that, whatever their size, they depend on three things.

1 They depend on what you mean by ''environment''—the physical environment of viruses, birth complications, or head traumas, for example, or the social/educational environment of parents, siblings, peers, and the wider community.

2 They also depend on what you are trying to explain because environmental factors that influence a person's lifetime risk for a disorder may be different from environmental factors that influence the course of a disorder—the duration of an episode or the intensity of symptoms, for example.

3 They depend on preexisting psychological qualities—self-defeating cognitions or feelings of vulnerability, for example, that make a person more susceptible to environmental factors.

MODELS OF ECOPATHOLOGY

Assumptions about the ecopathology-psychopathology connection can be divided into six models, as shown in Table 5.1. Let us start with the first model, which represents the assumption that ecopathology causes psychopathology.

TABLE 5.1   MODELS OF ECOPATHOLOGY

Category	Definition	Diagram	Examples
1. Proactive	Ecopathology causes psychopathology.	E → P	Head injury produces amnesia, complicated by depression. Abusive parenting produces chronic fearfulness.
2. Reactive	Ecopathology is caused by psychopathology.	E ← P	An incorrigible child elicits abusive punishment and emotional withdrawal in the parents, but their behavior has little influence on the child's abnormal disposition.
3. Transactive	Ecopathology and psychopathology are mutually caused.	E ⇄ P	A wife's paranoid suspiciousness elicits resentment and abuse in her husband, which in turn intensifies her paranoia, complicating it with depression.
4. Expressive	Ecopathology and psychopathology are two expressions of a common underlying cause.	E ↖ ↗ P	Behavioral peculiarities of a mother express in mild form the same pathological process more blatantly expressed in the schizophrenic disorder of her son.
5. Selective	Ecopathology is sought out as a "best fit" for psychopathology.	E—P	Psychopaths seek out antisocial environments while schizophrenics "drift" toward relatively less demanding conditions.
6. Inventive	Ecopathology is invented by psychopathology.	(E)P	The hostile "forces" of the paranoid delusion and the "dangers" of the agoraphobic fear are two examples.

Proactive Ecopathology

Proactive means actively promoting some effect. We use the term proactive to indicate environment-to-person causality. Proactive ecopathology is diagramed in Table 5.1 with an arrow that points from environment (E) to person (P). Proactive events exist on their own, regardless of the behaviors that they produce; they are ''independent variables,'' like the experimental treatments imposed by an experimenter regardless of the subject's reactions. A real-life example of proactive ecopatholgy is the uncontrollable cruelty of a drunken father toward an innocent child; the cruel parental behavior is neither elicited nor altered by the child's behavior. A nonsocial example of proactive ecopathology is high alcohol intake during pregnancy, which causes fetal brain damage and consequent mental retardation or hyperactivity.

Proactive ecopathology can *interact* with individual differences; that is, the impact of ecopathology depends on other factors, such as a preexisting vulnerability. As Allport says, ''The same fire that melts the butter hardens the egg'' (1937, p. 325). So, noxious conditions can produce various abnormal adjustments in some people, but they may also inure and immunize other people to hardship. One can easily imagine different effects of ecopathology for two persons: one sensitive, dependent, and insecure; the other thick-skinned, stubborn, and self-confident.

Reactive Ecopathology

Ecopathology may sometimes be the *effect* of psychopathology rather than its cause. Table 5.1 represents this "reverse causality" of *reactive ecopathology* with an arrow pointing from P to E. For example, the behaviors of an abnormal child may cause parental dysfunctions and family disruptions (Bell, 1968; Liem, 1974; Thomas, Chess, & Birch, 1968, pp. 79ff). Socially disruptive disorders such as schizophrenia, autism, psychopathy, and hyperactivity are especially likely to provoke parents to withdraw or retaliate, thus setting up a hostile environment. Reactive ecopathology is sometimes mistaken for a cause rather than recognized as an effect.

Transactive Ecopathology

When ecopathology is both proactive and reactive, this mutual causality is called *transactive*. In Table 5.1 arrows going in opposite directions connect the E and P. Irritating behavior of a hyperactive child, which elicits physical abuse from an unstable parent and in turn intensifies the child's antisocial behavior is an illustration of transactive ecopathology. In such cases, ecopathology and psychopathology feed on one another, producing a spiral of increasingly dysfunctional actions and reactions.

Transactive, like reactive, ecopathology underscores the important idea that people do not merely respond passively like so much clay to be shaped by events. This means that psychopathology may be reflected not only in the dysfunctional behavior of the person but also in the abnormal environments *created by* that person's behavior. Clearly then, rating scales, such as Axis IV of *DSM-III-R*, which supposedly measure the external causes of stress, may sometimes actually describe the *effects* of psychopathology.

Expressive Ecopathology

Now consider the possibility that ecopathology and psychopathology co-occur, not because one causes the other, but because each is independently caused by a *common* pathological process. Consider the example of a father's abusive behavior which seems to cause his son's aggressive behavior. In fact, both of their behavioral patterns might represent some common underlying pathology rather than reactions to each other's behavior. The common cause might be a genetically based antisocial disposition or a product of living in the same crime-ridden neighborhood. Common causality is represented in Table 5.1 by two arrows diverging from a common source.

Selective Ecopathology

There is yet another possible reason for the co-occurrence of ecopathology and psychopathology. People often *seek out* environments that constitute a "best fit" for their temperament and intelligence. The search for a best fit motivates healthy people with special interests in science or music to select specific college majors and to make specific vocational choices. This selection of a best fit may also explain the occasional similarity of psychopathology in husband and wife as due partly to assortative mating—selecting a spouse with similar traits (Merikangas, 1982). Unlike reactive ecopathology that is caused by psychopathology, selective ecopathology is found ready-made—for example, sadists find masochists.

Selective ecopathology isn't the by-product of a conscious self-destructive intent; people typically don't want new problems to complicate their lives. Then why are troubled people attracted by abnormal behaviors and maladaptive situations? There are many possible reasons. One is the natural appeal of others with similar or complementary qualities. For example, a schizotypal person may be attracted to a histrionic person because of shared unconventional attitudes and lifestyle. Another is the tendency to use others to compensate for personal weaknesses. For example, an anxious-dependent person might be attracted to a psychopath who seems decisive and confident. Finally, even harmful conditions are attractive if they promise gratification. For example, a psychopath might be drawn to dangerous situations that satisfy antisocial motives.

Inventive Ecopathology

Adverse environmental events may be magnified into personal threat by an oversensitive person, or even invented by a person with a morbid imagination. *Inventive* ecopathology, a frequent by-product of psychopathology, can sometimes affect behavior as forcefully as real events. Like nightmares, morbid and irrational fantasies, including delusions, can become substitutes for objective reality, often providing an "explanation" for personal distress—for example, when a patient erroneously blames parental abuse or indifference for causing feelings of inadequacy or vulnerability. Inventive ecopathology is compellingly illustrated by the reaction of a severely disturbed person with borderline personality disorder who, "speaking to her idealized attorney, devalued her therapist as 'sadistic, vicious, and full of rage.' When the flattered attorney, incensed at this depiction of the doctor, began to agitate for a new therapist for his client . . . [she] turned savagely on her bewildered lawyer, berating him for sabotaging her treatment" (Gutheil, 1985, p. 11).

We have now described six different models of ecopathology to explain the ecopathology-psychopathology co-relationship. The rest of this chapter is devoted to theory and research bearing on many of the points raised by our discussion. We begin with the most straight-forward assumption about the ecopathology-psychopathology connection—namely, that ecopathology causes psychopathology, in part by learning processes that can be illuminated by laboratory research on both animals and humans.

TRAUMATIC FRUSTRATION IN THE LABORATORY

Experiments on proactive ecopathology typically include manipulations that frustrate basic survival needs and sometimes produce lasting behavioral effects. These investigations usually rest on the assumption that abnormal behavior often develops out of traumatic environmental conditions that frustrate basic needs.

Need and Competence Frustration

All organisms need physical and social stimulation, among other things. Basic needs can be frustrated experimentally by physical confinement, food deprivation, painful stimulation, or social isolation. Need frustration is further heightened when organisms are prevented from coping effectively with such conditions (Mineka & Kihlstrom, 1978). Frustration of coping behaviors—what we call competence frustration—occurs when experimenters make environmental events unpredictable and uncontrollable.

Stimulus *unpredictability* refers to a random relationship between environmental stimuli and specific noxious events. Under such conditions, there are no reliable warning signals and therefore the organism cannot predict threatening events. For example, the amount of stomach ulceration produced in stressed rats given periodic electric shocks while they are physically confined depends largely on whether or not the rats can predict when the shocks will occur: the more unpredictable the shocks, the more extensive the ulceration (Weiss, 1977).

Regardless of their predictability, events may become uncontrollable. *Uncontrollability* exists to the extent that there is a random rather than systematic relationship between behavior and subsequent events it is designed to influence. When, under such conditions, normal behavior no longer "works," helplessness behaviors can develop. These can range from anxiety to despair, and are especially evident when normal coping behaviors devoted to reducing pain or increasing the sense of well-being become ineffective.

In sum, in order to produce symptoms of abnormal behavior in laboratory animals, experimental studies of proactive ecopathology will usually include unpredictability, uncontrollability, and high levels of need frustration (Mineka & Kihlstrom, 1978). A key question is their relevance, or generalizability, to human psychopathology. Do these laboratory manipulations represent the kinds of ecopathology that influence the development of human psychopathology? Are people with anxiety disorders or chronic depression, for example, the victims of objectively frustrating environments? Again, the answer seems to be that it depends, first, on the disorder, and second, on what aspect of a disorder you are trying to explain: its causes or its symptoms. The origin of some disorders—hysterical and anxiety disorders, for example—are often traceable to traumatic events, but this is not the case for others, such as schizophrenia and manic-depression. Of course, the symptomatic expression of all disorders will to some extent be affected by external conditions, and this is true even for highly heritable disorders.

Experimental Neurosis

Laboratory animals exposed to the helplessness-inducing ecopathological extremes described above typically pass through two behavioral stages—the first, an agitated stage called distress or protest, and the second, a passive stage called resignation (discussed later). In the distress stage the subject struggles against helplessness. Behavior is highly energetic, emotional, and, at least initially, disorganized. At some point, compulsive reactions—that is, rigidly stereotyped behavior—may develop. Because they typically reduce severe distress, compulsive reactions can become very hard to change, even though they also produce deleterious consequences. Both the disorganized and the rigid qualities of helplessness-induced protest behavior are laboratory versions of neurotic symptoms: hence the phrase experimental neurosis.

Anxiety Perhaps the most famous study of experimental neurosis was reported in 1921 by Shenger-Krestovnikova (Pavlov, 1927/1960). A harnessed dog was trained to salivate in the presence of a luminous circle which was always followed by food, and not to salivate in the presence of a luminous ellipse never followed by food. The repeated connection between the stimulus and its consequence transformed the circle into a positive conditioned stimulus (CS+), and the ellipse into a negative conditioned stimulus (CS−). With the dog reliably trained to respond to CS+ and not to respond to CS−, the experimental conditions were altered. The experimenter made the discrimination between CS+ and CS− more difficult by gradually equalizing the ratio of the major to minor axes of the ellipse, thus making it more circlelike. When the ratio of the axes reached 9:8, the dog's ability to discriminate became markedly impaired, leading to its emotional breakdown—violent barking, agitation, and an inability to perform even an easy discrimination.

Probably the earliest known study of this sort was done in 1799 on the celebrated "Wild Boy of Aveyron," a 12-year old feral child named Victor. One day, Victor's teacher and benefactor, Jean-Marc Itard (Lane, 1976), gave him a matching-to-sample task that required Victor to place paper cutouts next to identical samples located on a board. Gradually, Itard changed the stimuli so that Victor had to make finer and more difficult discriminations. As Itard explains: "At length, the multiplicity and the complications of these little exercises exhausted his attention and his docility. Then those emotions of impatience and rage which exploded so violently at the beginning of his stay in Paris, especially when he was locked in his room, reappeared in all their intensity" (Lane, 1976, p. 120).

Certain conditions involving extreme discomfort, frustration, and helplessness can produce experimental neurotic behaviors in laboratory animals that are remarkably similar to the symptoms of posttraumatic stress disorder of combat veterans—in particular, heightened vigilance, frequent startle reactions and aggressive outbursts to a wide variety of "threatening" stimuli, extreme physiological activation (elevated heart rate, sweating, shakiness), loss of competencies, and depression (Kolb, 1987).

Rigidity   Recall that rigid and persistent compulsivity may characterize the distress stage. Maier's work (1949) on the frustrative behavior of rats demonstrates this. Animals were first trained to jump from a platform to one of two windows, each covered by a stimulus card. When the animal jumped to the "correct" stimulus, the card gave way, allowing the rat access to safety and food; when it jumped to the "incorrect" stimulus, however, the card remained fixed in place and the animal fell into a net below. Under these highly distressing conditions, animals quickly learned to identify the safe stimulus.

Now the problem was made insoluble. This was done by making each stimulus equally often associated with reward or punishment, that is, by making random and therefore unpredictable the relation between the stimuli and their consequences. In addition, the rat was forced by an air blast to jump from the platform to one of the two stimuli. Thus the rat was subjected to conditions least conducive to life: severe need frustration induced by confinement and physical threat, and severe competence frustration imposed by unpredictability and uncontrollability. The result was a fixated "compulsive" reaction—inflexible jumping to one of the windows, the right or left one, regardless of the stimulus—that persisted even when the task was again made soluble. A compelling similarity exists between this inflexible behavior in rats and the compulsive behavior of neurotic humans—in particular, hand washing, cleaning, or checking compulsions (see Chapter 15).

Aggression   Curiously, animals given the opportunity to express their frustration aggressively may be less adversely affected by such experimental manipulations. For example, confined rats given unpredictable and uncontrollable shock develop fewer stomach ulcers if they have the opportunity to attack each other (Weiss, 1977). A human example of the "protective" function of angry emotion is the low levels of stress-related hormones observed in some people who use angry emotional behavior to defend against feelings of helplessness. In short, organisms can often defend themselves (at least temporarily) against need frustration by vigorous actions and emotions which may appear inappropriate or even self-destructive, yet provide a sense of mastery and security.

Resignation and Depression   But when the ability to cope is totally blocked—when even emotional and compulsive defenses against helplessness become ineffective—behavior can evolve into a *resignation* stage marked by apathy and passivity that some would describe as hopelessness. The hopelessness behavior of the resignation phase is analogous to symptoms of human depression, especially the most severe form. It is characterized by (1) passivity and slowed movements, (2) expectations of personal failure and helplessness, (3) reduced aggressiveness, sexuality, or appetite, and (4) changes in neurochemical patterns (Miller, Rosellini, & Seligman, 1977). Experimental research on these aspects of depression is discussed in Chapter 14.

Unlike laboratory animals, humans are rarely exposed to such objectively noxious conditions over which they have absolutely no control. They do, however, often *feel* a lack of control over their environment, and this recognition of helplessness and hopelessness, regardless of its objective reality, is often what counts. We do not know how often human psychopathology arises from ecopathological conditions, but we do know that people with few coping resources and low self-confidence are inclined to exaggerate dangers and be less able to escape real adversity by healthy coping through action or fantasy. Such people presumably would be the least able to react effectively to stress.

Evaluating the Evidence Serious questions have been raised about the validity of experimental psychopathology (Coyne et al., 1981). The fact that laboratory animals can be made "neurotic" by exposing them to ecopathology doesn't tell us to what extent human neurotic disorders are thereby explained; some may be but some may not. Moreover, laboratory experiments do not adequately represent the subtle variety of provocations and resources available in the real world. Stress manipulations are, for ethical reasons, relatively mild in human research and relatively extreme in animal research, raising questions about whether either adequately represents real world events. In addition, experimental work rarely evaluates individual differences in vulnerability that might explain why not everyone is adversely affected by ecopathology. Finally, when laboratory work treats behavior solely as a "dependent variable"—that is, as the reactive by-product of events that cannot be influenced by the behavior—the significance of ecopathology other than the proactive type cannot be illuminated.

Nevertheless, laboratory research on experimentally induced abnormal behaviors has had an enormous impact on theorizing about environmental causes of psychopathology, and especially traumatic events including rape, combat, child abuse, and other life-threatening dangers. So, the final question is not about the validity of the proactive model of ecopathology, but rather its applicability both to short-term reactions and to the development of enduring vulnerabilities.

CONDITIONED FRUSTRATION: ENVIRONMENTAL CONTROL OF ABNORMAL BEHAVIOR

Abnormal behavior often suggests a desperate person victimized by threatening conditions. Close inspection, however, may fail to reveal any external threat, thus making the behavior seem that much more irrational. How then can we explain such "desperation" in the context of seemingly benign conditions? In some cases, the answer may lie in hypersensitivity, emotional instability, and malignant imagination that can transform essentially innocuous events into threatening ones. In other cases, the answer may be much simpler; perhaps there is a conditioned, or learned, connection between information in the current environment and *past* trauma. Abnormal behavior might still be irrational, but it would then appear "pathological" only because the observer is unaware of the individual's learning history. In this view, many kinds of abnormal behavior are merely the by-products of normal learning mechanisms programmed by abnormal environmental conditions. Let us take a closer look at how such mechanisms could work, starting with the acquisition of anxiety-related behaviors.

Behavior Control through Classical Conditioning

In the language of classical conditioning, anxiety can start out as an "unconditioned" response (UCR) to a threatening *unconditioned* stimulus (UCS), that is, one that naturally elicits a reaction without learning. Like withdrawal from painful shock, anxiety in the context of abuse, abandonment, or loss of support is an unconditioned response to unconditioned stimuli. The psychologically significant UCS–UCR event—the anxiety reaction—is capable of powering the conditioning of innocuous events. Specifically, if an innocuous event (S) reliably predicts a significant UCS–UCR event, then S will become a conditioned stimulus, or CS. This means that when a CS, or something similar to the CS, is perceived, the organism reacts strongly in *anticipation* of the UCS–UCR event, that is, with a conditioned reaction.

A frightening experience in a churchyard, for example, might transform the psychological meaning of related stimuli. Thus, formerly innocuous stimuli— even positive stimuli like church bells—might come to elicit discomfort or phobic fearfulness, depending on the intensity of the original experience and other psychological factors. In short, the conditioning model makes clear that although a strong reaction to innocuous stimuli may seem "irrational," it may have a hidden psycho-logic with a straightforward explanation.

The psycho-logic of the conditioning paradigm is given in Figure 5.1. The innocuous stimulus (S) develops, by association with a noxious event (UCS–UCR), into a conditioned signal (CS); this signal triggers two components of defensive behavior: (1) *emotional* or expressive reactions and (2) *instrumental* reactions, so called because they have practical significance in bringing relief. Figure 5.1 shows schematically how an escape reaction develops eventually into an effective avoidance response that prevents an unpleasant emotional reaction. It is important to understand that, in humans, learned avoidance responses are often purely *cognitive*; that is, they involve conditioned changes in thinking and fantasy. Such changes, like the development of a delusion, may be quite abnormal and therefore deleterious, yet persist if they defend against unpleasant experiences.

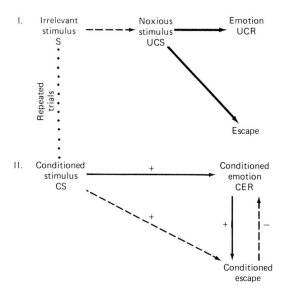

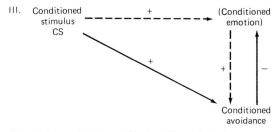

FIGURE 5.1   *Two-factor model of conditioning. Phase I shows a psychologically insignificant stimulus reliably preceding and therefore predicting an aversive event composed of noxious stimulus and defensive reaction. Defensive reaction includes a motivating emotional component and a motivated instrumental component. In Phase I, the defensive reaction is "unconditioned," meaning that it is already built in by instinct or prior experience. Thus, the aversive "unconditioned stimulus" (UCS) and aversive "unconditioned response" (UCR) cause the transformation of the insignificant stimulus (S) into a conditioned stimulus (CS). By Phase II, the CS can "substitute for" the UCS to elicit the defensive reaction, the emotional component of which is now called a "conditioned emotional response" (CER). The figure shows the CS reliably (solid horizontal " + " arrow) guiding, and the CER strongly (solid vertical " + " arrow) motivating, the instrumental component of the defensive (conditioned escape) reaction. (Note: "+" indicates a facilitating effect while "−" indicates an inhibitory effect. A solid arrow indicates a strong effect while a dashed arrow indicates a weak effect.) By Phase III, the instrumental component, reliably controlled by CS, comes to inhibit (solid vertical "−" arrow) the emotional component. Thus, from Phase I to III, the defensive reaction has changed from primarily "instinctive," sensory, and emotional to conditioned, anticipatory, and instrumental. In pathological conditions, the emotional component manifests as anxiety and disorganized behavior while the instrumental component manifests as rigid and fixated behavior.*

CSs need not start out as innocuous stimuli. Many are emotionally significant yet typically cause no anxiety unless they come to be associated with a traumatic UCS. For example, tape-recorded combat sounds that provoke no anxiety in most people can, through conditioning, elicit intense reactions in veterans with posttraumatic stress disorder (Kolb, 1987).

So far, we have concentrated on *external* UCSs, that is, powerful laboratory or real-world events imposed on otherwise normal individuals. However, UCSs may arise from *within* the person—for example, from spontaneous panic attacks or from nightmarelike fantasies. This raises an interesting point. Perhaps classical conditioning can be driven not only by *objective* threats, but also by *imagined* threats created *by* persons with special sensitivities or a morbid imagination.

In short, our discussion raises two separate questions that are still debated by investigators. For what kinds of psychopathology is a classical conditioning mechanism relevant, and what drives the mechanism: external events operating on the person (proactive ecopathology) or internal events created by the person (inventive pathology)? In subsequent discussions we will discover that cognitive factors—including the way one perceives and interprets external events—are critically important to the development of many types of abnormal behavior.

Behavior Control through Instrumental Conditioning

Organisms develop emotional reactions to CSs that predict aversive conditions. Also, they can learn to escape and avoid UCSs that are signaled by CSs. This instrumental learning—that is, learning based on the *consequences* of behavior—enables mastery of frustrating conditions and therefore is highly reinforcing; the more intense the frustration, the more intense and resistant to change is the instrumental behavior. For example, a phobic person's avoidance of objects is *reinforced* (strengthened) by the consequent decrease in anxiety and increase in a sense of security. Since persistent avoidance prevents the organism from learning that the CS no longer "means" noxious UCS, neurotic avoidance "protects" against extinction of the classically conditioned emotional reaction to the CS (Mowrer, 1947). This can explain the seemingly irrational resistance of neurotic behavior to change despite its heavy cost to the affected person. Indeed, it can also explain why forcing a person to confront an otherwise avoided CS is a major approach to treating anxiety disorders (see Chapter 15).

In sum, experimental research suggests that many forms of neurotic behavior can be explained simply as a matter of either (1) anxiety acquired through classical conditioning, or (2) inappropriate avoidance behaviors acquired through instrumental conditioning (see Figure 5.1). Moreover, there is growing evidence that biological factors influence the readiness to develop conditioned reactions. For example, the potential importance of genetic factors is illustrated by results of a study done by Royce and Covington (1960). These investigators reported that strain differences in mice determined whether and how fast they learned a conditioned avoidance response to shock and how fast it extinguished. One additional noteworthy finding was that some strains of animals *never learned* the response, suggesting a kind of "invulnerability" to these traumatic conditions.

The study suggests that ignoring individual differences, including biological differences, may sometimes impede the ability to predict how organisms will react to external events, even when external events are traumatic. Other studies similarly show that ignoring individual differences in *cognitive* factors—selective perception and biased thinking—can also lessen the ability of observers to predict behavior on the basis of external events. Environmentalists often argue, quite rightly, that such cognitive factors arise by prior learning shaped by external events. Nevertheless, evidence discussed in Chapter 7 suggests that cognitive factors and prior learning may also be influenced by hereditary predispositions.

Behavior Control through Modeling

By observing the behavior modeled by others, we learn a great deal about the world and how to behave. *Modeling* occurs when an observer mimics the behavior of another person, or model. The probability of a modeling effect depends on many factors—among them the love, fear, dependency, interest, and admiration the observer has toward the model. The effect of a model may not only be imitation (modeling). An observer may learn to behave in ways quite different from the model's behavior as, for example, the child of an alcoholic who resolves to become a teetotaler.

Sometimes a model's behavior seems sufficient to explain why an abnormality develops—for example, phobic behavior learned vicariously (described in Chapter 15, pp. 406–409). But in other cases a modeling explanation seems less straightforward. Why, for example, does *only one* child in a family acquire abnormal behavior modeled by a parent? One obvious possibility is that the modeling effects of the other parent override those of the disturbed parent. Another possibility is that only one of the children has a predisposition to acquire the modeled abnormal behavior.

How important are modeling effects to explaining environment-behavior correspondence? One estimate of their importance is the degree of *resemblance* between adopted children and their adoptive parents. Note that the question is not whether parents can produce reactions in situations, but rather how effective parents are in shaping enduring dispositions that correspond to those of the parents. Consider one study that used a questionnaire to assess the resemblance in occupational interests of parents and their teenage adoptive or biological children (Grotevant, Scarr, & Weinberg, 1977) . Overall, the correlations were rather modest (Table 5.2), but more interesting, they practically vanished when the genetic overlap between parents and children was eliminated through adoption.

TABLE 5.2 PROFILE CONTOUR CORRELATIONS FOR INTEREST STYLES*

Pair	Biological	Adopted
Father-son	.29	.13
Mother-daughter	.24	.13
Father-daughter	.19	.06
Mother-son	.24	.07
Brother-brother	.33	—
Sister-sister	.34	—
Child-child	.25	.08

*The six categories surveyed in this questionnaire study included realistic, or practical, interests; investigative, or scientific, interests; and artistic, social, enterprising, and conventional interests.
Source: Grotevant, Scarr, & Weinberg, 1977, Table 9. Copyright © 1977 by the American Psychological Association. Reprinted by permission.

It would seem that a 50 percent genetic commonality between people may be required to produce even the modest correlations observed in Table 5.2. Modeling may be less important to creating long-term psychopathological vulnerabilities than are genetic, traumatic, and other factors; however, if the observer is strongly dependent on the potential model, the chance for modeling abnormal behavior is probably vastly increased. For example, laboratory-raised monkeys who are normally unafraid of snakes can develop what looks like a snake phobia—including agitation and intense avoidance behavior—after merely observing an adult model reacting fearfully to snakes (Mineka et al., 1984; see Chapter 15, pp. 408–409, for a discussion of model-induced observational learning of anxiety behavior.)

FRUSTRATIVE CONDITIONS IN THE REAL WORLD

Clinical investigations of psychopathology have long recognized the power of irrational and self-destructive cognitions—for example, pathological guilt and depression driven by imagined rather than actual transgressions. We should therefore consider how such subjective factors can modulate the effect of real-world ecopathology.

Cognitive Appraisal versus Objective Conditions

In the real world, the relation between objective threat and psychopathology often depends on how things seem to a person. Thus, subjective conditions determine whether external conditions are perceived as threatening.

During World War II, airmen, civil defense people, and civilians were exposed to considerable objective danger during bombings and air combat. There were, however, surprisingly few psychological casualties, especially if some sense of personal responsibility, group mission, and community or national purpose was present. Exposure to expressions of patriotism and acts of courage inhibited distress, while social isolation was associated with higher rates of psychopathology. Another circumstance that seemed to prevent psychopathological outcomes was the abundance of opportunities to make use of skills. Those who would use their talents were relatively free from distress while those overworked at boring or personally irrelevant tasks were at higher risk.

Especially distressing were physical constraints such as confinement to foxholes and psychological constraint such as assignment to insignificant tasks. Risk for traumatic neurosis was greater among noncombatant military personnel than among combatants operating in the same combat zone, presumably because of the relatively greater sense of personal control felt by the combatants. Collectively, these findings (see Baker, 1980; Rachman, 1978) point to *perceived* competence or competence frustration as determinants of the affective impact of life-threatening events.

People are surprisingly resilient when threats are real rather than imagined. For example, few people brought to first aid posts during the London bombings sustained any serious psychological reaction beyond the first few hours, and virtually none with civil responsibilities, such as policemen or firemen, became psychological casualties. British researchers also observed that of the few people suffering traumatic reactions, most had prior problems that appeared to be magnified by the subjective sense of personal threat. Struck by surprisingly modest rates of anxiety-related forms of psychopathology in one of the most devastating conditions imaginable, the Hiroshima explosion, Rachman (1978) says, ''I can think of no psychological theory, naive or sophisticated, commonsensical or scientific, that would have predicted the prompt return of the Hiroshima survivors, or their extraordinary psychological resilience'' (p. 39).

Traumatic Ecopathology

Concentration Camp Effects   Some traumatic conditions can challenge the psychological defenses of even resilient people. Eitinger and Strom (1973) did a fifteen-year follow-up on 498 Norwegian ex-prisoners of Nazi concentration camps and a matched group of controls, comparing them on the frequency of fourteen medical and psychiatric conditions. Results shown in Figure 5.2 indicate that frequency of psychosis is relatively small and statistically insignificant, suggesting that environmental factors that come into play after childhood, even traumatic ones, need not push people over the psychotic threshold. (The effect of such conditions during childhood is a separate matter.) In contrast, there are striking elevations in diagnoses of ''neurosis and nervousness''; that is, depression and anxiety, and also of ulcers, in the ex-prisoner group.

Neurotic symptoms and personality disorder persisting even long after objective threat is eliminated are often associated with other traumatic conditions such as kidnapping (Terr, 1983) and childhood sexual abuse (Browne & Finkelhor, 1986), especially incest (Gelinas, 1983). One study of female psy-

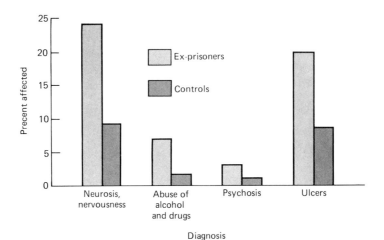

FIGURE 5.2   Psychological disorders in Norwegian ex-prisoners of Nazi concentration camps and controls, 1945–1966. (After Eitinger and Strom, 1973)

chiatric inpatients revealed a strikingly high percentage (72 percent) of reported experiences of physical and/or sexual abuse, often perpetrated by a family member (Bryer, Nelson, Miller, & Kroll, 1987). A particularly severe and debilitating reaction to trauma is posttraumatic stress disorder.

Posttraumatic Stress Disorder   This disorder is elicited by *unexpected* life- or ego-threatening traumas involving profound helplessness. A relatively high prevalence of posttraumatic stress disorder is associated with combat experiences. A recent epidemiological investigation found prevalence rates of 1 percent for the general population, about 3.5 percent for nonwounded Vietnam veterans, and 20 percent for wounded Vietnam veterans (Helzer, Robins, & McEvoy, 1987; see also Roberts, 1988).

A patient with posttraumatic stress disorder experiences chronic nervousness, hyperalertness, and exaggerated startle reactions. In Vietnam veterans affected with the disorder, there may also be flashbacks of painful experiences and violent outbursts against even loved ones who are misperceived, in hallucinatory fashion, as the threatening "enemy." Pervasive "psychic numbing" can also be part of the pattern; that is, estrangement from people and an inability to be intimate and caring (Andreasen, 1980). Psychic numbing also shows up in loss of energy, diminished appetite, and flagging interest in formerly engaging experiences. There may also be crying spells and intense feelings of guilt and self-condemnation.

The essential feature is the development of characteristic symptoms following a psychologically traumatic event that is generally outside the range of usual human experience. The characteristic symptoms involve reexperiencing the traumatic event, numbing of responsiveness to, or reduced involvement with, the external world; and a variety of autonomic, dysphoric, or cognitive symptoms (American Psychiatric Association, 1980, p. 236).

Posttraumatic stress disorder can manifest itself shortly after the traumatic event, or months and even years later. In some cases, a person may have been living a productive and uneventful life until some event triggers the disorder, as illustrated by the following example.

> Mr. A was born in 1936 in Indonesia to a Dutch family. In 1942, the entire family was interned in a Japanese concentration camp. His father and older brother were placed in the men's section, where the father eventually died of malnutrition. Mr. A was placed with his mother and sister, and together they survived. Mr. A lived in Holland for 8 years after the war, and became a writer and linguist, and actually worked in Japan for 1 year with no ill effects. He was well until 1971, when an assignment took him to the site of his camp. There was no trace of it. At that point, after 25 years of successful adaptation, he began to suffer chronic anxiety and nightmares (Krell, 1988, p. 383).

Such a delayed form of posttraumatic stress disorder strongly implies a breakdown of compensatory defenses that may have given a misleading impression of "normal" adjustment in a vulnerable person burdened by painful memories. These memories may be reactivated by stimuli directly related to the original trauma—as illustrated in the vignette—or by symbolically relevant situations such as imprisonment or death of a loved one.

What is the nature of the posttraumatic reaction? One aspect, clearly reflected in the distressing repetitive fantasies of the patient, is the close call with annihilation. According to the psychodynamic view, this "repetition compulsion" in fantasy is an exaggerated version of a natural tendency to reduce the psychological impact of stressful events through mental reiteration when other defenses like repression are no longer effective. Persistent morbid preoccupations are therefore pathological versions of a common tendency in adults to think obsessively about what they might have done, or in children to repeat especially disturbing events in play.

In some cases, however, guilt plays a large role. Guilt may be a reaction to a sense of unworthiness compared to those who didn't survive; or it may be a reaction to having had selfish hopes and fantasies of survival to the disadvantage of others. As Fenichel (1945) says: "All military psychiatrists know the depressive features in traumatic neuroses of soldiers whose 'buddy' was killed while they themselves were saved [and where] they had hoped that if 'somebody's number is up,' it may be another fellow and not they themselves" (p. 125).

Studies have yielded evidence of predispositions to the disorder in the form of prior or co-existing psychopathology, especially dissociative and antisocial personality traits, alcoholism, and nonbipolar depression (Speigel, Hunt, & Dondershine, 1988). In addition, the patients often have first-degree relatives with elevated rates of various mental disorders (Davidson et al., 1985). Evidence of psychopathology in patients and their relatives supports the clinical impression that posttraumatic stress disorder can represent the breakdown of the psychological defenses of vulnerable people, those who are rigid, guilt-ridden, or otherwise disturbed (Andreasen, 1980; Trimble, 1981). Nevertheless, normal or even "healthy" people can be seriously affected, though there is no objective basis to determine exactly how much or what kind of trauma is required in these cases.

CONVENTIONAL PROVOCATIONS AND PSYCHOPATHOLOGY

That extreme ecopathology is associated with elevations in clinical casualties, even in relatively normal people, is not too surprising. But what about the association between abnormal behavior and more conventional provocations? Paykel (1974) found that most clinical depression was *not* associated with unemployment, poor health, family, marriage, or legal problems. While depressed people reported significantly higher rates of negative life events, many of these events were typically *mundane,* sometimes even trivial, rather than traumatic. Lazarus (1981) makes this point nicely:

> And how can we respond knowledgeably to the implications of a poetic statement by Charles Bukowski in the "Shoelace" that:
>> It's not the large things that send a man to the madhouse. . . . No, it's the continuing series of small tragedies that send a man to the madhouse . . . not the death of his love but a shoelace that snaps with no time left.
>
> Although I believe it is true that people can be distressed over what seem at the moment to be trivialities, they are not really trivial at all in meaning, since they symbolize things that are very important to the person. The shoelace might break, but a major part of the psychological stress created thereby is the implication that one cannot control one's life, that one is helpless in the face of the most stupid of trivialities, or even worse that one's own inadequacies have made the obstacle occur in the first place. This is what brings the powerful, stressful, and pathogenic message that breaks one's morale. In any case, how is one to evaluate such a momentous issue in the traditional style of laboratory stress research? There is no way (Lazarus, 1981, pp. 181–182).

On average there is only a small association between mental illness and life stresses such as those listed in Table 5.3; in fact, only from 1 to 9 percent of the differences between well and sick people can usually be predicted from the differences reported by them in quality of environment—for example, stressful versus nonstressful conditions (Rabkin & Struening, 1976). But even this modest correlation between quality of environment and behavior is subject to many competing interpretations. By examining the timing of the environmental stresses and the concomitant symptoms, it becomes possible to untangle causal from noncausal factors.

The proactive ecopathology model assumes that external stress factors *precede* changes in symptomatic behavior. When, on the other hand, changes in external events and symptoms occur simultaneously, causality is ambiguous. When external events follow behavioral changes, the proactive assumption

TABLE 5.3   SOCIAL READJUSTMENT RATING SCALE

Rank	Life event	Mean value* (LCU)
1	Death of spouse	100
2	Divorce	73
3	Marital separation	65
4	Jail term	63
5	Death of close family member	63
6	Personal injury or illness	53
7	Marriage	50
8	Fired at work	47
9	Marital reconciliation	45
10	Retirement	45
11	Change in health of family member	44
12	Pregnancy	40
13	Sex difficulties	39
14	Gain of new family member	39
15	Business readjustment	39
16	Change in financial state	38
17	Death of a close friend	37
18	Change to different line of work	36
19	Change in number of arguments with spouse	35
20	Mortgage over $10,000	31
21	Foreclosure of mortgage or loan	30
22	Change in responsibilities at work	29
23	Son or daughter leaving home	29
24	Trouble with in-laws	29
25	Outstanding personal achievement	28
26	Wife begin or stop work	26
27	Begin or end school	26
28	Change in living conditions	25
29	Revision of personal habits	24
30	Trouble with boss	23
31	Change in work hours or conditions	20
32	Change in residence	20
33	Change in schools	20
34	Change in recreation	19
35	Change in church activities	19
36	Change in social activities	18
37	Mortgage or loan less than $10,000	17
38	Change in sleeping habits	16
39	Change in number of family get-togethers	15
40	Change in eating habits	15
41	Vacation	13
42	Christmas	12
43	Minor violations of the law	11

*Mean value of an item indicates its seriousness in life change units (LCUs), i.e., relative significance and time required for adjustment as judged by raters. The sum of LCUs across events checked by a respondent is treated as a measure of life stress. The correlation between LCU and disease can then be determined to assess the role of stress. For example, if an individual with an LCU greater than 300 gets sick, it is more likely to be a serious disorder like cancer or schizophrenia than if LCU is less than 100 (Holmes, 1979).

Source: Reprinted with permission from the *Journal of Psychosomatic Research,* vol. 2, T. Holmes and R. H. Rahe, "The Social Readjustment Scale," Table 3, p. 216, 1967, Pergamon Press PLC.

can reasonably be rejected. Grant, Yager, Sweetwood, and Olshen (1982) focused on the co-relation between life events and symptom self-reports given every two months for a three-year period by seventy-two outpatients (previously diagnosed as having affective, schizophrenic, personality, or other disorder) and ninety-four control subjects. Reliable co-occurrences of stress and symptoms were found for about half the patients and controls, but less than 10 percent of these were separated in time. Even if all of these instances of stress and symptoms separated in time involved external events *preceding* symptomatic increase rather than vice versa, the proactive effect, overall, would seem rather weak.

A more detailed analysis of this study suggests that the modest correlation between external events and symptoms represents a strong association for a few individuals rather than a modest one for everyone. This makes good sense if we assume that some "reactive types" are very susceptible to external provocations while most others are not.

Moreover, because people often influence events to which they in turn react, "stress" or "trauma" should not necessarily be thought of merely as an effect of ecopathology. Even when uncontrollable outside events do occur—a car accident, for example, or an untimely death of a relative—their effects on the person will depend on subjective factors that interact with them. That is why objectively minor events—unrequited love, a low grade, a lost ring—or even trival events—that broken shoelace—can sometimes provoke intense and irrational behavior. In short, we need to consider both the magnitude *and the meaning* of event-behavior relations. Evidence that stressful events are frequently experienced prior to the occurrence of episodes of abnormal behavior is theoretically ambiguous and of uncertain usefulness. As Mechanic (1974) says "since the illnesses of many individuals do not appear to be preceded by identifiable stressors, and since many people who are under stress do not become ill, meaningful statements must specify the conditions under which stress affects the occurrence of illness and consider how stress interacts with biological, psychological, and behavioral factors" (p. 88).

Inferences about causality are on safest ground when they are based on experimental research—for example, experiments showing that ecopathology produces experimental neurosis in animals. Inferences about causality are far less secure when, as is often the case with research on humans, they are based on correlations between ecopathology and psychopathology. Moreover, an inference may be quite different, depending on how the correlation is "dissected" by nonexperimental research methods. The "dissection" can start from the psychopathology side of the correlation; the investigator first selects instances of abnormal behavior and then seeks evidence of ecopathology. Or the "dissection" can start from the ecopathological side of the correlation; the investigator first selects instances of proactive ecopathology and then seeks evidence of psychopathology.

To appreciate just how different an inference about causality can be when based on one or the other approach to "dissecting" a psychopathology-ecopathology correlation, imagine that we want to test the hypothesis that ecopathology is an important cause of acute-onset schizophrenic breakdowns. If 40 to 50 percent of such cases were associated with recently occurring adverse circumstances (Cooper, 1978), we would be impressed by environmental factors. On the other hand, if only 1 percent of all people exposed to exactly those environmental factors developed acute schizophrenic disturbances, we might be more impressed by vulnerability factors in the person.

In sum, the critical question is not so much whether specifiable events are associated with abnormal behavior; clearly, often they are. Rather, it is the psychological significance of those events, or, in the language of Table 5.1, the extent to which they are proactive, reactive, expressive, selective, or imaginary. Answers will require attention to cognitive and psychodynamic, and conditioned and heritable aspects of dysfunctional behavior.

RESILIENCY AND VULNERABILITY

Most people are resistant to psychopathology, even under extreme conditions. This suggests that we should pay attention not only to ecopathology-psychopathology co-occurrences, but also to normalcy in the context of ecopathology—that is, *resiliency*—and psychopathology in the context of benign conditions—that is, *vulnerability*.

Resiliency

Resiliency is the capacity to bounce back from the potentially disorganizing effects of adversity (Garmezy, 1983). It is frequently marked by certain traits, including autonomy, self-confidence, friendliness, reflectiveness, and self-control. A striking example of resiliency in the face of misfortune is provided by the remarkably healthy emotional development of dwarfs, whose short stature, abnormal appearance, and medical complications would seem to make them candidates for chronic psychosocial stress. Nevertheless, the evidence suggests that ''by adulthood most of these subjects had learned that the important issue in life was how to relate to others. Therefore they had mastered the ability to set others at ease and had developed a pleasant interpersonal style. . . . The important point is that a chronic disease which results in an obviously different body shape than other people does not automatically lead to a psychological disorder'' (Ford, 1983, p. 46).

Resiliency can be appreciated by taking a developmental perspective. Most developmental theories of psychopathology give exalted significance to the ''formative years.'' Early childhood experiences are said to have an everlasting impact on later development. A complete test of the special significance of early experience, however, requires that we compare children exposed to three types of environmental conditions: (1) continuously negative, (2) early negative and later positive, and (3) early positive and later negative. Results of studies comparing the continuously negative and early negative/later positive conditions indicate that deprivation and/or abuse has an adverse impact on competence and personality development, but that rescued children can show dramatic improvement (Clarke & Clarke, 1976).

Consider a study of identical twins reared by a cruel stepmother who kept them in a small, unheated closet much of the time, and in a cellar at other times (Koluchova, 1976a,b). When rescued at age 7, they were malnourished, fearful, and unable to walk or speak and had estimated IQs in the 40s. Fortunately, these children were placed with two exceptionally good caretakers, and they improved dramatically in intellectual and social functioning. The steadily increasing scores of annual IQ tests up to age 14 are shown in Figure 5.3.

The biological parents had been judged to have had near-average intelligence, and therefore the children's final IQ scores are close to that expected had they been reared normally. Their emotional and social development followed a similar positive pattern: they became cheerful and self-confident, active in sports and games, and popular with peers. No eccentricities were noted, and even their understandable fear of the dark largely disappeared in time. They did well in school, even excelling in some subjects like arithmetic, reading, and music. In short, the twins bent but did not break. What accounts for their capacity to bounce back from pathology to normalcy? For one thing, they had each other; research on monkeys suggests that companionship provides a buffer against what, for a singleton, would have been a far more crippling experience (Suomi & Harlow, 1977). In addition, the twins showed no sign of brain damage at the time of rescue. Had they been neurologically impaired, normal function would have been less likely.

Studies of rescued children raise fundamental questions about inner strengths and weaknesses. Why are psychopathological effects of early disadvantage sometimes reversible? Do the conditioned abnormal reactions extinguish over time, or are their effects "diluted" by the accumulation of other,

FIGURE 5.3   IQ change in a set of abused and deprived identical twins rescued at age seven. (Based on Koluchova, 1976b)

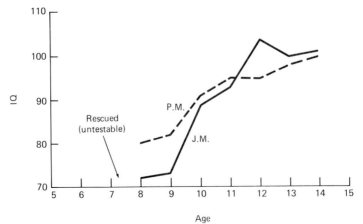

more positive, experiences? Or, as the evidence on child abuse suggests, do they get pushed "underground," transformed into a vulnerability that is defended against by compensatory processes? We could approach the same problem from the opposite perspective by asking why psychological dysfunction occurs in advantaged and benevolent environments. All these questions boil down to *vulnerability* and *resiliency,* two sides of a hypothetical coin (sometimes called "ego strength") that has great value in theories of psychopathology.

Vulnerability

Some people, by virtue of their biological or social backgrounds, are at greater risk than others for disorder. This greater risk refers to *vulnerability,* or underlying predisposition, and not only to the actual disorder. Whereas a behavioral disorder obviously indicates realized risk, the *absence* of a disorder may indicate either no risk or a latent predisposition as yet unexpressed. Vulnerability bears the same relationship to behavioral disorder as ability does to performance: just as high ability may never be realized in great accomplishments, vulnerability may never be realized in abnormal behavior.

In medicine, there are provocative tests that utilize certain chemical substances to challenge the physiological coping capacities of the organism and thus yield measures of its vulnerability (or resiliency). One example is the large dose of glucose used in the glucose tolerance test for diabetes mellitus, a disease involving defects in the body's ability to eliminate blood sugar. After fasting overnight, the patient takes a large load of glucose and the rate of metabolism is observed.

Figure 5.4 gives glucose tolerance curves for three groups of medical students, none of whom had been diagnosed as diabetic. The normal controls had no parental history of diabetes; another group had one diabetic parent; a third group had two diabetic parents. Thirty minutes after glucose administration, the curves for the three groups begin to diverge. Those with one or more affected parents rid themselves of glucose at a slower rate than the normal controls. The test results suggest that some people genetically predisposed to diabetes are vulnerable to developing the disorder even though, under normal day-to-day conditions, they currently show none of the symptoms of diabetes.

Provocative tests designed to stress the person and thereby expose preexisting vulnerabilities are also available for some forms of psychopathology. A sampler of these provocative tests as well as some useful nonprovocative tests for vulnerability to disorder is shown in Table 5.4. Such tests, however, raise at least one obvious question: Do people who perform like patients with the disorder already exceed some important threshold in the disease process (Hanson, Gottesman, & Meehl, 1977)? In other words, we do not know whether these resemblances are actually early or mild signs of the disease itself or are expressions of risk factors that increase the probability of disease—for example, hypertension is not itself a heart disease, but it is one of its precursors.

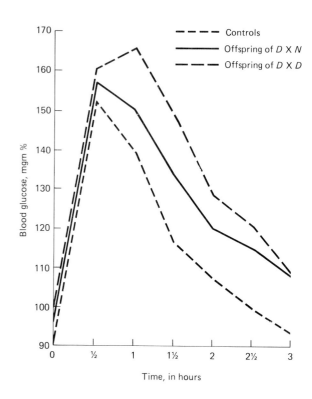

FIGURE 5.4   Glucose tolerance curves for offspring of diabetic (D) and nondiabetic (N) matings. (From Neel et al., 1965).

The Ecopathology-Psychopathology Correlation

When does ecopathology cause, aggravate, or merely reflect psychopathology? Frank (1965) reviewed forty years of research on the hypothesis that early social experiences, especially those related to maternal behavior, have a powerful influence on the development of psychopathology. He found much evidence inconsistent with this hypothesis, in particular for schizophrenia, but even for neurosis and psychopathy. Although ecopathology was found to be associated with psychopathology, ecopathology occurred quite often among normals as well. Furthermore, no special ecopathological feature was reliably found to be associated with one or another category of psychopathology.

Frank's review ends with a penetrating distinction between what the family "does to" the child and what the child "does to" the family. "The important variables in the development of psychopathology might be factors which the child brings to the family, the functioning of the nervous and metabolic systems and the cognitive capacity to integrate stimuli," Frank says. He then asks "whether the proclivity towards fantasy distortion of reality might not be *the* factor in the development of psychopathology..." (1965, p. 201). The clear implication here is that expressive and inventive ecopathology is sometimes misidentified as proactive ecopathology.

TABLE 5.4   A SAMPLER OF PROCEDURES FOR LOCATING THOSE WITH VULNERABILITY TO PSYCHOPATHOLOGY

Disorder	Technique	Partial result	Comment
		Schizophrenia	
Buchsbaum and Rieder (1979)	Biochemical test for low monoamine oxidase (MAO)	Low MAO subjects manifest more schizophreniclike pathology	Theory is that low MAO levels in schizophrenics might also occur in preschizophrenics.
Latham et al. (1981)	Pursuit eye tracking	45% of first-degree relatives of schizophrenics have disordered horizontal and vertical pursuit eye movements.	May indicate an oculomotor defect marking a predisposition to schizophrenic behavior
Chapman et al. (1980)	Questionnaire asking about anhedonia and perceptual aberrations	High scorers exceed controls on several psychoticlike experiences.	May be a marker for psychosis in general rather than schizophrenia in particular
Hartmann et al. (1981)	Newspaper ad: "Do you have frequent nightmares?"	Elevated on schizophrenia and psychopathic deviancy scales of the MMPI	Nightmares may be associated with a defect in neural systems that use dopamine as a neurotransmitter.
		Bipolar disorder	
Depue et al. (1981)	Questionnaire tapping mood swings and dysregulation	High scorers had more bipolar pathology in structured interviews and in roommates' ratings. High scorers also had more relatives with affective disorder.	Assumes that those at high risk for bipolar disorder manifest same (but milder) symptoms as clinically diagnosed cases.
		Psychopathy	
Widom (1977)	Newspaper ad for charming, aggressive, impulsive people who are also fun-loving	Respondents to ad had scores on the MMPI like clinical psychopaths.	Unobtrusive measure that can detect noninstitutionalized cases.
		Psychophysiologic disorder	
Pincus and Tucker (1978)	Overbreathe for three minutes until dizzy. Select those who display hyperventilation syndrome.	77% of hyperventilators had history of "medical" disorders that could not be verified; only 26% of controls.	May account for particular choice of symptoms; e.g., specific bodily weakness under stress. May be a mechanism for producing Briquet syndrome.

That general qualities of the environment—lack of social support, family stability, or educational opportunities—correlate modestly at best with psychopathology suggests that, *on the average,* ecopathology plays a relatively small role in the genesis of many kinds of abnormal behavior. Yet the opposite conclusion is suggested by laboratory work on conditioning, modeling, and "experimental neurosis," and clinical evidence on the effects of child abuse. This apparent inconsistency can perhaps be resolved with three supportable assumptions. First, specific ecopathological events—especially the traumatizing kind—typically affect *certain behaviors of some people.* Second, such events may have subtle or indirect effects, depending on the compensatory processes that underlie the balance between vulnerability and resiliency. Third, such events are often poorly correlated with the general quality of the environment; they occur in "good" as well as "bad" settings, making the overall quality of the environment a surprisingly poor predictor of psychopathology.

THE PROBLEM OF UNPREDICTABILITY

Predicting abnormal behavior from knowledge about the environment is often difficult for other reasons. First, the sheer number of possible causes, both past and present, that have to be taken into account is often overwhelming. Suppose we make a conservative estimate that ten factors combine in some unique way to produce pathologies. If each of these ten factors can be scored "present" or "absent," then there are 2^{10}, or 1024, possible combinations. Moreover, if we require that they occur in a certain order, the number is much larger than that. A more complicated and realistic hypothesis might assume that there are twenty such causal factors, each with three possible classifications (severe, mild, absent); this assumption would generate more than 3 billion combinations! No wonder that psychologists, like historians, often must start from effects and work back to presumed causes. Unfortunately, such after-the-fact reconstructions can misidentify presumed causes or overestimate their importance.

The sheer number of potential causes is not the only impediment to developing predictive theories. There may be unknown critical events that, practically speaking, will never be identified. Consider a 10-year-old boy who suddenly becomes noticeably timid and submissive. Perhaps a fierce scolding prompted him always to conform in order not to lose his mother's love. Although the fear of losing love may have been an issue for him for a long time, expressing that fear may be precipitated by a series of seemingly insignificant events. On the fateful day, perhaps he felt slightly ill, had been accidentally knocked down on the playground, and learned that he had failed a test. The scolding that followed was not a cause in the usual sense. Rather, it was more like the straw that broke the proverbial camel's back.

In short, the difficulty with theorizing about causality is that events insignificant in themselves may collectively lead to disorder, and no convincing causal sequence can be reconstructed. Although theories may identify the "big" causal factors that occur with sufficient frequency or potency, we may never be able to devise any theory that can handle individual human beings in all their uniqueness, and this may be true for both abnormal and normal variations in human behavior. Finally, behavior disorders occur in people who often come from families with few or no other members who are similarly affected. This suggests that influences unique to the individual and not shared with other family members play an important role in behavior disorders.

Two types of causal events that uniquely affect individuals can be described. One type, *systematic causality*, involves unique but nonchance influences on behavior. For example, one child in a family may be chosen as the scapegoat; perhaps the relatively less attractive or behaviorally awkward child is singled out for ridicule or punishment. In contrast, *unsystematic causality* includes unique but random events like contracting a disease or suffering a head trauma. Random events are basically unpredictable, a matter of good or bad luck. They bear no systematic relationship to enduring characteristics.

Meehl (1978) discussed twenty factors, four of which appear in Table 5.5, that block rapid progress in psychopathological theory. All converge on the conclusion that both systematic and unsystematic causes for many forms of psychopathology may be nearly impossible to ascertain, thereby limiting what can be assumed with confidence about the origins of psychopathology.

The discussion of systematic versus unsystematic causality and the unpredictability of behavior concludes our analysis of the environment concept as it bears on psychopathology. On the theoretical level, we have seen that a causal connection is only one of many interpretations of an ecopathology-psychopathology co-occurrence. Empirically, we have much evidence that (a) the correlation is often rather modest; (b) it is limited, in part, by vulnerability and resiliency; and (c) the actual connection between environment and behavior may frequently be *unpredictable* because the underlying events are often too numerous, complex, or unsystematic. All this means that we should be cautious about interpreting the ecopathology-psychopathology correlation. This is true whether the environment is defined as a specific event

TABLE 5.5 MEEHL'S OBSTACLES TO PROGRESS IN PSYCHOPATHOLOGY*

Factor	Problem
Divergent causality	In complex systems, small differences can mean a lot (e.g., a slight deviation from equilibrium can cause an avalanche).
Unknown critical events	Critical events never observed or recorded
Feedback loops	Person's behavior affects behavior of others. Untangling the causal sequences may be nearly impossible.
Random walk	Individually minor, but determinative events cumulate. Example: After suitor is refused date, he is involved in an auto accident through no fault of his own. Becomes depressed as a result.

*Meehl (1978) lists twenty obstacles. This is only a partial list.
Source: Copyright © 1978 by the American Psychological Association. Adapted by permission.

(stress or traumatic incident, for example) or as a general influence (quality of family life, for example).

Our discussion of ecopathology—in particular, the expressive, selective, and inventive types—suggests that certain factors operate within the person—in particular, cognitive traits that predispose to psychopathology. But there are other inner factors that must be considered. These will be discussed in the next two chapters, on psychodynamic and genetic determination, which further develop our psychopathological perspective.

SUMMARY

Our appreciation of psychopathology is enhanced by an environmental perspective on abnormal behavior. Consequently, we began by analyzing the more specific concept of *ecopathology,* or adverse external events that are associated with psychopathology, dividing it into six categories, only three of which represent interpersonal causality: *proactive,* or environment-to-person; *reactive,* or person-to-environment; and *transactive,* or mutual causality. We then described laboratory research showing how manipulations of need and competence frustration—confinement, unpredictability, and uncontrollability, in particular—can produce the disorganized, compulsive, and depressive behavioral abnormalities of ''experimental neurosis'' in animals. We also saw how similar, though less extreme manipulations—imposing near-impossible discriminations, for example—can produce similar effects in humans. We also described the pathological effects of real-world traumatizing events on human behavior, and the *learning mechanisms,* including classical conditioning, instrumental conditioning, and observational learning, that can explain the transformation of situational reactions into lasting dispositions and behavior disorders.

At the same time, we noted the marked variability and even *unpredictability* of animal and human behavior in both laboratory and real-world settings. For example, our discussion of the .10–.30 correlation between events (ranging from no stress to stress) and behavior (from normal to symptomatic) suggests a number of things. First, ecopathology may have a strong impact on especially vulnerable people. Second, the behavioral manifestation of that impact may not show up for months or even years, suggesting the importance of compensatory defenses that can break down during a stressful period occurring at a later time. Third, the trigger for psychopathological reactions may come from innocuous, or *non*ecopathological, events—a broken shoelace, for example—which raises questions about the role of predispositions and the inner world of *inventive* ecopathology.

Our evaluation of ecopathology thus helps to explain the surprisingly *low predictability* of behavior given external events, the frequent association of behavioral abnormality and *normal* environments, suggesting *vulnerability,* and, conversely, the existence of normalcy in spite of bad environments, suggesting *resiliency.*

Psychodynamic Facet

OUTLINE

Irrational and self-destructive behaviors that persist despite their negative consequences represent a paradox of human nature. Psychodynamic theories attempt to resolve this paradox by assuming that behavior is organized by a rich and often conflict-ridden inner life of unconscious meanings whose connections to current events may be ambiguous. Thus, even "irrational" behavior can have a hidden psycho-logic, but one that, in some important ways, is quite different from the psycho-logic proposed by conditioning and cognitive models.

> Instead of seeing merely a groomed American in a business suit, travelling to and from his office like a rat in a maze...I visualize...a flow of powerful subjective life, conscious and unconscious; a whispering gallery in which voices echo past events, currents of contending complexes, plots and counterplots, hopeful intimations and ideals. To a neurologist such perspectives are absurd, archaic, tender-minded; but in truth they are much closer to the actualities of inner life than are his own neat diagrams of reflex arcs and nerve anastomoses. A personality is a full Congress of orators and pressure-groups, of children, demagogues, communists, isolationists, war-mongers, mugwumps, grafters, log-rollers, lobbyists, Caesars and Christs, Machiavellis and Judases, Torries and Promethean revolutionists. And a psychologist who does not know this in himself, whose mind is locked against the flux of images and feelings, should be encouraged to make friends, by being psychoanalyzed, with the various members of his household (Murray, 1940, pp. 160–161).

This chapter deals with psychodynamics, that is, the active, inventive, symbolic, conflict-ridden, and affectively charged aspects of mental life that, when abnormal, characterize the psychopathology of symptom and personality disorders. Our discussion is purposely selective, emphasizing a few of the "basics" while minimizing theoretical debate. Consequently, this will be much more than just a "Freud chapter," even though we start with some of Freud's basic ideas. Because Freud is the intellectual source of the psychodynamic approach, and because his writings have had such a profound influence on contemporary Western culture, we believe that no textbook of psychopathology can ignore classic psychoanalytic theory regardless of its shortcomings and failures.

MOTIVATIONAL ASPECTS OF BEHAVIOR

Many behavior disorders seem to have their roots in childhood frustrations of basic needs for pleasure, security, and social affiliation. The classic psychoanalytic approach to the psychodynamics of frustration—in particular, the frustration of pleasure striving—involves three components of personality, what Freud called the id, ego, and superego (Freud, 1923/1960).

Three Components of Personality

Id Human beings strive for pleasure because it constitutes a powerful inner signal of well-being. Freud gave the name *libido,* or "life energy," to the hypothetical energy that drives pleasure-seeking behaviors. Later, he incorporated libido into a broader concept of unconscious motivation called the *id*. The id is that part of personality that includes purely selfish and irrational libidinal and aggressive impulses that become bound up in emotionally significant, yet entirely unconscious, memories laid down during early childhood (Brenner, 1957; Erdelyi, 1985). In psychoanalytic theory, some types of psychopathology represent the abnormal influence of id motivation over the ego, that part of personality whose task it is to control the id.

Ego Expressing id tendencies in selfish, pleasure-seeking, impulsive behavior can lead to adverse consequences such as rejection, shaming, or physical punishment. Partly in response to the inevitable frustrations of id-motivated behavior, the ego aspect of personality emerges during infancy and childhood. The ego has the capacity to anticipate with anxiety the dangers of id tendencies, and to defend against them.

Defense against the unbridled expression of anxiety-ridden selfish impulses includes inhibiting them, blocking them from consciousness (repression), and channeling them (sublimation) in ways that are socially acceptable yet at the same time personally gratifying—for example, telling jokes about sex. Ego development is thus a psychological "solution" to the problem of frustration, enabling the instinctive tendencies toward pursuing pleasure (what feels good) to be satisfied indirectly through expedient behavior (what works).

Note that both the id and the ego characterize the *self-serving* aspects of personality. The difference between these selfish tendencies is that the id is blindly impulsive, whereas the ego is cunning and pragmatic. If ego defenses against unbridled id motivation are chronically deficient, behavior will have a frankly selfish and often antisocial quality. If, on the other hand, defenses against id tendencies are excessive—if *intrapsychic conflict* is severe—behavior will have an inhibited and compulsive quality. Finally, if defenses begin to fail, anxiety and other neurotic symptoms can occur (Freud, 1926/1959).

Superego According to psychoanalytic theory, an important consequence of socialization is that ego defense against id motivation becomes increasingly influenced by an appreciation that selfish striving is often "wrong" or "bad." This moral component of personality, called the *superego,* includes conscience and something called the ego ideal. *Conscience,* or the sense of "right" and "wrong," is not merely knowing the rules intellectually, but also the capacity to *feel* them. The *ego ideal* refers to idealized versions of parental characteristics, the internalized models of "good" behavior. Psychoanalytic theory explains certain forms of psychopathology, especially those involving guilt-ridden behavior, as the result of an overly severe or irrational superego.

Like the ego, the superego has its roots in early socialization when a child's cognitive abilities are immature, thinking is naive, and misapprehensions are common. With time, more mature thinking comes to predominate and the superego, in normal people at least, becomes more realistic; behavior becomes more considerate and ethical, and consequently less selfish and egocentric.

Normally, superego-inconsistent behavior can produce guilt, shame, and depression. In some neurotic conditions, such feelings are chronic, intense, and seemingly irrational. The hapless ego, caught between a frustrated id and an irrational infantile superego, struggles by the use of pathologically exaggerated defense mechanisms to preserve security and self-esteem. In psychopaths—adults with deficient superegos—impulsive, expedient, and remorseless behavior is the rule because the ego is unconstrained by empathy and conscience.

Personality Development

Events during early childhood are widely believed to influence later personality. Classic psychoanalytic theory reflects this assumption, in part, in its psychosexual theory of personality development (see Table 6.1).

Psychosexual Aspects Many psychologists believe that personality develops in stages—age-specific time periods within which distinctive psychological patterns emerge—and that the developments at each stage influence what happens at subsequent stages. Freud added something new to this idea by arguing that the stagelike development of personality is psychosexual. By psychosexual, he meant the enduring psychological by-products of conflict between stage-specific kinds of libidinal striving and certain socialization practices of parents.

TABLE 6.1 OUTLINE OF EARLY PSYCHOSEXUAL STAGES

Zones of pleasure	Modes of maximal pleasure	Classes of relevant parental behavior	Positive achievements (gratification)	Negative achievements (frustration)
Oral	Incorporation	Nursing	Trust, security, optimism, vitality	Mistrust, insecurity, pessimism
Anal	Retention Elimination	Discipline, especially toilet training	Autonomy, pride, confidence	Shame, doubt, rigidity
Genital	Intrusiveness (male) Inclusiveness (female)	Sex-relevant role modeling and training	Initiative, purpose, ethical sense	Guilt, sentimentality, superficiality

Source: Derived from Erikson, 1960.

According to this view, during the highly self-centered first five years of life, "erogenous zones" of the body provide particularly intense libidinal pleasure—the mouth during the "oral stage" of infancy, the anus during the "anal stage"—roughly from years 1½ to 3—and the genitals during the "phallic" or "oedipal stage"—roughly from years 3 to 6. Zone-specific pleasure striving is satisfied by certain self-stimulating behaviors such as sucking, defecating, and masturbating, and also by interpersonal behaviors such as cuddling, wrestling, dominating, soliciting, and competing. Furthermore, each of these zone-gratifying behaviors becomes more intense, prominent, and subjectively pleasurable during its relevant psychosexual stage—masturbation during the phallic stage, for example.

A central idea is that social consequences, taboos, and punishments that make zone-specific strivings anxiety provoking can have lifelong psychopathological effects. In other words, Freud's theory explained why neurotic patients seem irrationally conflicted, inhibited, and guilt-ridden about pleasure striving and expressing affection.

Lifelong psychopathological effects of early frustration have been documented—we discussed some of these in Chapter 5. Nevertheless, there is little evidence to support psychoanalytic assumptions regarding the causal significance of psychosexual stage-specific frustrations for specific types of psychopathology. For example, frustration of anal stage strivings—as estimated by rating the difficulties over toilet training—does not increase the risk for developing so-called "anal (compulsive) personality patterns," including traits such as frugality, obstinacy, and orderliness.

Other Aspects Revisions of psychoanalytic theory have de-emphasized the significance of libidinal motivation while giving greater emphasis to other types of innate motivation. These include (a) instrumental strivings to understand, influence, and master the environment (White, 1963), (b) prosocial strivings to become part of a social community (Adler, 1927), and (c) attachment needs—that is, dependency on primary caregivers for the development of a sense of self and feelings of self-confidence (Winnicott, 1965). Neurotic preoccupation with achieving or avoiding failure, for example, might reflect inferiority feelings initially stirred up by parents who ridiculed or ignored early expressions of self-assertiveness. Likewise, neurotic dependency, competitiveness, or sexual inhibitions could be the long-term consequence of the early frustration of positive social feelings.

In sum, the classic psychoanalytic model of psychosexual development emphasizes the key role of libidinal strivings whose frustration can produce *conflict* by forcing an irrationally conscientious ego to mobilize sometimes symbolic inhibitory defenses. The result, according to the model, is certain neurotic disorders involving phobic, compulsive, and hysterical symptoms. Revisions of the model emphasize various innate tendencies—not just for libidinal pleasure, but also for security, affiliation, and personal growth—whose frustration can elicit compensatory efforts by a weak ego that struggles to defend against its own *deficiency* (Kohut, 1977). The result is certain personality disorders involving borderline, histrionic, and schizoid traits.

FRUSTRATIVE ASPECTS OF BEHAVIOR

Because it is experienced as a threat to personal survival, the frustration of basic needs produces anxiety and depression, unpleasant feelings that are defended against. The source of frustration can be external or internal.

Sources of Frustration

Social and Physical Environment Table 6.2 lists some major categories of frustration. Whether a child becomes frustrated or not depends on many factors such as dependency, sensitivity, and imagination; rarely is it merely a matter of what the parents do or fail to do. For example, disappointment with a parent may result as much from childish idealizations as from objective parental inadequacy. In addition, parental behavior may be a *reaction* to negative

TABLE 6.2 CATEGORIES OF FRUSTRATION

1. Family Discord or Conflict
   a. Capricious discipline
   b. Parental separation
   c. Parent absence
   d. Parent death
   e. Parental inadequacy
   f. Temperamental conflict
2. Danger from Physical Environment
   a. Accidents
   b. Being alone
   c. Darkness
   d. Animals
3. Loss of Support
   a. Nourishment
   b. Companionship
   c. Respect
   d. Attention
4. Traumatic Mistreatment
   a. Cruel punishment
   b. Sexual abuse
5. Disappointment
   a. Betrayal
   b. Deception
6. Inferiority
   a. Physical defect
   b. Intellectual deficiency
   c. Social difference

Source: Adapted from Murray, 1938, pp. 291–292.

characteristics of the child. For example, evidence indicates that many abused children have congenital physical stigmata or behavioral deficiencies that can provoke parental maltreatment (Friedrich & Boriskin, 1976).

According to psychodynamic theories, the adverse effects of early childhood frustration go "underground" as ego development moves the child away from rampant selfishness toward greater objectivity and self-control. While "underground," frustrations in the form of affectively charged memories continue to influence behavior, sometimes giving it a compulsive and symbolic quality. Thus, a psychodynamic perspective might explain an inordinate preoccupation with collecting certain objects as a substitute for a child's frustrated needs for love and security.

During adulthood the "underground" residue of early frustration can re-emerge in the form of pathological symptoms. This happens under special conditions involving internal stresses such as puberty and disease, and external stresses such as rejection, failure, or anxiety-provoking sexual opportunities. The symptoms of a reactivated conflict may be in the form of emotional outbursts or destructive behaviors, like suicides that occur in the context of shattered relationships. Symptoms of reactivated conflict can also occur in the form of stereotypical reactions called *repetition compulsions,* inappropriate and habitual ways of defending against anxiety. A classic example is the *transference* behavior of neurotic patients. Emotional attachment to the therapist often is so strong that, in the mind of the patient, the therapist becomes a parent-equivalent. Thus, the patient "acts out" (transfers to the therapist) childish patterns of never-outgrown thoughts and feelings about the parents, and these are typically characterized by dependency, ambivalence, and possessiveness. A person in the grip of a transference reaction is, in a sense, stuck in the past.

Studies of animal behavior have frequently supported a widespread belief in the long-term behavioral consequences of early deprivation, abuse, isolation, or abandonment. Scott (1968) describes a study illustrating the lifelong effects of punishment during infancy. Puppies were punished for playful behavior with females and rewarded for attacking males. As adults, these dogs attacked males approaching a female in heat, yet they showed none of the overt sexual behavior that normal male dogs typically show toward the female. On the basis of these and other data, Scott (1968) says: "Such results confirm impressions from clinical data that strong early inhibitory training can have important effects on sexual behavior in human beings. . . . Although experimental data are lacking, it is very likely that over-conscientious parents have in the past severely punished their children for actions which appeared to be sexual, and there is every reason to expect that the effects of such inhibitory training might be long-lasting" (pp. 106–107).

In a different experiment, Hunt (1941) subjected 24- and 32-day-old infant rats to a fifteen-day irregular feeding schedule (frustration). A nonfrustrated control group was also used. All animals were then given five months of unlimited feeding followed by five days of feeding frustration. Compared to the

32-day rats (late-onset infantile frustration) and control rats (no infantile frustration), the 24-day (early-onset infantile frustration) animals hoarded more food and ate faster, but only during the five days of adult frustration. (No rats hoard food when it is freely available.)

In sum, the long-term maladaptive effects of early frustration can be documented experimentally. What we still do not know, however, is to what extent experimental neuroses provide valid models of typical human neurotic disorders. The fact that animals can be made neurotic does not necessarily mean that human neuroses are thereby explained.

Cognitive Immaturity   Although external sources of frustration (Table 6.2) are obvious, internal sources—high levels of need and cognitive immaturity, for example—are often subtle and difficult to determine. In theory, these can magnify the effects of social events to produce "complexes," largely unconscious, irrational, and anxiety-ridden residues of frustrating childhood experiences that promote transference behavior and other symptoms.

Psychoanalytic theory assumes that abnormal behavior reflects a *prelogical* style of thinking characteristic of early childhood. What qualities of prelogical thinking (what Freud called "primary process") can contribute to the frustration of the child and, when erupting later, can sabotage the capacity for objective and rational thinking? Here are a few examples.

An egocentric child, insensitive to external perspectives, behaves as though personal experience were the only standard. A 2½-year-old boy, noticing the anatomic difference between him and his mother, asks: "Did it died?" According to classic psychoanalytic theory, little boys must deal with the possibility of "castration" while little girls must deal with the "fact" of castration. In any case, a prelogical mind is clearly capable of inventing some rather bizarre explanations for events both misperceived and grossly misunderstood, and according to theory, some of these inventions—about castration, for example—can have long-term consequences for personality development.

Naive children can develop fantastic misinterpretations, especially about adult sexual behaviors. A glimpse of the apparent "brutality" of sexual intercourse between their parents (what is called the "primal scene" in psychoanalytic writings) may generate fantasies that serve as the nucleus of neurotic preoccupations. The very young child has trouble separating real and imaginary events. Bad thoughts toward a parent can elicit anxiety because they are emotional equivalents of bad acts, and bad acts elicit punishment. This perceived equivalence of mental activity and physical reality, called "magical thinking," can sometimes be observed in the playful regressions of adults who find themselves in emotionally exciting situations. A bowler arching his body as if to control the path of a ball well out of reach is expressing a magical feeling of mind over matter.

Normally, prelogical thinking is appropriately expressed in fantasy and play, conditions in which there is minimal constraint to think objectively and rationally. We usually outgrow many prelogical beliefs, but if we do not, they can become chronic and pervasive, increasing the risk for psychopathology.

Significance of Frustration

What is the long-term significance of the frustration of basic needs? How is it related to adult psychopathology? These questions can be separated out into more specific ones, the first of which concerns the source of painful experience.

Subjective and Objective Frustration   As we have seen, the source of frustration can be *subjective,* invented by a sensitive child with a rich imagination; recall the example of the false assumption about ''castration'' made by the naive child on the basis of observed anatomic sex differences. On the other hand, the source may be *objective*—for example, an insensitive parent makes castration threats.

A major shift in Freud's views about the causes of neurotic behavior reflected some ambiguity about the relative importance of subjective and objective sources of frustration. At first, Freud proposed a ''seduction hypotheses'': that neurosis is caused by the repression of frustrating experiences arising from sexual overstimulation by parents. The repressed ''complexes''— prelogical memories arising out of the clash of childish needs, frustrating experiences, and anxiety—would remain stagnant because they would be cut off from the ''educational'' influence of further personality development. Later, certain life situations could reawaken these dormant, affectively charged complexes to influence behavior, for example, to create repetition compulsions.

The ''seduction hypotheses'' was based on the erotic fantasies of patients caught up in transference reactions with their therapist. These fantasies came to light through the use of *free association* whereby the patient is asked to report without censorship anything that comes to mind.

Freud subsequently came to doubt the seduction hypothesis because, for one thing, he could not believe that sexual abuse by parents was so prevalent (Freud, 1900/1953). His new hypothesis was that the erotic fantasies represented frustrated infantile *wishes* rather than frustrating parental misconduct. The new hypothesis was the foundation of the *oedipal theory* of psychosexual development. In a nutshell, this theory emphasized the lifelong pathological consequences of an overblown and frustrated erotic attachment of the child to the parent of the opposite sex.

With the historical shift from seduction hypothesis to oedipal theory, the concept of memory as a passive mechanism for storing objective information was changed to a concept of memory as a process for creating experience in order to gratify unconscious motivation. This change transformed a limited hypothesis about the behavior of neurotics into a powerful theory about the creative and self-destructive tendencies of human nature.

Causal and Expressive Frustration   We have just discussed one major question regarding the source of childhood frustration: external events or imagination. A second major question concerns the long-term significance of frustrations, whatever their source.

One view is that frustrations have *causal* significance; they can produce a kind of permanent psychic flaw. This flaw weakens personality, making an otherwise normal person more susceptible to later problems in much the same way that exposure to an allergen during childhood makes a person permanently vulnerable to developing the allergy. The personality flaw might exist as a general insecurity and emotional immaturity or as a repetition compulsion driven by specific frustrations. In either case, fixation in the past forces a person constantly to misinterpret contemporary situations and therefore to react irrationally and compulsively. In short, early frustration is *neurotogenic*: it causes self-centeredness and neurotic symptoms.

An alternative view is that early frustrations have *expressive* significance; they are signs of the early development of neurotic sensitivity, like the bud is an early developmental sign of a flower. Frustration does not ensure neurotic personality development; rather, neurotic personality development ensures frustration. Therefore, basic problems with security, love, control, and so forth will burden both the child and the adult.

In sum, there are two sources of frustration—objective and subjective—and two concepts of significance—causal and expressive. Psychodynamic theory uses different combinations of these four possibilities to explain different disorders. Its emphasis on objective sources of frustration—parental behavior in particular—is consistent with theories that emphasize environment-driven conditioning; on the other hand, its emphasis on subjective sources of frustration—conflict-ridden prelogical processes—means that it can be thought of as a cognitive model as well.

UNCONSCIOUS ASPECTS OF BEHAVIOR

In the psychoanalytic model, human behavior is not just conditioned reactions to objective stimuli. It has subjective and symbolic aspects that can obscure its meanings. It is *subjective* to the extent that personal needs and idiosyncratic interpretations predominate—for example, a hypochondriac's inordinate apprehension about "disease," a paranoid's delusion of "persecution," or a depressive's masochistic "guilt" for a broken relationship. It has *symbolic* aspects when it represents something as other than what it appears to represent—for example an animal phobia or compulsive ritual that, in disguised form, represents conflict with a parent. The meaning of any behavior with subjective and symbolic aspects will be obscure, especially when it reflects experiences that are distant from current conscious experience—in other words, remote both in time (early childhood) and in "space" (unconscious mind).

Unconscious Influence

The psychoanalytic view of human cognition just described shares with other, less controversial theories the basic assumption that conscious experience is constructed by active and selective mechanisms guided by knowledge and needs operating mostly from outside of conscious awareness (Dixon, 1981; Erdelyi, 1974; Kihlstrom, 1987).

The influence of unconscious thought processes can be illustrated by certain neurological conditions that appear to bring about the uncoupling of conscious and unconscious intention. Normally, reflective conscious awareness is a function of left hemisphere-dominated language capacities. On the other hand, the right hemisphere, in a mostly nonverbal manner, perceives, understands, intends, and acts, but it generally does so apart from normal conscious awareness. In other words, it seems to follow somewhat different cognitive rules.

Split Brains and Unconscious Behavior   When fibers connecting the left and right hemispheres of the brain are severed, their normal influence on each other is diminished if not eliminated. The mute and largely unconscious right hemisphere expresses itself through actions of the left hand, just as the largely conscious left hemisphere expresses itself through actions of the right hand. The decoupling of unconscious motivation (right hemisphere) from conscious and voluntary (left hemisphere) control produces some fascinating and unexpected behaviors (Geschwind, 1981). One "split-brained" patient, whose fibers connecting the left and right hemispheres had been severed, found his left hand (right hemisphere) around his own throat trying to choke himself. Another patient's left hand slammed a dresser drawer on the patient's right hand. Still another patient was mortified by attacks on his wife which he carried out only with his left hand. These bizarre examples illustrate the multifaceted, competitive, and unconscious qualities of mental life to which Freud insisted we pay attention.

Unconscious information can have complex and systematic effects on conscious behavior. A physician may make a valid medical diagnosis during an epileptic "absence," or lapse in normal conscious awareness (Blumer, 1975). Individuals with damage in certain areas of the visual cortex can detect and even discriminate between stimuli they cannot "see," that is, between stimuli that they are not consciously aware of (Dixon, 1981). Others with lesions in brain regions devoted to consolidating new memories can learn laboratory tasks—they show improved performance with practice—even though they do not recognize the tests or realize that they have taken them before (Rozin, 1976). Other studies show that subjects develop an unconscious preference for even meaningless stimuli depending on their familiarity. For example, preference for one of a pair of meaningless geometric stimuli has been shown to depend on the number of times it has previously been presented even though subjects are totally unaware of this relation between preference and familiarity (Kunst-Wilson & Zajonc, 1980; Zajonc, 1980).

Subliminal Perception   Subliminal stimuli whose intensity or duration is insufficient for conscious registration can nevertheless have psychological influence (Kihlstrom, 1987). For example, emotionally significant subliminal stimuli presented to one eye can influence the detection and interpretation of neutral stimuli presented simultaneously to the other eye (Dixon, 1981). By the same token, a subliminal stimulus that registers as a hostile act can make a consciously perceived, or *supraliminal,* stimulus seem sinister.

Subliminal stimuli are, by definition, unconscious. But stimuli need not be subliminal to have unconscious effects. *Supra*liminal stimuli may have unconscious effects if they are not noticed. For example, unattended stimuli that are threatening—words like "injury," for example—can disrupt performance on laboratory tasks, especially in chronically anxious subjects (Mathews & MacLeod, 1986). The effects of unconsciously perceived stimuli may show up hours or even days later in word associations, waking preoccupations, and dreams despite complete lack of insight. What has been registered but apparently "repressed" may emerge later in distorted or symbolically elaborated form.

In sum, research strongly supports the idea that many stimuli that influence our behavior are unconscious because they are (a) subliminal, (b) supraliminal but unattended, or (c) supraliminal and attended but unappreciated (Bowers, 1984).

Symbolic Unconscious

These observations are relevant to two psychodynamic assumptions: (a) that unconscious needs are highly motivating and (b) that unconscious needs can affect the symbolic aspect of mental life as in symptoms and "Freudian slips," and influence what events are attended to and what events get pushed into the unconscious. We turn now to a fuller description of these symbolic and defensive aspects of unconscious cognition.

Parapraxes A parapraxis is loosely defined as a behavioral "error" or "slip." A person intends to do something but, inadvertently, does something else or fails to do it entirely. In psychoanalytic theory, such errors have frequently been analyzed for hidden meanings. Let us consider the famous example of a special type of parapraxis, a Freudian slip of the tongue, described in *The Psychopathology of Everyday Life* (1901/1960). According to Freud, he and another man were having a conversation while traveling by train. To underscore a point, Freud's companion quoted in Latin a passage from Virgil's *Aeneid,* but omitted the word *aliquis,* which means "someone" or "something." Freud supplied the missing word and then responded to the man's challenge to prove that the omission was motivated.

At Freud's suggestion, the man gave many associations to the omitted word, including: a-liquis (suggesting no fluid); new accusations of ritual child sacrifice leveled at Jews; a series of saints including St. Simon of Trent (murdered as a child), St. Augustine (who made negative comments about women, and whose name appears on calendars), and St. Januarius (another calendar name, and another reference to blood in that once a year his blood is supposed to liquefy in a phial located in a Naples church); and, finally, a woman with disturbing news. (Before going on, can you figure out what the man was pre-occupied with?)

From the associations, Freud inferred the man was concerned that a certain lady was no longer having her menstrual period. Omitting the key word *aliquis* was a symbolic expression of a subjective concern: "no liquid." This concern had intruded itself in the form of momentary "forgetful-ness"—in this case, an example of repression. Freud believed that all such slips were subjectively motivated. Sometimes, the motivation is obscure, as it was in the aliquis incident. But sometimes it is quite transparent—for example, when a manipulative patient says "I'll play (instead of pay) you later, doctor," or another highly vulnerable patient expresses "a foetal, I mean feeble, attempt at individuality."

Few psychologists believe that all parapraxes are Freudian slips. Clearly, many if not most are *unmotivated* momentary and innocuous errors of speci-fiable cognitive mechanisms. For example, replying with great irritation to a lazy student, a professor blurts out: "You have *t*asted the whole *w*orm!" This type of slip of the tongue, called a *spoonerism,* involves exchanging the initial consonants of intended words. This anticipatory speech error occurs because of the complexities of speech mechanisms, and not because the personal meanings of the words produce anxiety and avoidance. Nevertheless, as we have seen, psychoanalytic theory raises the possibility that similar errors of speech and other defects of so-called "normal" behavior *sometimes* may ex-press the hidden motivation of inner conflict.

Research designed to elicit spoonerisms has yielded evidence that certain experimental techniques can arouse concerns that bias the type of speech error elicited. In one study, male subjects with high scores on a test of sex anxiety were especially prone to errors like reading "fine body" when the stimulus *bine foddy* was presented by a seductive female examiner (Motley, 1980, 1985; see Figure 6.1). Such findings are consistent with the psychoanalytic emphasis on motivational influence on thinking, but they do not speak to the more basic and controversial assumption that such errors originate in repressed infantile frustrations that endure over a lifetime (Grunbaum, 1984).

Symptoms   According to psychoanalytic theory, certain types of symptoms such as hysterical paralysis, agoraphobia, and compulsive checking are *sym-bolic*. In other words, they have specific though unconscious *meanings* that are discoverable through the techniques of psychoanalysis. For example, one might learn through a process of free association that an agoraphobia repre-sents an unconscious conflict about sexuality; feared outdoor situations might symbolize personally threatening sources of sexual opportunity.

In theory, a symbolic symptom is a condensed expression of three compet-ing aspects of personality: desires (id), defenses (ego), and moral sentiments (superego). Thus, a compulsive hand-washing ritual could be interpreted as the condensation or "compromise formation" forged out of aggressive id im-pulses, inhibitory ego tendencies, and expiatory superego influences. In short,

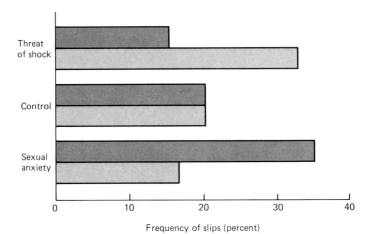

Frequency of slips (percent)

FIGURE 6.1 Freudian slips induced experimentally. The subjects (undergraduate males) all saw the same sequence of word pairs displayed on a screen. In one experiment ("threat of shock") the subjects were warned they would receive an electric shock from electrodes attached to the body. No shocks were given; nevertheless, the subjects' anxiety preferentially elicited spoonerisms related to electricity (gray bars). "Cursed wattage" for "worst cottage" is an example. In another experiment ("sexual anxiety") the presence of a woman monitoring the experiment preferentially elicited spoonerisms with sexual content (black bars). "Fast passion" for "past fashion" is an example. The results support the hypothesis that slips of the tongue reveal hidden anxieties. (From "Slips of the Tongue" by M. J. Motley, p. 118. Copyright © 1985 by Scientific American, Inc. All rights reserved)

a symbolic symptom is a *pathologically creative solution* to the problem of conflict among strong and incompatible tendencies within the personality.

The idea that behavior can simultaneously express different, even incompatible tendencies of id, ego, and superego is not particularly radical or hard to understand. For example, emotional ambivalence may be expressed with smiling lips and unsmiling eyes. Barking laughter may express both anger and joviality. Sometimes laughter and crying are intermixed in the expression of joy, relief, and self-pity. Figure 6.2 shows how anger and fear can be expressed simultaneously in a compromise formation involving posture and facial expression (Lorenz, 1963/1966). According to psychoanalytic theory, phobic, compulsive, and other symptoms are cognitively sophisticated, symbolic versions of this general mammalian capacity to integrate into a single behavioral expression more than one impulse or idea.

Symbolic transformation of experience need not reflect neurotic conflict between incompatible tendencies within personality. In psychotic conditions, for example, it may reflect the effects of traumatic events and the childhood misunderstanding of those events. A classic illustration is the case of Daniel Schreber (1841–1911), a German judge who developed a paranoid psychosis.

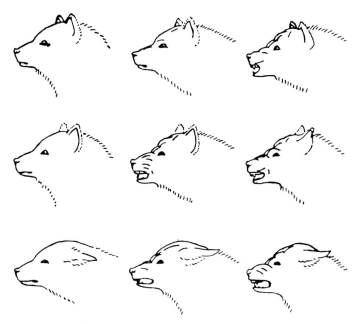

FIGURE 6.2   Combinations of aggressive and fearful expressions in the dog. Note the increasingly intense expressions of *aggressiveness* (top row, from left to right), *fear* (left column, from top to bottom), and their *combination* (diagonally, from top left to bottom right). (Source: Figure 3 from *On Aggression* by Konrad Lorenz, copyright © 1963 by Dr. G. Borotha-Schoeler Verlag, Wien; English translation copyright © 1966 by Konrad Lorenz, copyright © 1983 Deutscher Taschenbuch Verlag GmbH and Co. KG, Munchen, reprinted by permission of Harcourt Brace Jovanovich, Inc.)

He believed that rays from God caused "miracles," strange and unpleasant bodily sensations such as head compression and pain in the spine or trunk. The writings of Schreber's father make clear the objective basis of the son's delusions. The elder Schreber was a much admired pedagogue with bizarre ideas about the socialization of children. His sadistic disciplinary practices included the use of various apparatuses (see Figures 6.3 and 6.4) that forced young children, even babies, to comply with rigid and uncompromising rules of conduct. These bizarre practices clearly influenced the content of the son's delusions. As it happened, Freud overlooked the historical connection between the father's practices and the son's delusional fantasy. Unfortunately, Freud attempted to psychoanalyze the younger Schreber solely from his writings without consulting the published works of the father (Schatzman, 1973).

Implications

Mental life involves creative processes that are influenced by hidden motivation. But what is the nature of this hidden motivation? Psychoanalytic theory

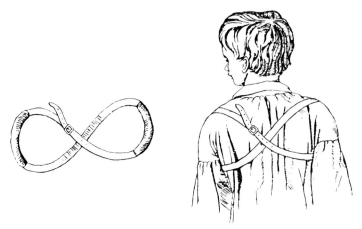

FIGURE 6.3 A shoulder harness worn continuously to regulate posture and condition an upright attitude. The shaded parts shown on the left are metal springs that press against the front of the shoulders. (From Schatzman, 1973, p. 67)

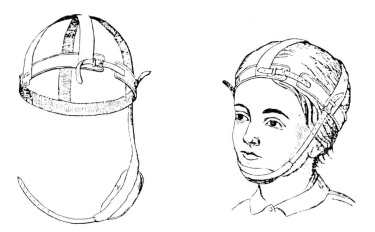

FIGURE 6.4 A harness for the chin. (From Schatzman, 1973, p. 79)

is most controversial and least confirmable scientifically when it argues (1) that hidden motivation is *repressed* and *symbolically transformed*, that is, disguised rather than merely obscure; (2) that the *repressed* and *disguised* aspects of motivation are of *infantile* origin; and (3) that the content of these repressed and infantile aspects is largely of a *sexual* nature.

Nevertheless, it seems true that objective events are prone to subjective transformations and this explains why behavior seems both frequently autonomous and inexplicable. What people know may not be manifest in their behavior, and the reverse is also true: behavior may provide a poor basis for inferring what individuals know (Blodgett, 1929; Bortner & Birch, 1970; Gelman, 1979). Also, what people know may be highly subjective and idiosyncratic, especially if it is rooted in infantile misunderstandings that continue unconsciously to influence adult thinking.

Consider a little boy of 2½, exuberant over newly mastering a tricycle, who explains joyfully: "I can pedal my feet...only boys have penises, not girls." One detects in the child a *personal* connection between feelings of competence and a newly emerging sense of masculinity in this otherwise inexplicable association of penis and pedaling. According to psychoanalytic theory, such personal connections need not always be outgrown. If repressed, they can remain active, serving as an unconscious source of idiosyncratic meanings that make the behavior of the adult neurotic seem so irrational and obscure. In short, what you see is often *not* what you get when you look below the surface. And the reason, according to psychodynamic theory, is largely due to the *defensive* aspect of mental life, which makes it difficult for an observer, including the person himself, to know what is really going on.

DEFENSIVE ASPECT OF BEHAVIOR

"Nature, despite all her progressiveness, is also a staunch conservative..." (MacLean, 1973, p. 20). Self-preservation and resistance to change are the rule at all levels of living function: molecular, chemical, physiological, behavioral, and cognitive. The organism's instinctive tendency is always to express self-organization, and to defend it if threatened.

Threatening impulses (to engage in forbidden behavior—for instance) or threatening experiences (of worthlessness or helplessness) generate anxiety and depression unless they are defended against. Excessive defensiveness is expressed in many forms—for example, (a) selective perception, denial, and changes in feeling, (b) aversions to people or situations that symbolize a dangerous repressed wish, (c) masochistic or self-destructive behavior to preserve a relationship that satisfies dependency needs, and (d) aggressive and egotistical self-assertion to avoid feelings of inferiority or inadequacy. Because these behavior patterns enhance the sense of security and effectiveness, they are very resistant to change despite their maladaptive consequences. At this point, some illustrative examples of defensiveness will be helpful before proceeding to a more formal classification of defense mechanisms.

Defensiveness Illustrated

A 9-year-old boy named Danny was brought to an outpatient mental health clinic because of his parents' concern about his anxiety and underachievement at school, which he seemed unable, or at least unwilling, to face squarely. Danny avoided any discussion of the family problems that were undermining his sense of security. As far as he was concerned, everything was "fine."

Consider the evidence that Danny's "happy face" was his way of denying threatening ideas and feelings. First, group therapy with his parents clearly revealed a shaky marriage unbalanced by excessive maternal dominance and paternal passivity. Second, Danny's dreams included symbols representing this imbalance. For example, in one dream, Danny is saved from falling off a cliff by a mother dinosaur while the father dinosaur sits quietly in the background. Third, while playing with a dollhouse, Danny took the mother doll and casually stuffed it head-first down the toilet. Fourth, Danny made a drawing, shown in Figure 6.5, that further demonstrated angry and insecure feelings about his mother. But again, Danny could not speak to the therapist about these signs of anxiety, anger, and insecurity. He would merely smile and clam up.

Danny's behavior illustrates the excessive use of the defensive processes that neutralize threatening ideas and feelings. In relatively formal settings in

FIGURE 6.5   "My Mother."

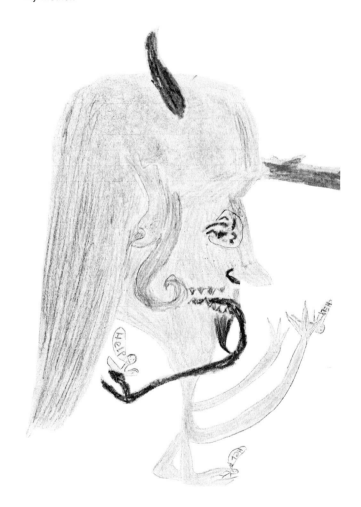

which he felt self-consciousness (therapist's office, for example), denials, smiles, and incommunicativeness were the rule. In settings conducive to play and fantasy (game room, for example), symbolic substitutions of otherwise defended ideas and feelings were more often the rule. In short, Danny's defensiveness, as expressed in his change-resistant repetitive behavior, distorted objective reality sufficiently to ward off painful ideas and feelings. He could expose these more directly only under special conditions—play, fantasy, dreaming.

The following example illustrates the power of defensive activity to alter reality in the service of personal motivation. Miss J., a 22-year-old woman self-referred for psychological testing, was given the Thematic Apperception Test (TAT). Each TAT card shows an ambiguous situation about which a story is to be constructed (see Chapter 4). With her first response to the first card, Miss J. grimaced in what might be called a compromise formation of exuberance and pain. Then she explained, "I hate it. I just hate it. I can't tell stories. (Why?) I can't do it unless I'm being cute. You'd better pamper me and tell me that I'm cute . . . you don't know what you are doing to me." The childish (or "regressive") quality of Miss J's defensive transference behavior is typical of the hysterical personality faced with a male authority figure. The "child" attempts to disarm the "parent" and neutralize the testing situation by turning it into a game. The defensive strategy is to appeal rather than reveal; the goal is love and support rather than respect and rapport. The bottom line of this defense is "Nothing serious is going on; I'm just fooling."

On the basis of this behavior, a psychoanalyst would make two predictions about Miss J.'s test data. First, they should show evidence of oedipal frustration, including longing for father and hostility toward mother. And, in fact, Miss J's TAT stories did strongly suggest loss, anger, and depression. She perceived males as appealing and desirable, yet exploitative and undependable. She perceived females less ambivalently as suspicious, angry, and unsympathetic. Her interpersonal relationships were described as unstable if not elusive, and ultimately meaningless.

Second, psychoanalytic theory would predict evidence of enhanced repression supplemented with denial of anger and depression. In fact, her initial denial did contrast sharply with her subsequent expression of those darker sentiments. A graphic representation of this dichotomy is illustrated by a remarkable set of drawings (Figure 6.6) made by another woman giving evidence of personality problems similar to Miss J's. The left side of Figure 6.6 shows the initial drawing of a childlike and playful cartoon girl. The hidden left hand suggests an undisclosed, possibly sinister dark side. After completing the picture, she tentatively canceled it with a lightly (ambivalently?) drawn wavy line. On the back of the paper, she drew the figure shown at the right.

Miss J.'s performance on the TAT nicely illustrates the classic psychoanalytic view that repression and unconscious preoccupation with oedipal frustrations can adversely affect cognitive function—producing, for example, perceptual blocks, memory failures, and a babe-in-the-woods naiveté (Schafer, 1954).

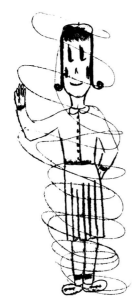 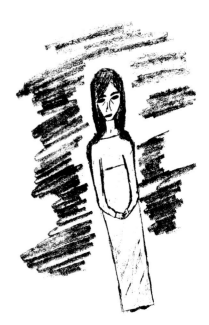

FIGURE 6.6   Two figure drawings illustrating the defensive hysteroid (left panel) and the defended depressive (right panel) sides of a character-neurotic personality.

Typically, Miss J. would become especially uncomfortable when shown a card with some sexual implication. Once she sighed, "How can I possibly tell you a story?... I can't think of anything that has to do with sex."

One TAT card, given near the end of the test, shows a bare-breasted woman lying on a bed with a sheet draped over the lower half of her body. In the foreground is a man covering his face with his arm as though in fatigue or remorse, the picture being purposely ambiguous. A typical story describes either an early morning domestic scene or a rape. When Miss J. looked at this card she first burst out into a nervous laugh that suggested disturbance over the sexual implications of the picture. But after beginning to develop a story about the man's drinking behavior, she stopped and said, "Oh, I can't think." Miss J. gave no indication that she had seen the partially naked woman. Yet her characteristic emotionality with respect to sexual matters was evident. When the examiner asked "Did you leave anything out?", she responded uncertainly, "...man, bottle, and some funny looking things that look like a tent." In response to the more specific question, "Is there only one person in the picture?", she studied the picture intently and after a few seconds exclaimed, "Oh! There's a female there, with a sheet over her or something... I'm sorry, I *didn't see that at all!*"

The failure of a woman with superior IQ to see a salient feature of visual information—a sort of "negative hallucination"—is hard to explain without reference to psychodynamics. If motivation can radically alter conscious perception, it can certainly affect thinking and interpersonal behavior, transforming personality in a pathological direction. The result is rigidity, subjectivity, emotionality, inefficiency, and self-deception. But why do people persist in such painful and self-destructive ways?

A study by Forrest and Hokanson (1975) suggests a possible solution to this "neurotic paradox" of persistent yet punishing behavior. Twenty normal and twenty depressed college students were instructed to respond to aggressive behavior, specifically electric shock delivered by a person who was actually a confederate of the experimenter. By pressing any of three buttons, the subject could respond to the aggression by delivering a "reward" signal to the confederate or an electric shock either to the confederate (the aggressive counterresponse) or to himself (the self-punitive counterresponse). Subjects were asked to use all three types of counterresponse, but in varying amounts to be decided by them. Compared to the nondepressed subjects, depressed subjects more often used the self-punitive (shock) mode of response, and also showed either diminished or relatively less physiological arousal (anxiety) after self-punishment than after aggressive reactions. In short, self-punishment was subjectively *reinforcing* to depressive subjects despite the pain.

The results of this study support the psychodynamic view that dysfunctional, even self-destructive, behavior may be positively reinforcing if it prevents or substitutes for an even more negative consequence. Depressive self-punishment may ward off the threat of rejection and loss; masochistic pain-seeking may compensate for fear of separation and the inability to feel in normal relationships. What appears to be "error" from the perspective of the observer may be perfectly "correct" from the perspective of the subject, even though the underlying psycho-logic is completely unconscious.

Defense Mechanisms

In the psychoanalytic model, internal dangers involve impulses, affects, and ideas—for example, the frustrated oedipal motives of early childhood. Ego *defense mechanisms* enable a person to cope with such internal dangers. They may be repressed so that they are not recognized at all, but there are other possibilities. They can be *projected,* experienced as coming from an external source—for example, a paranoid person unable to recognize that the hostility he "perceives" in others is his own. Inner threat can be *denied* (through pretense and pollyannaish naiveté), or *intellectualized* (making it remote with the use of abstract explanations). These and other ego defense mechanisms reduce anxiety but at the cost of producing behavior that has a compulsive and irrational quality.

Psychodynamic theories describe two general kinds of psychopathology that are associated with inner threat, one involving a *strong id* that threatens an otherwise normal ego, and the other involving a *weak ego*. Let us take a closer look at these two from the perspective of defense mechanisms.

Id Impulse Regulation According to the conflict model of classical psychoanalytic theory, the basic threat to personality is the potential eruption of id impulses. An essentially normal ego is driven to take action by mobilizing *impulse-regulating* defenses that are specialized for inhibiting and controlling the manifest expression of the "uncivilized" part of personality (id). Repression is the basic regulatory defense, but there are others (see Table 6.3). These others are devoted to reinforcing the inhibitory function of repression by transforming forbidden impulses into more acceptable behavior—for example, hostility into "biting" sarcasm (Schafer, 1954).

An overreliance on repression and related regulatory defenses—that is, intense *intrapsychic* (id versus ego) *conflict*—shows up in various forms of so-called neurotic behaviors—for example, a constricted, inflexible, or compulsive pattern in some people, and a naive and unsophisticated pattern in others. In addition, repression is implicated in certain so-called psychosomatic symp-

TABLE 6.3   SAMPLER OF REGULATORY DEFENSES*

Type	Explanation	Examples
Repression	Blocking the awareness of threatening impulses, ideas, or feelings associated with anxiety (e.g., harm, abandonment) or guilt (moral transgression)	Inability to perceive or recall threatening experiences or forbidden desires—in particular, those from early childhood; appearing to be naive, that is, unknowing or inhibited
Isolation	Isolation of a feeling (anger) from its appropriate referent (parent) so that it is experienced only in a different context (when alone)	An unemotional talk with a boss (unconscious father figure) is followed some time later by inexplicable rage
Intellectualization	An intellectualized form of isolation, a retreat from feelings to abstract concepts, principles, theories	An unconsciously frustrated patient calmly agrees with the therapist's hypothesis that he must be angry with his father and that this anger probably stems from his oedipal conflicts
Reaction formation	Transforming unconscious but dangerous impulses, feelings, or ideas into conscious but acceptable opposites—for example, anger into "affection" or erotic impulses into "aggression"	A mother's unconscious hostility toward her child is transformed into relentless "concern" about its well-being, including compulsive checking for dirt, broken glass, or other "dangers"
Undoing	Unconscious hostility turned into "good deeds"; a form of expiation and thus a moral version of reaction formation (an example of especially strong superego influence over ego defense)	Excessive helpfulness and even altruistic behavior with people unconsciously hated
Displacement	Impulses unconsciously felt toward one person expressed toward someone else	Anger at the boss taken out on the spouse

*According to psychoanalytic theory (Schafer, 1954), regulatory defenses have three functions with respect to forbidden impulses: *inhibition* (main objective being anxiety avoidance), *gratification* (main objective being pleasure), and *expiation* (main objective being guilt avoidance). Thus, defense mechanisms reflect the influence of id, ego, and superego components of personality.

toms, fatigue, aches, mind wandering, insomnia, and anxiety, the consequences of the constant struggle to inhibit forbidden impulses. To illustrate, consider the following experimental study of repression.

Sommerschild and Reyher (1973) had male subjects imagine while under hypnosis that they were having a sexually provocative experience that included a highly arousing but frustrating encounter with a seductive older woman. The subjects were then instructed to forget (repress) the hypnotic experience. The intensity of their sexual impulses associated with this experience was later systematically varied by controlling certain stimuli in the post-hypnotic testing situation. Despite professed lack of awareness of the experience, subjects showed signs of unconscious motivation connected to it. When exposed to words that referred to the experience, subjects spontaneously reported anxiety and distress: heart thumping, coldness in parts of the body, shakiness, twitching, bladder and bowel sensations, shortness of breath. These distress-related symptoms indicated at least partial awareness or a weakening of hypnosis-induced repression; subjects whose amnesia for the hypnotically induced experience was greatest showed the fewest symptoms.

Ego Defect Compensation   While some defenses seem specialized for regulating unacceptable impulses, other defenses seem to compensate for ego *deficiencies* in seriously disturbed, highly vulnerable people. Such *compensatory* defenses (see Table 6.4) represent unconscious efforts to create a sense of self and personal adequacy while defending against feelings of emptiness, meaninglessness, boredom, hostility, and panic (Kohut, 1977). Nevertheless, compensatory defensiveness is typically associated with many undesirable things—in particular, compliant, combative, or avoidant relationships, pervasive suspiciousness and hostility, and the sense that one's behavior is artificial or unreal.

> Every analyst knows those patients, who, for example, often to the embarrassment of those around them tend to be overly enthusiastic, dramatic, and excessively intense in their responses to everyday events and who, analogously, romanticize and sexualize their relation to the analyst, giving at times the impression of an overtly reinstated display of Oedipal passions. In cases of... personality disorder, it is not difficult to discern the defensive nature—a pseudovitality—of the overt excitement. Behind it lie low self-esteem and depression—a deep sense of uncared-for worthlessness and rejection, an incessant hunger for response, a yearning for reassurance. All in all, the excited hypervitality of the patient must be understood as an attempt to counteract through self-stimulation a feeling of inner deadness and depression (Kohut, 1977, p. 5).

Compensatory defenses are especially characteristic of people with "borderline" psychopathology—in particular, the narcissistic, borderline, and antisocial personality disorders of *DSM-III-R,* Axis II. In these, behavior tends to be chaotic, destructive, and unstable as manifested by idiosyncratic and peculiar ideas, volatile relationships, drug abuse, excessive risk-taking, shoplift-

TABLE 6.4   A SAMPLER OF COMPENSATORY DEFENSES

Type	Explanation	Examples
Primitive denial	Adopting insensitive, aloof, and/or grandiose pretenses in fantasy and behavior to reinforce a sense of one's strength and importance	Believing that one has special "powers" or "talents"; denying the significance of a deficiency or failure that is clearly evident
Pseudovitality	Enhancing the sense of being alive by engaging excessively or irresponsibly in highly stimulating and emotionally arousing behaviors	Reckless sensation-seeking; provocative aggressive, or exhibitionistic behavior; self-mutilative or dramatic suicidal gestures
Primitive idealization*	Overidentifying with people misperceived as omnipotent, omniscient, all-loving, or all-good, thereby securing an enhanced sense of security, importance, or power	Believing that the therapist is all-powerful and has perfect insight; deifying and giving total and unquestioned allegiance to a cult leader
Primitive devaluation*	Attributing a hostile, degrading, or unforgiving attitude that helps to bolster fragile self-esteem by minimizing other people	Emphasizing other people's faults; mocking or minimizing their achievements, adopting a supercilious or disdaining attitude
Projection	Attributing "bad" aspects of oneself to others or situations without recognizing them in oneself	Misperceiving one's own weakness as an "external threat"—for example, paranoiac suspiciousness and avoidance

*Component of *splitting,* an infantile all-or-nothing way of thinking that dissociates "good" and "bad" aspects of self and others. Rather than appreciating the different and ever changing qualities of people, they are experienced as now and forever "all bad" or "all good." This dysfunctional style makes impossible a stable sense of self or stable relationships with others.

ing, promiscuity, and even suicide attempts. Consider the following two examples:

> A histrionic woman ... told a friend who called on the telephone that she had just slashed her wrists after taking an overdose of medication and that the paramedics were rushing to her home. This was blatantly untrue. Later, when the friend angrily confronted her with the lie, the patient replied, "What difference does it make? That's the way I felt at the time" (Ford, King, & Hollender, 1988, p. 556).

> ... husband presents wife with a dozen roses for their anniversary; unbeknownst to him, the florist inadvertently included only eleven; wife notices and upbraids husband mercilessly as a cheap uncaring bastard who thought he could get away with saving two dollars ... (Stone, 1988, p. 5).

Regulatory defenses, on the other hand, are more prominent in people with so-called "character-neurotic" psychopathology who tend to be inhibited, controlled, compulsive, and prudish. Some of these behaviors can seem a little "crazy," mainly in the sense of being irrational—for example, endless hand-washing to counteract an almost delusional belief that one is "contaminated." The "crazy" quality of behaviors associated with compensatory and regulatory defenses in borderline and neurotic people is, however, typically different from that of truly psychotic patients, as we will see (Chapter 10).

Both the borderline and neurotic types of psychopathology may co-exist in the same person. Therefore, the impulse-regulatory defense mechanisms emphasized by classical psychoanalytic theory (Table 6.3) may sometimes have a compensatory function while the compensatory defense mechanisms emphasized by revisions of the theory (Table 6.4) may sometimes have an impulse-regulatory function (see Table 6.5 for a comparison of neurotic and borderline types of psychopathology).

It is also worth noting that anyone can be "pathologized" by threatening opportunities that arouse forbidden impulses or traumatizing events that overwhelm coping capacities. In other words, excessive defensiveness may sometimes represent the situationally induced reactions of essentially normal people—like reactions of mothers of dying children (Mason, 1975)—just as it can represent the psychopathological dispositions of chronically troubled people.

Regardless of the developmental themes they emphasize, all psychodynamic theories assume that human existence involves some frustration of basic needs for security, pleasure, mastery, and self-expression. Accordingly, when frustration gets out of hand, especially during the vulnerable period of early childhood development, the risk for lasting psychopathology is increased. This dramatic view of a fundamental clash between human nature and culture resolving itself in behaviors with hidden meanings undoubtedly accounts for the continual attractiveness of psychodynamic theories. And, whatever their failings, they do focus our attention on basic human needs and the often defensive and idiosyncratic influences of mental life that compete with external events to control behavior.

TABLE 6.5   SUMMARY OF NEUROTIC AND BORDERLINE PSYCHOPATHOLOGY

Facet	Neurotic	Borderline
Clinical condition	Insecurity and anxiety	Vulnerability and depersonalization; derealization; emptiness
Associated qualities	Interpersonal relations marked by guilt and anger	Interpersonal relations marked by hostility and a mixture of intense idealization and devaluation
Theoretical condition	Frustration of impulses, especially the impulse to love; deep conflict between representations of impulses (id) and representations of social reality (ego; superego)	Defects in the capacity to organize and control impulses to master the world of objects and persons and to organize experience into a coherent sense of self
Pathological coping	Neurotic defense against impulse	Pseudoneurotic defense against inner weaknesses and disorganization

	Neurotic *compromise* symptoms:
	    Phobic fear of animals
	    Obsessive fear of dirt
	    Hysteric amnesia for sexual experience
		Borderline *compensatory* symptoms:
		    Paranoid pseudosuperiority (e.g., letter writing; delusions of significance)
		    Hysteroid pseudovitality
		    Sadomasochistic sensation-seeking

CRITICAL EVALUATION OF PSYCHOANALYTIC THEORY

From a scientific perspective, psychodynamic theories suffer from many shortcomings. We can list a few of them.

1 Some of their basic concepts, such as libido, are empirically *untestable,* while others, such as the causal connection between infantile experience and adult disorder, fare rather poorly when tested (Fisher & Greenberg, 1977; Kline, 1972). Often, it is the *least* controversial (least classically Freudian) aspects of the theory that survive scientific test. Motley's research (1980, 1985), for example, supports the *non*controversial idea that strong motivation including sexual anxiety can elicit parapraxes such as spoonerisms (see Figure 6.1). But that research does not address the controversial but fundamental assumption that such slips and other symptoms represent *repressed libidinal* or other preoccupations of *infantile origin.*

2 Psychoanalytic explanations often seem *circular,* as when hidden mechanisms inferred from behavior are used to explain that behavior—oedipal frustration is inferred from the patient's seductive behavior and then used to explain the seductiveness (as transference).

3 Psychoanalytic theory, despite its complexity, sometimes seems *simplistic* in its emphasis on a few core concepts—oedipal conflict, for example, or oral frustration. These core concepts describe fairly common experiences, yet they are used to explain any number of complex abnormal behaviors each of which may be rare.

4 Unbridled symbolic interpretations of personal statements about behavior often seem to have an *overly complex* and uncritical quality. And the validation of a therapist's interpretations is too often *unscientific,* based on the patient's acceptance (called insight) or even disagreement (called defensive resistance) rather than on scientific test.

5 There is a *tendency to pathologize*—in other words, to interpret behavioral deviations as symptomatic of hidden abnormalities. Looking for ambivalent feelings, hostile impulses, or neurotic complexes behind every hesitation or slip of the tongue—that is, assuming all slips are "Freudian slips"—is a good example of this unbridled application of theory.

Psychoanalytic theory has recently been subjected to especially vigorous criticism. Grunbaum (1984), for example, argues that the theory is "scientifically alive [but] hardly well" (p. 278). By "scientifically alive" he means that some aspects of the theory are potentially *falsifiable*—that is, if they are wrong, they can be proven wrong through scientific test. By "hardly well" he means that some aspects are not falsifiable, or, if falsifiable, they are often proven to be false if not just less credible than alternative interpretations. For example, the central concept that neurotic symptoms are typically caused by the repression of childhood frustrations fails two important clinical tests: (1) removal of repression through psychoanalytic treatment often produces at best only temporary remissions, and (2) behavioral treatment that ignores repression often produces permanent remissions.

Grunbaum also looks critically at the nonscientific arguments that have been devoted to validating (rather than falsifying) the fundamentals of psychoanalytic theory. For example, he makes clear how easily therapist bias and patient suggestibility can yield false evidence. Thus, therapists can see or select "evidence" to establish their hypotheses, while patients in the grip of transference attachments often "confirm" these hypotheses with obliging fantasies, selective memories, and cathartic emotional reactions. Even when a good case can be made for psychoanalytic interpretations of symbolic meanings, such methods cannot prove the *causal significance* of these meanings to neurotic symptoms no matter how appealing the arguments. Many of these critical points are recognized even by psychopathologists friendly to psychoanalytic theory (e.g., Taylor, 1984, p. 633).

Psychoanalytic theory cannot be ignored. Its formulations about conflict, repression, symbolic transformation of experience, and infantile origins have had an incalculable impact, not only on the historical development of theories about psychopathology, but also on our culture—especially the humanities, but also the social and behavioral sciences—and on day-to-day thinking. How often do we ask ourselves why we did or failed to do something, and how often do both the question and the answer reveal a tendency to slip into psychoanalytic thinking about hidden and devious meanings? Even psychologists who understand its shortcomings often use psychoanalytic concepts in discussing data and patients. The fact is, the psychoanalytic view of psychodynamics has provided what, for many people, remains an irresistible model of human nature.

Some aspects of the model will surely be discarded; others will continue to be defended as a matter of faith because, while unfalsifiable, they have appeal. Nevertheless, we believe that some will prove valid and continue to be useful either as explanations or as fuel for further research ideas. Obviously, psychoanalytic theory, like no other, represents a valiant attempt to grapple on the grand scale with deep questions about human nature—in particular, its selfish, defensive, unconscious, symbolic, creative, and unpredictable aspects. The challenge, then, is to extract that which is worthwhile and to integrate this with defensible concepts. This chapter represents one way of trying to do this.

SUMMARY

No presentation of psychopathology would be complete without considering *psychodynamics,* conflict-ridden mental mechanisms. The psychoanalytic model of psychodynamics includes frustration, repression, and symbolic expression. In this model, neurotic forms of abnormal behavior reflect the pathological exaggeration of *intrapsychic conflict,* the conflict of opposing tendencies within the personality. This dynamic quality of the psyche arises from the universal conflict between a child's biological motivation for sensual gratification and self-enhancement and the inhibitory forces of culture manifested in the parents' socialization practices.

According to psychoanalytic theory, psychological residues of this conflict are laid down gradually in the form of complex affectively charged memories and fantasies. Because they threaten the sense of well-being, these anxiety-ridden "complexes" are driven underground, made unconscious by repressive cognitive operations. The resulting tension between needs and inhibitions and between personal inadequacy and compensatory striving is expressed in *symptom neuroses* such as phobia and hysteria (Axis I disorders) and the *character neuroses* such as avoidant and compulsive personality disorders (Axis II disorders). Thus, psychopathology is viewed as a disguised *repetition* of infantile, affect-laden preoccupations suppressed and sublimated in symbolic form by defense mechanisms.

The unique contribution of psychoanalytic theory is its emphasis on the unconscious, pleasure-oriented (selfish), conflict-ridden, and inventive qualities of mental life. The developmental antecedents of these qualities are the inherited liabilities wired in by evolution and the acquired liabilities programmed in by socialization. Although some aspects of the theory have received empirical support, many other aspects are either untestable or untenable. Two major questions about psychodynamic causality have yet to be confirmed scientifically: To what extent do the subjective aspects of mental life rather than objective social reality determine infantile frustrations? And to what extent do these early frustrations cause or merely reflect the pathological development of personality?

Genetic Facet

OUTLINE

ENVIRONMENTALITY
  Shared and Unshared Influences
  Gene-Environment Interaction
  Identical Twins Reared Apart
WHAT'S INHERITED?
SUMMARY

GENETIC THEORIES

It seems clear that people as well as all other species differ in a variety of traits. Genetic theories arose to account for the differences among and within the species. Historically major milestones in explaining these differences and how they arose include Darwin's theory of evolution in 1859, Mendel's theory of genetic transmission in 1865, and Watson and Crick's discovery in 1953 of the genetic code in the double helix of deoxyribonucleic acid (DNA). The first two are more immediately relevant to psychopathology and will be accented in what follows.

Darwin's Theory

From Charles Darwin we learned that the diversity of life can be encompassed by a theory of *natural selection* (Mayr, 1978). Natural selection is a two-step process. First, chance events produce mutations or novel recombinations of existing genes. Second, if these random genetic changes are favorable, they lead to greater numbers of fit offspring who survive to disseminate the new mutation throughout the population.

Physical Evolutionary Connections   Darwinian theory proposes that life evolved from a common ancestor, suggesting that we can learn much by observing other species. Indeed, many otherwise incomprehensible physical and behavioral phenomena can be explained only by reference to our ancestry. Contemporary examples of our ancestry are seen in *atavisms,* the reappearance of features normally characteristic only of more primitive species (Hall, 1984). One of the most striking of these is hypertrichosis (excessive hairiness). Although human beings have as many hairs as apes, ours are shorter and thinner. Hypertrichosis, a reversion to the ancestral form, is caused by a gene mutation that "releases" our otherwise dormant hereditary legacy.

Behavioral Evolutionary Connections   Does reference to our evolutionary ancestry have implications for psychopathology? We think so. For example, animals threatened by a predator from which there is no escape lapse into a catatoniclike posture, a condition called *tonic immobility.* Tonic immobility can be produced in the laboratory by pinning an animal's limbs or wings firmly against its body (Gallup & Maser, 1977). In the natural environment, tonic immobility is the last of four distinct stages of an instinctive behavioral response to life-threatening events: freezing when a predator is at a distance, flight when it draws closer, struggle if about to be captured, and tonic immobility if there is no chance for escape (Ratner, 1967, and see Figure 7.1).

Catatonic schizophrenics are mute and assume bizarre postures analogous to the tonically immobile animal. Recovered patients report that during the catatonic state they were without "will," unable to make a voluntary movement. Failure of will can be interpreted as a human version of a primitive immobility mechanism. A further parallel between tonic immobility in animals and catatonic posturing in humans is that antipsychotic drugs diminish both. Moreover, animal strains can be bred for susceptibility to tonic immobility, perhaps paralleling the finding that catatonic schizophrenia can run in families.

Darwin's theory was weakest when it came to describing the specific means by which genetic information is transmitted from one generation to the next. Mendel's theory was able to provide a statistical model of genetic transmission that could explain why only some people in certain families are abnormal while others are normal.

Mendel's Theory

In 1865, Gregor Mendel reported a series of experiments on the common garden pea. He started with true-breeding plants—for example, tall plants that, if crossed with other talls, always produced tall offspring. He showed that when such talls were crossed with dwarf plants, the heterozygous offspring, called *hybrids,* were always tall. But when these hybrids were crossed, three-quarters of the offspring were talls and one-quarter were dwarfs.

FIGURE 7.1 A diagram of Ratner's (1967) hypothesis of tonic immobility. (*Psychopathology: Experimental Models* by Jack D. Maser and Martin E. P. Seligman. Copyright © 1977. Reprinted with permission of W. H. Freeman and Company)

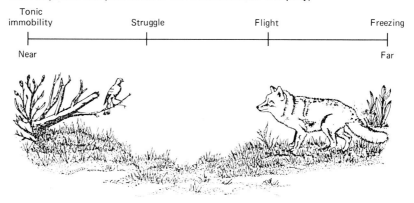

Mendel devised a theory to explain this outcome. The theory included (1) a hereditary factor—now called a gene—responsible for transmitting tallness or shortness, and (2) dominance of the tallness factor over that of shortness (the recessive factor). With these two ideas, the statistical distribution obtained in the offspring of the hybrids fit the binomial formula: $(T + t)^2 = (TT + 2Tt + tt) = 1$, where uppercase T is tall and lowercase t is short. Thus, offspring of hybrids produce on the average one-quarter of offspring that are pure tall (TT), one-half who are hybrid tall ($2Tt$), and one-quarter who are dwarf (tt).

Mendel's work implies that (1) inheritance is particulate—genes behave as particles that *segregate,* or separate independently, when transmitted from one generation to the next; [We now know of a major exception to the segregation theory; namely, that when genes are physically proximate (linked) to each other, they tend to be transmitted as a unit. We take up linkage later in the chapter.] (2) genetic factors account for both similarities and differences between generations; and (3) mathematical models can be used to describe genetic phenomena and to predict results of new breeding experiments.

A fourth conclusion of Mendel's work is that there is a difference between *phenotype*—visible characteristics such as height and color—and *genotype*—the underlying genetic constitution. Typically, the correspondence between the two is neither perfect nor obvious. For example, in Mendel's experiments, phenotypically tall plants could have the TT or the Tt genotype. The phenotype-genotype distinction turned out to be important because it showed that phenotypic dissimilarities between parents and offspring were entirely predictable from genetic theory. Applied to psychopathology, Mendel's theory could account both for normal children of abnormal parents and for abnormal children of normal parents. For example, phenotypically normal parents could each be carrying one copy of the same abnormal recessive gene. An abnormal offspring could have inherited the defective gene from each parent and thus have a double dose.

GENES, CHROMOSOMES, AND BEHAVIOR

For Mendel, the unit of heredity was entirely hypothetical. Now we know that the unit, or *gene,* is a sequence of DNA that directs the cell to make a certain combination of protein "building blocks" called amino acids. The arrangement of genes is analogous to beads on strings, the strings being the *chromosomes* (Figure 7.2). The nucleus of each human cell contains twenty-three pairs of chromosomes, for a total of forty-six. Of the twenty-three pairs, twenty-two are called *autosomes*; the other pair are sex chromosomes, identical in females (XX) and different in males (XY). Each parent contributes one member of each chromosome pair, or half of the total, encased within the egg or sperm. Each gene from one parent is normally at a fixed location along a chromosome so it can pair with its counterpart from the other parent. Genes occupying the same chromosome locus, but differing in molecular structure, are said to be alleles, or alternate forms to each other.

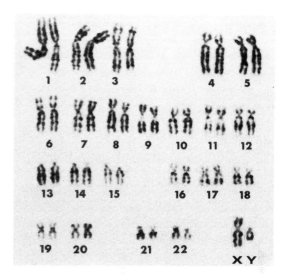

FIGURE 7.2   Normal human chromosome karyotype.

Chromosome Abnormalities

Sometimes pieces of a chromosome in the egg or sperm break off, with adverse effects on the organism. Four types of chromosomal abnormalities caused by breakage are shown in Figure 7.3. The last column illustrates what happens when the normal chromosome intertwines with the rearranged chromosome with which it is paired and possibly exchanges genetic material. These chromosomal abnormalities produce hundreds of disorders, many of which cause mental retardation. For example, the bottom portion of Figure 7.3 illustrates a *translocation* in which a fragment of one chromosome attaches to a different chromosome. An offspring may inherit from one parent a normal chromosome and from the other parent the corresponding normal chromosome plus the fragment. The consequence is an offspring with *three* copies of the specific genetic material—normal plus translocated chromosomes from one parent and a normal chromosome from the other parent. If the extra material comes from chromosome 21, the result is a disorder called Down's syndrome, formerly called mongolism.

Regulatory and Structural Genes

Genes can be classified according to their functions. Regulatory genes control the turning on and off of the structural genes that actually manufacture proteins. Regulatory genes are thus analogous to orchestra conductors; they don't make the sounds but they control their tempo and volume. The importance of regulatory genes in humans is just beginning to be appreciated; indeed, many disorders are now viewed as arising from faulty regulatory rather than faulty structural genes.

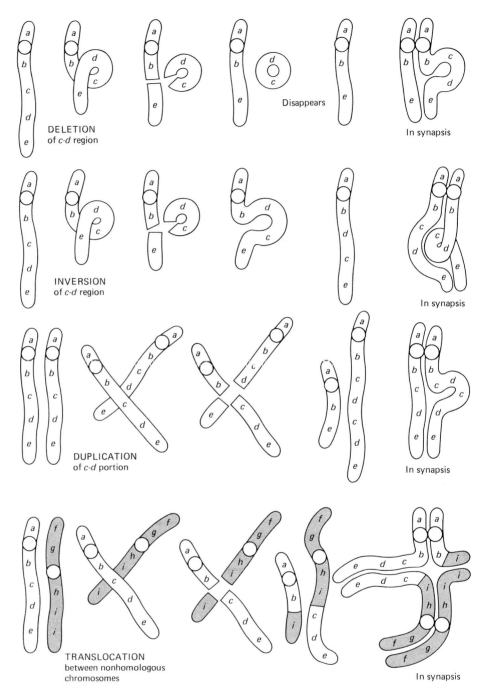

FIGURE 7.3 Types of chromosome rearrangements. *(From D. J. Merrill, Evolution and Genetics, New York: Holt, Rinehart & Winston, 1962)*

The number of regulatory genes is not known, but estimates of the number of structural genes in humans range from 50,000 to 100,000, about two-thirds of them identical for everyone (Vogel & Motulsky, 1979). These similarities extend across species. For example, more than 95 percent of the structural genes of humans and apes are identical (King & Wilson, 1975). Even similar disorders in different species can arise for the same reason; for example, Down's syndrome occurs in both the human and the chimpanzee and is caused in both instances by an extra copy of the same extra genetic material.

In some instances the onset of regulatory gene activity may not occur until adulthood. For example, Huntington's chorea is a lethal dominant genetic disorder with average onset during mid-life. It produces disfiguring writhing movements and progressive mental deterioration. Recently, a region of chromosome 4 has been found to contain the Huntington gene (Gusella et al., 1983), and one expects that its precise location and the specific nature of the abnormality will be revealed soon.

Sex Chromosome Disorders

The X and Y sex chromosomes are also shown in Figure 7.2. The Y chromosome is associated with the development of maleness in mammals. One of its genes and a homologue gene present on the X chromosome are both required to induce the undifferentiated gonads to develop into testes instead of ovaries during embryological development (Ferguson-Smith, 1988). Although each cell in the normal female (XX) also contains two copies of this critical gene, one of the two X chromosomes is inactivated, so that the necessary double dose required for differentiating the gonads into testes is absent. The testes secrete the sex hormone testosterone that is responsible for the masculinization of the brain and external anatomy. In the absence of testosterone, the embryo develops into a female.

Turner's Syndrome Individuals born with only one X and no Y chromosome (XO) can survive, but the absence of at least one X is incompatible with life. Those with Turner's syndrome have only one X chromosome (this XO pattern occurring only once per 2500 female live births). Turner's individuals usually come to medical attention because of failure to menstruate and very short stature (see Figure 7.4). Many have a webbed neck and shieldlike chest. Their ovaries are abnormal and they rarely can bear children (Vogel & Motulsky, 1979). People with Turner's syndrome display a form of "space-form blindness" that shows up specifically as difficulty reading maps, solving jigsaw puzzles, and copying designs. This is all the more remarkable because they have little or no deficit in verbal abilities (Money & Ehrhardt, 1972). Affected persons often have a poor self-concept and are not very popular with peers (McCauley et al., 1987). Nevertheless, with estrogen supplements they develop secondary sexual characteristics and typically can lead relatively normal lives as adults, marrying and perhaps adopting children.

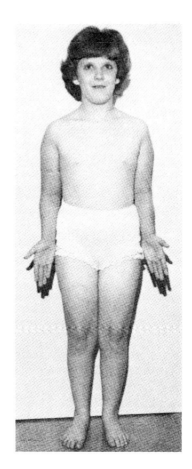

FIGURE 7.4   A 14-year-old female with Turner's syndrome (XO) who is 4 feet, 7 inches tall. (From J. J. Nora & F. Clarke Fraser, *Medical Genetics: Principles and Practice.* Philadelphia: Lea & Febiger Publishers, 1981)

Turner's syndrome often is caused by nondisjunction of the X chromosome before conception. Nondisjunction means that two copies of a particular chromosome failed to disjoin and go into separate sex cells, or gametes. Consequently, one gamete has two copies while another has no copy of the chromosome. In Turner's syndrome the abnormal gamete missing the X unites with a normal gamete containing twenty-three chromosomes.

The disorder can also arise by nondisjunction during early divisions of a normal zygote; that is, the fertilized ovum. When examined under the microscope, some body tissues will be normal and other tissues will be abnormal. The tissues derived from normal cell lines will all be normal, but the cell that lacks the X chromosome will give rise to tissues that will also lack the chromosome. Individuals with such a mixture of normal and abnormal tissues are called *mosaics*.

Klinefelter's Syndrome   Other sex chromosome nondisjunction abnormalities occur—for example, females with three X chromosomes (XXX; 1 per 1250 female births) and males with Klinefelter's syndrome (XXY; 1 per 850 male births). Klinefelter males have been investigated intensively because they are overrepresented in psychiatric and correctional institutions. They have a distinctive body build that borders on the feminine—for example, they have wide hips. Though about 2 inches taller than their brothers, they have small testes, a deficiency of sperm, and lowered sex drive as a result of diminished production of male hormone. This does not always prevent pleasurable sexual intercourse, however, and a minority have satisfactory heterosexual relationships. Treatment typically involves the administration of androgens, which leads to more virilization.

XYY Syndrome Occurring in about 1 per 900 male births, XYY syndrome is caused by nondisjunction of the Y chromosome or by the fertilization of one egg by two sperm (Warburton, 1987). The syndrome has received an inordinate amount of publicity, much of it erroneous. These males, on the average quite tall and often with acne, have been alleged to be extremely aggressive and dangerous. Stories that killers—for example, Richard Speck, convicted of murdering eight nurses in Illinois in 1966—had the XYY syndrome have proved false. Nonetheless, XYYs are overrepresented in prison populations (Nora & Fraser, 1981). Although not distinctively aggressive, XYYs do have abnormal electroencephalograms and lower IQs (Witkin et al., 1977) suggesting an underlying neuropsychological immaturity (see Mednick et al., 1982). These impairments, together with a failure to reflect before acting, may be responsible for their overrepresentation in prisons.

Intellectual Deficits There are often correlations between chromosomal abnormalities and deficits in intellectual function. Figure 7.5 shows IQ results from a ten-year follow-up of all newborns with sex chromosome abnormalities in two large Denver hospitals (Pennington et al., 1982). Between the ages of 4 and 5 these children were compared to their chromosomally normal siblings. The intelligence scale had verbal and performance (nonverbal) components.

The girls with the XXX pattern have both low verbal and performance IQs, with the verbal being slightly lower than the performance IQ. The other two groups show selective deficits in either verbal or performance IQ. The XXYs have normal performance IQs, but are verbally deficient. When they were about 9 years old, 27 percent had specific reading deficits, suggesting some continuity between their preschool deficiency in verbal IQ and their later reading impairment. The Turner (XO) cases showed only nonverbal IQ deficits, consistent with their space-form blindness. Surprisingly, the mosaics, those with sex chromosome anomalies in only some tissue, display few deficits relative to their normal siblings. This suggests that normal cells may be capable of compensating for functions deficient elsewhere.

TYPES OF INHERITANCE

Chromosome aberrations usually alter many genes simultaneously and thus produce many effects. Disorders due to aberrations in single genes, on the

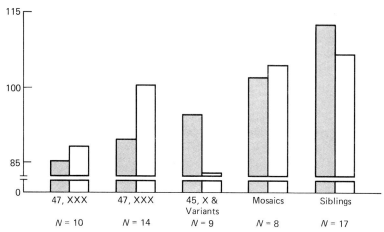

FIGURE 7.5   Mean verbal and performance IQs of 4-to 5-year-old children with sex chromosome anomalies and sibling controls. Hatched is verbal IQ, white is performance IQ. (From Pennington et al., *Child Development,* 1982, *53,* p. 1187)

other hand, are located in a tiny region of a chromosome and more often tend to produce specific dysfunctions.

Single-Gene Inheritance

Four types of single-gene inheritance exist: dominant, recessive, recessive sex-linked, and dominant sex-linked. The specific mode of heredity can often be revealed by inspecting pedigrees, or family trees, in which some relatives have the disorder. Pedigrees showing these different modes of transmission appear in Figure 7.6.

FIGURE 7.6   Examples of dominant, recessive, sex-linked recessive, and sex-linked dominant inheritance. Squares represent males and circles represent females. Empty symbols indicate absence of the trait and blackened symbols indicate its presence. The numerals at the side of the pedigrees refer to the generation of the family, and an arrow when present indicates the affected individual who was first identified (proband, or index case). A horizontal line directly connecting two adjacent individuals in a pedigree indicates mating and the vertical lines extending down from the horizontal lines point to the offspring of the mating. Sometimes the spouses are not included because they are presumed normal. Siblings are represented in the order in which they are born, from left to right. Slashes through a circle or square indicate that the individual is deceased. (A) The Huntington pedigree is from J. F. Gusella et al. A polymorphic marker genetically linked to Huntington's disease. Reprinted by permission from *Nature,* Vol. 306, p. 235. Copyright © 1983, Macmillan Magazines Ltd. (B) Inheritance of blue eye color. (C) The recessive X-linked pedigree for hemophilia in Queen Victoria's family. (From F. Vogel and A. G. Motulsky. *Human Genetics*: *Problems and Approaches* 2nd ed., 1986, p. 120) (D) The pedigree of dominant X-linked bipolar affective disorder. (From M. Baron et al., Genetic linkage between X-chromosome markers and bipolar affective illness. Reprinted by permission from *Nature,* 1987, Vol. 326, p. 291. Copyright © 1987 Macmillan Magazines Ltd.)

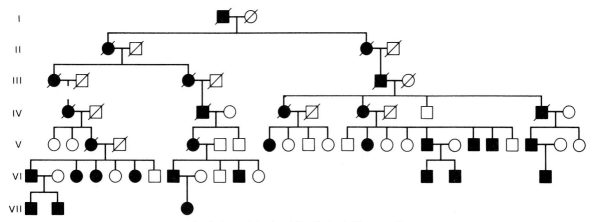

A. Autosomal dominant Huntington's Disease pedigree

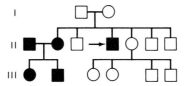

B. Autosomal recessive inheritance for blue eye color

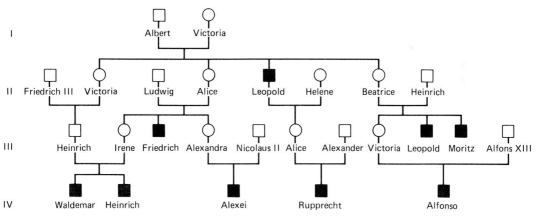

C. Recessive X–linked inheritance

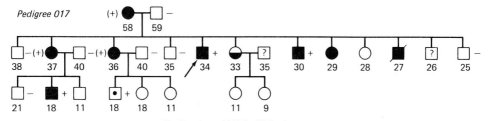

D. Dominant X–linked inheritance

Dominant Inheritance   With dominant autosomal inheritance (not involving the sex chromosome), certain facts are evident: (1) only affected parents can have an affected child; (2) both sexes are equally likely to have the disorder, and (3) the trait does not skip generations. Huntington's disease is caused by an autosomal dominant gene. In the especially unlucky family in Figure 7.6*A*, twenty-one of twenty-eight children in generations II to V have the disorder, although statistically only about half the offspring should have had it.

Recessive Inheritance   In recessive transmission the abnormal gene must be received from both parents for the trait to be expressed in the offspring. The example in the middle of Figure 7.6 points up the following conditions: (1) all children of two parents with blue eyes will have blue eyes; (2) brown-eyed carrier parents can have blue-eyed children; and (3) the trait can appear to skip generations because phenotypically brown-eyed carriers can mate with each other and have a blue-eyed offspring (here the trait is absent in generation I but present in generation II). In interpreting this pedigree, one can assume that the parents of generation I each carried one gene for the trait in question.

The forms of inheritance thus far described do not involve genes on the sex chromosomes. We now turn to inheritance that is associated with sex.

Sex-Linked Recessive Inheritance   Sex-linked recessive inheritance refers to the presence of certain traits or disorders that are associated with a gene on the X chromosome. There are two types of sex-linked inheritance, dominant and recessive. Recessive sex linkage means that the aberrant gene will produce an abnormal phenotype in males because males lack a normal X chromosome to compensate for the defective gene. However, recessive sex linkage produces an abnormality in females only if the gene is present on both X chromosomes. Dominant sex-linked inheritance means that the aberrant gene will be expressed in males and females.

The pedigree for a bleeding disorder called hemophilia A (see Figure 7.6*B*) is consistent with sex-linked recessive inheritance. The pedigree reveals that (1) only males have the trait (this is the first clue that the trait could be sex-linked); (2) not all male siblings of affected individuals have the trait (because in half the cases a carrier mother transmits her normal X chromosome to the child); and (3) fathers never pass the sex-linked abnormal gene to their sons (because they transmit a Y and not an X to their sons). Hemophilia, and color blindness too, are much more frequent in males precisely because they are sex-linked recessive disorders and affected females require the presence of the defective gene on both of their X chromosomes, a fairly rare event.

If a sex-linked trait or disorder involves a dominant instead of a recessive gene, the picture is somewhat different for males and females. (1) Heterozygous women express the trait if one of their two X chromosomes has the defective gene. (2) No sons of affected males express the disorder unless their mother happens to have the disorder. (3) On average, half the children of affected women will have the disorder and it will be independent of the children's sex. A pedigree of dominant sex-linked inheritance for one form of bipolar affective disorder is shown in Figure 7.6. Evidence that it is due to a gene on the X chromosome derives from the fact that a gene for color blindness is close to the gene for the disorder on chromosome 21. The plus (+) or minus (−) signs to the side of each person indicate whether or not that person is color blind. Note the strong tendency for color blindness to segregate with the affective disorder. This does not mean that color blindness causes bipolar disorder, but rather that physical proximity of the gene causing color blindness and the gene for the affective disorder makes them segregate together.

Patterns of inheritance are often less clear-cut. Sometimes a gene is not *penetrant,* which means that the individual has the gene but the trait is not expressed. This can occur for a variety of reasons, the main ones being that other genes may compensate for the defect, or a critical environmental factor that normally promotes expression of the trait is absent. A good example of incomplete penetrance comes from the discovery of an autosomal dominant gene for another form of bipolar disorder on chromosome 11 in the Old Amish (see Chapter 14, pp. 369-370). The data indicate that only about 63 percent of the people carrying the aberrant gene eventually express affective disorder. This means that other factors—genetic and/or environmental—influence the likelihood that the disorder will be manifested.

Multifactorial Inheritance

Certain familial diseases do not conform to simple dominant-gene or recessive-gene inheritance. For example, the rate of schizophrenia is 44 percent for identical co-twins of schizophrenics (it should be 100 percent for a disorder determined entirely by genes) and 7.3 percent for siblings of schizophrenics (it should be 50 percent or 25 percent, depending on whether genetic transmission is dominant or recessive). Although 7.3 percent may seem low, it is more than eight times greater than the rate in the general population (0.85 percent), implying some genetic determination. It may be that genes at several locations along the chromosomes as well as environmental factors are involved in schizophrenia. To cope with the problem of multiple genetic or environmental factors affecting a trait, multifactorial models of inheritance have been developed (Carter, 1977).

Multifactorial Model Illustrated   The multifactorial model capitalizes on the statistical fact that many simultaneous influences, each contributing a small amount to a trait, tend to approximate a normal, bell-shaped distribution. Figure 7.7 graphically illustrates the essence of the multifactorial model.

Suppose that five genes and five environmental factors each contribute equally to the risk for developing a disorder—the higher the number of genetic and/or environmental factors the higher the risk. Suppose also that a score of 8 or greater is required for the disorder to be evident in the phenotype. Thus,

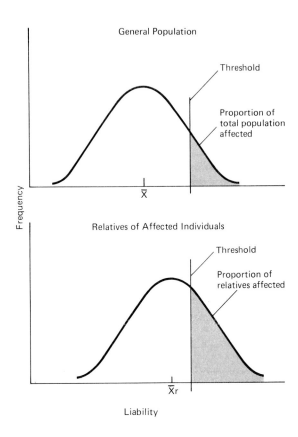

FIGURE 7.7 Multifactorial threshold model of liability. The top figure gives the distribution of the hypothetical liability in the general population. Note that only a small proportion of the general population is affected. The lower figure gives the hypothetical liability distribution for the relatives of affected individuals. Note that a greater proportion of relatives are affected and that the mean of the liability distribution is shifted to the right.

even if one has all five genetic factors, one must also have at least three environmental factors for the disorder to be expressed.

We expect that the risk in relatives of affected individuals will vary with their degree of genetic relationship. Leaving aside identical twins, first-degree relatives share only half their segregating genes, that is, those genes that are not identical in all members of the species. Thus, an ordinary sibling of an affected individual would have, on average, half the genetic risk as an identical twin. Since first cousins share only one-eighth of their segregating genes, their genetic risk would be only one-eighth. The same might roughly be true for the environmental factors as well.

Sex-Limited Multifactorial Traits By adding the concept of different thresholds for the sexes, the multifactorial model can also account for sex differences in the frequency of some disorders. For example, stuttering shows a familial pattern in which males are more often affected, but the incidence of stuttering in offspring is far greater if the mother rather than the father is the parent who stutters (Kidd, 1983). Table 7.1 gives probabilities of stuttering for all first-degree relatives in a study involving nearly 600 stutterers and more

TABLE 7.1 PROBABILITY OF STUTTERING AMONG FIRST-DEGREE RELATIVES OF ADULT STUTTERERS

	Sex of proband*	
Relative	Male	Female
Father	.18	.20
Mother	.04	.12
Brothers	.19	.23
Sisters	.04	.13
Sons	.24	.36
Daughters	.09	.18

*Proband refers to the individual first ascertained in each family.
Source: From K. K. Kidd (1983), p. 203. "Recent progress in the genetics of stuttering." In C. C. Ludlow and J. A. Cooper (Eds.), *Genetic Aspects of Speech and Language Disorders.* New York: Academic Press.

than 2000 relatives. You can see that the relatives of affected females, especially the male relatives, are at greatest risk for stuttering.

To account for the sex difference, suppose that females needed a total score of 9 to become stutterers while males needed only 8. Then, on the average, an *affected* female would have a higher total score than an *affected* male. If the higher total score required to express the disorder arises solely from the genetic side, then the relatives of affected females will be at increased risk for having the disorder also because those originally affected females must have been carrying a greater genetic loading for the trait initially.

HERITABILITY

Heritability is an index of the degree to which genetic differences among individuals in a population can explain corresponding differences in their phenotypes. Heritability coefficients can range from .00 to 1.00, where .00 indicates that genetic differences make no contribution to phenotypic differences, and 1.00 indicates that genetic differences alone (and no environmental differences) determine phenotypic differences. In fact, most traits of behavioral or psychopathological significance fall somewhere between these two extreme values.

Response to Selection

The heritability of traits is one reason that offspring resemble their biological parents. It also explains why some traits respond to genetic selection. In fact, the heritability index was originally developed by agricultural geneticists to predict the extent to which a trait would respond to genetic selection. A simple example of genetic selection will clarify how the heritability index is derived. If a farmer's cows average 1200 pounds and the farmer wanted to increase average weight in the next generation, he would select for breeding only the heaviest cattle. If selected mating pairs averaging 1500 pounds produced offspring weighing 1350 pounds as adults, the heritability index would equal .50 because the offsprings' weight would fall halfway between the herd's average weight of 1200 pounds. and the average weight of those selected for breeding. Had the offspring weighed 1275 pounds, the heritability index would have been .25. Although breeding experiments are not deliberately performed with humans, we can nevertheless ask questions about the heritable basis for the resemblance between offspring and parents from informative matings that occur "naturally," such as a schizophrenic with a normal person. Heritability indexes can also be derived for people of the same generation, such as siblings or cousins, using the same principles as those applied to parents and their offspring.

Measures of Similarity

Heritability estimates are derived from either correlations or concordances among relatives for the trait of interest. Correlations are used for traits that are continuous—height or IQ—and concordances are used for traits that can only be scored as present or absent, like schizophrenia or blue eyes. Unfortunately, a major obstacle to explaining trait similarity is that the underlying environmental and genetic factors often co-vary. For example, siblings reared together are more similar than first cousins, not only because they are genetically more alike, but also because their rearing environments are more alike.

To cope with this problem, investigators try to untangle the normal covariation of genetic and enviromental factors by studying (1) genetically unrelated people reared together, which yields an estimate of environmental influence, or (2) genetically related people reared apart, which provides an estimate of genetic influence.

Correlational Example   Table 7.2 provides IQ correlations for people of different degrees of genetic relatedness reared together or apart. Clearly, as genetic relatedness increases, IQ correlations increase, but the genetic or environmental basis of such a relation is ambiguous unless we have measures permitting us to estimate the two influences separately. That genetically identical twins reared apart correlate more highly than any other group reared together constitutes strong presumptive evidence for genetic factors. It would appear that environmental influences are also important, however, because genetically related people who are reared apart are generally less similar than those reared together.

The correlation of .30 for unrelated siblings reared together in Table 7.2 is derived from studies of young children, typically less than 13 years old. Studies of genetically unrelated older teenagers and young adults reared together since early childhood indicate average sibling correlations of around zero (Loehlin, Horn, & Willerman, 1989). These observations suggest that by young adulthood, shared family environmental influences on intelligence decline with increasing age of the siblings.

TABLE 7.2 FAMILIAL CORRELATIONS FOR IQ AS A FUNCTION OF DEGREE OF GENETIC
RELATEDNESS AND BEING REARED TOGETHER OR APART

Relationship	Degree of genetic relatedness	Reared together	Reared apart
Monozygotic twins	1.00	.85	.67
Dizyotic twins	0.50	.58	—
Siblings	0.50	.45	.24
Parent-offspring	0.50	.385	.22
Half-siblings	0.25	.35	.22
Cousins	0.125	—	.145
Unrelated children	0.00	.30	—
Adoptive parent-child	0.00	.18	—

Source: From T. J. Bouchard, Jr., & M. McGue (1981). Familial studies of intelligence: A review. *Science,*
212, 1055–1059. Copyright © 1981 by the American Association for the Advancement of Science. T. W.
Teasdale & D. R. Owen, Heredity and familial environment in intelligence and educational level—a sibling study.
Nature, 1984, *309,* 620–622, provided the correlation for half-siblings reared apart.

Concordance Example For discontinuous or qualitative categories—the
presence or absence of schizophrenia, for example—a popular but inexact
method for estimating heritability utilizes concordance rates. Concordance is
an index of the extent to which pairs of genetically related individuals are
alike—either for the absence or for the presence of disorder. Heritabilities are
estimated by looking at concordance rates for relatives of different degrees of
genetic relatedness—e.g., identical and fraternal twins. For example, if 60 percent of identical twin pairs are concordant for a disorder compared with 30
percent of fraternal twin pairs, the heritability of the disorder is .60 deriving
from the formula $h^2 = 2$ (identical concordance − fraternal concordance).
Heritability, symbolized as h^2 (not h), is twice the difference between the identical and fraternal concordance rates. The difference in concordance rates
must be doubled to estimate the heritability for the entire genome because the
two types of twins differ only by 50 percent in degree of genetic overlap. Corresponding corrections must be made when other degrees of genetic relatedness are compared to each other. For example, if concordance rates for
grandparent-grandchild versus parent-child were compared the difference
would have to be multiplied by four because their difference in genetic overlap
is only 25 percent (50 percent − 25 percent).

Although concordance rates are widely used for heritability estimates, they
can be misleading if investigators ignore the base rate of disorder in the general
population. To see how the base rate in the general population could affect
heritability estimates, imagine a study of criminality in a high crime rate area.
Many might be criminals for reasons other than heredity. If the population
rate, or *base rate,* for criminality were 33 percent, for example, a 33 percent
rate of criminality for siblings of criminals would be "normal." On the other
hand, if the base rate for criminality were only 10 percent, a 33 percent rate
among siblings of criminals would clearly be elevated. If this elevation were

sustained even when the siblings were reared apart (as when siblings are reared in different homes), that would point to genetic factors. Unfortunately, many early studies used concordances to calculate heritability without providing base rate figures. Consequently, we must often discuss concordance rates in later chapters without being able to estimate heritability.

Heritability for Multifactorial Traits   Figure 7.8 provides a recent summary of risk for schizophrenia in relatives of affected individuals in nine studies that could take base rates into account (McGue, Gottesman, & Rao, 1983). The base rate for schizophrenia, 0.85 percent, appears at the bottom of the figure. Comprehensive analyses of the concordances indicated a .69 heritability for schizophrenia. This means that 69 percent of the variance in liability underlying the development of schizophrenia is due to familial factors that are believed to be genetic. We say "believed" because the study of relatives reared apart usually is required to determine decisively the proportion of variance due solely to hereditary factors.

All heritability estimates fluctuate from sample to sample. Generally, if there is relatively little environmental variation in the sample under study, her-

FIGURE 7.8   The rate of definite schizophrenia in the relatives of definite schizophrenics as a function of degree of genetic relatedness. These data were used to estimate the heritability of schizophrenia. (After M. McGue, I. I. Gottesman, & D. C. Rao, The transmission of schizophrenia under a multifactorial threshold model. *American Journal of Human Genetics*, 1983, *35*, 1161–1178)

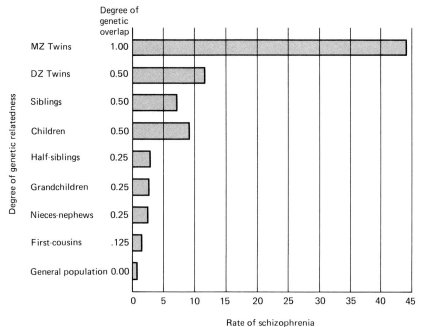

itability values tend to be higher because there is not enough environmental variation to produce differences. Correspondingly, if there is little genetic variation in the sample, heritability values tend to be lower. Precise estimates of heritability are almost impossible to achieve from any one study because chance sampling factors or ascertainment biases usually result in the particular sample deviating from the general population in the average amount of environmental or genetic variation. Only when several independent heritability estimates appear to be relatively consistent can much confidence be placed in them.

ENVIRONMENTALITY

Environmentality, the extent to which a trait is influenced by nongenetic factors, is the complement of heritability. The environmentality index thus indicates the proportion of behavioral variability among individuals that is caused by environmental factors. These nongenetic factors may include physical causes—for example, head trauma or viral infection that affects the brain—or social causes such as maternal deprivation or familial cultural factors. We can get a rough idea of the extent to which environmental factors may influence IQ differences by looking at the identical twins reared apart in Table 7.2. They correlate 0.67, leaving 0.33 as due to environmental factors (including error in measurement of IQ).

Shared and Unshared Influences

Environmental factors can be separated into two broad classes. One class involves *shared* experiences that promote similarity—siblings attending the same school, for example; the other involves *unshared* experiences that promote dissimilarity—a birth injury affecting only one sibling, for example.

Behavior-genetic strategies are among the most powerful for evaluating the importance of shared environmental influences. Any correlation that consistently exceeds the degree of genetic overlap between relatives is evidence for shared environmental influences. For example, if a correlation is much greater than .50 for siblings (who have in common only 50 percent of their segregating genes), shared environmental factors are making those siblings more similar than their 50 percent overlap in genes would warrant in genetic theory. A realistic example of this comes from family studies of juvenile delinquency in which siblings are much more concordant than would be predicted on genetic grounds alone, suggesting the importance of shared family environmental factors.

In recent years, studies of genetically unrelated teenagers and older adults reared together have questioned whether shared environmental influences during childhood have lasting effects on later personality traits or IQ. For example, genetically unrelated pairs of adult adoptively related siblings who had been reared together correlate about zero for IQ (Loehlin, Horn, & Willerman,

1989; Kent & Plomin, 1987) and perhaps only about .05 for various personality traits (Loehlin, Willerman, & Horn, 1987). This absence of a positive IQ correlation by the late teenage years is in striking contrast to the .30 IQ correlation for unrelated pairs reared together when tested as children (Table 7.2).

The implication is that being reared in the same home has no impact on later IQ resemblance and perhaps only a negligible impact on personality trait resemblance in the absence of a genetic connection between the pairs. Given the pervasive and almost irresistible belief that childhood experiences in the home indelibly shape personality and intelligence, these data come as a profound surprise and force us to reevaluate beliefs about the lasting effects of early social experiences. Having said this, we know that growing up together does have an impact on some important outcomes. For example, unrelated pairs of adults reared together from early childhood resemble each other in their ultimate educational attainments despite an absence of IQ resemblance (Teasdale & Owen, 1984). Obviously, familial ambitions for the children can influence the extent to which pairs reared together are motivated to remain in school.

The absence of a correlation among unrelated adults reared together does not necessarily imply a lack of environmental influence, but rather that environmental events may influence each member of a pair differently. One environmental hypothesis is that as teenage siblings extend their social networks beyond the immediate family, they choose different friends who have divergent influences on them. This hypothesis may have some merit, but one should keep in mind that they still live in the same family and usually have attended the same schools. Moreover, without hypothesizing that teenagers are more susceptible to influence by peers than by parents and siblings, it seems unreasonable to suppose that peer influences should be any more powerful than parental influences.

The unshared environmental influences that promote *dissimilarity* are more difficult to identify, yet they could be important for producing differences between relatives. Even for highly heritable disorders such as schizophrenia, relatives are more often discordant than concordant. One possible explanation for dissimilarity is gene-environment interactions: different effects of environmental events on people with different genotypes.

Gene-Environment Interaction Let us illustrate the concept of gene-environment interaction by looking at Figure 7.9, which describes potential outcomes for two different genotypes. In comparison to the "unreactives," the outcome for the "reactives" depends much more strongly on the quality of the environment. Most of those with a disorder in a "good" environment have the unreactive genotype. Their disorder has arisen for reasons other than a deleterious experience. Those affected in the "bad" environment are more likely to have a reactive genotype that potentiated their inherited liability (Kendler & Eaves, 1986).

One concrete example of a gene-environment interaction comes from a study of pairs of young adopted children reared together (Loehlin, Willerman,

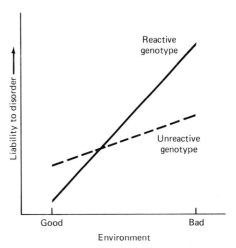

FIGURE 7.9   Gene-environment interaction illustrated. The "unreactive" genotype shows only a small increase in liability for disorder in a "bad" environment. But the "reactive" genotype shows a large increase.

& Horn, 1982). The adoptee rated as *better* adjusted by the adoptive mother had the more maladjusted biological mother, an observation that runs counter to common sense. But the evidence was rather compelling. For example, biological mothers of the better-adjusted adoptees had been much more likely than the biological mothers of the less well adjusted children to endorse items indicating that the mothers cried more easily and were more sensitive than most people. Presumably, being reared in "good" adoptive homes was especially beneficial to the adoptees with sensitive biological mothers. The picture changed ten years later when a follow-up of the adoptees showed that the "sensitive" ones had fared much worse (Loehlin, Willerman, & Horn, 1987). Apparently, the "good" home environment was no longer able to buffer sensitive children from the new problems arising during the teenage years. Consequently, their sensitivity made them especially vulnerable.

Identical Twins Reared Apart

Adopted children have two sets of families. The biological set provides the genes while the adoptive set provides the social/educational environment. Therefore, correlations between adoptees and their adoptive relatives yield estimates of social/educational environmental influence, while correlations between adoptees and their biological relatives yield estimates of genetic influence. We shall discuss the results of adoption studies in many later chapters, but here we will mention an unusual form of adoptive relationship—twins who are separated and reared in different homes.

Identical twins reared apart, especially if separated early in life and reared in different adoptive homes, are rare but invaluable because they allow for simultaneous estimates of genetic and social environmental influences. If identical twins reared apart are as similar to each other as those reared together, it indicates that different social/educational environments have little impact on the trait in question.

Studies based on identical twins reared apart have consistently contradicted the widespread belief that the family environment shared by siblings has an overwhelming impact on the development of adult personality and psychopathology. As an example, Table 7.3 gives adult identical and fraternal twin correlations on the Multidimensional Personality Questionnaire for identical and fraternal twins reared apart, as well as for typical contrast groups of identical and fraternal sets reared together (Tellegen et al., 1988). The questionnaire was carefully designed to measure different personality traits. The three traits presented here (Positive Emotionality, Negative Emotionality, and Constraint) are similar to extraversion-introversion, neuroticism or anxiety, and impulsivity, respectively.

Except for Positive Emotionality, the correlations for identical twins reared together and apart differ only slightly in magnitude, suggesting that being reared together has at best a small influence on their personality resemblance by adulthood. On the other hand, corresponding comparisons among the fraternal twins indicate that being reared together has a modest influence on their degree of similarity. For two of the three traits in the table, however, the identical twins reared apart are more similar to each other than the fraternal twins reared together. In short, while the evidence for genetic influences on personality is compellingly demonstrated in these data, the role of shared environmental influences in making people growing up together more alike in personality is somewhat more limited and confusing. Nevertheless, results such as these challenge environmental explanations for resemblance of people reared together.

One of the sets of separated identicals included in the study had been reunited at age 24. The twins discovered that they used the same brand of toothpaste, a virtually unknown Swedish import. The coincidence is instructive.

TABLE 7.3   CORRELATIONS FOR THE HIGHER ORDER SCALES OF THE MULTIDIMENSIONAL PERSONALITY QUESTIONNAIRE FOR MZ AND DZ TWINS REARED APART OR TOGETHER

MPQ scale	Kinship			
	MZA	DZA	MZT	DZT
Positive Emotionality (extraversion)	.34	−.07	.63	.18
Negative Emotionality (neuroticism)	.61	.29	.54	.41
Constraint (impulsivity)	.57	.04	.58	.25
Number of Twin Pairs	44	27	217	114

Source: From A. Tellegen, D. T. Lykken, T. J. Bouchard, Jr., K. J. Wilcox, S. Rich, and N. L. Segal, (1988). Personality similarity in twins reared apart and together. *Journal of Personality and Social Psychology, 54,* 1031–1039. Copyright © 1988 by the American Psychological Association. Reprinted by permission.

Had they not been exposed to the toothpaste, liked its taste, and made a special effort to obtain it, they would not have been concordant. Trying something new (extraverts desire variety), liking the same flavor, and making an effort to obtain the toothpaste, all could have been based on genotypic similarities. It is difficult to assess just how rare such coincidences are, but they have not been observed among fraternal twins reared apart (Lykken, 1982; Lykken, Tellegen, & Iacono, 1982), suggesting that genotypic influences on behavior can be both subtle and profound.

A pertinent demonstration of the importance of genes in psychopathology comes from an earlier study of thirty-four of these sets of separated identical twins (Gottesman, Bouchard, & Carey, 1984). The twins were moderately similar on all scales of the Minnesota Multiphasic Personality Inventory, a questionnaire sensitive to psychopathology (see Chapter 4); they were especially close on the scales tapping antisocial and psychotic tendencies.

WHAT'S INHERITED?

Any inherited trait must ultimately arise from the presence, absence, alteration, or timing of genetic events. Except for certain physiological syndromes involving mental retardation, however, no unequivocal connection exists in psychopathology between genotype and phenotype. What seems inherited is a disposition, or liability, to respond or transform internal and external experiences abnormally.

Symptoms do not unequivocally point to the nature of a specific underlying genetic impairment. Indeed, specific symptoms may differ considerably from patient to patient, yet the etiology of the underlying disorder may be identical for all of them. This is clear for the genetically identical Genain quadruplets, who were all concordant for schizophrenia, yet differed remarkably in the specific symptoms they displayed (see Chapter 12, pp. 335–337). Some schizophrenics have a good premorbid history and show mainly paranoid symptoms while others have a poor premorbid history and symptoms suggestive of lifelong impairment. Yet relatives of both types of schizophrenics have elevated risks for developing all forms of schizophrenia (McGuffin, Farmer, & Gottesman, 1987).

Conversely, a disorder can have different underlying genetic etiologies, as has been established for bipolar disorder (manic-depression). A bipolar disorder can be produced by a genetic defect either on chromosome 11 or on the X chromosome. Moreover, there are other causes for manic-depression; not all cases can be explained by defects on these two chromosomes.

Because of recent methodological advances, molecular biologists can now identify DNA sequences that constitute specific genes. One of these advances uses restriction enzymes that cut specific sequences of DNA from the rest of the chromosome according to some rule—for example, cutting the sequence CATTAGG into CAT and TAGG using the rule: "cut immediately after a CAT sequence." (A typical sequence is many times longer.) If one family member had a CATTAGG sequence while another had a CTTAGGCAT sequence, the restriction enzyme following the CAT-recognition rule would cut the DNA of the second person at a different point; the fragment of the second person would be longer. The cut fragments are called restriction fragment length polymorphisms, or RFLPs (pronounced ''rifflips'').

This difference in RFLP lengths is important. DNA has a net negative charge so that when exposed to an electrical field between electrodes, longer DNA fragments will migrate more slowly than shorter ones to the positive electrode. Now, suppose that the relative with the shorter fragment has a disorder, while the relative with the longer fragment does not. If this concordance between fragment length and presence/absence of disorder is consistent across many relatives of the family, the restriction enzyme has probably identified a DNA sequence that either determines the disorder or is very near to one that does. Investigators have used RFLP methodology to locate genes for one form of manic-depressive disorder (chromosome 11) and one form of schizophrenia (chromosome 5). These studies will be discussed later.

Diagnosable disorders may themselves depend on their conjunction with other independent dispositions such as emotionality or low intelligence that potentiate the expression of the disorder. For multifactorial psychopathologies it may be only a unique combination of factors, no one of which is remarkable, that results in the disorder.

It should be clear that the genetic approach requires different techniques from more than one discipline. Figure 7.10 outlines how the genotype (at the bottom of the figure) codes for biochemical products that in turn influence various metabolites, brain biochemistry, and development of nonbrain structures that may indirectly affect the brain.

Favorite subjects for behavior-genetic studies are identical and fraternal twins reared together or apart, and unrelated children reared together. With these types of subjects we can investigate, in ways that are impossible otherwise, the specific role of the social and biological environment in shaping behavior. Surprisingly, these behavior-genetic methodologies are among the most persuasive in establishing *environmental* effects on certain traits. For example, the fact that identical twins are not always concordant for schizophrenia is definitive evidence that nongenetic factors influence the expression of the disorder. Without the data on identical twins, some investigators might still be arguing that genetic factors are solely responsible for the disorder.

SUMMARY

Genetic and chromosomal events figure in many forms of psychopathology. Genetic impairments can arise from gene mutations and chromosomal rearrangements. Mutations can be dominant, recessive, or sex-linked. Dominant mutations produce abnormalities whether or not the gene from the other parent is normal. Recessive mutations require that the corresponding gene from the other parent also be abnormal. Sex-linked genes are found on the X chro-

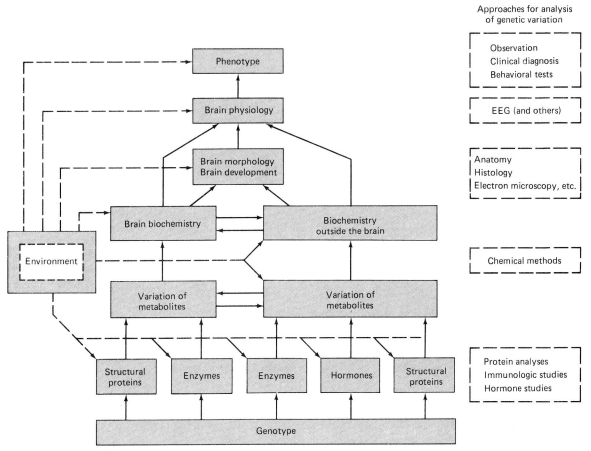

FIGURE 7.10   Levels at which genetic variability in brain function could be investigated. (From F. Vogel and A. G. Motulsky, *Human genetics—Problems and approaches* (2nd ed.). New York: Springer Verlag, 1986, p. 585)

mosome and, where recessive, X-linked abnormalities occur with much greater frequency among males.

Chromosomal abnormalities occur during cell division when either the chromosomes do not separate properly or the order of the genes on the chromosomes is rearranged. Consequently, the offspring inherits an abnormal number of chromosomes or ones that do not sequence genes properly. Many behavioral abnormalities are associated with chromosome abnormalities, including some forms of mental retardation and learning disability.

In recent years more complex models have been developed to account for otherwise inexplicable patterns of disease transmission. For example, schizophrenia is heritable (e.g., identical twins are concordant for the disorder 44 percent of the time and fraternal twins show a 12 percent concordance). Although the fraternal twin rate is more than 12 times greater than expected from the incidence of the disorder in the general population, the ratio of 44 percent to 12 percent does not conform to any simple genetic models. The applicable multifactorial model advances the idea that many genetic and environmental factors combine to produce the disorder when both genetic and environmental liabilities exceed a certain threshold. Studying identical twins reared apart or genetically unrelated adopted children reared together allows us to investigate the relative influence of genes and environment on multifactorial traits. Newer methodologies using restriction fragment length polymorphisms are beginning to identify the specific genetic components in some of these multifactorial traits.

Neurophysiological Facet

OUTLINE

This chapter on brain-behavior relationships adopts a fundamental assumption of the physiological model of psychopathology: namely, that abnormal behaviors often arise from known or discoverable abnormalities of specific brain structures. Consider a young man with a history of severe dyslexia who read at only a fourth-grade level despite years of special tutoring. He also had a history of clumsiness and delayed onset of speech. An autopsy following his accidental death revealed preexisting abnormalities in those regions of the left hemisphere that underlie language capacity. The cause of the abnormality appeared to be improper migration of certain brain cells during weeks 8 to 20 of fetal life (Galaburda & Kemper, 1979; Kemper, 1984; Galaburda et al., 1985). Autopsies of other severely dyslexic patients have revealed similar abnormalities of brain structure. Not all reading disturbances can be traced to such causes, but the evidence highlights the value of studying brain structure and function in the genesis of many kinds of behavioral abnormality. This chapter provides an overview of brain structures that seem important in the development of psychopathology.

BRAIN EVOLUTION AND STRUCTURE

The brains of all modern vertebrates can be divided roughly into three layers (MacLean, 1973). The innermost is called the reptilian layer because it is most prominent in reptiles. It presumably mediates the most instinctive of functions: vegetative processes such as the regulation of body chemistry, sleep-wakefulness, hunger, and the like—and reflexive or highly stereotyped behaviors, in particular, those involving feeding, fleeing, fighting, and mating. MacLean believes that the human brainstem, our reptilian legacy, continues to mediate these vegetative, reflexive, and stereotyped aspects of human behavior.

The other two layers of the human brain are called mammalian because they became prominent during mammalian evolution, roughly 200 million years ago, and because they provide the basis for the more flexible and cognitively sophisticated manner by which mammals carry out survival behaviors. In particular, the paleomammalian layer is involved in emotional and social behavior, and in learning and memory. The neomammalian outer layer, or neocortex, mediates conscious perception, language, and imagery.

Corresponding regions of the brain among evolutionarily ancient and modern mammalian species seem to subserve similar functions, such as vision, memory, and appetite. This is illustrated by the fact that lesions made in comparable brain structures of humans, monkeys, cats, and rats often produce remarkably similar behavioral deficits. It now appears that the "specialness" of the human brain is in the specific regions devoted to language-related functions, and in more and a greater variety of neural tissue (Kolb & Whishaw, 1985). The otherwise many similarities between the brains of higher and lower mammals is good news for reseachers because it indicates that lower animals can be used to study many behavioral dysfunctions observed in humans—for example, anxiety, depression, and amnesia.

Reptilian Structures

The core reptilian part of the brain is uniquely responsible for vegetative physiological functions that are vital to life: heart rate, respiration, sleep-wake cycles and alertness, appetite, and instinctually fixed behavioral mechanisms—for example, reflexive withdrawal from noxious stimuli. Major structures of the reptilian part of the brain are shown in Figure 8.1.

Reptilian brain function in humans is revealed by a condition known as *anencephaly,* or "brainlessness." Liveborn anencephalic infants lack most if not all mammalian brain structures. Nevertheless, they often can maintain vegetative and other basic "reptilian" functions. Indeed, these infants can even learn primitive conditioned responses (Berntson et al., 1983). One anencephalic boy was able to regulate his body temperature and maintain respiration, and displayed near-normal fear and startle responses. The hospital notes are quite instructive.

> If we handled the patient roughly, he cried weakly, but otherwise like any other infant; and when we coddled him, he showed contentment and settled down in our arms. When a finger was placed in his mouth, he sucked vigorously. When he was held supine on the extended hands and dropped 2 inches, he would throw his arms out in fear and then flex them when he again came to rest. He would sleep after feeding and awaken when hungry, expressing his hunger by crying (Nielsen & Sedgwick, 1949, p. 394).

Basal Ganglia The basal ganglia of the reptilian brain (Figure 8.1) control posture, muscle tone, and the initiation of movement. In humans the basal ganglia affect the earliest stages of movement initiation, "the stages when, by processes not yet understood, an abstract thought is translated into a concrete motor action" (Evarts, 1979, p. 179). A defect in this "translation" is evident

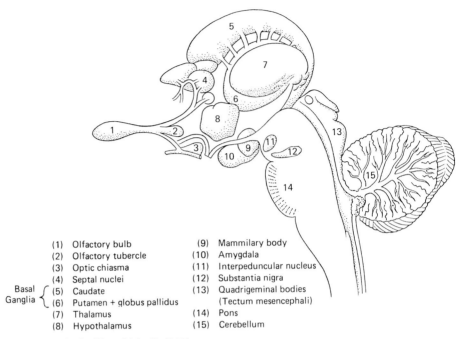

(1)	Olfactory bulb	(9)	Mammilary body
(2)	Olfactory tubercle	(10)	Amygdala
(3)	Optic chiasma	(11)	Interpeduncular nucleus
(4)	Septal nuclei	(12)	Substantia nigra
(5)	Caudate	(13)	Quadrigeminal bodies
(6)	Putamen + globus pallidus		(Tectum mesencephali)
(7)	Thalamus	(14)	Pons
(8)	Hypothalamus	(15)	Cerebellum

Basal Ganglia { (5), (6) }

FIGURE 8.1   The reptilian brain. (From Valzelli, 1981)

in patients with Parkinsonism, an abnormality of the basal ganglia characterized by rigidity or staccatolike movements. These patients sometimes seem to be "frozen," often reporting that they cannot generate the "idea" of moving.

Cerebellum   The cerebellum, lying near the base of the brain, is part of the motor system in all vertebrates. Although it constitutes only 10 percent of the brain's weight, the cerebellum contains more than half the brain's neurons, suggesting its importance for overall functioning. Normally, the cerebellum smooths movements initiated by other motor centers in the brain. In contrast to basal ganglia damage that leads to tremors while *at rest,* cerebellar damage leads to tremors and discoordination *during movement.* The cerebellum generally is involved in modulating and executing motor activities, and also plays a role in balance and in eye movements.

In recent years it has become clear that the cerebellum also participates in important learning functions by virtue of its extensive interconnections with other regions of the brain. It can be shown that destruction of certain regions of the cerebellum prevents the acquisition of classically conditioned responses and probably interferes with long-term memory (Thompson, 1986).

Hypothalamus   A small and complex structure, the hypothalamus regulates basic vegetative functions that include hormone activity, appetite, body temperature, and physiological events that are associated with stress and emotion. Via connections to the rest of the brain, the hypothalamus prepares the organism for action as well as for sleep. Hypothalamic abnormalities are implicated in severe depression, retarded growth in emotionally deprived children, some forms of amenorrhea (loss of menses), and disturbances in sleep and appetite.

Because of its connections to higher neocortical structures, the hypothalamus is responsive to "mental" events—in particular, it translates affective experiences involving anger, apprehension, disappointment, and the like into vegetative abnormalities such as insomnia, loss of appetite, and deviant hormone patterns. In short, the hypothalamus is like a bridge between body and mind, the somatopsychic "direction" involving bodily influences on mental life, and the psychosomatic "direction" involving mental effects on bodily functions.

Ventricles   Within the brain are fluid-filled interconnected cavities called ventricles (Figure 8.2). Special cells lining the ventricles continuously manufacture cerebrospinal fluid (CSF) which flows within and around the brain and spinal cord, bathing and cushioning them from shock.

Ventricular enlargement can arise from atrophy of brain tissue or from obstruction of CSF flow, causing the ventricles to expand. In infants, such obstructions produce a greatly enlarged head, a condition known as obstructive *hydrocephaly,* or "water on the brain." Ventricular enlargement without concomitant hydrocephaly is frequent in schizophrenics. Its specific cause is unknown, but it is believed to arise from atrophy of cortical tissue, which reduces the overall pressure within the skull, allowing the ventricles to enlarge.

FIGURE 8.2   Lateral or side view of the ventricles of the brain. .

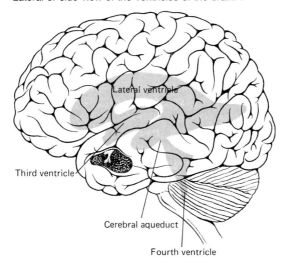

Lateral ventricle

Third ventricle

Cerebral aqueduct

Fourth ventricle

Paleomammalian Structures

The paleomammalian part of the human brain is the evolutionary by-product of millions of years of mammalian evolution. It is composed of the amygdala, hippocampus, septum, cingulate gyrus, and other structures that surround the reptilian core and are themselves enveloped by the neomammalian surface, or neocortex (see Figure 8.3). These tightly interconnected paleomammalian structures are, along with the hypothalamus, collectively called the *limbic system*.

The pivotal role of the limbic system in learning and memory has been greatly clarified by experiments in monkeys. If the amygdala and hippocampus are surgically destroyed, an animal cannot learn a new association between a stimulus and a reward (Mishkin & Appenzeller, 1987). It is therefore not surprising, given the structural and functional similarities between human and primate brains, that human memory disorders like Alzheimer's disease and Korsakoff's syndrome come from damage to limbic structures.

One of the historically most important cases of amnesia is that of H.M. who underwent surgery to remove both hippocampi—one on each side of the

FIGURE 8.3   The limbic brain. (From Valzelli, 1981)

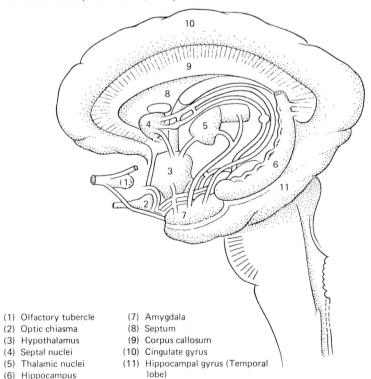

(1) Olfactory tubercle
(2) Optic chiasma
(3) Hypothalamus
(4) Septal nuclei
(5) Thalamic nuclei
(6) Hippocampus
(7) Amygdala
(8) Septum
(9) Corpus callosum
(10) Cingulate gyrus
(11) Hippocampal gyrus (Temporal lobe)

brain—as a treatment for intractable epilepsy. Although H.M. had an IQ of 118, after the operation he could not recall any new experiences. For example, he could not remember pictures seen even two minutes earlier, especially if he was involved in a distracting task during the interval. He would reread the same newspaper with no sense of familiarity, and did not even recognize people with whom he had extensive contact since the operation.

The role of the limbic system in mediating pleasurable and unpleasurable experiences has been demonstrated in the classic work of Olds and Milner (1954) who showed that electrical stimulation of certain limbic sites is intensely rewarding. Some stimulated animals even ignored life-sustaining food while pressing a bar for hours apparently for the pure pleasure obtained. Microinjections of cocaine into these sites seem to have similar effects (Goeders & Smith, 1983), suggesting that the neural substrates of strong cravings and addictions may also involve the limbic system (see Chapter 19).

Abnormalities of the limbic system are also suspected in some forms of affective disorder. For example, people with depression often show diminished appetite, aberrant sleep patterns, reduced capacity for pleasure, and a lack of motivation (see Chapter 13). Limbic abnormalities may also figure in some schizophrenic symptoms such as the lack of motivation and emotional blunting (Chapter 12).

Neomammalian Structures

Geography of the Brain All discussions of brain anatomy and function typically use a standard vocabulary for locating brain areas and structures on the left or right side, in the front or back, or on the under or upper side. Location is important, particularly in the neocortex, because functions often differ for corresponding regions located on opposite sides of the brain. Therefore, discussions about the neocortex will sometimes seem like a geography lesson. We begin our lesson with a brief bit of terminology aided by Figure 8.4. (Although, for simplicity, Figure 8.4 shows only the left hemisphere, our discussion applies to both sides of the brain.)

In both hemispheres, the *anterior* region is closer to the forehead or front. When we say that A is anterior to B, we mean that A is closer to the forehead along an imaginary plane running from front to back. The *posterior* region is closest to the back of the head along that plane, so B is posterior to A. The *lateral* or *temporal* regions are closest to the ears. Finally, the top is *dorsal* while the bottom is *ventral*. When the mammalian brain is bisected, the plane extending through the midline from front to back is the *medial* or *sagittal* plane. If a plane divides the brain into front and back instead of left and right, it is said to be a *transverse* plane.

The neocortex refers to the outermost layers of the brain, with about 90 percent consisting of six layers of neurons called *gray matter,* beneath which are fatty-covered or myelinated fibers called *white matter* that carry information between neurons in different regions. Functions of the neocortex can be in-

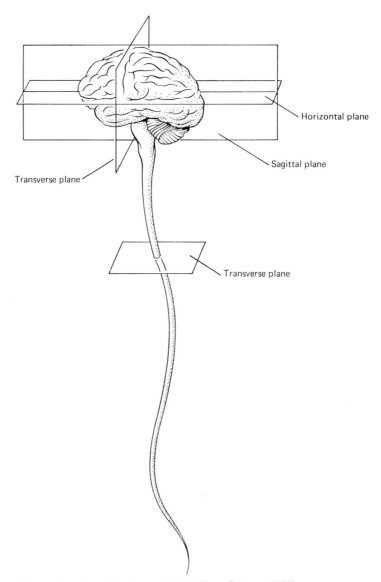

Horizontal plane

Sagittal plane

Transverse plane

Transverse plane

FIGURE 8.4   Planes of sections of the human brain. (From Carlson, 1980)

ferred from the changes in behavior that occur when a neocortical zone is either stimulated or damaged. It has become clear that the components of any complex cognitive task are parceled out to precisely localized areas of the brain for analysis; the results of this analysis are then integrated to produce a coherent perception or a coordinated movement (Kosslyn, 1988; Posner, Petersen, Fox, & Raichle, 1988). For example, analyses of sounds and meanings of words are carried out in different areas of the brain.

Regional Zones *Primary zones* are responsible for the preliminary mapping of sensory input from eyes, ears, skin, and other sources of "raw data" about the body and the external world, and for motor output—specific movements of discrete parts of the body. Electrical stimulation of the primary zones of the cortex produces isolated sensations of light, color, sound, and touch, or involuntary movement, depending on the site of stimulation. Likewise, damage to primary zones produces specific sensory or motor defects such as blindness or paralysis. Adjacent *secondary sensory zones* abstract, elaborate, and integrate primary sensory data into complex recognitions, such as objects, words, and melodies, while *secondary motor zones* integrate elemental acts into organized and coherent sequences.

Tertiary zones, collectively known as "association cortex," modify and combine information from different secondary zones. Not surprisingly, damage to tertiary zones produces deficits in imagery, reasoning, and planning. In short, tertiary cortex is the great integrator, combining specific sensory-based information from diverse sources to produce the abstract and rulefully organized problem-solving patterns that are so distinctively human.

Lobes The neocortex is conventionally divided into four large areas or lobes (see Figure 8.5). The *frontal lobe* extends from the anterior pole back to the first deep indentation, called the central fissure. Research on brain-damaged patients suggests that the frontal cortex has many important functions, including the planning and execution of movement, the control and expression of emotion, and the organization of certain aspects of personality.

Anterior frontal damage can produce impulsivity and a lack of initiative, called the *environmental-dependency syndrome* (Lerhmitte, Pillon, & Serdaru, 1986). People with this syndrome often respond reflexively to specific environmental stimuli. One patient with the syndrome saw a tongue depressor and began to conduct an examination of the physician's throat. Curiously, when confronted by the doctor, she defended herself by claiming that it was done voluntarily.

The frontal lobe area near the central fissure controls movement, and damage there will result in poor motor coordination. It is in this posterior frontal area that the different functions of the corresponding left and right sides of the brain also become evident. Damage to the left side will impair the motor sequencing of speech, causing slurring, a syndrome known as *Broca's aphasia* (*a* means "absence of," while *phasia* means "language"). Corresponding damage to the right side produces *aprosodia,* an abnormality in expressing affective and rhythmic aspects of language—for example, speaking in a robotlike monotone.

The *occipital lobe* in the posterior portion of the brain detects, identifies, and synthesizes visual information. Damage to its primary cortical zone causes blindness or, if more localized, tiny blind spots called *scotomas.* Adjacent secondary cortex elaborates primary sensations into visual forms and meaningful units. Damage to secondary visual cortex does not result in actual blindness,

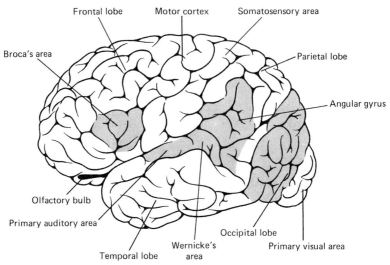

FIGURE 8.5 Map of the human cortex shows regions whose functional specializations have been identified. Much of the cortex is given over to comparatively elementary functions: the generation of movement and the primary analysis of sensations. These areas, which include the motor and somatic sensory regions and the primary visual, auditory, and olfactory areas, are present in all advanced species. Several other regions (dark areas) are more narrowly specialized. Broca's area and Wernicke's area are involved in the production and comprehension of language. The angular gyrus is thought to mediate between visual and auditory forms of information. These functional specializations have been detected only on the left side of the brain; the corresponding areas of the right hemisphere do not have the same linguistic competence. The right hemisphere, which is not shown, has its own specialized abilities, including the analysis of some aspects of music and of complex visual patterns. (From Geschwind, *Scientific American,* 1979, p. 186)

but in impairments in properly perceiving the meaning of visual stimuli. This impairment is called *visual agnosia* (*gnosia* means "knowing"). For example, one patient with damage to secondary visual cortex, when shown a drawing of eyeglasses, called the image a bicycle.

Much of the *temporal* lobe is concerned with detection and analysis of auditory information. The superior portion of the *left* temporal is, in most people, specialized for language comprehension. Damage here often leads to problems in understanding spoken or written language. Patients with such damage cannot properly analyze the meaning of letters and other symbols that they can easily see. The role of the temporal lobe in language function is illustrated by an educator who suffered a stroke, a sudden obstruction of blood flow, in that region of the brain. When presented with the visual stimulus "DIX," he could not read the letters as a word but responded "509," its correct value as a Roman numeral (Gardner, 1974). Clearly, his primary occipital zone for seeing visual stimuli was intact, but the secondary temporal zone enabling him to extract conventional linguistic meaning from the visual stimuli was impaired.

While damage to left temporal cortex usually impairs language comprehension and verbal memory, damage to the corresponding *right* temporal cortex more typically impairs comprehension of the affective aspects of language—for example, the ability to recognize an angry tone in an otherwise neutral sentence.

It has also become clear that the temporal lobe is part of a complex visual system that originates in subcortical structures that distinguish different kinds of information—for example, shape and location. Initially, this information goes to the occipital lobe and then to either the inferior temporal lobe or the parietal lobe, depending on the nature of the original information (Livingstone & Hubel, 1988).

Analysis of shape, including outline and internal pattern, is handled by the occipital-temporal system. Thus, patients with damage to this system cannot say what an object is, although they know where it is (Kolb & Whishaw, 1985). On the other hand, location in space appears to be mediated by the occipital-parietal system. Patients with damage in this system can recognize an object, although they cannot say where it is. Normally, the functions of the two visual systems are so smoothly integrated that their distinctiveness goes unrecognized.

An important function of the parietal lobe—in particular, the primary zone, or anterior region running parallel to the central fissure—is to analyze sensory data from the body. This *somatosensory* information is synthesized by parietal cortex into feelings of touch and texture. Injury to this area of the brain can result in failure to identify parts of the body (somatagnosia) or objects held in the hand but not seen (astereognosia).

The left half of Figure 8.6 maps the parts of the body that are represented in different regions of the parietal lobe. The extent of cortical representation does not correspond to the actual size of the body parts but rather to their significance—specifically the precision with which sensations in these body parts need to be identified. A good deal of tissue is devoted to the tongue, for example, which is vital to speech, and to the thumb which is vital to tool use. The right half of Figure 8.6 represents the motor cortex located in the most posterior portion of the frontal lobe just in front of the somatosensory cortex. Here, too, the amount of motor cortex devoted to any one part of the body corresponds to the precision needed for the complex motor acts that require the use of that body part.

The tertiary zone of the posterior parietal cortex is specialized for integrating visual and somatic information into abstract ideation. Posterior parietal damage can cause impaired spatial orientation like losing the ability to get from one familiar place to another, right-left confusion, and *neglect syndrome,* one of the most puzzling of all impairments. Some patients with damage to the right parietal cortex ignore the left visual world entirely; indeed, they even seem unable to imagine the left half of scenes they are asked to visualize. When asked to draw a clock face, one patient crowded all the numerals onto the right side. Not at all distressed by this, he could see no reason for any concern, a reaction typical of patients with neglect syndrome (McFie & Zangwill,

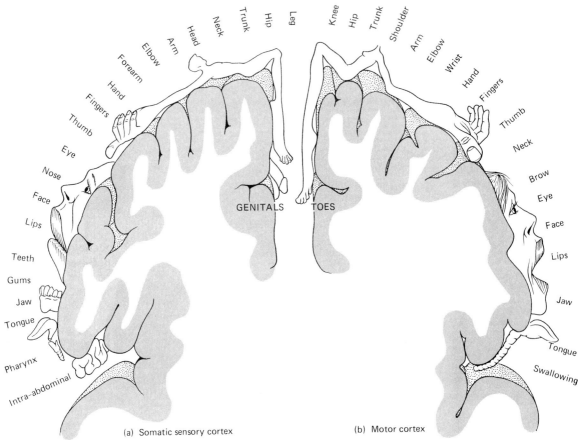

(a) Somatic sensory cortex   (b) Motor cortex

FIGURE 8.6   Somatic sensory and motor regions of the cerebral cortex are specialized in the sense that every site in these regions can be associated with some part of the body. In other words, most of the body can be mapped onto the cortex, yielding two distorted homunculi or little men. The distortions come about because the area of the cortex dedicated to a part of the body is proportional not to that part's actual size but to the precision with which it must be controlled. Only half of each cortical region is shown: the left somatic sensory area (which receives sensations primarily from the right side of the body) and the right motor cortex (which exercises control over movement in the left half of the body). (From Geschwind, *Scientific American,* 1979, p. 182)

1960). Drawings by another patient with neglect syndrome appear in Figure 8.7. Patients with damage to the right parietal lobe also may ignore body dysfunctions as well—for example, a left-side paralysis. Neglect syndrome also can occasionally occur with left hemisphere impairment, but that is usually much less severe (Weintraub & Mesulam, 1987).

Lateral Asymmetry

Our descriptions of the tertiary functions have made clear that the human brain is laterally asymmetrical, that is, the two sides differ in function. Yet,

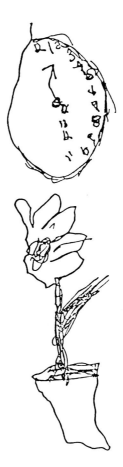

FIGURE 8.7   Examples of neglect on drawing test. (From Strub and Black, 1977, p. 36)

until 1861, this asymmetry was unknown. Then a report by the distinguished neurologist Paul Broca changed that view. He had observed an old man who had lost his speech. After the man died, an autopsy revealed damage to the posterior portion of the left frontal lobe, leading Broca to hypothesize and later confirm this region's responsibility for speech production. This anatomical region, located in the posterior portion of the left frontal lobe, is now known as *Broca's area* (see Figure 8.8)

A decade later, another distinguished neurologist, Carl Wernicke (pronounced VER niki), reported that language comprehension is also localized in the left hemisphere, specifically in the posterior left temporal cortex. Wernicke's observations gave rise to the distinction between receptive and expressive aphasia (Figure 8.9). Damage in Wernicke's area impairs *comprehension* (receptive aphasia), while damage in Broca's area impairs speech *production* (expressive aphasia). While patients with Wernicke's receptive aphasia can speak fluently, often that speech is gibberish because they cannot retrieve

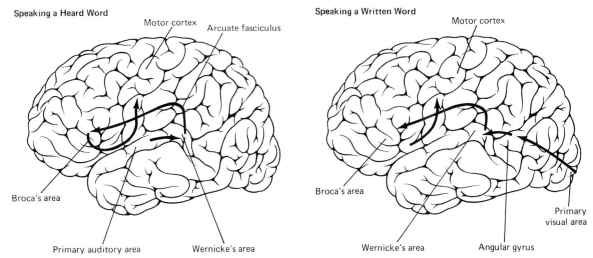

FIGURE 8.8   Linguistic competence requires the cooperation of several areas of the cortex. When a word is heard (upper diagram), the sensation from the ears is received by the primary auditory cortex, but the word cannot be understood until the signal has been processed in Wernicke's area nearby. If the word is to be spoken, some representation of it is transmitted from Wernicke's area to Broca's area, through a bundle of nerve fibers called the arcuate fasciculus. In Broca's area the word evokes a detailed program for articulation, which is supplied to the face area of the motor cortex. The motor cortex in turn drives the muscles of the lips, the tongue, the larynx and so on. When a written word is read (lower diagram), the sensation is first registered by the primary visual cortex. It is then relayed to the angular gyrus, which associates the visual form of the word with the corresponding auditory pattern in Wernicke's area. Speaking the word then draws on the same systems of neurons as before. (From Geschwind, *Scientific American,* 1979, p. 190)

the proper phonemes. They can no longer distinguish the sound units of speech, something like the way native Japanese speakers cannot distinguish the "l" and "r" sounds of English. Recovered patients say that while they were aphasic, spoken language sounded like rustling leaves.

Curiously, until the twentieth century there were few reports of corresponding deficits associated with right hemisphere damage. Now we know that the right hemisphere mediates the perception of complex geometric patterns, sense of direction, music appreciation, and the mental rotation of shapes.

Table 8.1 summarizes cognitive functions that are cortically lateralized. The left hemisphere is specialized for language and other *sequential,* or serially ordered types of information processing, such as deriving meaning from a sequence of words that are read or heard. In contrast, the right hemisphere is specialized for processing *simultaneous,* or "holistic," information—for example, recognizing faces and other configurations, the details of which are all available at the same instant. In normal people, the flow of information between the hemispheres is usually too rapid and efficient to disclose these component processes, but they can be revealed by experiments on split-brain patients (discussed in Chapter 6).

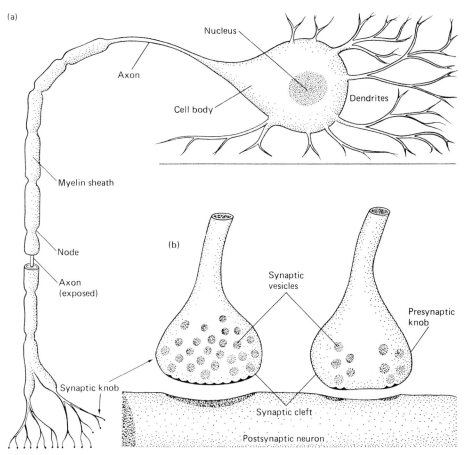

FIGURE 8.9   (a) Typical neuron with many short dendrites and one long axon. (b) Schematic example of a synapse. (From Snyder, 1980)

MICROSTRUCTURE, BIOCHEMISTRY, AND BEHAVIOR

One can examine brain-behavior relationships by looking at the psychological effects of anatomically discrete stimulation or damage in the brain, or by looking at the microstructure, the fine detail of neural anatomy and function. Evidence suggests that defects in microstructure underlie many forms of psychopathology and that correcting these defects may be the most effective means of treating some disorders.

The brain is composed of billions of interrelated cells, or *neurons*, that are specialized for conducting electrical signals. The activity of these neurons constitutes the electrochemical basis of behavior. Theorists have long speculated that some forms of psychopathology are at least partly determined by aberrations of neuronal function. An appreciation of the hypothesis of neuronal

TABLE 8.1 SUMMARY OF DATA ON CEREBRAL LATERALIZATION*

Function	Left hemisphere	Right hemisphere
Visual system	Letters, words	Complex geometric patterns Faces
Auditory system	Language-related sounds	Nonlanguage environmental sounds Music
Somatosensory system	?	Tactual recognition of complex patterns Braille
Movement	Complex voluntary movement	?
Memory	Verbal memory	Visual memory
Language	Speech Reading Writing Arithmetic	Emotional and rhythmic aspects of language
Spatial processes		Geometry Sense of direction Mental rotation of shapes

*Functions of the respective hemispheres that are predominantly mediated by one hemisphere in right-handed people.
Source: Slightly modified from *Fundamentals of human neuropsychology,* 2nd Edition by Brian Kolb and Ian Q. Whishaw. Copyright © 1980, 1985 W. H. Freeman and Company. Reprinted with permission.

disregulation, or "faulty wiring," requires a modest understanding of neurons and the connections between them.

Neurons

Neuronal Structure   Neurons have many forms, depending on their function and location. A typical neuron is shown in Figure 8.9. Its *dendrites* are branched, or arborized, structures that receive information from other neurons. Information is conducted from dendrites through the cell body to a common final pathway, the *axon*. When neuronal conduction reaches the axonal *terminal knobs,* these structures release a chemical "messenger" called a neurotransmitter.

The axon of many neurons, like the one in the figure, is surrounded by a sheath composed of a fatty substance called *myelin*. Myelin acts as a biological insulator, suppressing electrical activity except at the nodes of Ranvier where bare axon is exposed. This arrangement of myelin and nodes of Ranvier facilitates the speedy conduction of neural information by permitting electrical signals to leap by induction from node to node. *Multiple sclerosis* is a disease involving the widespread loss of myelin, thus impairing neuronal transmission and causing both profound sensory deficits such as blindness and motor deficits such as tremor and weakness.

Action Potential   What is the nature of the electrical signal conducted by a neuron? This is a complex question with more than one answer. Therefore, to keep things simple, we will focus on only one type of electrical signal. Simply put, this signal is a discrete electrical event produced by the sudden movement of ions—in this case, atoms with either a net positive or negative charge depending on the "deficiency" or "excess" of electrons in the outer shell. The neuronal membrane, which separates the inside of the cell from the extracellular environment, controls ionic movement. A relatively high concentration of sodium ions (Na^+)—sodium atoms minus one electron—exists outside the neuron. Inside the neuron is a relatively higher concentration of potassium ions (K^+).

If we record the electrical difference between the inside and the outside of a resting neuron, as shown in Figure 8.10, we find the cell more negative inside than outside, approximately −70 millivolts more negative. This polarization of inside versus outside is called the *resting potential* difference.

A dramatic change occurs when this resting state is disrupted by a depolarizing event in which positive ions enter the neuron (see Figure 8.11). Initially, the membrane's capacity to keep the inside and outside separate is compromised, and a sudden influx of sodium ions through the membrane changes the inside of the neuron from a relative difference of −70 millivolts to +50 millivolts.

The increase of positivity from the influx of sodium ions is quickly reversed by two somewhat different mechanisms, one that rids the neuron of excess potassium ions and another that rids the neuron of excess sodium ions. After less than three milliseconds, the initial resting potential of −70 millivolts is restored. The influx of sodium ions can be recorded as an "action potential," or

FIGURE 8.10   Schematic drawing of the method for recording the membrane potential of an axon. (From Carlson, 1980)

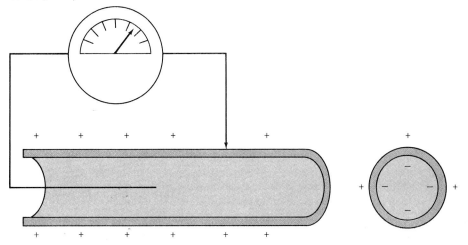

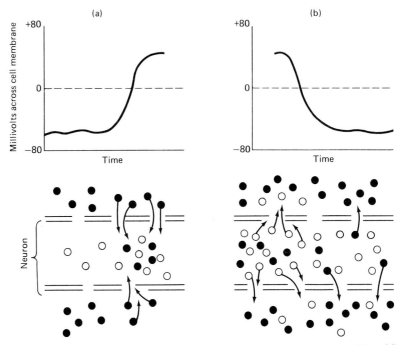

FIGURE 8.11 Propagation of a neural signal (action potential) separated into two phases. Top of figure shows electrically recorded signal; the bottom shows ionic events responsible for the signal. *(a)* Influx of positively charged sodium ions (dark circles) changes the normal −70 millivolts resting potential to a +40 potential (spike). *(b)* Efflux of positively charged potassium ions by repulsion of like-charged sodium ions quickly restores the −70 millivolts resting potential. Within 3 milliseconds, the two phases of the action potential are essentially completed.

an electrical signal. The signal moves down the neuronal cable in only one direction, from the dendritic to the axonal end of the cell.

Neurotransmitters When the action potential nears the end of its journey, it causes the release of neurotransmitter molecules from their storage vesicles in the axonal terminals. Released neurotransmitter molecules move into the synaptic cleft—the tiny space between the end of one neuron and the beginning of the next—that separates the terminal knobs of the presynaptic neuron from dendritic receptors of the postsynaptic neuron.

Dozens of neurotransmitters are known or suspected. Figure 8.12 provides a convenient reference to stages in the synthesis and degradation of four neurotransmitters prominent in contemporary theories about the biochemistry of psychopathology: dopamine (DA), norepinephrine (NE), serotonin (5-HT), and acetylcholine (ACh). Dopamine and norepinephrine are called *catecholamines* because they contain a catechol structure. Except for acetylcholine, each of the neurotransmitters shown in Figure 8.13 is synthesized from an amino acid, a chemical building block of protein. In addition, each neurotransmitter can be degraded by enzymes, biological catalysts that facilitate chemical events without themselves being altered. One degradative

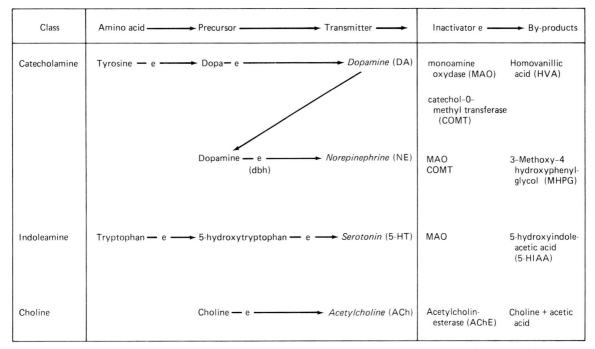

FIGURE 8.12   Metabolic pathways for three classes of neurotransmitter: catecholamine (represented by dopamine and its derivative, norepinephrine), indolamine (represented by serotonin), and acetylcholine. Enzymes (e) are required for synthesis and breakdown of chemical bonds.

enzyme, called monoamine oxidase (MAO), operates within the catecholamine neuron, while another degradative enzyme, catechol-o-methyltransferase (COMT), operates in the synaptic space.

Consider MAO for a moment. Because monoamine oxidase degrades catecholamines, any drug that increases MAO activity should tend to reduce catecholamine levels. Conversely, any drug that inhibits MAO should tend to increase catecholamine levels. Such drugs have concomitant effects on mood. MAO facilitators such as reserpine can induce depression. MAO inhibitors such as iproniazid can reduce depression. In fact, the reciprocal effects of MAO facilitators and MAO inhibitors were an important basis for the initial, and evidently too simplistic, catecholamine hypothesis that depression arises from a deficiency of catecholamines and mania from an excess (see Chapter 13).

Enzymes degrade neurotransmitters into by-products that appear in cerebrospinal fluid, blood, or urine. Finding these by-products can provide indirect evidence of neurotransmitter metabolism, and can be used to assess the psychopathological significance of a specific neurotransmitter system. For example, certain forms of severe depression appear to be associated with low levels of MHPG, the metabolic by-product of norepinephrine.

Synaptic Dynamics

Three Fates for Neurotransmitter Three possible "fates" of the neurotransmitter molecule after its release into the synapse are shown in Figure 8.13. First, it may *successfully cross* to a postsynaptic dendrite where it lodges in a special receptor, altering the probability that an action potential will be initiated there. The second and third fates involve inactivation of the neurotransmitter molecule. Thus, it may either be returned to the presynaptic neuron, an action called *reuptake,* or it may be *degraded* by enzymes in the synapse (just as it can be degraded by intraneuronal enzymes).

Postsynaptic Neural Events How does a neurotransmitter influence the probability that an action potential will occur at the postsynaptic neuron? The postsynaptic membrane contains "pores" that are sensitive to neurotransmitter molecules. When an appropriate molecule arrives at a postsynaptic membrane, it fits into the receptor site of the pore. The resulting receptor-transmitter complex then alters the pore. Now either one of two effects can occur: (a) *excitatory*: the pore allows sodium ions to rush through, thereby increasing the chance for depolarization, or (b) *inhibitory*: the pore permits chloride ions (Cl^-) to rush in and potassium ions to rush out; the net result is even greater relative negativity inside the neuron, thereby decreasing the likelihood that it will fire. An example of an excitatory synapse is shown in Figure 8.14.

FIGURE 8.13 Three fates of a neurotransmitter molecule **(T)** at the synapse: transmission, metabolic degradation, or reuptake. In transmission, the molecule lodges in a receptor on the postsynaptic neuron. In metabolic degradation, the molecule is altered or broken down by enzyme action so that it is no longer a neurotransmitter. In reuptake, the molecule returns, unchanged metabolically, to the presynaptic neuron where it is stored.

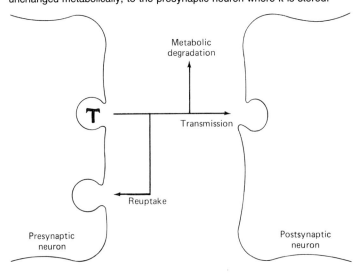

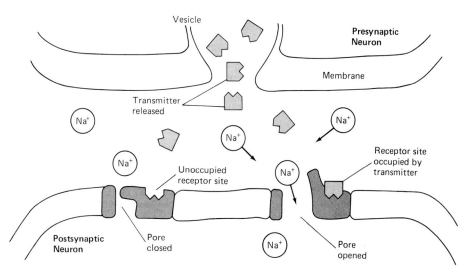

FIGURE 8.14 Excitatory synapse may employ transmitter molecules that open large channels in the nerve-cell membrane. This permits sodium ions, which are plentiful outside the cells, to pour freely through the membrane. The outward flow of potassium ions, driven by a smaller potential gradient, would be at a much slower rate. Chloride ions (not shown) may be prevented from flowing by negative charges on the channel walls.

Autoreceptors   There are also *pre*synaptic sites, receptors on the presynaptic neuron that are sensitive to neurotransmitter substance. Some presynaptic sites are responsive to the neuron's own neurotransmitter. These sites, called autoreceptors,

can also regulate the release of neurotransmitter. For example, if too much neurotransmitter collects in the synaptic space, those *autoreceptors* will inhibit further release; conversely, if too little neurotransmitter collects in the synaptic space, those autoreceptors will facilitate release. Their function can thus facilitate or inhibit the release of neurotransmitter, thereby complicating any predictions about the effects of drugs on the biochemistry of psychopathology. For example, while a drug that blocks reuptake might otherwise make available increased levels of neurotransmitter, autoreceptors may prevent the release of more neurotransmitter, thus producing no net effect on the level of neurotransmitter within the synapse.

Any factor that influences the production, storage, degradation, reuptake, or autoreceptivity of neurotransmitters can affect the likelihood that the postsynaptic neuron will fire. Genetic factors, for example, could produce a periodic insufficiency or excess of reuptake, either of which could alter postsynaptic events and therefore affect behavior.

Wiring Defect Hypothesis   In order to appreciate the problem of synaptic mechanisms of abnormal behavior, one must keep in mind two things. First, neurotransmitters are distributed in interacting and counterbalanced systems throughout the brain. Second, there are about 10 billion neurons in the brain, each with as many as 10,000 synapses, yielding a total of roughly 10^{14} connections. Since each connection may be firing or not, there is virtually no practical limit to the capacity and subtlety of information processing. Clearly, even a "small" abnormality of neural structure or synaptic function, multiplied by millions, could produce behavioral peculiarities which tend to attract social and medical attention. Genetic hypotheses about the causes of psychopathology typically imply some sort of a synaptic "wiring defect" that interacts with environmental influence to yield a liability or a disposition to aberrant behavior (for example, see Meehl, 1962).

Many investigators now subscribe to some version of the "wiring-defect" hypothesis, especially for those severe disorders not associated with obvious organic pathology. For example, consider the hypothesis that psychotic behavior is produced by disregulation within systems of dopamine neurons. This hypothesis is based on observations that (1) certain drugs like amphetamine and cocaine are dopaminergic, that is, they heighten dopamine function; (2) chronic use of such drugs can produce a paranoid psychosis, while relatively small doses can intensify psychotic symptoms; and (3) psychotic symptoms can be ameliorated with various antidopaminergic drugs, that is, drugs whose common effect is to block dopamine function—for example, by selectively inhibiting postsynaptic receptivity to dopamine. Table 8.2 summarizes abnormalities of synaptic function hypothesized as constituents of a wiring defect in psychopathology.

Maturation and Preparedness

During the course of fetal and infant maturation, a dramatic increase occurs in the treelike proliferation of dendrites, a phenomenon called *arborization*. Although the actual number of neurons decreases after birth, each surviving neuron develops many more arborizations, permitting more complex information processing. Figure 8.15 shows neocortical neurons and their arborization in the vicinity of Broca's area of a newborn child, a 3-month-old, and a 2-year-old. Clearly, the complexity of the neural interconnections increases dramatically with age.

Degree of neuronal complexity underlies the extent to which an infant can sense and react to stimulation, but many external events to which the brain can respond may have no enduring impact on later behavior. For example, young rats can learn a simple taste discrimination task perfectly, yet will not show any memory for the task two weeks later. Older rats taught the taste discrimination retain a memory for it over a long period of time. It also appears that the brain requires a certain level of maturation and experience before becoming sensitive to certain stimuli or events. For example, the stranger anxiety that is pronounced in 1-year-olds is not apparent in 5-month-old infants, presumably because their perceptual apparatus is not sufficiently

TABLE 8.2 POSSIBLE FACTORS IN THE HYPOTHETICAL "WIRING DEFECT" UNDERLYING PSYCHOPATHOLOGY

Hypothetical factors	Examples
Metabolic Factor	
Synthesis	An enzyme deficit could produce either an insufficiency or an excess of neurotransmitter. It could also produce "toxic" by-products that distort brain function and destroy neural tissue.
Degradation	Anything that affects the integrity of storage vesicles will expose the neurotransmitter to degrading enzymes within the neuron.
Membrane Factor	
Reuptake	Excess or deficiency in reuptake could have a major effect on postsynaptic activity. Influence over reuptake could account for the therapeutic effects of antidepressive drugs.
Sensitivity	Postsynaptic hypersensitivity might help explain psychotic behavior, given the evidence that antipsychotic medication blocks postsynaptic receptors. Defective activity of presynaptic autoreceptors could produce excess or deficient activity of postsynaptic neurons.

developed or the infant has not yet acquired a firm representation of his caretakers to recognize when a stranger has been introduced.

Brain Injury

Diaschisis   Reactions to traumatic brain injury that include shock, edema or swelling, changes in blood flow, and alterations in neurotransmitters are collectively called diaschisis (die-as-kih-sis). Diaschisis that may last for months from localized brain damage can adversely affect functions not directly involved in the trauma (Kolb & Whishaw, 1985). Much of the recovery that follows brain injury is due to the lifting of the diaschisis in undamaged areas. This improvement has often misled investigators into attributing recovery to neuronal plasticity in which a different part of the brain assumed the lost function. This does occur, but many times it is simply the lifting of the diaschisis that now permits the temporarily suppressed activities to resume normal function.

Early versus Late Damage   Brain injury occurring early in development appears to result in fewer specific behavioral impairments than injury occurring

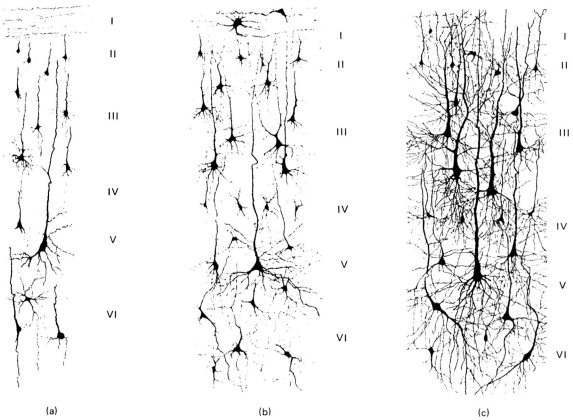

(a)   (b)   (c)

FIGURE 8.15   Postnatal development of human cerebral cortex around Broca's area showing an increase in interconnectedness of the dendrites with age (a: newborn; b: 3 months; c: 24 months). (From E. Lenneberg (1967). *Biological foundations of language;* New York: John Wiley and Sons, pp. 161–162. Original drawings from Conel, 1939–1959)

later. It appears either that the immature brain has less tissue irreversibly committed to specific functions or that its functions are less well localized.

Milner (1974) has argued, for example, that language initially develops in both hemispheres, with the left gradually assuming dominance and suppressing linguistic functions in the right. So, when damage to the left hemisphere occurs, the right hemisphere is freed to assume control. This idea would explain why relatively little linguistic loss follows left hemisphere damage in early childhood. Indeed, acutely injured 2- or 3-year-olds may not show any immediate signs of language disturbance following an injury.

Surprisingly, damage to the left hemisphere early in life produces later impairment in visual-spatial performance, normally thought of as a right hemisphere function. It is as if "crowding" both linguistic and spatial functions into the right hemisphere reduces the brain tissue available to carry out these spatial activities properly.

METHODS OF BRAIN-BEHAVIOR RESEARCH

In the days before sophisticated technology, brain-behavior relationships could be studied only in patients who had sustained accidental brain damage. The classic accident happened to Phineas Gage, a railroad foreman who survived after an iron bar with which he was tamping dynamite blasted through his left frontal lobe (Figure 8.16). Gage, a man of average intelligence and conscientiousness, was dramatically transformed. As J. M. Harlow, a contemporary observer, wrote in 1868:

> The equilibrium or balance between his intellectual faculties and animal propensities seems to have been destroyed. He is fitful, irreverent, indulging at times in the grossest profanity, manifesting little deference for his fellows, impatient of restraint or advice when it conflicts with his desires, yet capricious and vacillating, devising

FIGURE 8.16 Bust and skull of Phineas Gage, showing the hole in the frontal bone made by the iron rod blown through his head. (By permission of the Warren Museum, Harvard Medical School, Boston, Mass.)

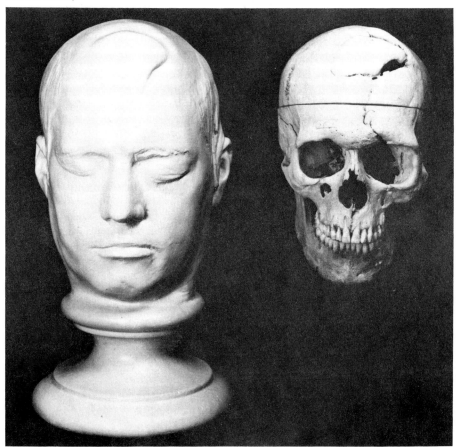

many plans of operation, which are no sooner arranged than they are abandoned in turn for others appearing more feasible. A child in his intellectual capacity and manifestations, he has the animal passions of a strong man (Blumer & Benson, 1975, p. 153).

Case histories like Gage's can be valuable as a resource for study. But so little is usually known about the preexisting character and intelligence of the typical patient—factors that greatly influence the behavioral consequences of an organic condition—that generalizations from the single case must be guarded. Furthermore, accidents often produce lesions whose boundaries are not clearly specified. For example, a penetrating injury can compress tissue or produce diaschisis that alters brain circulation outside the immediate area of the insult. Without autopsy, it can be extremely difficult to localize the anatomical consequences of an injury. Since the time of Gage, however, many new techniques have become available to evaluate the anatomical and functional consequences of an injury while the patient is alive.

Neurological Tests

Here we describe a few of the methods currently used to assess brain anatomy and function. Table 8.3 provides a more comprehensive but still incomplete listing of these techniques

Electroencephalograph (EEG)   In the 1920s Hans Berger first amplified and recorded spontaneous electrical activity in the intact human brain using electrodes pasted to the scalp. His EEG has inspired continuing investigations of electrical activity in sleep, waking, and psychopathology.

The brain generates waves with distinctive frequencies and amplitudes (see Figure 8.17). Different states of mind are reflected in different EEG wave characteristics. Generally, a combination of slower frequency and higher amplitude is associated with less consciousness and with disorganized and dulled responsiveness to external stimulation. A combination of fast frequency and low amplitude is associated with alertness and organized responsiveness.

Computerized Tomography (CT Scan)   The CT scan uses X rays beamed from one side of the head to the other as the machine rotates about the axis of the body. Sensing plates react differentially as the beam passes through tissue of varying density. A computer uses the data from the rotations to reconstruct the density patterns of planes of tissue at different levels of the brain.

Magnetic Resonance Imaging (MRI)   The MRI is one of the most extraordinary biomedical advances for visualizing the living brain. The images produced by this device are almost as good as an unobstructed view. The basis of the technique is described in Table 8.3. It takes advantage of the fact that atomic nuclei align themselves along a particular axis when in the presence of

TABLE 8.3   METHODS OF STUDYING BRAIN-BEHAVIOR RELATIONSHIPS

Technique	Rationale
FORTUITOUS EVENTS	
Accidents, stroke	Correlate site of accidental brain lesion with behavioral abnormality.
Autopsy	Correlate anatomical defects with prior behavioral abnormalities.
CONTROLLED CONDITIONS	
Experimental Lesions	
Ablate specific areas of brain	Assumes that behavior changes resulting from removal of brain tissue implies that area is involved in normal function as well.
Electrical stimulation of brain tissue	Behavior produced by stimulation of specific area indicates brain region subserving behavioral function.
Electrical Activity	
EEG	Aberrant tissue underlies aberrant electrical activity.
Evoked potential	Correlate specific forms of sensory stimulation with specific forms of brain electrical activity.
Microelectrodes	Record from specific neurons, not larger neuronal tracts.
X rays of Tissue	
Roentgenography	Used to visualize radiopaque tissue; e.g., skull, calcification, fracture.
Contrast X ray	Radiopaque dye injected into brain via cerebral arteries or air injected directly into brain ventricles.
Pneumoencephalography	Inject air into lumbar region of spinal column. Air moves up to brain and can be visualized on X ray. Blockage of circulation and displacement of arteries or ventricles can be observed.
Computerized tomography (CT scan)	Like a conventional X ray, except sensors rotate about the patient's head. Using a computer to integrate the signals, it is possible to provide a view of the brain at many levels, instead of the single level view provided by the typical X ray.
Magnetic Resonance Imaging (MRI)	In the presence of a strong static magnetic field certain atomic nuclei (e.g., hydrogen) will spin aligned along a specific axis. If a brief radio-frequency pulse is introduced, the spin will be perturbed as a function of the species of nuclei and the frequency of the radio-wave pulse. The nuclei themselves will emit characteristic radio waves when the pulse is turned off as they return to their original orientation in the static magnetic field. The time it takes to return to the previous state also depends on the tissue in which the nuclei reside, and this "relaxation time" is used by the MRI to produce a distinctive image. MRI is especially suited for distinguishing white from gray matter because gray matter contains more water and, hence, more hydrogen.
Metabolic Activity of Brain	
Regional cerebral blood flow (rCBF)	Radioactive Xenon ($_{133}$Xe) is inhaled with air. Scintillation counters surrounding the skull detect particles as they are emitted from various regions of the brain. More active cortical regions will utilize more oxygen, and the emitted isotopes will be concentrated there.
Positron emission tomography (PET)	A compound tagged with a positron-emitting element such as carbon-11 is inhaled or injected. The positrons emitted collide with an electron and release gamma ray photons, which bounce off in nearly opposite directions. Coincidence detectors at opposite sides of the head register simultaneous events and a computer reconstructs the spatial distribution of the collisions. Metabolically more active brain regions have more positrons emitted.
Neuropsychological Tests	Brain lesions often produce behavioral impairments. Neuropsychological tests work backward by specifying the behavioral impairment and then inferring the underlying brain damage.

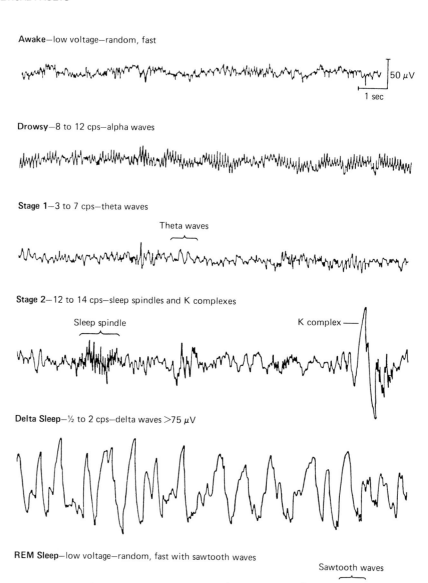

Awake—low voltage—random, fast

50 μV

1 sec

Drowsy—8 to 12 cps—alpha waves

Stage 1—3 to 7 cps—theta waves

Theta waves

Stage 2—12 to 14 cps—sleep spindles and K complexes

Sleep spindle

K complex —

Delta Sleep—½ to 2 cps—delta waves >75 μV

REM Sleep—low voltage—random, fast with sawtooth waves

Sawtooth waves

FIGURE 8.17 EEG wave forms. (From P. Hauri & W. C. Orr (1982). *The sleep disorders.* Kalamazoo, MI: Upjohn Co., p. 41)

an ultrastrong magnetic field. When a radiofrequency pulse is introduced, the nuclei are perturbed and then characteristically return to their earlier alignment in the static magnetic field while emitting radio waves themselves. The time it takes for them to return to their previous alignment, called the relaxation time, is used by MRI sensors to form images. Relaxation times depend on the tissue in which the atomic nuclei are embedded and therefore can be used to distinguish various types of tissue in the brain or elsewhere in the body.

Figure 8.18 compares images of horizontal cuts roughly three-quarters of an inch above the ear obtained by CT scan and by MRI for a normal person. The detail in the MRI is truly remarkable. MRI is especially successful in distinguishing white from gray matter because gray matter contains more water and therefore more hydrogen, which is an especially good resonator (Martin & Brust, 1981).

Regional Cerebral Blood Flow (rCBF) rCBF techniques make use of the principle that more active areas of the brain are associated with greater blood flow to provide more oxygen. The patient inhales a mixture of oxygen and radioactive xenon. The xenon-oxygen mixture moves preferentially to the metabolically most active brain regions where the radiation from the xenon is sensed by surrounding scintillation counters. A picture of metabolically active and inactive surfaces of the brain can then be reconstructed by computer from the numbers of particles emitted. In contrast to the static image of brain anatomy provided by CT scan, the rCBF method provides a dynamic picture of brain function (see Figure 8.19).

Positron Emission Tomography (PET) PET represents a new advance because, unlike rCBF, which works only at the surface of the brain, the PET technique can reconstruct metabolic activity at any level. Like the CT scanner, the PET scanner has sensors that rotate about the patient's head. However, this is where the similarity ends. With PET, inhaled or injected ra-

FIGURE 8.18 CT versus MRI scan. Notice the high resolution for the MRI picture *(b)* of a normal human brain compared with that for the CT scan *(a)*. The horizontal plane of the MRI picture is slightly higher, so that a point-by-point comparison of the two pictures cannot be made.

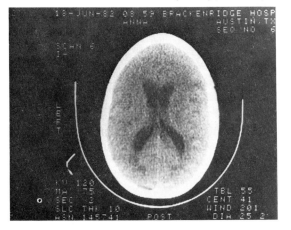

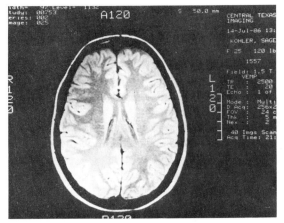

(a)   (b)

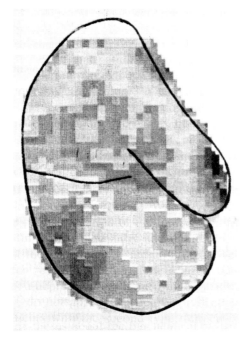

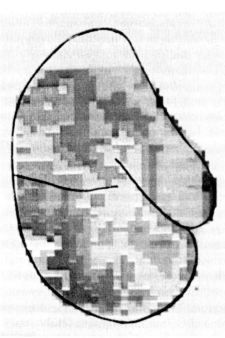

FIGURE 8.19 rCBF. Resting pattern of nerve-cell activity in the left and right hemispheres of the normal cerebral cortex was revealed by measuring regional blood flow, which is closely coupled to metabolic rate and hence to functional activity. The images were generated by a computer from data obtained by detecting the passage of the radioactive isotope xenon 133 through the cortex. Each pixel, or picture element, represents a square centimeter of cortex. Images suggest that in a resting state the frontal areas are notably active. (From N. A. Lassen, D. H. Ingvar, & E. Skinhoj, "Brain function and blood flow," p. 63. Copyright © 1978, October, by *Scientific American*. All rights reserved.)

dioactive substances preferentially enter metabolically more active brain tissue. The radioactive substance emits particles, called positrons, that immediately collide with electrons. The annihilation of these two particles produces gamma ray photons, and these are what the sensors detect. From the pattern of photon hits, a computer reconstructs the location of actual collisions. Unlike the CT scan which represents planes of structural density, the PET scan represents planes of metabolic activity. A PET scan of the brain of an epileptic person is shown in Figure 8.20.

Neuropsychological Tests

Neuropsychological tests represent a different approach to understanding brain function. Instead of assessing brain anatomy and activity, neuropsychological tests focus on cognitive and affective behaviors that are assumed to be correlated with brain abnormalities. Initially, neuropsychological tests were simply more reliable versions of clinical procedures employed routinely by neurologists. For example, a neurologist might have a patient forcefully shake hands with each hand. A markedly weaker grip on one side might indicate injury to the contralateral, or opposite, side of the brain. Instead of relying on subjective judgments of grip pressure, psychologists employed a hand dynamometer to measure pressure more precisely. With quantitative precision available, statistical norms were developed for left-right differences that could be applied uniformly from one laboratory to the next.

Similarly, neurologists had described the behavioral deficits produced by established brain lesions. Subsequently, psychologists devised more objective tests of these behavioral deficits that could be applied uniformly to patients. These tests were eventually combined into batteries, because no single one could assess all aspects of brain function. First, these test batteries were validated by showing that they could document *known* brain damage—for example, a patient with damage in the left posterior temporal lobe would show a deficit on a test of sound perception. Next, the batteries could be used on patients with *suspected* brain lesions, on the assumption that people with test performance like that of patients with established brain injury might have similar brain damage.

In theory, all psychological tests are neuropsychological because the brain is involved in all performance. But unlike other psychological tests, standard neuropsychological tests are especially designed to detect brain injury and even the locus of impairment.

Halstead-Reitan Battery The first comprehensive neuropsychological test battery was devised in 1947 by Ward Halstead and later elaborated and validated by Ralph Reitan (Reitan & Davison, 1974). Each of the original tests could distinguish between patients with and without frontal lobe injury. It was subsequently shown, however, that the tests could also distinguish injuries in other parts of the brain. There are now seven tests in the battery, each de-

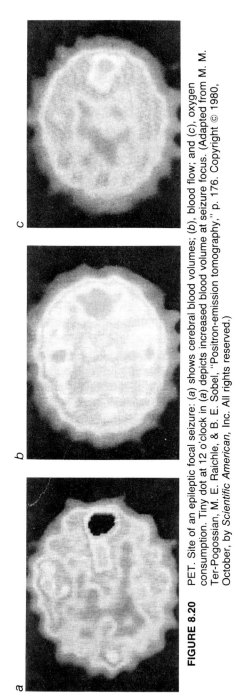

FIGURE 8.20 PET. Site of an epileptic focal seizure: (a) shows cerebral blood volumes; (b), blood flow; and (c), oxygen consumption. Tiny dot at 12 o'clock in (a) depicts increased blood volume at seizure focus. (Adapted from M. M. Ter-Pogossian, M. E. Raichle, & B. E. Sobel, "Positron-emission tomography," p. 176. Copyright © 1980, October, by *Scientific American*, Inc. All rights reserved.)

signed to access a different neuropsychological function. A summary of the tests is given in Table 8.4.

Another test frequently used with the battery is *Trail Making, Parts A and B*. On Trail Making A, the subject must connect a sequence of numbered dots as quickly as possible. On Trail Making B, the subject alternates connecting a numbered dot with a letter, going from 1 to A to 2 to B and so on. Failures on Part B suggest left frontal damage, particularly when performance on Trail Making A is unimpaired.

Usually, a Wechsler intelligence test also is administered to estimate the general level of intellectual functioning. The general level of intelligence may be especially important for predicting school performance or whether the person can return to work. The Wechsler tests are divided into verbal and

TABLE 8.4   THE CURRENT HALSTEAD-REITAN BATTERY

Tests	Stimuli and responses	Processes
Category test	208 slides; *S* picks one of four stimuli according to some principle; seven different subtests; buzzer for incorrect choice, chime for correct.	Nonverbal abstracting, problem solving, learning.
Tactual-performance test—Time	Formboard with ten forms that *S* must replace while blindfolded: first with preferred hand, second with nonpreferred, and third with both.	Tactual-spatial speed, learning with unfamiliar stimuli; problem solving.
Tactual-performance test—Memory	After performing test as described above, *S* is asked to draw from memory the forms and their location.	Incidental memory for forms.
Tactual-performance test—Location	(Same as above.)	Incidental memory for spatial location.
Rhythm test	Thirty pairs of auditory stimuli (beats) presented (e.g., .../.. ...); *S* must declare same or different.	Short-term auditory memory, attention.
Speech-sounds perception test	Sixty nonsense words (ee digraph) presented by tape recorder. *S* must choose one of four written alternatives for each.	Receptive language (phoneme discrimination) and attention.
Finger-tapping test	A lever attached to a counter is depressed as rapidly as possible with preferred-hand index finger, then with nonpreferred hand. Five trials with each hand.	Motor speed and variability.
Impairment index	The ratio of number of tests on which *S* falls above a cutoff point to the total number of tests.	Level of impairment; .5 and above impaired.

Source: From O. A. Parsons, and R. P. Hart, "Behavioral disorders associated with central nervous system dysfunction," p. 847. In H. E. Adams & P.B. Sutker (Eds.), *Comprehensive handbook of psychopathology.* Copyright © 1984 and reprinted by permission of Plenum Publishing Corporation.

nonverbal tests (see Chapter 4). Since the verbal tests tap predominantly left-hemisphere functions while the nonverbal ones draw heavily on right-hemisphere capacities, discrepancies between verbal and performance test scores could indicate damage to one or the other side of the brain.

The Halstead-Reitan battery and other currently popular batteries have some limitations. For example, the tests are sensitive primarily to cortical rather than subcortical damage. The only common behavioral symptom of subcortical damage on these tests is "a certain slowness and proneness to fatigue, which is equally manifested in all spheres" (Luria, 1980, p. 365). Thus, neuropsychological tests cannot identify all forms of brain injury.

Neuropsychological Assessment Overview Neuropsychological assessment serves many purposes. It is commonly employed to evaluate the presence or absence of cortical damage, to localize the damage if possible, and to provide a specific description of information-processing deficits. It also can be used to chart the course of improvement or deterioration in psychological functioning. Therefore, it may be useful in counseling family and patients, especially with respect to their occupational and social future.

Finally, neuropsychological assessment is used to examine scientific questions about brain-behavior relationships. Some of the "big" questions are the effects of early versus late injury, if and how the brain reorganizes after damage, and which brain sites are related to particular psychological functions. Another question concerns the relationship of lateralized damage to left- and right-handedness. Early left-hemisphere damage can often produce a switch of handedness from right to left. If early damage involves the language areas, that function too can switch to the right hemisphere.

With this discussion of brain-behavior relationships behind us, we shift our focus to specific disorders that are accompanied by known or suspected underlying organic abnormality.

SUMMARY

In the course of evolution, humans have acquired something like "three brains in one." The ancient "reptilian" part controls reflexive and vegetative functions, including respiration, body temperature, sleep-wake cycles, and appetite. The paleomammalian part subserves many of the distinctively mammalian functions necessary for personal and species survival, including emotional expression, social behavior, curiosity and play, and cognitive learning and memory. The neomammalian neocortex is largely responsible for the the elaboration of sensory and motor functions into higher intellective processes that in humans include language, imagery, and other complex and abstract capacities.

Many neurological and psychological functions are lateralized to one side of the neocortex or the other. For example, hand movements are under contralateral control; that is, the left hand is controlled by the right hemisphere and vice versa. Lateralized psychological functions include the processing of language (left hemisphere) and spatial analysis (right hemisphere). The behavioral effects of damage to these hemispheres, however, depend on the age at which the damage is sustained. Left-side damage in early childhood typically impairs nonverbal functioning more than verbal; in adults left-sided damage more often affects only verbal functioning. The prevailing explanation is that right-hemisphere verbal functions normally present to some degree in children assume control after damage to the left hemisphere, dominating and "crowding out" normal right-hemisphere nonverbal functions.

Information is transmitted throughout the brain by neurons and the chemicals they produce, called neurotransmitters. Theories about the mechanisms of psychosis, depression, and other types of psychopathology hypothesize corresponding abnormalities of neurotransmitter storage, secretion, degradation, or reuptake. But other physiological theories propose structural changes in the neuron or disease processes that disrupt normal communication among neurons.

Knowledge about brain-behavior relationships is increasing rapidly with the advent of noninvasive ways of assessing brain function. These new techniques include CT and PET scans, measures of cerebral blood flow, and neuropsychological tests designed to evaluate localized aspects of brain function.

Disorders and Treatments

Organic Disorders

GENERAL ASPECTS OF ORGANIC DISORDERS

The main focus of this chapter is on psychological disorders caused by more or less specifiable brain abnormalities. By understanding some established neurological causes of behavioral abnormalities, it may also be possible to shed light on other disorders whose mechanisms are unknown. A good illustration of how this latter objective may be achieved is by studying what may first appear as an intermittent explosive disorder producing irrational violence.

A woman with a history of several psychiatric hospitalizations and many episodes of rage and assault "found herself with a bloody stick next to an unconscious man and surmised that she was responsible for the assault even though she recalled no details." The same patient "once held her psychiatrist at knife-point for several hours and was then amnesic for the event" (Mesulam, 1981, p. 177). Remorse was so severe after this last episode that she brought the psychiatrist a vial of her blood. Her roommate had observed two other personalities in this woman: a childish little girl and an angry adult. These additional personalities, combined with the assaults and the subsequent amnesia, led to a diagnosis of a dissociative state with multiple personality.

Both her neurological examination and CT scan were negative, but her EEG revealed abnormal spiking in both temporal lobes, suggesting temporal-lobe epilepsy. Irrational violence is rare among temporal-lobe epileptics, but some find even mundane experiences so affectively charged with personal meaning that they respond with pathologically excessive emotions. This patient's outbursts were probably related to the epileptic activity, but it was unclear whether seizures occurred during the assaults, and if they did, whether they were the sole cause of the attacks. How would her behavior have been interpreted if there were no detectable EEG abnormality? This question raises an important issue, to which we now turn.

Etiology of Organic Disorders

Functional/organic distinction. In almost all behavioral abnormalities, the affected person experiences pathologically altered perceptions, thoughts, memories, or emotions. If there are no detectable neurological abnormalities, the usual assumption is a *functional* disorder, implying that the patient has no known organic abnormality. For example, had this assaultive woman with multiple personality been free of a known neurological dysfunction, her disorder would have been considered purely functional. When neural abnormality is known or suspected, however, the diagnosis is *organic* disorder, or "organicity." Organic disorders involve structural damage to brain tissue, neurotransmitter abnormalities, or metabolic aberrations elsewhere in the body that disturb brain function.

In short, an organic disorder would, in principle, be detectable if we could remove the brain from a living patient without altering it and perform the proper metabolic and neurological tests. These tests applied to the brain of a patient with a truly functional disorder would reveal no such *physical* abnormalities.

Types of injury. In general, brain injuries of sudden onset such as a stroke (abrupt loss of blood supply due to blocking or bursting of a vessel) or a penetrating head wound are more easily recognized because they produce dramatic behavioral changes. Neurological abnormalities of gradual onset, arising from slowly growing tumors or degenerative brain conditions, are less quickly identified because they produce insidious behavioral changes. Patients often adjust well to the initial damage, but further tumor growth or deterioration eventually brings on recognizable behavioral deficits. Diagnosis is usually more difficult if brain damage occurs prenatally or in infancy; the behavioral repertory of infants is fairly limited anyway and a previously normal base line for comparison is often lacking. Many of the disorders to be described produce symptoms that depend on the location, timing, and type of injury, as well as on individual factors like sex, age, and personality. In describing these disorders, it is good to keep in mind that the case examples given may differ dramatically from other cases with the same diagnosis.

Clinical Aspects of Organic Disorders

Organic disorders typically reveal themselves by cognitive deficits of thinking, perception, memory, or attention, and noncognitive changes including loss of motivation and diminished control of impulses and emotions. Lipowski (1980) arranges organic clinical symptoms into five broad classes: (1) cognitive and intellectual impairment; (2) changes in emotionality and impulsiveness; (3) disturbances of alertness and wakefulness; (4) compensatory symptoms that protect the individual from consciously acknowledging the extent of the impairment; and (5) reactive symptoms that typically exaggerate previously existing personality traits. Table 9.1 provides a summary of commonly observed clinical disturbances in organic psychopathology.

Coping with Brain Damage

One should keep in mind that behavioral abnormalities following brain damage depend not only on the cause and location of the physiological pathology, but

TABLE 9.1 CLINICAL MANIFESTATIONS OF ORGANIC PSYCHOPATHOLOGY

Cognitive and intellectual impairment

1. Memory—defects especially pronounced for recent events.
2. Abstraction—difficulty in generalizing, reasoning logically, and planning actions.
3. Responses to novel situations—especially impaired under time pressures.
4. Attention—defects in sustaining or appropriately shifting attention.
5. Spatiotemporal orientation—disoriented as to time and location.
6. Judgment—impairments in anticipating the consequences of one's actions, especially in social contexts.
7. Calculations—impaired ability to calculate.
8. Body image—distortions of body image leading to misperceptions of one's own body.

Altered emotionality and impulsivity

1. Inappropriate apathy, euphoria, and irritability.
2. Mercurial or unpredictable emotional displays.
3. Poor social appreciation of the consequences of emotional outbursts.

Disturbances of alertness and wakefulness (vigilance)

1. Clouding of consciousness—patient may appear to be in a twilight state.
2. Hyperarousal may be present in withdrawal reactions, e.g., to alcohol withdrawal.
3. Hallucinations and delusions accompanying a dreamlike state.
4. Alterations in alertness during the day, with more alertness during the morning.

Compensatory and protective symptoms

1. Coping strategies to avoid novelty so as to prevent catastrophic anxiety in response to adaptive failures.
2. Denial of defects; invention of implausible excuses to explain performance failures.
3. In contrast to patients with nonorganic psychopathologies, organic psychopathologies are associated with attempts to conceal rather than exaggerate defects.

Reactive symptoms

Patients react to their symptoms with the gamut of functional psychopathologies. Characteristic personality traits are exaggerated. The moderately suspicious may become paranoid; the nurturant may become excessively indulgent.

Source: After Lipowski, 1980, pp. 1365–1367.

also on the patient's preexisting coping capacities. As Birch (1964) reminds us, "We never see an individual whose disturbed behavior is a direct consequence of his brain damage. Instead we see individuals with damage to the nervous system which may have resulted in some primary disorganization, who have developed patterns of behavior in the course of atypical relations with the environment" (p. 8); consequently, it is often impossible to distinguish the direct physiological expression of damage from the patient's attempt to cope. Bizarre behavior in brain-injured patients may have less to do with the specific nature of the damage than with their attempts to reduce anxiety.

Imagine finding that you are unable to copy a square or repeat five digits you have just heard. Anxiety and loss of self-esteem could be overwhelming. Patients experiencing this catastrophic anxiety may unintentionally fabricate implausible stories to rationalize their deficiencies and memory gaps, or they may compulsively perform rituals to avoid novelty or complexity (Goldstein, 1975). They may even deny their disability; for example, a truly blind patient may insist that she can see objects presented by the interviewer, or that she could see them if the light weren't so poor (Critchley, 1979). Clearly, clinicians and relatives must be especially sensitive to aspects of the patient's psychological condition in addition to the impairment caused by the specific injury.

Now that we have discussed some general clinical aspects of organicity, we turn to specific organic disorders. We start with a few of the many varieties of epilepsy, focusing especially on those which may be helpful in explaining aspects of psychopathology that appear so irrational as to be otherwise incomprehensible.

EPILEPSY

Epilepsy refers to a collection of disorders of brain physiology which have as their most conspicuous feature paroxysmal bursts of neuronal firing. A major diagnostic distinction lies between generalized and focal seizures. Generalized seizures disrupt function throughout the brain, whereas focal seizures affect more limited or localized regions of the brain. Quite often, a focal seizure can spread to produce a generalized seizure. Here we look at two of the major generalized forms and then discuss temporal-lobe epilepsy as representative of a focal form.

Generalized seizures are not, by and large, associated with elevated rates of psychopathology. Exceptions are excesses of depression and suicide secondary to the demoralization and adverse interpersonal consequences of epilepsy (Hermann & Whitman, 1984). Focal seizures, however, are more often associated with psychopathology, and many people with focal seizures have been mistakenly diagnosed as having other psychiatric conditions before their epilepsy was recognized.

Petit Mal Epilepsy

Petit mal seizures, a type of generalized epilepsy, tend to begin in childhood and often remit later in life. They usually start with an "absence," an interruption of consciousnes and a blank stare that lasts five or ten seconds, with or without twitching about the eyes and extremities. Ongoing activities are interrupted but posture is maintained. If the seizure occurs while the patient is talking, the sentence may be interrupted mid-word and resumed after the absence, thus indicating that the motor speech program remained intact despite this major physiological perturbation. Although petit mal is generally not associated with other neurological or mental abnormalities (Westmoreland, 1980), absences can adversely affect interpersonal and occupational functioning. Figure 9.1 shows a typical EEG pattern associated with petit mal seizures. Synchronous and generalized spike-and-delta wave discharges occur at three cycles per second.

Grand Mal Epilepsy

Another form of generalized seizure occurs in grand mal epilepsy. Typically, a grand mal seizure begins with an abrupt loss of consciousness; a *tonic,* or continuous stiffening of the body; and an "epileptic cry" caused by the forced expiration of air. This stiffening is followed by diffuse trembling for a minute or two, and then an alternating stiffening and relaxation called *clonus* (see Figure 9.2).

The tonic and clonic stages of the convulsion are associated with specific EEG waveforms. Generalized spiking occurs during tonus. In clonus, the stiffenings coincide with the spikes, and the relaxations with slow waves. In the immediate postictal (after-the-seizure) phase, the EEG slows and the patient falls asleep, awakening later with a headache. Figure 9.2 shows an EEG tracing during a grand mal seizure.

In contrast to generalized types of epilepsy in which the cause of the seizure is often found in subcortical structures with widespread projections throughout the cortex, focal seizures arise from abnormal activity in subcortical structures having more limited cortical projections, or from abnormal activity in a specific region of the cortex itself. While generalized seizures produce widespread derangements in virtually all aspects of functioning, focal seizures produce more specific behavioral dysfunctions.

Temporal-Lobe Epilepsy

Variously termed psychomotor, limbic, or temporal-lobe epilepsy (TLE), this form of epilepsy includes (1) *subjective feelings* such as disturbing, repetitive thoughts, mood alterations, panic attacks, irritability, and an inappropriate sense of familiarity (*déjà vu*) or unfamiliarity (*jamais vu*); (2) *automatisms,* either simple aimless repetitive movements like lip smacking and buttoning and unbuttoning one's clothes, or more complex activities like searching for a missing piece of paper; and (3) *postural changes* that typically involve bizarre positions like those sometimes found in catatonic schizophrenia (Pincus & Tucker, 1978). When automatic behaviors are present, TLE is called

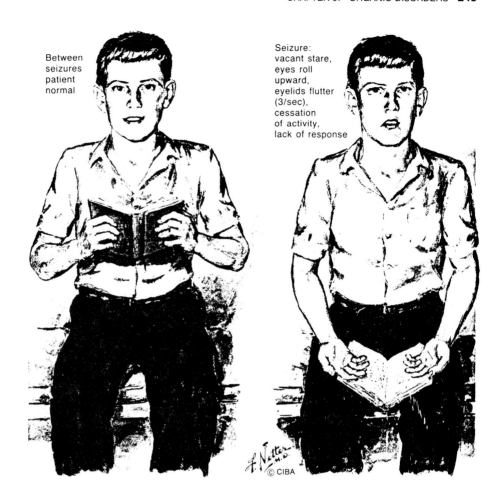

Between seizures patient normal

Seizure:
vacant stare,
eyes roll
upward,
eyelids flutter
(3/sec),
cessation
of activity,
lack of response

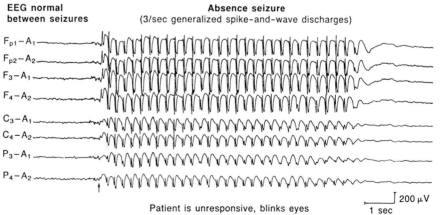

FIGURE 9.1 Generalized 3-hertz spike-and-wave discharge in a 10-year-old with petit mal absences. (From Westmoreland, 1980)

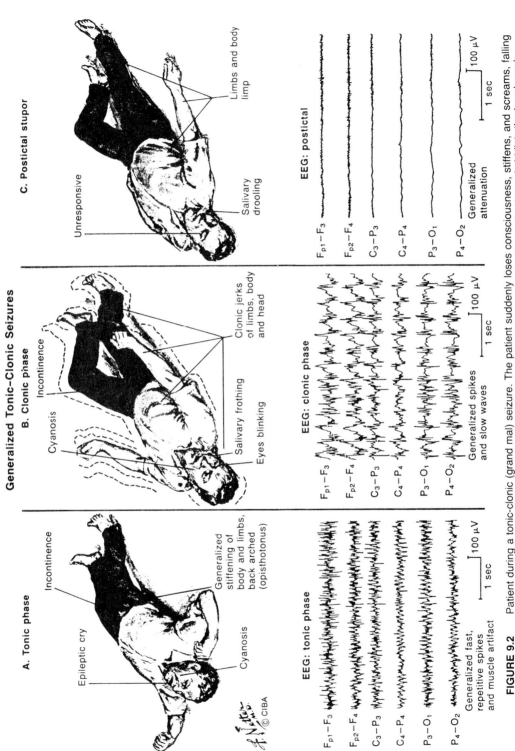

Generalized Tonic-Clonic Seizures

A. Tonic phase

Incontinence

Epileptic cry

Cyanosis

Generalized stiffening of body and limbs, back arched (opisthotonus)

EEG: tonic phase

$F_{p1}-F_3$
$F_{p2}-F_4$
C_3-P_3
C_4-P_4
P_3-O_1
P_4-O_2

Generalized fast, repetitive spikes and muscle artifact

1 sec | 100 μV

B. Clonic phase

Incontinence

Cyanosis

Salivary frothing

Eyes blinking

Clonic jerks of limbs, body and head

EEG: clonic phase

$F_{p1}-F_3$
$F_{p2}-F_4$
C_3-P_3
C_4-P_4
P_3-O_1
P_4-O_2

Generalized spikes and slow waves

1 sec | 100 μV

C. Postictal stupor

Unresponsive

Salivary drooling

Limbs and body limp

EEG: postictal

$F_{p1}-F_3$
$F_{p2}-F_4$
C_3-P_3
C_4-P_4
P_3-O_1
P_4-O_2

Generalized attenuation

1 sec | 100 μV

FIGURE 9.2 Patient during a tonic-clonic (grand mal) seizure. The patient suddenly loses consciousness, stiffens, and screams, falling to the floor. In the tonic phase (left) his torso is arched and he cries out. In the clonic phase (middle), the head, neck, arms, and legs display rhythmic, rapid, and forceful contractions. The EEG recording, showing rhythmic sharp waves and muscle artifacts during tonic phase, spike-wave discharges during clonic phase, and reduced activity during the postical stupor.

psychomotor epilepsy. During psychomotor seizures, patients may reflexively incorporate features of the environment into their activities. For example, if a pencil is nearby, they might pick it up and start scribbling.

TLE has captured the interests of many investigators because of its controversial but oft-reported associations with schizophrenia, hysteria, and dissociative disorders (see Fedio, 1986, for a review of the controversy). About one-third of those with temporal-lobe epilepsy have mistakenly been hospitalized for these psychiatric conditions (Bear & Fedio, 1977).

Many temporal-lobe epileptics routinely attach overly intense affective significance to even mundane experiences. This has suggested that an overactive limbic system sparks the connection of emotions to otherwise trivial events (Bear & Fedio, 1977). It has been claimed that TLEs are more likely than others to keep detailed diaries as a reflection of the intensity of their feelings, but this has been difficult to verify (Hermann & Whitman, 1984). It does appear, however, that psychoses are overrepresented among such people.

The EEG typical of TLE usually shows a clustering of anterior temporal spikes (see Figure 9.3), but half or more of these patients display a normal EEG on any one testing occasion. Drugs such as metrazol that can reduce seizure thresholds, and hyperventilation or sleep deprivation are usually employed to help validate an otherwise uncertain behavioral diagnosis of TLE.

The placement of electrodes can influence whether or not epileptic foci are detected. When Jennie, a teenager who had murdered two children, underwent a neurological examination, neither a routine EEG nor recordings made directly from the cortical surface or from within the amygdala revealed any signs of epileptic discharge. One electrode, however, was placed in the hippocampus deep inside the temporal lobe. When investigators played a tape recording of a baby's cry, Jennie went into a vicious tantrum accompanied by epileptic hippocampal discharges. Presumably, a baby's crying had also triggered the epileptic activity which had set off her violence earlier. Mark and Ervin (1970) summarized the results of their studies of Jennie and others:

> Violent irrational behavior may be the only overt symptom of brain disease, especially when the abnormalities are deep within the brain and do not register on brain wave recordings from the scalp, or even from the outer surface of the brain itself (p. 121).

Cases of such violence are undoubtedly exceptions to the general observation that most people with TLE show no signs of psychopathology (and that most violent people show no signs of TLE). We do not yet know what distinguishes TLE patients with and without psychopathology, but the question remains a conspicuous target for research.

Auras

Many epileptics with focal abnormalities have specific sensations or experiences just before the observable seizure, and these auras may signal an impending attack. Auras can range from simple sensations such as hot or cold

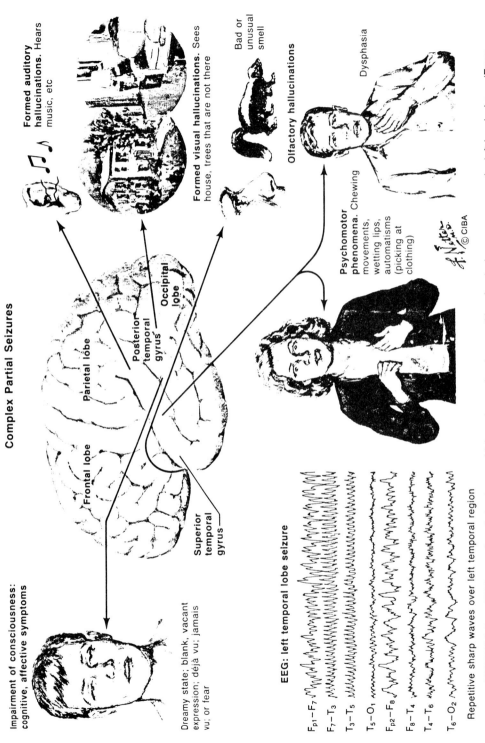

Complex Partial Seizures

Impairment of consciousness: cognitive, affective symptoms

Dreamy state; blank, vacant expression; déjà vu; jamais vu; or fear

Formed auditory hallucinations. Hears music, etc

Formed visual hallucinations. Sees house, trees that are not there

Bad or unusual smell

Olfactory hallucinations

Dysphasia

Psychomotor phenomena. Chewing movements, wetting lips, automatisms (picking at clothing)

Frontal lobe

Parietal lobe

Posterior temporal gyrus

Occipital lobe

Superior temporal gyrus

EEG: left temporal lobe seizure

$F_{p1}-F_7$
F_7-T_3
T_3-T_5
T_5-O_1
$F_{p2}-F_8$
F_8-T_4
T_4-T_6
T_6-O_2

Repetitive sharp waves over left temporal region

FIGURE 9.3 EEG recording during temporal-lobe seizure, showing repetitive, focal, sharp waves over the left hemisphere. (From Westmoreland, 1980)

246

flashes, strange odors, or gastrointestinal symptoms to more complex manifestations, including visual and auditory hallucinations or forced thoughts that cannot be resisted. Some people have learned to recognize that the aura marks the onset of their seizure and have devised techniques for aborting the full-blown seizure. For example, Efron (1957) reported a patient who had a complex aura preceding her seizures. The aura included depersonalization, hallucinations, and peculiar head movements. If a strongly unpleasant odor was present early in the aura, however, the seizure could be averted, presumably because the odor activated a neural inhibitory system. Through repeated coupling of the noxious odor with a silver bracelet, she eventually could inhibit her impending attack merely by looking at the bracelet.

The underlying damage is usually in structures within the temporal lobe, often in the amygdala. It is not clear why the amygdala is especially vulnerable to injuries, but many experts believe that it has a very low seizure threshold and may be damaged more easily during the birth process when there is often great pressure on the temporal region of the head. Other consequences of epileptic discharge from the anterior temporal lobe include complex "automatic" behaviors such as lip smacking, seemingly aimless but compulsive searching, and blank staring. Discharges in the posterior temporal lobe usually produce vertigo and auditory or visual disturbances (Schomer, 1983).

Mechanisms and Treatment

Epileptic seizure occurs with the synchronous paroxysmal firing of many neurons, followed by a period of hyperpolarization during which the neurons become unresponsive to further stimulation. Hyperpolarization arises from the firing of other inhibitory neurons that prevent the paroxysm from recurring. Thus, most seizures are self-limiting. During the epileptic seizure itself, the balance between neuronal excitation and inhibition is somehow lost and excitation becomes dominant (Martin, 1981). Genetic forms of epilepsy reflect certain inherited alterations in either excitatory or inhibitory neuronal mechanisms that in some way bring about lower seizure thresholds.

Treatment of epilepsy ranges from surgery and drugs to behavioral therapies and family counseling. The mainstays of treatment are drugs, twenty or more of which are helpful for controlling seizures. When drugs fail, surgery is considered. A split-brain operation is the last resort for patients with intractable epilepsy, but other relatively less serious operations can be performed. Patients who do not respond to drugs are eligible for surgery only if the foci of their seizures lie in well-defined and surgically accessible places that permit excision without disrupting important physical, emotional, and cognitive functions. Three major questions about epileptic seizures remain unanswered: why they start, why they spread, and how they stop (Pincus & Tucker, 1978).

Epilepsy does not exist as a diagnosis in the *DSM-III-R*. Given its association with mental disorder, the reasons for this decision are not entirely clear. Perhaps its obvious neurological basis and the fact that it is only occasionally associated with psychopathology were responsible for the decision. We now turn to psychopathologies that, with the exception of Parkinson's disease, are represented in the *DSM-III-R*. These psychopathologies are invariably associated with mental and behavioral symptoms.

ORGANIC PROBLEMS INVARIABLY ASSOCIATED WITH PSYCHOPATHOLOGY

DSM-III and *DSM-III-R* divide organic psychopathologies into two broad categories: (1) *organic brain syndromes,* constellations of psychological and behavioral signs that lack a known specific etiology—for example, dementia—and (2) *organic mental disorders,* which have a specific etiology, for—example, multi-infarct dementia caused by a succession of individually small strokes. Although both categories indicate a disease process, the "syndrome" diagnosis pleads etiological ignorance, while the "disorder" diagnosis presumes some knowledge of cause. Table 9.2 provides an abbreviated listing of the two categories and their major subtypes.

Delirium

Delirium is typically a rapid-onset confusional state in which all aspects of cognitive function are disturbed in gross but fluctuating ways. Perception, atten-

TABLE 9.2   CATEGORIES FOR ORGANIC BRAIN SYNDROMES AND ORGANIC MENTAL DISORDERS

Organic brain syndromes

Delirium and dementia—global cognitive impairments; delirium is more transitory.

Amnestic syndrome and organic hallucinosis—only selective areas of cognitive impairment.

Organic delusional syndrome and organic affective syndrome—have features resembling schizophrenic or affective disorders, but suggestive of underlying organic brain damage.

Organic personality syndrome—a marked change in personality, e.g., emotional lability, temper outbursts, no clouding of consciousness.

Atypical or mixed organic syndrome—a residual category for any unclassified organic syndrome.

Organic mental disorders

Primary degenerative dementias—disorders indicating widespread and profound loss of global intellectual functions. Follow a progressively deteriorating course. Appear because of destruction of brain tissue and not because of metabolic derangements in other organs.

Multi-infarct dementia—a stepwise deterioration in intellectual functioning, with "patchy" performances. Suggestive of successive small strokes and focal, as opposed to global, brain damage. There must be signs of cerebrovascular disease.

Alcohol organic mental disorders—class of disorders caused by alcohol intoxication or withdrawal.

Barbiturate, opioid, or hallucinogen organic mental disorder—class of disorders due to specifiable substances.

Source: Abbreviated list from *DSM-III.*

tion, memory, and psychomotor activity are all abnormal. Delirious patients are disoriented and hallucinate, have heightened or lowered vigilance, and sleep fitfully. Psychological testing is useless because the patient is confused or unresponsive. The most distinguishing laboratory test for delirium is an EEG characterized by an excess of slow wave frequencies that suggest diminished alertness. Delirium occurs most often in later life, when the aging brain succumbs to disease or trauma or has diminished capacity to cope with medications.

The course of treatment depends on discovering the underlying cause. In the meantime, however, patients can be protected from injury and reminded of where they are and what is happening in order to help allay the additional anxiety that arises from their confusion.

Dementia

Called the "quiet epidemic," dementia affects a million or more Americans over age 65. With increasing life expectancy, dementia will affect even more people as times goes on. Dementia is diagnosed when the behavioral symptoms suggest global cognitive and memory impairments accompanied by progressive deterioration in social and occupational function. Dementia is not a single disease but the final common path for various neural and metabolic derangements. In contrast to delirium, it is more often morbid rather than self-limiting, involving impoverished more than disorganized thinking, alertness rather than clouded consciousness, and a nearly normal capacity for attention until its final stages (Lipowski, 1980). In dementia, preexisting personality traits often become exaggerated to the point of caricature; the mildly distrustful may become paranoid, the boastful grandiose, and the submissive extremely dependent.

During the early stage of dementia, the patient has failures of recent memory, becoming evasive and providing implausible explanations for behaviors and events in a desperate effort to avoid the catastrophic anxiety that would result from consciously acknowledging newly acquired intellectual limitations. As the disorder progresses, impairments become more global, affecting all spheres of cognitive function. Ironically, the potential for catastrophic anxiety diminishes as intellect declines.

Amnestic Syndrome

In contrast to the general cognitive defects in dementia, those defects associated with amnestic syndrome—in particular, defects in short-term and long-term memory—are specific. Short-term memory losses are especially noticeable. If distracted by other stimuli, amnestic patients will forget virtually anything they just said or has just happened to them. While impairments in long-term memory may be severe, they are typically less striking than the short-term memory losses. The syndrome frequently arises from alcohol abuse, but electroconvulsive therapy (ECT), used for the treatment of depression, can produce the syndrome temporarily.

Another common feature of amnestic syndrome is *confabulation,* when the patient attempts to compensate for gaps in memory by inventing confused and implausible "explanations." Although the extent to which the confabulation is a conscious act is unclear, in some patients it may represent an attempt to conserve their self-concept and dignity. Other patients are apathetic and lack any insight about their defects. Still others vehemently deny the defect in spite of clear evidence to the contrary.

Amnestic syndrome is usually a symptom of *Korsakoff's disease.* The disease typically arises from chronic alcoholism, induced by a thiamine deficiency that damages three brain areas in particular: the thalamus (a subcortical structure involved in relaying sensory information), tissue near the ventricles, and the frontal cortex (Squire, 1982). Administration of thiamine can stabilize the progressive memory disturbance but cannot reverse it. Given the apparent gaps in their memory, patients with Korsakoff's disease do surprisingly well on general intelligence tests that emphasize abstraction and reasoning, but they do poorly on tests that emphasize rote learning and the recall of recent events.

Amnestic memory impairment is illustrated in Figure 9.4 (Albert, Butters, & Levin, 1979). In the study, patients were compared with normal controls matched for age and education. Asked to identify pictures of famous faces from the 1930s to the 1970s, normals recognized the faces with virtually per-

FIGURE 9.4   Identification of famous faces from the 1930s to the 1970s by patients with alcoholism-induced Korsakoff's syndrome (K) and normal controls (NC). (From M. S. Albert, N. Butters, and J. Levin, (1979). Temporal gradients in the retrograde amnesia of patients with alcoholic Korsakoff's disease. *Archives of Neurology, 36,* 211–216. Copyright © 1979, American Medical Association.)

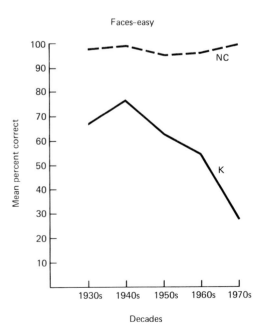

fect accuracy, but the Korsakoff patients showed a decline in accuracy as the pictures grew more recent. Obviously, memories for events before onset of the disorder were spared. We now know that the Korsakoff patients' problem actually comes from a failure to encode new information properly rather than from a specific disturbance in memory. Thus, the reason these patients do so poorly with respect to recent events is that they did not effectively encode the more recent information. Indeed, Korsakoff patients learn slowly, but once they have learned something, they forget at a nearly normal rate.

Organic Psychiatric Conditions

We provide here a brief overview of several organic brain syndromes. The brain syndrome diagnosis makes no presumptions about specific etiology other than a neurological basis that often cannot be clearly specified. Nevertheless, we will give some of what are believed to be the most frequent causes for the syndromes to be described.

Organic Affective or Mood Syndrome This syndrome is characterized by a mood disturbance that resembles either mania or depression. The syndrome typically reflects an abnormality of neural function caused by toxic factors associated with drugs, metabolic factors associated with abnormal levels of hormones, or viral agents. But whatever the cause, an endocrine dysfunction appears central. For example, the constellation of depressive symptoms—disturbed mood, sex drive, appetite, and sleep—suggests something endocrinologically awry (Sachar, 1981). Reserpine, a drug used to treat hypertension, has been known to trigger the syndrome.

Organic Personality Syndrome The chief feature of this syndrome is a drastic change in personality style, especially in the area of impulse control and drive. Propriety gives way to lust or apathy. Emotions fluctuate rapidly, jocularity lacks authenticity, and poor impulse control can lead to antisocial behavior. The syndrome most often is due to a focal lesion in the frontal lobes. Because such lesions can have a variety of causes—trauma, stroke, tumor, infection—treatment depends on the specific cause.

Tourette's Disorder In 1885, Gilles de la Tourette described a strange disorder characterized by *tics*—"jerky" movements and grimaces—other bizarre mannerisms, and often explosive utterances of obscenities (Comings & Comings, 1985). The disorder is quite rare, striking no more than one in 2000, with three out of four cases being male.

The onset of Tourette's disorder occurs typically before age 8. It can vary considerably in severity. The severest, and fortunately the rarest, form can produce an irresistible impulse to mimic at lightning speed everyone the patient encounters. Sacks (1985) vividly describes a particular episode in a 60-year-old woman while she walked down a crowded street.

This woman not only took on, and took in, the features of countless people, she took them *off*. Every mirroring was also a parody, a mocking exaggeration of salient gestures and expressions, but an exaggeration in itself . . . a consequence of the violent acceleration and distortion of all her motions. Thus a slow smile, monstrously accelerated, would become a violent, milliseconds-long grimace. . . . In the course of a short city-block this frantic old woman frenetically caricatured the features of forty or fifty passers-by, in a quick-fire sequence of kaleidoscopic imitations, each lasting a second or two . . . . The woman who was becoming everybody, lost her own self . . . . Suddenly, desperately, the old woman turned aside, into an alley-way which led off the main street. And there, with all the appearances of a woman violently sick, she expelled, tremendously accelerated and abbreviated, all the gestures, the postures, the expressions, the demeanours, the entire behavioural repertoires, of the past forty or fifty people she had passed (pp. 117–118).

Tourette's appears to have a familial component, with MZ twins fully concordant about 53 percent of the time versus 8 percent for DZ twins. If the co-twin is counted as concordant even if only tics are present, the rates increase to 77 percent for MZ twins and 23 percent for DZ twins (Price et al., 1985). About 2 percent of nontwin first-degree relatives are similarly affected. While a 2 percent incidence seems low, this is forty times the general population rate.

About half of Tourette victims report obsessions and compulsions often severe enough to qualify for a diagnosis of obsessive-compulsive disorder (Frankel et al., 1986). High rates of obsessions and compulsions also are found in their non-Tourette first-degree relatives, suggesting that some cases of obsessive-compulsive disorder are genetically linked to Tourette's syndrome (Pauls & Leckman, 1986).

The pathophysiology of Tourette's is unknown, although many believe it represents an abnormality of basal ganglia function that causes an overproduction of dopamine. Indeed, the condition can often be treated successfully by haloperidol, a dopamine-depleting drug that is also used for schizophrenia. We'll say more about Tourette's disorder in Chapter 15.

ORGANIC MENTAL DISORDERS ASSOCIATED WITH AGING

With increasing life expectancy, society must cope with a higher frequency of age-related disabilities. Some people die while they are still capable of independence while the less fortunate die only after suffering for years. Neuronal degeneration is an expected feature of aging. Postmortem examination of the aged brain typically reveals degeneration whose severity correlates with the severity of the dementia before death (Tomlinson, Blessed, & Roth, 1968).

Alzheimer's Disease

The most common form of primary degenerative dementia is called Alzheimer's disease (AD). When originally described in 1907, AD was thought to occur only in those younger than 65 years of age. But now we know that at least half of the 2 to 5 percent of people over 65 with degenerative dementia have AD.

Clinical Description   Reisberg (1983) has proposed a fairly uniform sequence for the global deterioration observed in AD. Early signs such as forgetfulness are often attributed to inattention, but when a person gets lost going to a new place and loses verbal fluency, this excuse can no longer be sustained. Somewhat later the person becomes unaware of current events or cannot recall aspects of personal history. Eventually, the individual may forget the spouse's name and retain only a sketchy knowledge of past life. By this time, the patient, clearly unable to survive without assistance, is unaware of the surroundings and cannot report the season of the year. The patient may be delusional—think a close family member is an imposter, for example—talk to imaginary companions, have compulsive rituals, and become quite agitated without warning. Speech is usually impoverished, and ideas cannot be retained for more than a few seconds. The last stages of AD involve a loss of the capacity to feed oneself, inability to walk, and incontinence.

Etiology   Neuropathological signs of AD are observable throughout the cerebral cortex and in many lower brain centers. The most distinguishing signs in the cortex include neuritic or senile *plaques* and neurofibrillary *tangles*. Senile plaques are composed of degenerated nerve terminals that have been replaced by a starchlike protein called amyloid. Neurofibrillary *tangles* are derived from filaments within the neuron that have become chaotically organized. The function of amyloid is not entirely known, but amyloid is abundant in people with AD, not only in neural tissues but also within cerebral blood vessels (Wurtman, 1985).

The number of plaques and tangles in the brain correlates with the severity of the dementia (Roth, 1986). Behavioral deterioration becomes manifest when a high number of plaques has been exceeded. If the number of plaques remains lower, the widespread collapse of those brain functions associated with cognition and memory does not seem to occur.

Autopsies of patients with AD reveal that neurons throughout the cortex and limbic system have been lost, especially those neurons that contain choline acetyltransferase (Coyle, Price, & Delong, 1983). This enzyme is necessary for the manufacture of acetylcholine, an important neurotransmitter implicated in normal memory function. Indeed, the basis for one unproven experimental therapy for AD involves an attempt to increase the amount of brain acetylcholine in affected people.

A significant fraction of AD runs in families. Relatives of patients are more likely to have the disease and succumb earlier than those in the general population (Heston et al., 1981). Figure 9.5 gives the cumulative risk of AD in first-degree relatives of patients with AD (Mohs et al., 1987). Rates for AD rise precipitously after age 65, and by 90 years of age 50 percent of the relatives are expected to have AD. This proportion of affected relatives is higher than re-

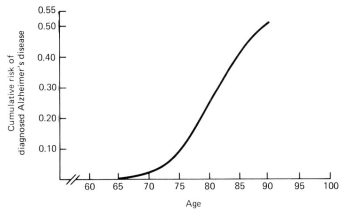

FIGURE 9.5 Cumulative incidence of Alzheimer's disease by age in the first-degree relatives of Alzheimer's patients. Note that by age 90, 50 percent of the first-degree relatives are predicted to develop the disease. (After R. C. Mohs, J. C. S. Breitner, J. M. Silverman, and K. L. Davis (1987). Alzheimer's disease: Morbid risk among first-degree relatives. *Archives of General Psychiatry, 44,* 405–408. Copyright © 1987, American Medical Association.)

ported in any previous study because the investigators took into account the fact that many elderly people are missed because they often die from other causes before developing noticeable AD. These data indicating a 50 percent risk thus suggest that AD is transmitted as an autosomal dominant disorder. The diagnosis of AD can be made with assurance only at autopsy, however, and one must be cautious about inferring the disease when people are alive, even if the course of debilitation appears to be typical for AD. A recent study of clinically diagnosed people with AD found that only half actually had AD at autopsy (Homer et al., 1988). About a third had multi-infarct dementia marked by cerebrovascular deterioration that symptomatically resembled AD.

Evidence now suggests that some familial cases of AD arise from an abnormal gene located on chromosome 21 (St. George-Hyslop et al., 1987). Figure 9.6 provides a five-generation pedigree of one family of twenty-three cases of AD used to locate the defect on that chromosome. The investigators used restriction fragment length polymorphisms (see Chapter 7, p. 195), and found that relatives who were concordant for the disease tended to co-inherit the same polymorphism, implying a genetic basis to familial AD. Other evidence suggests that some cases of familial Alzheimer's disease are due to a gene or genes at another location, but the specific location has not been identified (Schellenberg et al., 1988). Recent evidence also indicates that about half the people with Alzheimer's disease have a membrane abnormality of their blood platelets, raising the possibility that the conspicuous behavioral symptoms of Alzheimer's disease may arise from an abnormality originating elsewhere than in the brain (Zubenko, Huff, Beyer, Auerbach, & Teply, 1988). The upshot is

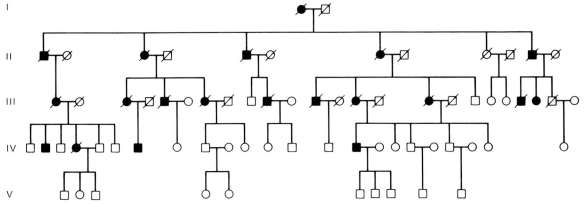

FIGURE 9.6 Pedigree of a family with Alzheimer's disease. (After P. H. St. George-Hyslop, R. E. Tanzi, R. J. Polinsky, J. L. Haines, L. Nee, et al. (1987). The genetic defect causing familial Alzheimer's disease maps on chromosome 21. *Science, 235,* 885–890. Copyright © 1987 by the AAAs. (See p. 182 on how to read pedigrees.)

that the genetic causes of familial Alzheimer's disease may be heterogeneous, which will hamper the search for a specific mechanism. To make things even more complicated, the possibility of a viral etiology for some cases cannot be excluded.

Alzheimer's disease is almost invariably present in people with Down's syndrome by the time they reach 40 years of age. This Alzheimer-like brain neuropathology in people with Down's syndrome was the main reason investigators looked to chromosome 21 for the defect in AD. Curiously, the families of AD cases seem to have a significant excess of people with Down's syndrome. The pedigree in Figure 9.6 happens to include a person with Down's syndrome.

Treatment A drug called THA was hailed as a promising treatment for AD in one recent study (Summers et al., 1986). You will recall that people with AD have a deficiency of acetylcholine. THA presumably blocks the enzyme that destroys acetylcholine, thus making more acetylcholine available for neuronal transmission. Unfortunately, the Summers et al. study has severe methodological flaws that prevent firm conclusions; therefore we must await further research (see *New England Journal of Medicine,* 1987, *316,* pp. 1603–1605, for critiques of the original study).

Pseudodementia

Some demented elderly patients appear nearly normal on various neurological tests. The most likely explanation is that they are only mildly demented. Some, however, have *pseudodementia,* a disorder that looks like dementia, but is actually a secondary consequence of another psychiatric condition. Often these patients behave nearly normal outside of the hospital, but appear confused when examined. The intellectual deficits in pseudodementia can occur as a result of depression, and may be treated successfully with antidepressant drugs (Wells, 1978). Since such deficits are not prominent in younger depressed individuals, pseudodementia caused by depression is a puzzle.

The diagnosis of pseudodementia must be made cautiously, however, because better diagnostic tools may reveal previously hidden organic deficits that indicate a true degenerative dementia. For example, one patient diagnosed with pseudodementia was later found with a new-generation CT scanner to have frontal lobe atrophy (Caine, 1981). It has been suggested that the tendency to become demented when depressed may indicate a proneness to dementia so that, upon follow-up, after successful treatment of the depression, the patient may begin to display signs of a genuine dementia (Clarfield, 1988).

Parkinson's Disease

Clinical Description In 1817, James Parkinson first described a disease now known to affect 1 percent of the over-50 population. The symptoms of Parkinson's disease include progressive loss of voluntary movement, muscular rigidity, slowness, and aberrant postural control that often produces a distinctive shuffling gait (Dakof & Mendelsohn, 1986). One of its most striking motoric symptoms is *festination,* the tendency to accelerate the tempo of movement, speech, or thought in a dramatic and involuntary manner. For example, after initiating a slow walk, such individuals soon find themselves nearly running.

Mechanisms and Etiology There are two major natural etiologies of Parkinsonism: a more frequent idiopathic type whose ultimate cause is unknown, associated with aging, and a rarer type caused by a viral encephalitis epidemic in the 1920s. Parkinsonism can also be caused by MPTP, a compound used to illegally manufacture a synthetic heroin. Whatever the etiology, however, Parkinsonism involves a decrease of dopamine-rich pigmented cells in the substantia nigra, a major part of the basal ganglia (Figure 9.7).

> Post-encephalitic Parkinsonism, as opposed to idiopathic Parkinsonism, tended to show less in the way of tremor or rigidity . . . but much severer states of "explosive" and "obstructive" disorders, of akinesia [literally, without movement] and akathisia [cruel restlessness], push and resistance, hurry and impediment . . . . Many patients were swallowed up . . . in states of Parkinson akinesia so profound as to turn them into living statues—totally motionless for hours, days, weeks, or years on end . . . all aspects of being and behavior—perceptions, thought, appetites, and feelings, no less than movements—were brought to a virtual standstill by an active, constraining Parkinsonian process (Sacks, 1974, pp. 32–33).

Some patients suffering from postencephalitic Parkinsonism have been mistakenly diagnosed as catatonic schizophrenics. Indeed, aspects of their behav-

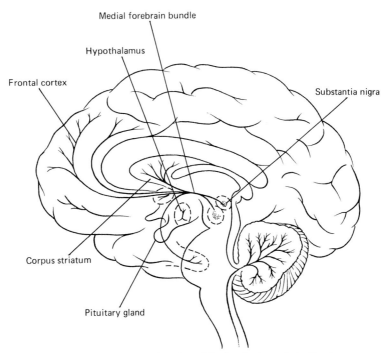

Medial forebrain bundle

Hypothalamus

Frontal cortex

Substantia nigra

Corpus striatum

Pituitary gland

FIGURE 9.7   One set of dopamine-rich tracts has its cell bodies in the substantia nigra, a structure in the midbrain. Ascending fibers enter the corpus striatum, a structure involved in regulating motor activity, to form the nigrostriatal tract. Depletion of dopamine in this tract is associated with the etiology of Parkinsonism. (Adapted from illustration by Albert Miller, from "The chemistry of the brain," by Leslie Iverson. Copyright © 1979, September, by *Scientific American.* All rights reserved.)

ior bear a remarkable resemblance to that disorder. Sacks (1974) put it this way:

> Some of these patients showed automatic compliance . . . maintaining (indefinitely, and apparently without effort) any posture in which they were put or found themselves, or "echoing" words, phrases, thoughts, perceptions or actions in an unvarying circular way, once these had been suggested to them (pp. 33–34).

Not only is the initiation and monitoring of motor activity impaired in all forms of Parkinsonism, but intentions can actually give rise to their opposites. Thus, willing a movement only produces a more profound loss of movement, or *akinesia*. The basal ganglia are implicated in the behavioral symptoms because they are particularly important for initiating movement in the absence of sensory guidance, that is, when a person initiates a movement based on a memory trace rather than from an external stimulus (Evarts et al., 1984).

It thus becomes possible to understand why patients otherwise disabled with Parkinsonism have acted heroically and nearly normally in situations where survival needs or emotional arousal were prominent. One severely disabled patient typically confined to a wheelchair raced into the water to rescue someone, only to collapse promptly after the emergency was over. Another could move normally while climbing stairs, yet became immobile after reaching the top (Sacks, 1974). In these cases the movements involved were probably sensory-prompted rather than willed in the absence of sensory guidance.

Many features of Parkinsonism can be reproduced by administering a drug that depletes dopamine neurons. Animals given the drug display virtually all the motor features of the disease, including moving normally if a predator is introduced or if dropped into cold water (see Marshall, Levitan, & Stricker, 1976). Parkinson symptoms can also be a debilitating side effect of neuroleptic antipsychotic treatment, because these drugs work by blocking the uptake of dopamine in the postsynaptic neuron.

Treatment   Parkinsonism is usually helped by L-dopa, a chemical precursor of dopamine (see Chapter 8). Unlike dopamine, L-dopa can pass through the blood-brain barrier and once in the brain, can be converted to dopamine and utilized by those cells still functioning in the substantia nigra. Originally it was hailed as a miracle drug because it could arouse patients with chronic immobility and painfully distorted posture to near normal activity. Unfortunately, L-dopa eventually loses its effectiveness, because the dopamine neurons continue to degenerate unabated and there remain few functional cells on which the drug can work. Nevertheless, L-dopa can provide a better life for the majority of patients, at least for a few years.

Having briefly surveyed some organic syndromes and disorders, we now turn to the behavioral effects of brain lesions caused by traumatic head injury.

HEAD INJURY

Traumatic head injuries are quite common. Despite their high prevalence, head injuries have consequences that are difficult to evaluate without some preinjury base line. Rare studies with a preinjury base line suggest that certain types of people are accident-prone. For example, previously hyperactive and impulsive children are more likely to sustain mild head injuries (Rutter, 1981). Without the base line, one would have overestimated the frequency of hyperactivity and impulsivity caused by mild head injuries rather than resulting from it.

Mild head injuries usually result in no obvious impairments, but severe head injuries usually cause loss of consciousness. Loss of consciousness typically results in an *anterograde* amnesia for events that follow an injury, but it may also produce a *retrograde* amnesia for events prior to the injury. Both anterograde and retrograde amnesia tend to diminish with time after trauma. Figure 9.8 shows the diminution of retrograde amnesia between six and sixteen months after a traumatic head injury (Barbizet, 1970). This patient remained

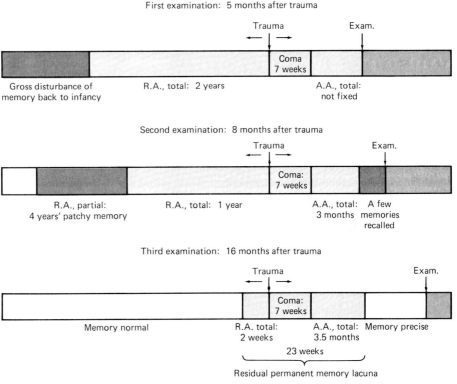

FIGURE 9.8 Development of posttraumatic amnesia. Mr. G, 40 years old, cranial trauma on Oct. 17, 1963; R. A., retrograde amnesia: A.A., anterograde amnesia. (From *Human memory and its pathology* by Jacques Barbizet. Copyright © 1970 W. H. Freeman and Company. Reprinted with permission.)

permanently amnesic for the twenty-one weeks following the injury, but showed dramatic improvement in memory for events prior to the trauma.

The extent of amnesia predicts subsequent psychiatric and intellectual disability. Table 9.3 gives frequencies for various degrees of disability following penetrating head injuries; the more severe the posttraumatic anterograde amnesia, the more probable and severe the subsequent disability. Penetrating brain damage can also result in personality changes in the absence of intellectual impairments.

A congenial and supportive environment appears to promote recovery from brain injury (Finger & Stein, 1982). In brain-injured children, the more adverse the social climate, such as high family discord, the less likely a favorable recovery (Rutter, 1981). A simplified overview of the behavioral consequences of penetrating brain injury by site of damage appears in Table 9.4. The most important points here are that left-hemisphere injury more often produces intellectual deficits, while right-hemisphere injury leads to affective, behavioral, and somatic problems, and that frontal lobe damage is most like to produce deterioration in personality and social functioning.

TABLE 9.3   DURATION OF POSTTRAUMATIC AMNESIA RELATES TO PSYCHIATRIC AND GENERAL INTELLECTUAL DISABILITIES

Duration of posttraumatic amnesia	No. of patients	Percentage with severe psychiatric disability	Percentage with severe intellectual disability
< 1 hour	329	12	2
< 7 days	131	24	3
> 7 days	210	34	11

Source: From Lishman (1978).

Two personality disorders resulting from frontal damage are well known (Blumer & Benson, 1975). Which type the patient suffers appears to depend on the precise location of the injury. The first type, called *pseudodepressive,* is distinguished by apathy and indifference. Although pseudodepressives have lost their spontaneity and do little actively to shape their environments, they often respond appropriately to direct commands. The "pseudo" prefix signifies a depression different from typical depression. These patients, for example, do not appear worried or preoccupied with guilt like other depressives. Patients with the second type, termed *pseudopsychopathic,* have symptoms quite similar to those with organic personality syndrome, displaying unwarranted impulsivity and euphoria. Lacking tact and restraint, they often act without anticipating consequences. Although the behavior of the frontal pseudopsychopath can resemble that of the true psychopath, the premorbid history reveals no lack of restraint, impulsivity, or trouble with authority so characteristic of the true psychopath. Indeed, when a previously normal adult starts showing generalized signs of uninhibited psychopathic behavior, there is a fair chance of drug abuse or recently acquired frontal damage.

LINGUISTIC IMPAIRMENTS

Because the currency of human interchange is language, impairments in reading, speaking, and understanding language produce educationally and socially

TABLE 9.4   SIMPLIFIED TABLE OF SYMPTOMS FIVE YEARS AFTER A PENETRATING INJURY ACCORDING TO THE LOCATION OF THE DAMAGE

Symptom	Hemisphere		Lobe			
	Left	Right	Frontal	Parietal	Temporal	Occipital
Intellectual impairments	*			*	*	?
Behavioral (e.g., criminality)		*	*	*	*	
Somatic complaints (e.g., headaches)		*	*			?
Frontal-lobe syndrome		*	*			

Source: Substantially simplified from Lishman (1978).

debilitating handicaps. Not only do such handicaps make it difficult to learn much of what is considered culturally important, but affected individuals are often isolated from much social interchange. The *DSM-III-R* includes the diagnosis of some developmental language disorders in children, but says little about aphasias acquired in adulthood.

Aphasias

Aphasias are disorders of language that arise abruptly in a previously normal individual. The disorders can be either expressive and/or receptive. The *expressive* types involve no loss of language comprehension but rather are marked by impaired and sluggish speech that is often described as nonfluent. In contrast, *receptive* aphasias involve little loss of speech fluency but rather impaired language comprehension. To some extent a disorder of one function is associated with milder impairments in the other function, but we will treat them here in accordance with the primary difficulty and leave aside other consequences.

Wernicke's Aphasia   Those with this form of *receptive* aphasia cannot separate the continuous flow of speech into appropriate acoustic segments, sometimes even speaking in gibberish as a secondary consequence. They also have difficulty in understanding written language, presumably because they cannot retrieve from memory the sounds corresponding to the letters or words they are reading. Typically, the site of damage is in the posterior portion of the superior left temporal lobe, though the exact spot can vary. One patient with Wernicke's aphasia of moderate severity described a picture of children stealing cookies while their mother was washing dishes in the following way:

> I would say that the little boy was hooking some cookies and was going to fall off, his girl wanted a piece of the cookies too . . . . His mother was washing clothes and spilt on the . . . up over the, the "shring" . . . (Naeser, 1982, p. 56).

It is clear that the patient got the gist of the picture, but the linguistic representations of the picture could not be retrieved properly from memory. Although speech is fluent, there are word substitutions—"hooking" for stealing, "girl" for sister, and "clothes" for dishes. Experiments on patients with Wernicke's aphasia reveal that they lose linguistic distinctions such as the difference between "p" and "b" sounds, necessary for language comprehension and therefore expression. Unable to analyze phonemes (the smallest meaningful speech segments), the patient cannot always comprehend the meaning of words heard, spoken, or written. For example, a patient with Wernicke's aphasia may lose the ability to write because he cannot generate the phonemes that would eventually be transformed into letters.

Broca's Aphasia   The control of speech production is in the left posterior-inferior portion of the frontal lobe. Damage in this region produces an *expressive* aphasia arising from the inability to handle the "kinetic melody," the rapid sequencing of articulations for producing speech sounds (Luria & Hutton, 1977). The speech apparatus, like the motor system generally, requires successive activation and inhibition of neurons that control small muscle groups. Broca's aphasia results from damage to the neural center which controls those muscle groups. A patient with damage here speaks telegraphically and without fluency or correct articulation. To illustrate, consider the following response by a patient with Broca's aphasia to the picture of the children stealing cookies while the mother washed dishes.

> Well...mess...ush "sagga...dder" cookie, uh-oh, fall down...wife spill water...and un "dis...ez...and, us "tsups" and saucer and plate...I, un...no...done...(Naeser, 1982, p. 56).

Articulation errors—"tsups" for cups and "sagga...dder" for scatter—vividly reveal the impairment in rapid sequencing of speech sounds. Other impairments, especially in organizing sequences of words into sentences, are also evident. Usually Broca aphasics speak in the present tense, with an excessive use of nouns and a deficiency of *s* sounds for plurals. Nevertheless, comprehension is usually good, if not perfect, and the patient may recognize linguistic mistakes, although correcting them is difficult.

Spontaneous Recovery

Some recovery of function in traumatic aphasic disorders does occur, but it is unlikely to be complete. The linguistic competence of an intact right hemisphere may be what determines the extent to which spontaneous recovery will occur (Kinsbourne, 1971). Kinsbourne injected a temporarily "paralyzing" drug into an artery supplying either the left or right hemisphere in three aphasic patients with damage to the left hemisphere. They showed no further speech deterioration following the left hemisphere injection, yet they became completely aphasic when the right hemisphere was anesthetized. The implication is that further improvement depends on the extent to which residual language capacities of the right hemisphere can assume more than its typically minor linguistic responsibility.

In tracing the course of recovery from aphasia, Kertesz (1979) found that younger patients appeared to show better recovery than older patients. This finding is in keeping with a twenty-year follow-up of brain-injured soldiers. Teuber (1975) observed that those injured at a younger age showed somewhat greater recovery than those injured when older (although almost all the injuries occurred in soldiers under 30). Virtually none of the aphasics returned completely to normal language function, however.

One general principle is that younger organisms have greater reserve capacity to cope with all forms of brain damage. Schallert (1983), for example, has shown that rats lesioned in early life have complete behavioral recovery in the weeks following an experimentally produced lesion, but in old age the original behavioral deficits reemerged. *Dementia pugilistica* (punch-drunkenness) appears to show the same pattern. Prizefighters may suffer brain damage during their careers yet show few cognitive deficits. A decade later, however, they develop dementia because of the brain's failing capacity to compensate, though no new injury has been inflicted (Roth, 1986). Thus the capacity to cope with injury appears to depend on the age and resiliency of the brain that originally sustained the damage.

Speech Therapy

There is surprisingly little solid evidence that conventional language therapy can importantly influence recovery from aphasia. On the negative side is a British study that randomly assigned aphasic stroke patients to rehabilitation or no-rehabilitation groups (Lincoln et al., 1984). Twice-weekly speech therapy was begun in the tenth week following the stroke and continued for twenty-four weeks. Objective tests at the end of speech therapy showed no differences between treated and untreated patients. They concluded that a great deal of linguistic improvement usually occurs spontaneously in the first weeks following injury, and speech therapy may have been mistakenly credited for recovery during that time.

The Lincoln et al. study was criticized on grounds that two hours of treatment per week is inadequate as a test of speech therapy (Wertz et al., 1986). A more intensive speech therapy program involving eight to ten hours per week was instituted by Wertz et al. After randomly assigning patients to treated and untreated groups, they found significant beneficial effects for speech therapy. The patients in the Wertz study were younger and somewhat less severely disabled by their strokes, so that we are unsure whether the intensity of therapy, their relative youth, or their initially less disabling speech problems figure in these contradictory findings. At present we can only await further studies that consider these different possibilities.

In this chapter we have provided only an overview of the clinical consequences of brain dysfunction. New reports in the scientific literature appearing almost weekly are revealing that many behavioral abnormalities are associated with previously unrecognized brain dysfunctions. With the advent of increasingly sensitive noninvasive imaging techniques one can confidently predict that these new discoveries will continue.

SUMMARY

Many behavioral abnormalities are produced by some form of organic brain dysfunction. Sometimes psychopathology can be produced by epilepsy, a heterogeneous group of disorders characterized by violent bursts of neuronal firing. Its two major forms are generalized and focal. Generalized forms produce diffusely disturbed brain electrical activity, while focal forms affect only limited areas of the brain. The behavioral symptoms of focal temporal lobe, or "limbic," epilepsy can resemble some features of psychotic and dissociative disorders. Specifically, limbic epileptic activity can spark intense affective and dissociative experiences that alter perception and memory and prompt impulsive, irrational actions.

Many forms of organic disorder are related to degenerative changes associated with aging. Alzheimer's disease, one of the most frequent and debilitating of these conditions, produces a dementia characterized by global deterioration in all aspects of cognitive function. Because the American population is living longer, Alzheimer's disease can be expected to affect an increasingly large number of people, thus constituting a major public health problem.

Other disorders considered in this chapter include Parkinsonism, which produces an inability to will movements, and Tourette's disorder, characterized by many vocal and motoric tics.

The consequences of traumatic brain injury also are described. These injuries can produce changes in personality that resemble some features of depression and psychopathy if they occur in the frontal lobes. Damage to language areas of the brain can produce aphasias, or loss of language involving the inability to speak, comprehend spoken language, or read, depending on the specific location of the damage.

Finally, the chapter considered the question of recovery from brain injury, especially the finding that aging is associated with less resiliency to recover from a brain insult. We also considered in this context the effectiveness of therapy for language disorders, a topic that remains controversial.

Psychosis

A psychosis is primarily a *cognitive* condition, a dysfunction of perception and thinking in which the ability to distinguish fantasy from reality breaks down and thinking becomes disorganized, irrational, and peculiar. A psychotic condition sabotages those psychological functions that normally give direction and meaning to a person's life. That is why we say that the psychotic person is out of touch with reality.

PSYCHOTIC BEHAVIOR

Psychotic symptoms are essential features of schizophrenia, schizoaffective disorder, and paranoia, but they are also associated with other disorders (see Figure 10.1), including affective disorder, multiple personality (Kluft, 1987), borderline personality disorder (Stone, 1980), posttraumatic stress disorder (Mueser & Butler, 1987), epilepsy (Pakalnis et al., 1987), alcoholism (Berger & Tinklenberg, 1977), and kidney disease (Jefferson & Marshall, 1981). Psychotic symptoms are not essential to the diagnosis of these latter disorders because (a) the symptoms are often mild, isolated, and transient, and (b) they are secondary consequences of an essentially nonpsychotic process. For example,

FIGURE 10.1   Causes of psychotic behavior.

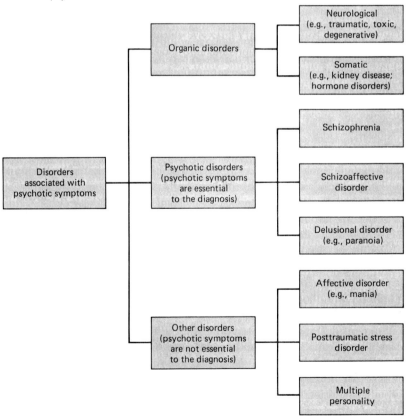

the extreme swings of mood associated with manic-depressive disease can disrupt otherwise normal cognitive functioning but the disorder can be diagnosed in the absence of psychotic symptoms.

We will first consider psychotic symptoms per se regardless of the underlying disorder, and then ask how specific forms of psychopathology and ecopathology affect the expression of the psychotic symptoms.

The best-known disorders associated with psychotic behavior are schizophrenia and affective disorder. Because they have been so highly researched, we will devote two chapters to each. Here, we will provide a framework for those chapters, first by describing psychotic and related symptoms (see Table 10.1), and then by discussing research on the psychopathological distinctiveness of disorders that are associated with psychosis.

Psychotic Symptoms

Psychotic symptoms can be classified into three types: (a) perceptual dysfunction, or impaired "reality testing," (b) disorganized thinking, or "thought disorder," and (c) bizarre beliefs, or delusions.

Impaired Reality Testing The capacity for perceiving reality correctly can be seriously compromised in psychotic disorders. The patient who said that part of a razor blade held by his mother "seemed to spread into

TABLE 10.1 CHARACTERISTIC SYMPTOMS OF PSYCHOTIC DISORDERS

Symptoms	Description	Examples*
Psychotic		
Impaired reality testing	Inability to apprehend reality and distinguish reality from fantasy	Clouding of consciousness, depersonalization, derealization, hallucination, magical thinking, lack of insight
Thought disorder	Deficiencies in the organization and communication of thought at an appropriate level of abstraction	Fragmentation, condensation, idiosyncracies, hyperabstraction, concreteness, blocking
Delusion	Pathological storylike interpretations of the relationship between individual and external events	Delusions of grandeur, persecution, reference
Nonpsychotic		
Emotional dysfunction	Pathological excess, deficiency, or disorganization of emotion	Apathy, ambivalence, anger, euphoria, depression, or panic
Motor dysfunction	Pathological excess, deficiency, or disorganization or movement	Awkwardness, rigidity, grimacing, statuesque posturing, mannerisms, stereotypy, perseveration

*See text for illustrations.

me . . . . Later a cat jumped in and out of me . . . I ejected it'' (Freeman, 1969, p. 89) perceived reality quite incorrectly. Impaired reality testing also includes *lack of insight*, or failure to perceive just how abnormal one's behavior is, *derealization*, or the perception that the environment is alien and unfamiliar, and *hallucinations*, or sensory experiences of objectively nonexistent events. A classic description of some of these experiences was written by Emil Kraepelin, one of the founders of modern psychiatry.

> *Hallucinations of sight* begin with variegated rings in front of their eyes, plays of colour, fiery rays and balls, seeing sparks, everything looks awry and wrong. . . . On the wall appear white figures, reflections, the mother who is dead. . . . *Smell and taste* frequently share in the morbid condition. Evil smelling substances are scattered about; there is a smell of sulphur; of corpses. . . . A patient smelled human souls; another felt the devil standing behind her, ''it stank.'' . . . By far the most frequent are *hallucinations of hearing*. At the beginning these are usually simple noises, rustling, buzzing, ringing in the ears . . . [and] the *hearing of voices*. Sometimes it is only whispering . . . a secret language, ''taunting the captive''; sometimes the voices are loud or suppressed, as from a ventriloquist . . . (quoted by Hamilton, 1967, pp. 14, 15, 19).

Thought Disorder The capacity to sustain attention to a set of ideas and to think clearly about them is also compromised in psychotic disorders. The breakdown of this capacity, called *thought disorder*, can occur at different levels of cognitive control. Disorganization only at higher levels of integration, where connections are made between general ideas and topics rather than specific thoughts, is sometimes called ''flight of ideas,'' especially when the patient communicates in rapid-fire speech. The patient may begin talking about conditions in the hospital and then, associating to the idea of authority, shift to a discussion of the CIA and then, associating to covert movement, shift to the automotive industry and then, associating to economics, to the difference between capitalism and communism, and so on. Even if the specific thoughts associated with each of these general ideas are expressed rationally, the overall picture appears to be disorganized because the ideational shifts are unpredictable. But the disorganization occurs not because the connections among ideas are random, but because they are private, idiosyncratic, and hard to follow.

When cognitive disorganization occurs at the level of *specific thoughts*, we speak of ''loose associations''—for example, a patient discussing flowers remarks that the pistil is the flower's only protection against insects, or another patient remarks, while shaking hands with the therapist, that both of them are sure to get the shakes. Even if such a patient remains loosely on one topic, this lack of conventional connection among specific thoughts gives the impression of cognitive disorganization.

Thought disorder at the general level of ideational control, or ''flight of ideas,'' is clearly evident in the *affective* psychoses, especially in mania and in agitated depression. Thought disorder at the more specific level of "loose associations" is prominent in *schizophrenic* psychosis. Both general and specific thought disorders are prominent in those "mixed" psychoses called *schizoaffective* (described below). Cognitive disorganization can be quite severe in psychoses, with patients losing control even of the basic cognitive rules of grammar that normally organize sounds into coherent words and words into coherent sentences. For example, one patient wrote "Now to eat if one cannot other one can—and if we cant the girseau Q. C. Washpots prizebloom capacities—turning out—replaced by the heard patterns my own capacities—I was not very kind to them" (Critchley, 1979, p. 57). The appearance of such an agrammatical "word salad" makes it sometimes difficult to tell whether the underlying condition is really a psychosis or an organic aphasia (see Chapter 9, pp. 261–262).

Disorganized thinking may partly arise because the psychotic patient is easily distracted by irrelevant events or ideas. As an illustration of the distractibility factor, consider the following patient-therapist interaction. The therapist cracks his knuckles at the same moment that the patient comments that his breakfast egg looked poisoned. Instantly, the patient comments that calcium is missing from his diet and his bones are too thin (Freeman, 1969, p. 53).

The thought disorder of distractible patients may be complicated by weirdly inventive rhymes and playful rearrangements of ideas that are kicked in by chance events—for example, when a patient, observing a man named Mr. Gathercole pass by, says: "You should be a pole or a Jack Tar; we can't all gather from that." Asked if she knew the name of the man, the patient replied: "No, I don't listen like that . . . I listen to the king" (Freeman, 1969, p. 123); is this a subterranean reference to Old King Cole? Disorganized thinking may also occur because the patient is distracted by the sound of a word, and the sound provides the link to the next idea. An example of this *clang* type of association is a patient's response to a Rorschach card: "And this *mist* here kind of suggests that they live in a *myst*ical world" (Solovay et al., 1986, p. 489).

Disorganized thinking may also occur when attention wanders because the patient's thinking is insufficiently regulated by external events. This happens when a socially detached patient withdraws into a private world of thought. This private world can be rich in hallucinatory fantasy or impoverished with vague or amorphous thoughts. The special combination of impoverished ideation and apathy in some patients, however, suggests a severe motivational deficit—a kind of existential emptiness which patients sometimes describe as "being dead inside."

Thought disorder may be marked by idiosyncratic associations and meanings and by condensations in perception and thinking. An *idiosyncratic association* is a highly subjective connection between two images or ideas that don't belong together. For example, a patient interprets a Rorschach card as "a man shedding his skin" or a "beetle crying" (Solovay et al., 1986, p. 490). *Idiosyncratic meanings* are often observed—calling a ballpoint pen a "paperskate" or a television set a "news vessel," for example (Andreasen, 1986, p. 478), or calling Brutus "an Italian" or saying that Egypt is located "between Assyria and the Congo" (E. Bleuler, 1911/1950, p. 19) or asking for "a little more *allegro* in the treatment" (Rosenthal, 1970, p. 94).

When meanings become vague and distinctions among them blurred, thinking becomes uncritical and peculiar. To illustrate, consider a hyperabstract and illogical comment of a patient who explained that "Parents can be anything, material, vegetable, or mineral, that has taught you something. Parents would be the world of things that are alive, that are there. Rocks, a person can look at a rock and learn something from it, so that would be a parent" (Andreasen, 1986, p. 478).

Idiosyncratic *condensations* are subjectively determined inventive combinations of two or more ideas within one expression or even a single word. For example, a patient created a forced and incongruent perceptual composite out of two details of a Rorschach card in "two potatoes with eyes and a mouth trying to climb up some kind of pipe or pole" (Solovay et al., 1986, p. 492). Sometimes the condensation occurs with a novel word, or *neologism*. One patient explained "insinuendo" as follows: "insinuation toward innuendo, the implication of reincarnation throughout negativism" (Rokeach, 1964, p. 131). Compare this bizarre but comprehensible neologism of the psychotic patient with the meaningless neologisms of the organically impaired aphasic patient— for example, "I want to buy gum in the flark," or "Put the yerts in the sellows" (Kaufman, 1981, p. 116). In both cases word usage is idiosyncratic and bizarre, the difference being that the psychotic extends and distorts word meanings in playful and reckless disregard for convention, while the aphasic has lost word meanings almost entirely.

The psychotic patient may be given to *hyperabstractions*, that is, thought and speech characterized by highly abstract, seemingly empty concepts. For example, in response to the question "What is a cupboard?" a patient replied: "An element of the conditions of life." Another patient said that both sledge (sleigh) and cart represented "the modification of appearance" (Zeigarnik, 1965, pp. 96–97). Note how much more abstract such an answer is than a more appropriate one to the effect that these are two types of primitive vehicles for transporting people or things.

On the other hand, *concrete thinking*, the opposite of hyperabstract thinking, may also be apparent, with the patient seemingly stuck in the concrete sensory qualities of objects. A knife, fork, and spoon may seem to belong together because they are hard or shiny. Concrete thinking is often expressed in bizarre literal-mindedness. For example, in response to a request to give someone his hand, the patient says: "Why should I give you my hand? I should then have to walk without a hand" (Zeigarnik, 1965, p. 120). Another patient said he was not unhappy. But asked if something was weighing heavily on his mind, he answered, "Yes. Iron is heavy" (E. Bleuler, 1911/1950, p. 19). Note how the concrete quality of the association deflects the patient's thoughts in an inappropriate manner. The result is an ''angularity'' of thought sometimes referred to as ''knight's move'' (Wing, Cooper, & Sartorius, 1974, p. 185).

Occasionally thoughts may be blocked. *Blocking* refers to a cognitive ''absence'' but without the loss of consciousness that characterizes petit mal epileptic absences. It is a kind of stop-action without content during which the patient seems fixed in position. The patient may come up with a ''crazy'' explanation for the blocking—for example, that the CIA is using special machinery to rob her thoughts.

Delusions Human beings are naturally motivated to reduce ambiguity and uncertainty by interpreting information in terms of what they already know. Interpretations and beliefs that are irrational and resist refutation by objective reality are called *delusions*. Dominated by fantasy and subjective needs, delusions indicate a severe form of egocentricity.

The delusion of *reference* is the patient's idea that he or she is being influenced by external forces. Sights and sounds may be interpreted as ''messages,'' perhaps inserted into the mind by special machinery controlled by hostile agents. A patient may have the delusion that his thoughts are ''broadcast'' to others as though his mind were a radio transmitter. Thought insertion and thought broadcast are delusional expressions of the psychotic dissolution of the normal barrier between private and public events. *Magical* thinking, the delusional belief that one's thoughts alone can control physical events, also illustrates the dissolution of the ''barrier.'' As one patient said, ''Whenever I think of speed, the police appear'' (Freeman, 1969, p. 57).

The delusion of *grandeur* carries the person to extreme heights of power and influence. These delusions often include an encompassing ''solution'' to scientific, philosophical, or social problems. And the patient is frequently sure that these are solutions on the grandest scale with enormous implications for revealing the deepest truths of human nature and for influencing the survival or destruction of the world and the universe beyond. Figure 10.2 shows a hyperabstract, pseudomathematical delusional ''solution'' to an obscure question about mental mechanisms.

The delusion of *persecution* is a frank expression of personal vulnerability articulated in fantasies of being victimized. For example, a patient was preoccupied with fears of retaliation from the ''bookies.''

> [They] were supposed to have gangster protection. . . . [Soon] he noticed strangers loitering about the hotel lobby. They seemed to be watching him and making little signs which referred to him. An automobile full of men stopped in front of the hotel entrance. He now felt sure that he would be kidnapped, tortured and killed. He barricaded himself in his room and arranged by telephone with a relative to flee the city the next morning. (From Norman Cameron, *Personality Development and Psychopathology: A Dynamic Approach*, p. 489. Copyright © 1963 by Houghton Mifflin Company. Used with permission.)

"MATHEMATICAL–PSYCHOLOGICAL DETERMINATION OF THE MEANING OF THE 'EGO'."

$(p \& q \& r) > s$

if: p, df.: $\exists (x): (x \in A) > (x \in B)$

q, df.: $C \subset D$

r, df.: "There is, at least, 1, 'ego', such that: that 'ego' thinks or assumes that s is T."

s, df.: $0 < \Delta (t) < \infty.,$

A, df.: "the class of 'egoes', which are 1-dimensional".

B, df.: "the class of 'entities'".

C, df.: "the class of the term, 'ego'".

D, df.: "the class of 'heuristical' (or, 'scientific–tropic) terms".

FIGURE 10.2 A delusional "solution" to an obscure psychological question.

A more exotic version of persecutory delusion appears in the "Capgras symptom," the delusional belief that a loved one has been replaced by a double.

A 47-year-old white woman fearfully explained that her husband had been switched and was not who he appeared to be. She believed that the imposter was trying to poison her food and kill her with gas from the kitchen range. She believed that the substitution first appeared two years before, when her husband went on a trip to Philadelphia and an imposter took his place (Walker & Brodie, 1980, p. 1295).

Delusions of persecution are most prominently associated with *paranoid* disorders. These include both a *paranoid personality disorder* associated with pervasive mistrust, hypersensitivity, and "cold" affect (see Chapter 3), and *paranoid psychoses* that run the gamut from pure *paranoia* with no thought disorder to paranoid schizophrenia where thought disorder occurs, and also to paranoid types of manic, depressive, and organic psychoses. Usually, delusions of persecution or delusional jealousy are typical in these disorders although other delusional concerns can occur. These may include the belief that one is secretly loved by a famous person (erotomania), delusions of grandeur (megalomania), delusions of bodily infestation (hypochondriacal psychosis), and pathological obsession with legal retribution (litigious monomania) (Munro, 1982).

Delusional behavior is a pathological version of the human tendency to invent stories that clarify ambiguity, explain danger, and absolve the self from fault (Sarbin, 1981). Delusions provide a personal sense of elevated importance if not outright superiority (Maher & Ross, 1984). Thus we can see how delusions could occur secondary to the psychological upheaval of schizophrenic, affective, and organic disorders.

Is there a *primary* delusional disposition which, if strong enough, could in itself produce delusions, even with very little provocation? Evidence relevant to this question comes from a study of adoptees with pure delusional disorder, that is, nonschizophrenic and nonaffective psychotic disorder marked by delusions. The evidence suggests that the biological, but not the adoptive, relatives of adoptees with pure delusional disorders such as paranoia appear to have an elevated risk for delusional disorder and for excessive feelings of jealousy and inferiority (Kendler & Davis, 1981; Kendler & Hays, 1981; Kendler, Gruenberg, & Strauss, 1981). At the same time, these biological relatives are *not* at greater risk for schizophrenia or for affective disorder (Winokur, 1977; Winokur, 1985). Therefore, it would seem that a heritable liability exists specifically for delusional thinking, but the evidence is slim and debatable.

Related Symptoms

Psychotic symptoms rarely exist alone. Additional symptoms typically coexist in a psychotic disorder. We will briefly describe some major emotional and motoric symptoms that may accompany psychotic symptoms.

Emotional Dysfunction A major correlate of psychosis—sometimes a cause, sometimes an effect—is an abnormality in the expression or control of emotion. This abnormality may be expressed in emotional *excess* (euphoria, rage, depression, and anxiety) or *deficiency* (apathy, detachment, and unresponsiveness), as well as unpredictability of mood and *uncontrollability* of temper. For example, a combination of sadness (an excess) and apathy (a deficiency) may accompany psychotic depression.

> [A patient] sat staring in front of her, silent, tearful and dejected, wringing her hands, rubbing her forehead and picking at her skin. She was the picture of a woman in profound grief. She rarely spoke. When she did she said that she had no feeling and no thoughts, that she was like a statue, a vegetable, lifeless. (From Norman Cameron, *Personality Development and Psychopathology: A Dynamic Approach*, p. 529. Copyright © 1963 by Houghton Mifflin Company. Used with permission.)

Unpredictable/uncontrollable emotionality is, however, more typical of certain types of schizophrenia.

> The patients are able to react to sad news with cheerfulness or even with laughter. These patients will often become sad or, even more frequently, irritated by events to which others would react with indifference or with pleasure. A mere "how-do-you-do" can upset them. . . . They will relate laughingly their torturing hallucinations, or portray themselves with a cheerful mien as unfortunate creatures (E. Bleuler, 1911/1950, p. 52).

Motor Dysfunction Psychotic disturbances are sometimes accompanied by awkward gait, muscular rigidity, passive flexibility (catatonia), bizarre grimacing, repetitive and purposeless movement (buttoning and unbuttoning, for example), odd mannerisms (flicking the head or saluting movements, for example), difficulty initiating or terminating actions, tremors, writhing, and dancelike movements. That some of these motor dysfunctions may have a neurological basis is suggested by evidence that the use or abrupt withdrawal of antipsychotic drugs may produce them (Jeste & Wyatt, 1984).

Some deviant motor behaviors are expressed in the form of *mannerisms,* as illustrated by the following description:

> Every conceivable stilted gesture occurs. Shaking hands is done very stiffly with the hand turned or only the little finger is presented; the hand may be shot forward quickly and withdrawn just as rapidly. Grimaces of all kinds, peculiar ways of shrugging the shoulder, extraordinary movements of tongue and lips, finger play, sudden involuntary gestures. . . . [T]he gait changes; a hospital patient, still intelligent and diligent, no longer walks but gallops. . . . [I]n eating, the spoon is held by its handle tip only or reversed. Before taking a mouthful of food, the patient knocks on the plate three times. The food is taken up on the fork and dropped back again seven times before it is taken into the mouth (E. Bleuler, 1911/1950, p. 191).

Others include uncontrollable repetitiveness. If the repetition is an autonomous mannerism, we speak of *stereotypy.*

> We find patients rubbing their right hands over their left thumbs, intently and energetically for decades . . . others beat on their beds rhythmically, clap their hands or perform all kinds of manipulations with their teeth, etc. (E. Bleuler, 1911/1950, p. 185).

If the repetition is situation-dependent, for example in response to a question, then we speak of *perseveration.* For example, in response to a question, a patient said: ''It's a presumptuous thing to respect someone . . . respect . . . respectable . . . respect . . . he didn't respect money of me but I didn't have it to give him'' (Freeman, 1969, p. 119).

Clinical Distinctions

Now that psychotic and related symptoms have been described, we can begin to explore their psychological meaning. We start with two clinical distinctions that will bring us closer to a major point of the chapter—to categorize the great variety of individual symptoms into a small set of disorders.

Negative, Positive, and Deficit Symptoms   This distinction calls attention to whether psychological processes such as attention, imagination, and feeling seem to be either absent or excessive. *Negative* symptoms include *avolition,* or the loss of capacity for effort; *apathy,* or blunted affect; *anhedonia,* or the inability to experience pleasure from bodily sensations or intellectual pursuits; *withdrawal,* or disengagement of attention from the physical and interpersonal environment; and *blocking,* or momentary absences of conscious thought (see Table 10.2). The more striking *positive* symptoms include hallucinations, delusions, thought disorder, and agitated behavior. Clinicians sometimes use the term florid—that is, fully expressed—to describe disorders marked by positive symptoms. A third category called deficit symptoms is sometimes distinguished from both negative and positive symptoms (Goldberg, 1985). This category includes odd mannerisms and inappropriate affect—laughing or crying out of context, for example.

TABLE 10.2   NEGATIVE SYMPTOMS

Affective Flattening or Blunting

    Unchanging facial expression
    Decreased spontaneous movements
    Paucity of expressive gestures
    Poor eye contact
    Lack of vocal inflections

Alogia

    Poverty of speech
    Poverty of content of speech
    Blocking
    Increased latency of response

Avolition-Apathy

    Poor grooming and hygiene
    Impersistence at work or school
    Physical anergia
    Subjective complaints of avolition-apathy

Anhedonia-Asociality

    Few recreational interests and activities
    Little sexual interest and activity
    Little ability to feel intimacy and closeness
    Few relationships with friends and peers

Attentional Impairment

    Work inattentiveness
    Inattentiveness during mental status testing

Source: From Andreasen, 1982, p. 786. (*Archives of General Psychiatry,* 1982, *39,* 784–788. Copyright 1982, American Medical Association)

Negative, positive, and deficit symptoms appear to have some value in distinguishing among different psychotic disorders. For example, when negative and deficit symptoms are particularly prominent in a psychotic disorder, chronicity and high heritability are also likely to be found (Andreasen & Olsen, 1982; Crow, 1980; Dworkin & Lenzenweger, 1984). Table 10.3 illustrates this in those cases of schizophrenic disorders where negative or positive symptoms predominate rather than appear roughly equally balanced. Negative and deficit symptoms are more characteristic of schizophrenia than of other psychotic disorders, such as mania and paranoia. Positive symptoms, on the other hand, have limited diagnostic usefulness in differentiating one disorder from another because they are present in all kinds of psychotic conditions and not just in schizophrenia (Carpenter, Strauss, & Mulch, 1973; Pope & Lipinski, 1978). Positive symptoms also have little if any value in predicting outcome (Bland & Orne, 1980). Finally, evidence that many positive symptoms have near-zero heritability (McGuffin et al., 1984) limits their usefulness for diagnosing, researching, or theorizing about specific disorders, such as schizophre-

TABLE 10.3 CORRELATES OF *DSM-III* SCHIZOPHRENICS WITH PREDOMINANTLY NEGATIVE OR POSITIVE SYMPTOMS

	Schizophrenia	
Correlate	Negative symptoms	Positive symptoms
Premorbid adjustment	Relatively poor	Relatively good
Impaired IQ	Yes	Little/none
Clinical impression	Deficiency	Disintegration
Rate of nonright-handedness	High	Low
Drug abuse	Little/none	Some

Source: Derived from Andreasen & Olsen, 1982.

nia, which are highly heritable (see Chapter 12). In short, positive symptoms are probably best thought of as *nonspecific* features of many psychoses.

Regressive and Defensive Aspects Certain psychotic symptoms are sometimes called *regressive* because of their apparent similarity to behaviors that are normal in children but bizarre in adults. For example, children are distractible, self-centered, and given to fantastic story-telling. The fact that bizarre regressive symptoms occur in adults, however, does not justify the view that psychosis is merely a regression, that is, a reversal of cognitive development. Most investigators have concluded, therefore, that psychosis is fundamentally a pathological condition involving defect and disintegration in which immature patterns of behavior may be expressed in ways that sometimes resemble the immature behavior of normal children. It is clear that despite many infantile behaviors, a psychotic person is not merely an adult whose psychological development has simply reversed (Buss, 1966; Cameron, 1938).

Psychotic symptoms are sometimes interpreted (and not without controversy) as a *defense* against underlying disintegration. A delusion, for example, can be a fantastic pretense through which the patient denies isolation and vulnerability and creates a false sense of self-importance. One patient, in an anonymous essay about the delusional defenses used by psychotic patients, wrote that "[the psychotic's] delusion . . . his philosophy, his rationalization, his intellectualization, is a kind of perverted sanity. It is a way of explaining himself and the world." Selye (1976) has written extensively about the universal occurrence of defensive adjustments that all organisms make under internally or externally induced stress. The psychotic condition seems to involve both a severe dysfunction and a bizarre attempt to adjust to, or cope with, that dysfunction.

DEVELOPMENT OF PSYCHOTIC DISORDERS

We have described the *cross-sectional* aspects of psychotic symptoms, that is, symptoms observed at one point in time. Now we turn to *temporal* aspects, the waxing, waning, and other changes in symptoms that occur as a psychotic disorder develops over time.

Temporal Features

Temporal aspects of psychotic disorders include age of onset, duration, course, frequency, and end state. Table 10.4 outlines some of these major temporal dimensions.

Age of onset refers to the age at which a psychotic episode first occurs. The ages of individual patients are usually lumped together into one of two periods: early onset, roughly the teens through the mid-thirties, and late onset, the mid-thirties through the fifties.

Rate of onset refers to the rate of development from the earliest diagnostic signs of the disorder. *Acute onset* is typically measured in days or weeks, while *insidious onset* refers to a slow, almost imperceptible evolution, typically over months and years. The distinction has practical significance; for one thing, acute onset is generally associated with a better prognosis than insidious onset. The *duration* of a psychotic disorder can be short-term, usually less than six months, or long-term, or chronic (see Table 10.5). Acute onset, short-term psychosis, called brief reactive psychosis in *DSM-III-R,* is typically associated with anxiety, confusion, emotional turmoil, and motivation to seek help. It can be as striking as it is short-lived. Sensory experiences are heightened with colors, sounds, and even bodily sensations intensified. Innumerable ideas and images, often deeply meaningful like revealed truths, come tumbling into consciousness with little organization or sense of control. The result is a kaleidoscopic hodgepodge of intensified experiences that can be both frightening and exalting.

Course refers to level and shifts of symptom severity. The course of the disorder may be episodic, with occasional or frequent shifts from severely abnor-

TABLE 10.4 TEMPORAL FEATURES OF PSYCHOTIC BEHAVIOR

Dimensions	Description
Age of onset for initial episode	Early (teens through mid-30s) vs. late (mid-30s through 50s)
Type of onset for typical episode	Acute vs. insidious
Duration of typical episode	Short term (less than 6 months) vs. long term
Course of a typical episode	Undulating vs. stable
Frequency (number) of episodes	Infrequent (less than 3) vs. frequent (3+) during a lifetime
End state of disorder	Recovery vs. continuing impairment to end of life

TABLE 10.5 THE PROCESS OF BECOMING CHRONIC

Chain of chronicity	Other alternatives

Person becomes ill

Chain of chronicity	Other alternatives
Peculiar behavior noticed by family and friends	Peculiar behavior unnoticed and eventually disappears
Peculiar behavior brought to the attention of clinic, physician, police, etc.	Peculiar behavior accepted by family and friends
Referral or commitment to a mental hospital	Treatment as an outpatient
Treatment on admission ward with minimal improvement	Treatment on admission ward, rapid improvement, and prompt discharge
Transfer to continued treatment ward	Remains on admission ward, continues to receive psychotherapy and individual attention
Regular employment at hospital job, loss of contact with family and outside, acquisition of institutional values	Remains in individual or group psychotherapy, retains contact with family and friends, frequent visits outside, no hospital employment

Source: From Sommer & Whitney, 1961. (*American Journal of Psychiatry, 118,* 111–117. Copyright © 1961, The American Psychiatric Association. Reprinted by permission.)

mal symptoms to normalcy. Conversely, the course may be nonepisodic, with severity remaining fairly constant or showing a gradual decline. While some association exists between acute onset and an episodic course, and between insidious onset and a nonepisodic course, many combinations are possible (Ciompi, 1980). The course of a psychotic episode will depend on such factors as premorbid traits, the duration of the episode, and whether the patient has continued medication (Rabiner, Wegner, & Kane, 1986). Because *frequency* refers to the number of psychotic episodes surrounded by extended periods of relative normalcy, the concept is not useful for describing an unremitting chronic disorder. A psychosis may develop only once or it may be episodic.

End state refers to the condition of the patient toward the end of life. Follow-up studies of patients with schizophrenic, affective, and other disorders associated with psychotic symptoms describe end state with terms like ''recovered'' or ''impaired.'' Figure 10.3 shows eight patterns of onset, course, and end state derived from a long-term follow-up of hospitalized schizophrenics (Ciompi, 1980). About half the cases showed acute as opposed to insidious onset, and about half showed the undulating as opposed to the nonundulating course. The two most typical patterns are acute onset/undulating/favorable outcome, and insidious onset/nonundulating/unfavorable outcome. However, many of the cases fit neither of these two categories.

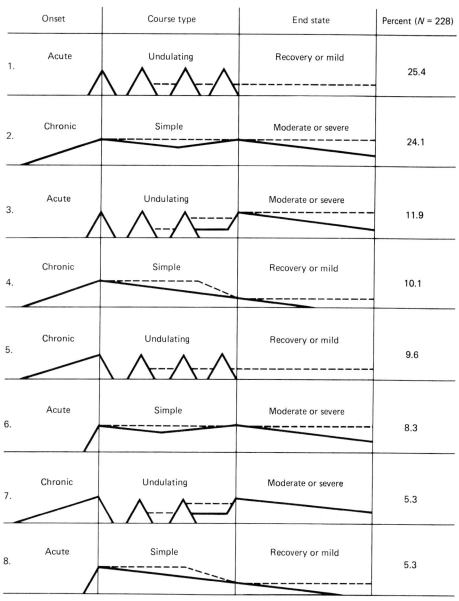

Onset	Course type	End state	Percent (*N* = 228)

1. Acute / Undulating / Recovery or mild — 25.4

2. Chronic / Simple / Moderate or severe — 24.1

3. Acute / Undulating / Moderate or severe — 11.9

4. Chronic / Simple / Recovery or mild — 10.1

5. Chronic / Undulating / Recovery or mild — 9.6

6. Acute / Simple / Moderate or severe — 8.3

7. Chronic / Undulating / Moderate or severe — 5.3

8. Acute / Simple / Recovery or mild — 5.3

FIGURE 10.3 Schematic representation of dynamic patterns of schizophrenic psychosis (Ciompi, 1980, p. 612). Dashed lines indicate alternative levels of behavioral severity within a temporal pattern. Insidious onset is indicated in the leftmost column by the term "chronic."

Temporal Categories

The somewhat predictable co-occurrence of temporal features suggests three major types of development for disorders associated with psychosis: chronic, cyclic, and reactive. A *chronic* pattern is expressed as a lifetime condition with early and insidious onset, unremitting deficiency symptoms, and minimal response to therapeutic intervention. The classic example is chronic schizophrenia (Chapter 11). A *cyclic* pattern involves a lifetime vulnerability to episodic disorganization regardless of external conditions. The classic example is the psychotic behavior associated with manic-depressive disorder (Chapter 13). A *reactive* pattern is expressed as an acute-onset, short-term, situation-induced disorder involving anxiety and emotional turmoil. The situation typically involves personal loss or life-threatening trauma like that associated with combat.

The chronic and cyclic disorders—typical of schizophrenia and affective disorder, respectively—seem to reflect fundamental differences in underlying psychopathology, as we will shortly see. However, we are not sure if the reactive category represents a distinct psychotic disorder. While some cases of reactive disorder appear to be variants of affective disorder, few, if any, are variants of schizophrenia (Fischer, Gottesman, & Bertelsen, 1985; McCabe & Stromgren, 1975).

Up till now, our discussion of the symptoms of psychosis has repeatedly suggested certain psychological distinctions, such as "flight of ideas" versus "loose associations," thought disorder versus delusions, positive versus negative symptoms, and process versus reactive development. These distinctions help to clarify the *multidimensional* nature of psychotic behavior.

But what about the idea that such behavior represents distinct types of psychopathology, as suggested by *DSM-III-R*? It is one thing to establish categorical distinctions on the basis of recognizable differences in behavioral patterns, but it is quite another to establish that such distinctions reflect correspondingly distinct types of underlying psychopathology.

Do behaviorally defined psychotic disorders—in particular the schizophrenic, manic-depressive (bipolar), and schizoaffective disorders of *DSM-III-R*—represent fundamentally different psychopathologies? Is schizophrenia, for example, basically a *cognitive* psychopathology with affective symptoms best viewed as merely the by-products of the more primary dysfunction? Likewise, is manic-depression basically an *affective* psychopathology with psychotic disturbances best viewed as secondary by-products? And do schizoaffective disorders represent the combined effects of the psychotic and affective types of psychopathology in more or less equal measure?

On the other hand, perhaps the categorically distinct psychotic syndromes of *DSM-III-R* are merely different behavioral expressions of a common psychopathology, what some investigators call "psychoticism." In this case, the behavioral differences might reflect differences in (a) severity of psychoticism and (b) personality traits and cognitive style. Evidence regarding the somewhat ambiguous distinction between schizophrenia and other psychotic disorders is taken up next.

SCHIZOPHRENIC, AFFECTIVE, AND SCHIZOAFFECTIVE DISORDERS

Affective and schizoaffective disorders can produce psychotic behavior like that of schizophrenia. However, because they often have reactive, cyclic, and affective features, these disorders seem fundamentally different from schizophrenia. Is this true? Let us start with a brief review of the clearest distinction—that between schizophrenia and affective disorder.

Schizophrenia versus Affective Disorder

Schizophrenia and affective disorder seem to have a different etiology and developmental course (see Table 10.6). The most compelling evidence for separating the two categories of disorder comes from family studies suggesting different etiologies (Loranger, 1981). In nine studies involving more than 150 manic-depressive MZ twins, and in twelve studies involving more than 500 MZ twins with schizophrenia, *not one* of the co-twins had the other disorder. However, there are now two reports of cases of identical twins where one twin has been diagnosed as schizophrenic and the other as manic-depressive (Dalby, Morgan, & Lee, 1986; McGuffen, Reveley, & Holland, A, 1982). Such exceptions to the general rule raise complicated questions about the diagnosis, classification, and theory of psychotic disorders, but these are well beyond the

TABLE 10.6 SOME TYPICAL DIFFERENCES BETWEEN SCHIZOPHRENIA AND AFFECTIVE (BIPOLAR AND UNIPOLAR) DISORDER

Dimension	Schizophrenia	Affective disorder
Premorbid adjustment	Poor*	Good
Type of onset	Insidious*	Acute, reactive
Age of onset	Early (teens to 20s)	Late (late 20s–40s)
Duration of behavioral impairment	Relatively long-term	Relatively short-term episodes (which may repeat through the life cycle)
Endocrine, biorhythm, and/or appetitive dysfunctions	Absent/minor	Prominent
Benefits from		
Antipsychotics	Yes	Yes
Lithium carbonate	No	Yes
Tricyclic antidepressives	No	Yes
Sleep deprivation	No	Yes
ECT	No	Yes
Biological relatives		
Higher liability for	Schizophrenia	Affective and anxiety disorders

*Many exceptions occur, so that good premorbid adjustment, acute onset, and even the remission of severe symptoms are not uncommon.

scope of the present chapter. Nevertheless, the preponderance of evidence still supports the argument that there is a *qualitative* difference in the hereditary liabilities for schizophrenia and affective disorders. Thus, the relatives of patients with manic-depressive disorder have a markedly elevated rate of affective disorder, but an unremarkable rate of schizophrenia; likewise, the relatives of patients with schizophrenia have a markedly elevated rate of schizophrenia but an unremarkable rate of manic-depressive disorder (Gershon et al., 1988).

Evidence of differences in timing and course also supports the argument that schizophrenia differs from affective disorder. Figure 10.4 shows the incidence for first admissions to hospitals in Britain. The admission rate for schizophrenia peaks earlier than the corresponding rate for affective disorder, and both rates show a decline after age 60 when the incidence of organic disorders associated with aging (not shown in the figure) begins to increase markedly.

Even in the realm of psychotic behavior where the two disorders may at first seem quite similar, the verbal behavior of the two can be distinguished. In manic thought disorder, fragmentation of thinking occurs largely around transitions between topics or general ideas; within a given topic, however, thought

FIGURE 10.4 First-admission rates per 100,000 per year over three years (1964–1966). (Slater & Cowie, 1971, p. 73, *The Genetics of Mental Disorder,* Oxford University Press. Reprinted with permission.)

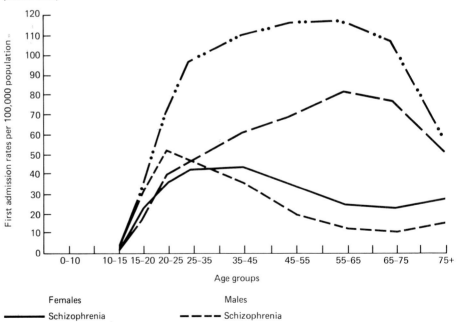

is more rational, organized, and clear despite its playfulness and flamboyance. By contrast, in schizophrenic psychosis fragmentation occurs even within topics (Hoffman, Stopek, & Andreasen, 1986). For these and other reasons, schizophrenia and affective disorder—even affective disorder with psychosis—are believed to be two distinct disorders.

The controversial case of Daniel Schreber can be used to illustrate how difficult it can sometimes be to distinguish between schizophrenia and other psychotic disorders. Recall that Schreber was a famous German judge who developed a psychotic disorder (see Chapter 6, pp. 158–159). Freud diagnosed Schreber as paranoid schizophrenic from writings suggesting bizarre delusional thinking that was both persecutory—divine forces were making him crazy, for example—and "schizophrenic"—his brain was softening.

There is good reason to suspect, however, that Schreber was suffering from an *affective* disorder rather than from schizophrenia (Lipton, 1984). First, hallucinations, delusions, and thought disorder can also characterize affective and organic psychotic states. Second, the familial, premorbid, and developmental aspects of Schreber's disorder are more consistent with psychotic affective disorder than with schizophrenia: (1) good-to-excellent premorbid adjustment reflected in positive personal qualities and notable achievements; (2) the late onset of reactive and remitting psychotic episodes marked by emotional turbulence and positive symptoms, suicidal behavior, and vegetative symptoms including insomnia and loss of appetite; (3) excellent recovery between episodes; and (4) relatives with affective, hysterical, and paranoid problems, but not schizophrenia. The diagnostic controversy over the Schreber case illustrates the potential value of family background and developmental features for distinguishing between disorders with overlapping symptomatology.

Schizoaffective Disorder

Many psychotic syndromes do not fit neatly into either the schizophrenic or affective disorder category because they have elements of both. One of these, the so-called schizoaffective disorder, has been defined over the years in different ways. During the 1960s, for example, researchers focused on certain characteristics of the schizoaffective disorder—in particular, acute onset, precipitating stress, emotional turmoil, short duration, and relatively normal personality development (Levitt & Tsuang, 1988). Currently, *DSM-III-R* requires (a) episodes that include psychotic symptoms such as hallucinations or delusions, and also mania or depression; and, at other times, (b) episodes of psychosis without mood disturbance. There is an additional requirement that the syndrome not satisfy the diagnostic criteria for either schizophrenia or an affective disorder (American Psychiatric Association, 1987).

There is a continuing debate about how to define and categorize schizoaffective symptomatology (Procci, 1976; Pope et al., 1980; Levitt & Tsuang, 1988); the evidence both supports and contradicts the three major hypotheses, namely, that it represents (1) a ''third'' type of psychotic disorder, behaviorally overlapping but etiologically distinct from the other two; (2) a mixture of the two others, perhaps one parent supplying the schizophrenic, and the other the affective, vulnerability; or (3) a variant of schizophrenia or affective disorder, depending on whether cognitive or mood dysfunction predominates.

In some ways, schizoaffective patients are like schizophrenics in their fragmented thinking and bizarre ideation, but in other ways they are like patients with affective disorder—for example, in their irritabilility, flightiness, and hyperresponsiveness to irrelevant stimuli (Holzman, Shenton, & Solovay, 1986). On laboratory tasks, the schizoaffective usually tests out in ways more characteristic of affectively disordered patients. For example, in contrast to schizophrenics, schizoaffectives usually display few signs of abnormal brain electrical activity and show few organiclike deficits on neuropsychological tests (Tutko & Spence, 1962; Walker, 1981). Schizoaffectives tend not to show the negative symptoms that are prominent in schizophrenia. Moreover, unlike schizophrenics, schizoaffectives and affectively disordered patients show an abnormally early onset of rapid eye movement (REM) sleep (Kupfer, 1976). Finally, schizoaffectives generally respond more favorably than schizophrenics to biological treatments used for affective disorder, especially lithium carbonate and electroconvulsive therapy (ECT) (Abrams, Taylor, & Gaztanaga, 1974; Pope et al., 1980; Procci, 1976). In sum, schizoaffective patients are more like schizophrenics in their fragmented thinking and loose associations, but more like affectively disordered patients in their flight of ideas, mood instability, brain function, and response to treatment.

Schizophrenic and schizoaffective disorders tend to have divergent kinds of outcome (Stephens, 1978). Schizophrenics more often display a chronic pattern of unremitting or progressive impairment and long-term or repeated hospitalization (Harrow, Carone, & Westermeyer, 1985). In contrast, schizoaffectives more often have shorter hospitalizations and better treatment response (Pope & Lipinski, 1978; Tsuang, Dempsey & Rauscher, 1976). Nevertheless, the many exceptions to these observations raise questions about their utility in arguing that schizoaffective disorder represents a distinct type of psychopathology.

Unfortunately, the question cannot yet be satisfactorily resolved by evidence on etiology. The biological relatives of *schizoaffectives* have an elevated risk for all three major psychotic disorders: schizoaffective, schizophrenic, and manic-depressive (Angst, Grigo, & Lanz, 1981; Fowler, 1978; Kendler, Gruenberg, & Tsuang, 1985). However, the biological relatives of *schizophrenics* have an elevated risk for schizophrenic and schizoaffective disorders, but not for manic-depressive disorder, while the relatives of *manic-depressives* have an elevated risk for schizoaffective and manic-depressive disorders, but not for schizophrenia (Gershon et al., 1988). All these observations suggest that, while schizophrenia and manic-depressive disorders are distinct, some schizoaffective disorders are variants of schizophrenia, while others are variants of manic-depression (Angst, Felder, & Lohmeyer, 1979).

In this chapter we have described the behavioral and developmental aspects of psychotic symptoms, and also the evidence for distinguishing among major categories of psychotic disorder. We concluded that the schizophrenic and manic-depressive categories probably represent distinct psychopathologies but that the theoretical status of the schizoaffective category remains uncertain.

In the next two chapters, we proceed to a more detailed look at schizophrenia. The evidence will suggest that the psychosis of schizophrenia is *primary;* that is, produced directly by the cognitive psychopathology of the schizophrenic illness, but that the psychosis of affective disorders (Chapter 13) is a secondary by-product of extreme fluctuations in mood—the primary pathology—that sabotages otherwise normal cognitive mechanisms.

SUMMARY

All psychoses involve a loss of contact with reality. The central features of psychotic disorders are disorganized or fragmented thinking, idiosyncratic meanings, delusions, and hallucinations. These are sometimes called "positive" symptoms, suggesting excesses, and these are distinguishable from negative symptoms like apathy and social withdrawal that suggest deficiency. Different combinations of positive and negative symptoms seem to be relatively more prominent in the different disorders. The *schizophrenic* type usually involves mixtures of positive and negative psychotic symptoms. While the depressive variant of *affective* disorder typically includes only negative symptoms, the manic variant usually shows only positive symptoms. *Delusional* disorder—for example, paranoia—is characterized by specific delusions, but does not show marked signs of other positive symptoms such as thought disorder.

While schizophrenic, affective, and delusional psychoses can each exist in relatively pure form, mixtures of all three frequently occur. For example, *schizoaffective* disorder is marked by positive psychotic symptoms and by the excessive mood swings of affective disorder. For this and other reasons it is difficult to determine whether schizoaffective disorder exists as a distinct entity or is actually a variant of schizophrenia or affective disorder. Our discussion underscores the necessity of going below the surface of behavioral symptoms, and sets the stage for more systematic treatments of the two major types of functional disorders—schizophrenia and affective disorder.

Schizophrenia: I. Psychological Aspects

Schizophrenia is marked by disorganization of thought and deterioration of affect and motivation. Its most florid expression includes defective reality testing, thought disorder, bizarre delusions, apathy, social withdrawal, mannerisms, and an absence of the prominent mood fluctuations of affective disorder. An awesome and enigmatic mental disorder, its bizarre and shifting symptoms sabotage the competence and self-esteem of patients and cause hardship and sadness to relatives and friends. Schizophrenia has huge social and economic costs—for example, somewhere between $20 and $30 billion annually in treatment and lost productivity in America, where roughly one in 100—more than 2 million people—will develop the disorder during a lifetime.

Because of the complexity of the problem and the scope of the research, we devote two chapters to schizophrenia. Chapter 11 describes historical and contemporary approaches to its clinical description and to research on underlying psychological deficits. Chapter 12 deals with its biological mechanisms and etiology.

SCHIZOPHRENIA AS PROCESS AND SYNDROME

A disorder can be viewed "cross-sectionally" as a syndrome of basic symptoms that co-occur at some point in time. A disorder can also be viewed longitudinally, with special emphasis given to *changes* in symptomatic behavior that develop over time. The longitudinal perspective on schizophrenia distinguishes between process and reactive psychoses (Garmezy, 1966).

A *process* psychosis is characterized by insidious onset, chronic impairment, and resistance to treatment, characteristics that suggest some kind of underlying organic abnormality. Most investigators tend to view schizophrenia as a process psychosis (although the old term "process schizophrenia" is generally no longer used).

A *reactive* psychosis, on the other hand, is characterized by acute-onset, short-lasting psychotic disorganization often occurring with affective turmoil in reaction to adverse external events as interpreted by the person. Most investigators no longer think of reactive psychosis as a type of schizophrenia, and the old term "reactive schizophrenia" has been replaced in *DSM-III-R* by the category "brief reactive psychosis."

Table 11.1 clarifies the difference between process and reactive types of psychosis. While the table remains neutral about the classification of reactive psychosis, evidence discussed in Chapter 10 suggests that most cases of reac-

TABLE 11.1   CHARACTERISTICS OF SCHIZOPHRENIA AND REACTIVE PSYCHOSIS

Factor	Schizophrenia	Reactive psychosis
Premorbid adjustment	Poor (e.g., schizoid, antisocial, deficient)	Normal
Onset	Insidious	Acute
Apparent importance of "stress"	Little or none	Some or much
Course	Chronic	Short term
Nonpsychotic adjustment	Marginal; impaired	Recovered
Implicit hypothesis	Endogenous factors (e.g., genetic etiology; organic pathophysiology)	Exogenous factors (e.g., learning plus stress) interacting with *possible* genetic vulnerability

tive psychosis are atypical expressions of affective disorder, or at least something other than true schizophrenia.

In the *DSM-III-R* classification system, schizophrenic disorder represents a synthesis of process and syndrome views; schizophrenia is defined as a set of basic behavioral symptoms (syndromal view) with an insidious and chronic development over time (process view). We will describe some of the history and research first on the process, and then on the syndromal, aspects of schizophrenia. This will provide a foundation for understanding the theories about the essential nature and origin of the disorder.

Schizophrenia as Process

Classic Description by Kraepelin   One of the great pioneers of modern psychiatry was the German psychiatrist Emil Kraepelin (1856–1926) (Figure 11.1). Kraepelin adopted Benedict Morel's term ''dementia praecox'' to describe the entity that we now call schizophrenia. By dementia, Kraepelin meant an *organic* disorder with *progressive deterioration* of thought, affect, motivation, and behavior. By praecox, or precocious, Kraepelin meant that the disorder has an early ''ripening''; it begins to show up relatively early in adulthood, sometimes as early as early adolescence. In short, Kraepelin's dementia praecox concept was synonymous with early-onset process schizophrenia.

According to this process view, the diagnosis of schizophrenia (dementia praecox) required that the clinician give special attention to certain essential developmental features, including the time and nature of onset, the duration of symptoms, and the eventual outcome of the disorder. No wonder that Kraepelin was disinclined to apply the diagnosis to a rapid-onset, short-term psychotic disorder. In fact, Kraepelin would reverse an early diagnosis of dementia praecox if follow-up showed remission or recovery.

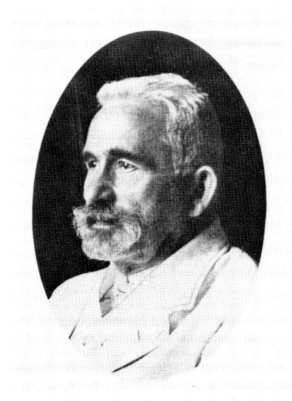

FIGURE 11.1   Emil Kraepelin (1856–1926), the German psychiatrist who pioneered the process view of schizophrenia (dementia praecox).

Course   In the light of many long-term follow-up studies, Kraepelin's emphasis on a chronic or deteriorating course seems to have been overly pessimistic. For example, Manfred Bleuler (1978) has carried out extensive work on outcome in schizophrenia. The following points summarize his and others' work on thousands of patients. First, only 10 percent of all schizophrenics remain continuously hospitalized. Second, after five years, the psychotic deterioration of the average patient tends to cease or even reverse; improvement occurs regardless of the specific criteria used to assess adjustment: hospitalization, earning capacity, or psychological condition, for example. Consider the observations of one prominent investigator. "Some of the patients who have hardly ever uttered coherent sentences start to speak or behave as if they were healthy on certain occasions, for instance, when on leave, at hospital festivities, or on the occasion of a catastrophe such as exploding bombs in wartime. I have seen improvements after 40 years' duration of a severe chronic psychosis. And, what is even more amazing, a schizophrenic may recover after having been psychotic and hospitalized for decades. Such a late, complete recovery is rare, but it occurs" (M. Bleuler, 1978, p. 633).

Bleuler believes that at least 25 percent of schizophrenic patients show permanent recovery with no need for drugs. Bleuler's concept of "recovery," however, does allow for the persistence of delusions and other cognitive disturbances, and this, along with other recent data (Crowe et al., 1986), suggests to some investigators that Bleuler may be overly optimistic.

Roughly 50 percent of improved schizophrenics regress or suffer varying degrees of continuous but milder dysfunction. For example, they "remain underactive, lack personal initiative, and have somewhat apathetic, colorless personalities" (M. Bleuler, 1978, pp. 634–635). After attending a meeting of Schizophrenics Anonymous, Roger Brown recounted a poignant experience. Brown tells us how the group leader

> began with an optimistic testimony about how things were going with him, designed in part to buck up the others. Some of them also spoke hopefully; others were silent and stared at the floor throughout. I gradually felt hope draining out of the group as they began to talk of their inability to hold jobs, of living on welfare, of finding themselves overwhelmed by simple demands. Nothing bizarre was said or done; there was rather a pervasive sense of inadequacy, of lives in which each day was a dreadful trial. Doughnuts and coffee were served, and then each one, still alone, trailed off into the Cambridge night.
>
> What I saw a little of at that meeting of Schizophrenics Anonymous is simply that there is something about schizophrenia that the antipsychotic drugs do not cure or even always remit on a long-term basis (Brown & Herrnstein, 1975, p. 641).

Some recovered but still dysfunctional schizophrenics show marked withdrawal and embarrassing social behavior (Creer & Wing, 1981). Withdrawal is expressed in avoiding people, spending long hours in isolation, showing little interest in external events, failing to initiate or even react to conversation, and doing things very slowly as if in a fog. Socially embarrassing behavior includes pacing late at night, expressing weird ideas, dressing or grooming in an exotic fashion, talking, laughing, or shouting spontaneously, or other odd behavior such as walking out of a room in the middle of a conversation. The characteristics most noticed by relatives who live with schizophrenics are isolation, underactivity, lack of conversation, few leisure interests, and slowness.

The fact is, confident conclusions about the long-term course in schizophrenia are complicated by variability in the results of studies that use different outcome measures of psychological, social, and vocational functioning. Nevertheless, the weight of the evidence seems to support Bleuler's relatively optimistic view over Kraepelin's more pessimistic view on the long-term course of schizophrenia. For example, a recent thirty-two-year follow-up study found that one-half or more of a group of hospitalized patients with *severe* schizophrenia—some hospitalized for as much as five years—were functioning well or had achieved at least significant improvement. Improvement included meaningful employment, stable friendships, and freedom from marked symptoms (Harding et al., 1987). These and similar findings cast doubt on Kraepelin's assumption that true schizophrenia inevitably involves long-term deterioration. Consequently, his insistence that a deteriorating course be used to validate an initial diagnosis of schizophrenia seems increasingly questionable.

To what extent are behavioral deterioration and relapse rates affected by the social environment? The behavior of hospitalized schizophrenics may be especially aggravated by stress in the environment. For example, schizophrenics display increased linguistic deficits especially when forced to communicate about personal matters (Shimkunas, 1972). And in some studies, relapse rates among hospital-discharged schizophrenics appear to be influenced by emotional turmoil in the family (Brown & Birley, 1968).

Research on family factors related to relapse has focused on expressed emotionality, or EE, including critical, hostile, or emotionally intrusive behavior toward the patient (Brown et al., 1966). In initial studies, the relapse rate for schizophrenics released to high EE conditions was very substantial (Vaughn & Leff, 1976), especially if the duration of exposure to high EE conditions was high (greater than thirty-five hours per week) and if the patient failed to continue to take medication. In fact, the data shown in Figure 11.2 suggested that overexposure to high EE conditions and failure to continue medication make relapse nearly a certainty (Vaughn & Leff, 1976).

In a follow-up study of twenty-five of these patients two years after discharge, Leff and Vaughn (1981) reported that a large percentage of high EE patients had relapsed *despite medication,* while none of the low EE patients taking antipsychotic drugs had relapsed. Nevertheless, low EE apparently does not guarantee sustained improvement because a large percentage of low EE patients will relapse if they stop taking medication. In short, the initial work suggested that both EE and medication are important to predicting relapse.

FIGURE 11.2   Relapse rates for 128 schizophrenic patients during a nine-month period. (Vaughn & Leff, 1976, p. 132)

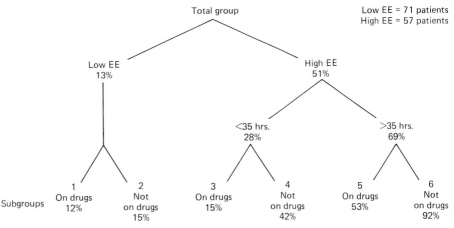

Recently, questions have been raised about the methodology of the earlier research, the size of the EE-relapse correlation, and thus the causal role of EE (Parker, Johnston, & Hayward, 1988). With regard to methodology, it has been noted that patients are obviously not randomly assigned to high or low EE environments, and typically there is no experimental control over patient drug-taking. Therefore, investigators cannot estimate the *independent effects* of EE versus drug compliance on the course of the disorder. Nor can they estimate the importance of the initial severity of the schizophrenia independent of drug and EE factors if, as is probably the case, severity of schizophrenia is associated with family patterns of high EE and tendencies not to comply with medication. So EE and medication "effects" found in some studies may to a large extent *reflect* rather than explain the course of schizophrenic disorder.

With regard to the EE-relapse correlation, four recent studies done in Europe and the United States have been unable to confirm earlier findings that it is substantial (see Hogarty, McEvoy, Munetz et al., 1988; Posner, Early, Reimer et al., 1988). At best, the EE-relapse correlation seems to be relatively small compared to the correlation between compliance/noncompliance with medication and relapse rate (MacMillan et al., 1986).

Nevertheless, we cannot entirely rule out the causal role of the EE factor because there is evidence that lowering EE can have positive effects on the course of schizophrenia. For example, when previously hospitalized schizophrenics returning to high EE families were given a family-oriented treatment designed to identify problems and develop family coping skills, there were sustained gains in terms of fewer relapses, lower drug dosage needed, and fewer positive symptoms in comparison to those in an individually oriented control treatment (Falloon et al., 1985) (see Figure 11.3). Perhaps family therapy promotes higher rates of release from the hospital and lower rates of symptom relapse more by encouraging compliance with antipsychotic medication than by promoting a supportive environment (Strachan, 1986). (For a review of the techniques, outcome, and theoretical implication of therapeutic interventions with schizophrenic patients, see *Schizophrenic Bulletin,* 1986, Vol. 12, No. 4.) One thing seems clear: there is no convincing evidence that EE has much to do with the etiology of schizophrenia; that is, the risk to developing schizophrenia in the first place (see Chapter 12).

Downward Social Drift   Consistent with a process view, schizophrenia is associated with so-called "downward social drift." That is, prior to hospitalization, the average schizophrenic has arrived at a lower socioeconomic status (SES) than either family background or the person's own educational achievements would predict. The evidence regarding downward social drift is as follows.

First, adult schizophrenics are concentrated in lower status occupations and in poorer neighborhoods than those typical of their biological parents (Faris & Dunham, 1939). This is true even for schizophrenic *adoptees,* regardless of the SES of rearing parents (Heston & Denny, 1968; Turner & Wagonfeld, 1967).

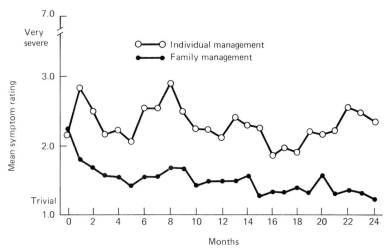

FIGURE 11.3   Average ratings for selected symptoms of schizophrenia over a twenty-four-month observation period. (From Falloon et al., 1985, p. 891. *Archives of General Psychiatry,* 1985, *42,* 887–896. Copyright © 1985, American Medical Association)

In contrast, *non*schizophrenic adoptees achieve *higher* SES than their adoptive parents (Wender et al., 1973). In short, it appears that the schizophrenic condition rather than the rearing environment determines the downward drift.

Second, a major discrepancy exists between the schizophrenic's achieved level of *education,* which is predictable from the biological father's SES, and achieved level of *occupation,* which is lower than expected. In other words, the schizophrenic's downward social drift is manifested more by reduced occupational attainment than by reduced intellectual capability (Dunham, Phillips, & Srinivasan, 1966). The schizophrenic "may function long enough to obtain a certain level of education, the real test comes when he enters the job market. Here his traits, attitudes, mannerisms, and verbal reactions become only too obvious and operate against his securing a position in the work force and—if he does secure some position—operate to restrict his advancement on the job" (Dunham, Phillips, & Srinivasan, 1966, p. 225). A reasonable conclusion is that failure to achieve occupationally appears to be a characteristic, rather than a cause, of schizophrenia.

Premorbid Adjustment and Prognosis   Kraepelin's process view of schizophrenia is supported by evidence (discussed in Chapter 12, pp. 319–320) that early signs of schizophrenia can be detected in premorbid adjustment, and that premorbid adjustment predicts outcome. A scale to estimate premorbid adjustment was devised by Phillips (1953). The items of the scale assess the capacity for heterosexual activity, sustained friendships, and meaningful work (see Table 11.2).

TABLE 11.2 THE PHILLIPS SCALE OF PREMORBID ADJUSTMENT IN SCHIZOPHRENIA (EXTREME ITEMS)

Area	Good	Poor
Recent sexual adjustment	Stable heterosexual relation and marriage	No sexual interest in either men or women
Social aspects of sexual life during adolescence and immediately beyond	Always showed a healthy interest in the opposite sex—with a "steady" during adolescence	No desire to be with boys and girls; never went out with opposite sex
Social aspects of recent sexual life—30 years of age and above	Married and has children, living as a family unit	Single, occasional same-sex contacts, no interest in opposite sex; single, interested in neither men nor women
Social aspects of recent sexual life—below 30 years of age	Married, living as family unit, with or without children	Single, never interested in or never associated with either men or women; asocial; antisocial; destructive, belligerent acting out against others
Personal relations: history	Always has been a leader, and always has had many close friends	Never worried about boys or girls; no desire to be with boys or girls
Recent adjustment in personal relations	Habitually mixed with others, was usually a leader	Antisocial, actively avoided contact, acted out against others

Source: Adapted from Garmezy (1966), Appendix B, pp. 464–466.

Positive correlations are found between Phillips scale scores and both duration of hospitalization and posthospital adjustment, but these correlations are surprisingly modest. The low correlations reflect an asymmetrical relationship between outcome and premorbid adjustments. In other words, while patients with the worst overall outcomes tend to have had poor premorbid adjustment, patients with the best outcomes have had *either* good or poor premorbid adjustment. Clearly, then, the process-reactive and poor versus good premorbid distinctions given in Table 11.1 are not completely interchangeable; too many patients show either a good premorbid but chronic/deteriorating pattern or a poor premorbid but remitting/recovering pattern.

So what can we conclude? The safest statement is that the development and ultimate outcome of schizophrenia are, at best, only roughly predictable from information about premorbid adjustment, symptom picture, and treatment responsiveness, but that no one of these is a powerful predictor in and of itself (World Health Organization, 1979). In other words, as Table 11.3 makes clear, premorbid adjustment is only one of many factors correlated with outcome. In fact, "it is the sheer number of favorable prognostic symptoms that provides the most powerful means of predicting remission. Accurate diagnosis finishes a poor second" (Vaillant, 1978, p. 638). Indeed, our ability ever to predict the outcome for a particular schizophrenic may always be severely limited by unknown chance factors (see Chapter 5, pp. 142–143).

Feighner et al. Criteria In 1972, investigators working at Washington Uni-

TABLE 11.3   PROGNOSTIC FACTORS

	Favorable sign	Unfavorable sign
Duration of onset	Six months or less from onset of disorder to hospitalization	More than six months from onset of disorder to hospitalization
Precipitating stress	Present	Absent
Age at first hospitalization	25 years or older	Younger than 25 years
Marital status	Ever married	Never married
Current age	Older	Younger
Social competence	Low score on Phillips Scale	High score on Phillips Scale

Source: Adapted from Bromet, Harrow, & Kasl, 1974, p. 204.

versity, St. Louis, published a set of criteria for diagnosing schizophrenia (Table 11.4). The so-called Feighner et al. criteria, named after the first author of the paper, included process factors. Thus, while section B in the table includes the familiar positive symptoms of hallucination, delusion, and communication disturbance, sections A and C include developmental and etiological features such as chronicity, premorbid adjustment, and pedigree.

TABLE 11.4   DIAGNOSTIC CRITERIA FOR SCHIZOPHRENIA ACCORDING TO FEIGHNER ET AL.

For a diagnosis of schizophrenia, A through C are required

A.   Both of the following are necessary:
   1. A chronic illness with at least six months of symptoms prior to the index evaluation without return to the premorbid level of psychosocial adjustment.
   2. Absence of a period of depressive or manic symptoms sufficient to qualify for affective disorder or probable affective disorder.

B.   The patient must have at least one of the following:
   1. Delusions or hallucinations without significant perplexity or disorientation associated with them.
   2. Verbal production that makes communication difficult because of a lack of logical or understandable organization. (In the presence of muteness the diagnostic decision must be deferred.)

C.   At least three of the following manifestations must be present for a diagnosis of "definite" schizophrenia, and two for a diagnosis of "probable" schizophrenia:
   1. Single.
   2. Poor premorbid social adjustment or work history.
   3. Family history of schizophrenia.
   4. Absence of alcoholism or drug abuse within one year of onset of psychosis.
   5. Onset of illness prior to age 40.

Source: Feighner et al., 1972. (*Archives of General Psychiatry*, 1972, *26*, 57–63. Copyright © 1972, American Medical Association)

The Feighner et al. criteria are the foundation out of which the Research Diagnostic Criteria (RDC) and the more widely used *DSM-III* and *DSM-III-R* criteria evolved. The appearance of Feighner et al. criteria represented a process view of schizophrenia and, more generally, a *medical model* of abnormal behavior, that is, an emphasis on biopsychological processes, diagnostic categories reflecting distinct mental illnesses, and medically oriented treatment (Klerman, 1978). This emphasis, reflected by the research described in Chapter 12, has an increasing influence on current theory, research, and treatment.

Schizophrenia as Syndrome

Another major pioneer of the study of abnormal behavior, Eugen Bleuler (1857–1939) (Figure 11.4), agreed with Kraepelin that psychotic disorders of the dementia praecox type have an organic basis and that the symptoms,

FIGURE 11.4   Eugene Bleuler (1857–1939), the Swiss psychiatrist who pioneered the syndromal concept of schizophrenia and coined the term.

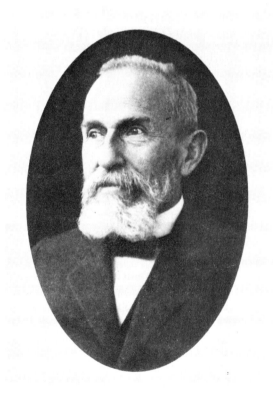

whether severe or mild, tend to persist for a lifetime. According to Bleuler: *"As yet I have never released a schizophrenic in whom I could not still see distinct signs of the disease; indeed there are very few in whom one would have to search for such signs.* . . .Therefore, we do not speak of *cure but of far-reaching improvements* and differentiate them from the severe deteriorations (in which the patient is wholly incapable of social relations) and from the mild deteriorations which include all the rest of the cases between the two extremes (Bleuler, 1911/1950, pp. 256; 258).

Nevertheless, Bleuler was less impressed than Kraepelin with the *diagnostic* significance of the course of a disorder, whether it be deteriorating or remitting. For this reason, Bleuler rejected the Kraepelinian view that a diagnosis of schizophrenia (Bleuler's term) should be revised when psychotic symptoms remitted and a reasonably productive lifestyle was reinstated. Bleuler therefore considered the seemingly "recovered schizophrenic" to be a beneficiary of good fortune rather than a victim of misdiagnosis.

Classic Description by Bleuler Bleuler emphasized four essential behavioral symptoms which were both necessary and sufficient for a diagnosis of the schizophrenic syndrome. These "fundamental" symptoms (Bleuler's "4 As") included: (1) *association disturbances* (ideation that is fragmented, tangential, circumstantial, and idiosyncratic), (2) *affective disturbances* (flat, wooden, or incongruous affects such as inappropriate mirth), (3) *ambivalence* (simultaneous or rapidly shifting love-hate sentiments regarding others), and (4) *autism* (withdrawal into fantasy). "Accessory" symptoms such as hallucination, delusion, and motor disturbances (catatonia) might often co-occur, but these symptoms were not necessary for the diagnosis. In fact, Bleuler used the term "simple schizophrenia" for cases that failed to display accessory symptoms.

Bleuler was especially interested in underlying cognitive mechanisms that might be inferred from clinical behavior. Kraepelin scorned the Bleulerian approach, which, like the psychoanalytic approach, he considered too speculative.

> Here we meet everywhere . . .the representation of arbitrary assumptions and conjectures as assured facts, which are used without hesitation for the building up of always new castles in the air ever towering higher, and the tendency to generalization beyond measure from single observations. I must frankly confess that with the best of will I am not able to follow the trains of thought of this "metapsychiatry," which like a complex sucks up the sober method of clinical observations. As I am accustomed to walk on the sure foundation of direct experience, my Philistine conscience of natural science stumbles at every step on objections, considerations and doubts, over which the lightly soaring power of imagination of Freud's disciples carries them without difficulty (Kraepelin, 1919/1971, p. 250).

Bleuler coined the term "schizophrenia" to represent the primary psychopathology underlying the patient's psychotic behavior. For Bleuler, the splitting (*schizo*) of mental life (*phrenia*) included the separation of (a) intention from action, causing passivity and avolition; (b) feeling from feeling, causing ambivalence; (c) feeling from thought, causing inappropriate emotion; and (d) thought from thought, causing associational loosening or disconnection. Bleuler considered associational disconnection to be the most direct expression of the hypothetical pathophysiology assumed to underlie schizophrenic behavior. Therefore, in his theory, disturbances of association are not only *fundamental,* that is, essential to making the diagnosis; they are also *primary*; that is, the most direct expression of the causal mechanism that explains the other symptoms.

Bleuler's theoretical distinction between primary symptoms indicating cause and secondary symptoms indicating effects prefigured the research on cognitive deficit that we take up later in the chapter. Now we look briefly at three sets of diagnostic criteria that treat schizophrenia as a syndrome of fundamental symptoms without suggesting that any of them might be primary.

International Pilot Study of Schizophrenia In the early 1970s, the World Health Organization (WHO) and the National Institute of Mental Health (NIMH) co-sponsored a nine-nation collaborative project to develop a set of diagnostic criteria for schizophrenia as a cross-culturally recognizable syndrome (Sartorius, Shapiro, & Jablonsky, 1974). Clinicians from mental health centers in each of nine Western, African, and Asian countries were trained to use the Present State Examination (PSE) (see Chapter 4, pp. 97–98, for structured interviewing). Diagnoses were done on more than 1000 patients initially screened to eliminate organicity, mental retardation, and drug abuse. Statistical procedures were used to identify the twelve variables that most clearly discriminated schizophrenics from nonschizophrenic patients (Carpenter, Strauss, & Bartko, 1973) and these are shown in Table 11.5. Notice that these items collectively represent a broad conceptualization of schizophrenia as a pathology of cognition and motivation like that suggested by Bleuler.

The International Pilot Study of Schizophrenia (IPSS) demonstrated that standardized methods can yield cross-culturally reliable diagnoses. It also suggested that previous reports of cross-cultural differences in the rates of schizophrenia reflect differences in diagnostic methods more than true prevalence. Additional evidence comes from a study of psychiatric diagnosis in New York and London (Cooper et al., 1972). Psychiatrists selected by the researchers used a standard set of narrow diagnostic criteria for distinguishing schizophrenia from affective disorder. With these criteria the project psychiatrists diagnosed as schizophrenic about 30 percent of all patients at hospitals in London and New York.

These rates for the diagnosis of schizophrenia among the specially trained psychiatrists compared well with the rates for nonresearch hospital clinicians in London who found 34 percent of the patients to be schizophrenic. However, they diverged rather dramatically from the 63 percent found by hospital clinicians in New York. Of the patients considered schizophrenic by the New York clinicians, 42 percent were diagnosed with *affective* disorder by the project investigators. The apparent overdiagnosis of schizophrenia by American clini-

TABLE 11.5   ITEMS FROM THE PRESENT STATE EXAMINATION (PSE) CORRESPONDING TO THE 12 SIGNS OR SYMPTOMS ESPECIALLY DISCRIMINATING SCHIZOPHRENIA FROM OTHER DISORDERS

Sign or symptom	PSE observation or question
Restricted affect	Blank, expressionless face. Very little or no emotion shown when delusion or normal material is discussed which would usually bring out emotion.
Poor insight	Overall rating of insight.
Thoughts aloud	Do you feel your thoughts are being broadcast, transmitted so that everyone knows what you are thinking? Do you ever seem to hear your thoughts spoken aloud (almost as if someone standing nearby could hear them)?
Waking early (−)*	Have you been waking earlier in the morning (one to three hours earlier than usual) and remaining awake?
Poor rapport	Did the interviewer find it possible to establish good rapport with patient during interview? Other difficulties in rapport.
Depressed faces (−)*	Facial expression sad, depressed.
Elation (−)*	Elated, joyous mood.
Widespread delusions	How widespread are patient's delusions? How many areas in patient's life are interpreted delusionally?
Incoherent speech	Free and spontaneous flow of incoherent speech.
Unreliable information	Was the information obtained in this interview credible or not?
Bizarre delusions	Are the delusions comprehensible?
Nihilistic delusions	Do you feel that your body is decaying, rotting? Do you feel that some part of your body is missing—for example, head, brain, or arms? Do you ever have the feeling that you do not exist at all, that you are dead, dissolved?

*(−) indicates that the *absence* of the criterion favors a diagnosis of schizophrenia.
Source: W. J. Carpenter, et al., A flexible system for the identification of schizophrenia. *Science,* 1973, *182,* 1275–1278. © AAAS.

cians has become less of a problem since *DSM-III* introduced clearer and more narrowly defined criteria that more closely fit the so-called European view.

Schizophrenia as *DSM* Disorder

The *process* concept of schizophrenia reflects the Kraepelinian focus on chronic, often progressive, impairment. The *syndrome* concept reflects the

Bleulerian focus on cross-sectionally defined fundamental symptoms. The *DSM-III-R* schizophrenia category reflects both the process and syndromal views. To appreciate this better, consider a little bit of history.

The diagnostic criteria of the *DSM-III-R* category represent a slight revision of the DSM-III criteria that had evolved from earlier versions rooted in the work of Feighner et al. Collectively, the effort to develop a modern working definition of schizophrenia was often guided by a basic scientific assumption—that the validity of a set of behavioral criteria constituting a working definition of a disorder should rest on five kinds of evidence (Robins & Guze, 1970): (1) developmental factors such as onset, course, and age; (2) laboratory findings such as differential drug responsiveness; (3) differences from other psychotic disorders; (4) outcome; and (5) family background.

Schizophrenia Conventionally Defined   The diagnostic criteria shown in Table 11.6 reflect this assumption about empirical evidence relevant to a working definition of a disorder like schizophrenia. For example, along with the major symptom-based criteria for detecting schizophrenia and for excluding organic and affective disorder, there are developmental criteria relating to duration and to premorbid and residual patterns.

Table 11.7 gives *DSM-III-R* criteria for variants or subtypes of schizophrenia. Although these subtypes can be diagnosed reliably at any one point in time, questions have been raised about their validity. For example, within a given schizophrenic episode, symptoms of supposedly different subtypes can be seen together. Across episodes, one subtype may change into another. "The fact that patients may be catatonic one week, paranoid the next month, and hebephrenic the next year discourages the use of traditional subtypes" (Carpenter & Stephens, 1979, p. 494). It is also true that the relatives of schizophrenics of whatever subtype have elevated risks for all types of schizophrenia; in other words, subtypes do not always seem to "breed true." In sum, despite questions about the validity of schizophrenia subtypes, the tradition of diagnosing them remains as durable as it is debatable (Kendler, Gruenberg, & Tsuang, 1988; Farmer, McGuffin, & Gottesman, 1987).

Paranoid versus Nonparanoid Subtypes   One such debate concerns the relation between paranoid and nonparanoid subtypes of schizophrenia. Are these two, in fact, really subtypes of the same disorder or is the nonparanoid type "real" schizophrenia while the paranoid type is basically a different disorder? There is quite a lot of evidence bearing on this question (Cromwell & Pithers, 1981; Kendler & Davies, 1981; Megaro, 1981; Silverman, 1964, 1967). The behaviors of paranoid and nonparanoid schizophrenics deviate in different, or even opposite, directions from each other on certain laboratory tests of perception and thinking. For example, paranoid schizophrenics have a greater than normal ability to recall incidental information compared with the less than normal ability of nonparanoid schizophrenics.

TABLE 11.6   DIAGNOSTIC CRITERIA FOR A SCHIZOPHRENIC DISORDER*

A. Presence of characteristic psychotic symptoms in the active phase: either (1), (2), or (3) for at least one week (unless the symptoms are successfully treated):

(1) Two of the following:
   (a) Delusions
   (b) Prominent hallucinations (throughout the day for several days or several times a week for several weeks, each hallucinatory experience not being limited to a few brief moments)
   (c) Incoherence or marked loosening of associations
   (d) Catatonic behavior
   (e) Flat or grossly inappropriate affect

(2) Bizarre delusions (i.e., involving a phenomenon that the person's culture would regard as totally implausible, such as thought broadcasting or being controlled by a dead person)

(3) Prominent hallucinations [as defined in (1)(b) above] of a voice with content having no apparent relations to depression or elation, or a voice keeping up a running commentary on the person's behavior or thoughts, or two or more voices conversing with each other

B. Deterioration from a previous level of functioning in such areas as work, social relations, and self-care.

C. Duration: Continuous signs of the illness for at least six months. The six-month period must include an active phase lasting at least one week (or less if successfully treated) during which there were psychotic symptoms from A, with or without a prodromal or residual phase, as defined below.

Prodromal phase: A clear deterioration in functioning before the active phase of the illness not due to a disturbance in mood or to a substance use disorder and involving at least *two* of the symptoms noted below.

Residual phase: Persistence, following the active phase of the illness, of at least *two* of the symptoms noted below, not due to a disturbance in mood or to a substance use disorder.

Prodromal or Residual Symptoms
1. Marked social isolation or withdrawal
2. Marked impairment in role functioning as wage-earner, student, or homemaker
3. Markedly peculiar behavior (e.g., collecting garbage, talking to self in public, or hoarding food)
4. Marked impairment in personal hygiene and grooming
5. Blunted, flat, or inappropriate affect
6. Digressive, vague, overelaborate, circumstantial, or metaphorical speech
7. Odd or bizarre ideation, or magical thinking (e.g., superstitiousness, clairvoyance, telepathy, "sixth sense," "others can feel my feelings," overvalued ideas, ideas of reference)
8. Unusual perceptual experiences (e.g., recurrent illusions, sensing the presence of a force or person not actually present)
9. Marked lack of initiative, interests, or energy

D. The full depressive or manic syndrome (criteria A and B of major depressive or manic episode), if present, developed after any psychotic symptoms, or briefly present relative to the duration of the psychotic symptoms in A.

E. Not due to any organic mental disorder, affective disorder, or mental retardation.

*The table presents a simplified summary of *DSM-III-R* criteria (American Psychiatric Association, 1987, pp. 194–195) that, in most respects, is quite similar to, or identical with, *DSM-III* criteria.

Source: Reprinted with permission from the *Diagnostic and Statistical Manual of Mental Disorders, Third Edition, Revised.* Copyright © 1987 American Psychiatric Association.

TABLE 11.7 DIAGNOSTIC CRITERIA FOR VARIANTS OF SCHIZOPHRENIC DISORDER

**1. Disorganized
(Hebephrenic) Type A type of schizophrenia in which the following criteria are met:**
  a. Incoherence, marked loosening of associations, or grossly disorganized behavior.
  b. Flat or grossly inappropriate affect.
  c. Does not meet the criteria for catatonic type (see below).
2. Catatonic Type A type of schizophrenia dominated by any of the following:
  a. Catatonic stupor (marked decrease in reactivity to environment and/or reduction of spontaneous movements and activity) or mutism.
  b. Catatonic negativism (an apparently motiveless resistance to all instructions or attempts to be moved).
  c. Catatonic rigidity (maintenance of a rigid posture against efforts to be moved).
  d. Catatonic excitement (excited motor activity, apparently purposeless and not influenced by external stimuli).
  e. Catatonic posturing (voluntary assumption of inappropriate or bizarre posture).
3. Paranoid Type A type of schizophrenia in which there are:
  a. Preoccupation with one or more systematized delusions or with frequent auditory hallucinations related to a single theme.
  b. *None* of the following: incoherence, marked loosening of associations, flat or grossly inappropriate affect, catatonic behavior, grossly disorganized behavior.
4. Undifferentiated Type A type of schizophrenia in which there are:
  a. Prominent delusions, hallucinations, incoherence, or grossly disorganized behavior.
  b. *None* of the criteria for any of the previously listed types.
5. Residual Type A type of schizophrenia in which there is:
  a. Absence of prominent delusions, hallucinations, incoherence, or grossly disorganized behavior.
  b. Continuing evidence of the disturbance, as indicated by two or more of the residual symptoms listed in criteria C for schizophrenia (see Table 11.6).

Differences in laboratory behavior reflect differences in clinical behavior. The paranoid schizophrenic is hypervigilant, conceptually rigid, and overintellectualized. The delusional ideas resist the influence of objective reality. The paranoid schizophrenic seems to be locked into a rigid and unshakable way of thinking by which any perception can be readily "explained." We might say that the "data" of the paranoid schizophrenic's personal experiences are *theory-driven,* that is, misinterpreted in the light of unshakable but equally erroneous assumptions.

In contrast, the nonparanoid schizophrenic is passive, impressionistic, disorganized, and unpredictable from moment to moment. The nonparanoid schizophrenic seems to be without general and enduring ideas about how personal experience should be organized. We might say that the ever-changing explanations, or "theories," of the nonparanoid schizophrenic are *data-driven.* Thus, from the clinical and laboratory perspective, paranoid and nonparanoid schizophrenia seem to involve different thought worlds (Megaro, 1981).

Despite evidence that different subtypes of schizophrenia may be significantly different in important areas of psychological functioning, investigators continue to search for a fundamental deficit that all subtypes of schizophrenia have in common.

PSYCHOLOGICAL DEFICIT IN SCHIZOPHRENIA

Bleuler's view that thought disorder is a core psychological problem of schizophrenia still dominates research on cognitive mechanisms of psychosis—for example, research on attention-deficit dysfunctions in schizophrenia. How can we understand both the florid symptoms of the psychotic episodes of schizophrenia (Chapman, 1966), and the subtler disturbances of thinking, or "cognitive slippage," that typify its prodromal and residual stages (Meehl, 1962)? Many investigators believe that a specific attention deficit lies at the heart of the schizophrenic disorder regardless of symptom severity.

To appreciate the cognitive aspect of schizophrenic psychopathology, we will first look at one of its more striking aspects—disorganized thoughts and speech—and then describe some of the more interesting research strategies for getting at underlying mechanisms. Our discussion, taking us from clinical behavior to basic mechanisms of information processing, will suggest that the psychopathology of schizophrenia is fundamentally *neuro*psychopathological. The next chapter, devoted to research on brain mechanisms and genetic etiology, will carry forward this theme of schizophrenia as a mental disease.

Language

Verbal Association Tests of simple verbal association show that schizophrenics deviate from normals in two diametrically opposite ways: either they choose rare and idiosyncratic associations or they choose common but inappropriate associations. Although schizophrenics can produce conventional associates (*up*: "down," *light*: "dark," for example), they often use infrequent ones (*up*: "there," *light*: "weight"). Many studies have found schizophrenics to be idiosyncratic in simple verbal association tasks, but this behavior is highly variable and situation-dependent.

Psychotic thinking is often controlled by stimuli and mental associations that are task-irrelevant. For example, schizophrenics seem especially vulnerable to selecting an incorrect answer from a set of alternatives that not only includes the correct answer, but a seductive incorrect answer, and an irrelevant answer (Chapman, 1958). In other words, schizophrenics seem distracted by ideas which, *in the given context*, are incorrect. For example, schizophrenics are prone to choose an alternative like **1** in the following example from Chapman and Chapman (1973, p. 129):

Robert said he likes rare meat. This means:

   1 He likes the kind of meat that is exceedingly uncommon.
   2 He likes a meat with bones in it.
   3 He likes partially cooked meat.

Alternative **1** expresses the strongest—that is, the most frequently used—meaning of the word *rare*. Within the context set by the master statement, however, the *weaker*, less frequently used word is called for, and therefore the stronger meaning is inappropriate.

This excessive yielding to strong and conventional, rather than to weaker but appropriate associations is observed in schizophrenics, but it is also observed in manics (Naficy & Willerman, 1980). Thus, excessive yielding to conventional but inappropriate meanings, while typically schizophrenic, is *not exclusively* schizophrenic. In other words, it reflects nonspecific factors like egocentricity, poor judgment, and carelessness, which are secondary to *more than one* type of psychiatric impairment.

Verbal Communication Most schizophrenics are syntactically competent, that is, their speech reflects the correct use of grammatical rules. On the other hand, schizophrenics are semantically deficient, often constructing and communicating meanings poorly. Research has repeatedly demonstrated failures of overall organization and an inability to appreciate another person's perspective, or egocentricity.

The disorganized quality of schizophrenic communication is expressed in the poor organization of sentences rather than in the poor organization within each sentence (Rutter, 1979). That is, schizophrenia involves a loss of the overall guiding intention that normally allows us to organize strings of sentences into coherent narratives. This kind of thing can also occur in mania, but it is less pervasive than in schizophrenia (Hoffman, Stopek, & Andreasen, 1986).

Figure 11.5*a* provides a model of verbal communication. Normally, the flow of sentences (at the bottom of diagram *a*) is controlled by higher-order intentions. These, in turn, are controlled by still higher, more general, ideas that constrain the general direction of the communication, not the specific form of the sentences. The specific form is controlled by lower intentional ideas.

Diagram *b* of Figure 11.5 illustrates the schizophrenic condition, in which hierarchical control breaks down. The higher-order intentional idea is lost when a sentence or the idea that controls it suggests some new, inconsistent idea. The result is a tangential change, or "knight's move," and a segmental rather than coherent flow of sentences. For example, to the question, "How are you this evening?" the schizophrenic might reply: "Keeping away from apples." In other words, the schizophrenic focuses on the *eve* part of evening, and, following a personal association to Adam and Eve, is swept away along an egocentric path of least resistance to an interpersonal irrelevancy (Shakow, 1977).

Attention

Everyone has experienced the effect of sleepiness on mental events: mind-wandering, distractibility, and intrusion of subjective fantasies. These and

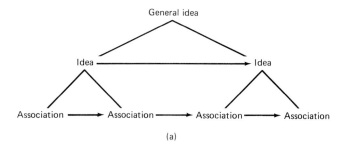

(a)

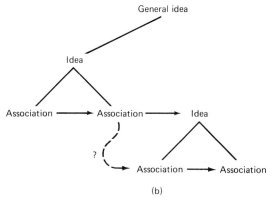

(b)

FIGURE 11.5 Hypothetical organization of the flow of verbal communication.
a. *Normal Situation.* Four specific ideas ("associations") are controlled by two more general ideas which in turn are directed "from above" by the most general idea (gist, notion, point). Control is top-down; i.e., the more general idea controls the more specific ideas. Any general idea elicited by a more specific association is suppressed. Thus, all the specific associations are consistent with their controlling ideas, which in turn are consistent with the overall general idea. This consistency (inner logic) of the speaker makes it easy for a listener to derive (re-create) that inner logic; i.e., to "get" the idea.
b. *Schizophrenic Situation.* New general ideas elicited by specific associations are *not* suppressed. The second association elicits a new idea, which takes over control and coordinates two new associations. These are mutually consistent but are inconsistent with the original idea and therefore are inconsistent with the first two associations. Top-down control has been replaced by bottom-up control. The result is a segmentalizing of set: two sets (controlling ideas) rather than one. If segmentalizing is momentary and there is a return to the original idea, we speak of cognitive slippage; it is difficult but possible for the listener to get the drift of such communication, with its incomprehensible associative links (indicated by dashed arrow and question mark). But if the segmentalization is more or less permanent, overall meaning may be lost to both speaker and listener.

other qualities are exaggerated in the thought disorder of acute psychotic conditions. Sights and sounds are very intensely experienced, as though brightness and volume "controls" were turned up to maximum. There is a concomitant increase in distractibility occasioned by an intensification of the experience of normally peripheral sights and sounds. Sensations and ideas come and go in a kaleidoscopic rush of experience. This state of heightened consciousness and disorganized thinking is elegantly described by a former patient.

> What I do want to explain, if I can, is the *exaggerated state of awareness* in which I lived before, during and after my acute illness. At first it was as if parts of my brain "awoke" which had been dormant, and I became interested in a wide assortment of people, events, places and ideas which normally would make no impression on me. . . .The walk of a stranger on the street could be a "sign" to me which I must interpret. Every face in the windows of a passing streetcar would be engraved on my mind, all of them concentrating on me and trying to pass me some sort of message. Now, many years later, I can appreciate what had happened. Each of us is capable of coping with a large number of stimuli, invading our being through any one of the senses. . . .It's obvious that we would be incapable of carrying on any of our daily activities if even one hundredth of all these available stimuli invaded us at once. So the mind must have a filter which functions without our conscious thought, sorting stimuli and allowing only those which are relevant to the situation in hand to disturb consciousness. And this filter must be working at maximum efficiency at all times, particularly when we require a high degree of concentration. What had happened to me in Toronto was a breakdown in the filter, and a hodge-podge of unrelated stimuli were distracting me from things which should have had my undivided attention (MacDonald, 1960, pp. 175–176).

This "faulty filter" mechanism is believed to produce odd associations, peculiar ideas, lapses of attention and other types of cognitive slippage. These are found not only in florid psychotic episodes, but also in the prodromal, morbid, and residual stages of chronic schizophrenia. Moreover, the "faulty filter" mechanism would presumably be primary in schizophrenia. In nonschizophrenic psychoses, an attentional dysfunction would be the result of something else—for example, a severe manic-depressive mood disorder. It is widely believed that a dysfunction of attention is a (if not *the*) primary cognitive defect in schizophrenia. We begin our discussion of the attentional dysfunction by focusing on reaction-time experiments.

Reaction Time Attention can be assessed from the speed of a response to a critical stimulus, and the loss of attentional capacity can be assessed from the inability to sustain speedy reactions across many trials. In a typical procedure, a subject sits in front of a screen where stimuli are displayed. The index finger of the preferred hand rests on a button, or "key." The subject is instructed to lift the finger off the key as quickly as possible in response to a critical stimulus—a light, for example. Attention can then be assessed in terms of reaction time (RT); that is, the time between onset of the critical stimulus and initiation of the reaction.

The classic work in this area is that of Rodnick and Shakow (1940). On each trial, the critical stimulus (light) is preceded by a warning bell. The subject is told to press a button at the sound of the bell and release it as soon as the light appears. The interval between warning signal (bell) and critical stimulus (light) is called the *preparatory interval*, or PI. Two features of the PI are important:

duration and predictability. On each trial, the duration of the PI can be short or long; across trials, the duration of the PI can be varied or held constant. If, within a set of trials, the PI is held constant, the onset of the critical stimulus can be predicted from the warning stimulus. However, if the PI is continually varied from trial to trial, the onset of the critical stimulus cannot be predicted. Schizophrenics typically produce slower RTs than nonschizophrenic controls. But more significantly, they also show a *crossover pattern*. Both characteristics are shown in Figure 11.6.

The crossover pattern refers to the relationship between RT and the two characteristics of the PI: predictability and duration. Schizophrenics show relatively *faster* RTs for regular, or predictable, trials of short duration, but they show relatively *slower* RTs to regular trials of long duration. The crossover pattern can easily be discerned in Figure 11.6. Compare the crossover pattern of the schizophrenics with the somewhat different pattern shown by the controls, who generally show shorter RTs, especially for regular trials.

The crossover pattern has been found for schizophrenics, but usually not for patients with other functional disorders or for normals. Interestingly enough, however, the pattern also occurs in college students with mild thought disorder, including those with elevations on the schizophrenia scale of the MMPI (Rosenbaum, Shore, & Chapin, 1988; Simons, MacMillan, & Ireland, 1982). If this crossover pattern were indeed a behavioral *marker,* an outward sign of a liability specifically to schizophrenia, we would expect the crossover

FIGURE 11.6   Mean reaction time for schizophrenics (*N* = 25) and normal controls (*N* = 10) depends on the duration and regularity, or predictability, of the preparatory interval. (From Rodnick & Shakow, 1940. *American Journal of Psychiatry, 90,* 214–255. Copyright © 1940, The American Psychiatric Association. Reprinted by permission.)

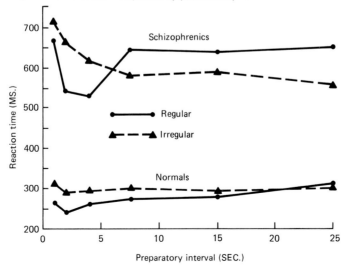

pattern to be associated with increased risk for developing schizophrenia—for example, in people who have a schizophrenic relative, or who later come down with the disorder. Unfortunately, reliable evidence bearing on these expectations is not yet available.

Reaction time and related research suggest that schizophrenics are unable to derive and maintain a stable idea, or "set," from task-related events. The result is a constantly shifting and disorganized series of ideas—what Shakow has called segmental sets—that are driven willy-nilly by inner needs interacting with task-irrelevant stimuli (Shakow, 1977). Let us take a closer look.

Distracted Attention Vulnerability to the distracting effects of task-irrelevant information can be demonstrated by the performance of schizophrenics on tests of apprehension span and continuous performance. Span-of-apprehension scores reflect an ability to detect accurately a target stimulus embedded in a briefly presented array of irrelevant stimuli. For example, Asarnow and MacCrimmon (1978) found that acute and remitted schizophrenics were much less able than normals to detect a target stimulus (a T or an F) within an array of five or ten letters, although the deficiency was not evident for a three-letter array or when only the target letter was presented. A similar deficit was also reported for fostered-away children of schizophrenics compared with fostered-away children of normals (Asarnow et al., 1978). Together, these findings for acute and remitted schizophrenics and for the offspring of schizophrenics suggest that a span-of-apprehension deficit might be a schizotypal characteristic; that is, a marker for a liability specifically to schizophrenic disorder. This hypothesis must be considered tentative because, as yet, there is no reliable evidence that nonschizophrenic psychotics in remisson and/or their normal relatives tend not to display the putative schizotypal pattern of attention deficit.

The continuous performance test assesses the patient's capacity to maintain attention to critical stimuli that occasionally appear within the context of continually changing irrelevant stimuli. For example, Asarnow and MacCrimmon (1978) asked subjects to signal when they detected a critical stimulus—the number 7—presented visually for 70 milliseconds on 20 percent of the trials (see Figure 11.7). In the distractor condition, subjects heard a voice reading digits. About every third trial the voice read the number 7, the critical digit.

Errors of two kinds were analyzed: errors of omission, or failures to detect, and errors of commission, or false positives. For both measures, and regardless of condition, acute schizophrenics did poorly and normals did well; in the distractor condition, remitted schizophrenics performed poorly, but in the nondistractor condition, they performed more like normals. Others have confirmed this marked effect of the distractor condition in the continuous performance test both for remitted schizophrenics and for the offspring of schizophrenics. Therefore, the continuous performance data provide further evidence of a susceptibility to distraction which, like the span-of-apprehension deficit, may characterize the schizotypal liability.

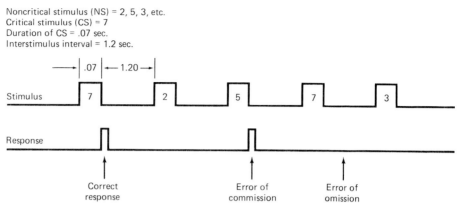

Noncritical stimulus (NS) = 2, 5, 3, etc.
Critical stimulus (CS) = 7
Duration of CS = .07 sec.
Interstimulus interval = 1.2 sec.

FIGURE 11.7 Schematic representation of continuous performance on one version of the CPT described in Asarnow & MacCrimmon (1978).

Sensory Memory   We have seen that schizophrenics are especially susceptible to the distracting effects of task-irrelevant information. Modern experimental techniques have also revealed an analogous deficit at an earlier stage of perception—specifically, the stage at which sensory information is made consciously memorable.

Visual, auditory, somesthetic, and other kinds of sensory information undergo a series of almost instantaneous transformations from concrete "thing" qualities to abstract idea, and from detail to gist. At each level, information is held in a memory "bin" and operated upon. Early on in this process, virtually all sensory information representing external and bodily events is held for a fraction of a second in a bin called the *sensory information store* (SIS). Every split second, selected aspects of SIS are subjected to cognitive operations which produce the more abstract spatial and verbal representations of conscious experience. A limited number of these representations can be held for a longer but still limited time in the bin called *short-term memory* (STM). STM ideas can be transformed into still more abstract and unconscious ideas, which are held more or less permanently in the bin called *long-term memory* (LTM). Figure 11.8 presents a simplified flow diagram of a response that is controlled by STM processes whose transformation of SIS information is, in turn, controlled by LTM.

Experiments have tested the hypothesis that schizophrenics have trouble transferring SIS information into memorable ideas or images that can be retained and communicated over time (Saccuzzo & Braff, 1981, Saccuzzo & Schubert, 1982). In a base-line condition, a critical stimulus, A or T, is projected for a fraction of a second. Poor-prognosis schizophrenics—those patients with the most severe and unremitting form of schizophrenia—require a longer exposure time to recognize the letter than do good-prognosis schizophrenics, manics, depressives, or normals (Saccuzzo & Braff, 1981; Braff & Succuzzo, 1985).

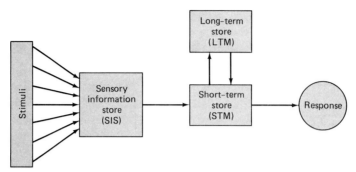

FIGURE 11.8 Schematic diagram of the transformation of a physical stimulus into a motoric response. The three components of transformation are sensory information stores (SIS), short-term memory (STM), and long-term memory (LTM).

In the *backward masking* condition, the critical stimulus is almost immediately followed by a *mask* stimulus—in this case an array of four Xs that degrades the mental image of the critical stimulus if projected quickly enough to the same location in the visual field. Compared with other psychiatric and normal subjects, poor-prognosis schizophrenics need about twice as much time—from the offset of the critical stimulus to the onset of the mask—to identify the target.

Figure 11.9 shows a schizophrenic pattern (above) and a normal pattern (below). Note that the schizophrenic requires more time (18 milliseconds versus 10 milliseconds) to view the letter under nonmasked conditions, and more time (120 milliseconds versus 70 milliseconds) to "protect" the letter from the

FIGURE 11.9 Backward masking paradigm. The figure shows the durations of stimulus (S), interstimulus interval (ISI), and mask for schizophrenics (upper) and normal controls (lower). Note that the schizophrenics require longer exposure (18 as against 10 milliseconds) of S in the nonmask condition, and a longer ISI (120 as against 70 milliseconds) in the backward masking condition. The stimulus is either an A or a T, while the mask is a set of Xs.

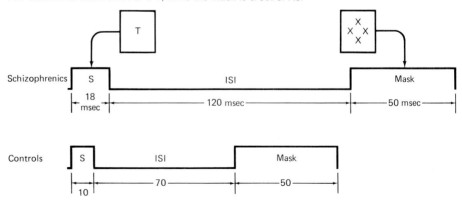

effects of the mask. This implies slower information processing to extract a conscious, and at least briefly memorable, image from a purely sensory visual "model" that is stored momentarily in SIS. The research suggests that "with a slowing down of information transfer in posticonic stages of information processing, the nature and quality of information that reaches the higher brain centers become altered. As a result, the individual not only loses critical information but also fails to perceive as others do" (Saccuzzo & Schubert, 1981, p. 310).

The fact that the adverse backward masking effect has been found for poor-prognosis schizophrenics, even when their symptoms are in remission, suggests that the effect may be a marker for the schizotypal liability rather than merely a feature of the psychotic state. Consistent with this hypothesis is the finding that subjects with schizotypal personality disorder perform like schizophrenics on the backward masking task (Saccuzzo & Schubert, 1981). Nevertheless, the hypothesis must remain tentative because there is as yet insufficient evidence that the pattern is reliably found in schizophrenics and their relatives, while less so in nonschizophrenics and their relatives.

Eye Tracking Attention deficit in schizophrenia can also be inferred from abnormalities in how well the eye tracks moving stimuli. Subjects in these studies attempt to follow the continuous rise and fall motion—that is, the sinusoidal movement—of a pendulum or a dot on a TV screen. Electrodes attached to the sides of each eye pick up tiny electrical signals, and eye movement is then measured by amplifying these signals. The result is a recording of *smooth pursuit eye movement* (SPEM), which normally conforms to the continuous movement of the stimulus.

Eye-tracking deviance appears to have a strong heritable component (Holzman et al., 1977). Moreover, schizophrenics and their relatives show elevated rates of deviant SPEM (Holzman, Levy, & Proctor, 1976). Instead of the normally smooth sinusoidal pattern, the record shows jagged irregularities, or "jumps," that are superimposed on poorly formed waves (see Figure 11.10a). When subjects with such a pattern are asked to detect changing numbers that appear on the moving pendulum, the pattern becomes somewhat less jerky (see Figure 11.10b). Some medications (lithium carbonate, for example) and aging are associated with deviant SPEM (Levy et al., 1983; Lipton et al., 1983). When these factors are eliminated or at least controlled statistically, deviant SPEM still occurs in schizophrenics and their relatives but *not* in affective patients and their relatives (Levy et al., 1983). Evaluating the SPEM data, Holzman and Levy (1977) comment that "SPEM dysfunctions implicate a neurophysiological substrate of impaired nonvoluntary attention in schizophrenia. This may be described as a failure of inhibitory, synchronizing, or integrating systems . . ."(p. 22).

These comments are consistent with the data on reaction time, masking, span of apprehension, and continuous performance, and also with data from EEG studies of the electrocortical evoked potential. EEG studies usually find

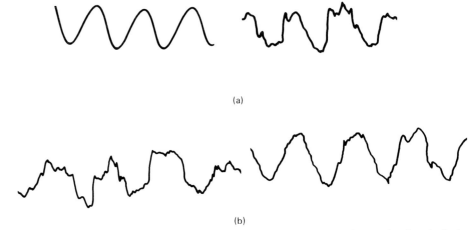

FIGURE 11.10 Two sets of SPEM. *a.* Normal (left) versus abnormal (right) pattern, the abnormal pattern typical of schizophrenics. *b.* Abnormal pattern (left) more "normalized" (right) during number reading. (Adapted from Holzman, Levy, & Proctor, 1976, pp. 1418–1419. *Archives of General Psychiatry,* 1976, *33,* 1415–1420. Copyright © 1976, American Medical Association)

that schizophrenics show an abnormally *high* amplitude in early components (less than 100 milliseconds), and an abnormally *low* amplitude in the late components (about 300 milliseconds), of a stimulus-evoked EEG response. This pattern, also observed in the children of schizophrenics, suggests impaired sensory information "filtering" (Friedman, Erlenmeyer-Kimling, & Vaughn, 1984). Unfortunately, a more exact characterization of this hypothetical impairment still eludes us.

Sensory Gating As we noted above, perception involves the detection, selection, and transformation of sensory information. Much of this goes on outside of conscious awareness. Nevertheless, certain aspects of this complex process can be studied with the aid of laboratory techniques. A good example is the earlier-described visual masking technique used to study the transformation of sensory information into short-term memories. Another technique uses the repeated presentation of sensory stimuli such as light flashes or clicks that elicit EEG patterns called *evoked responses.* You will recall that an EEG is a pattern of spontaneous "brain waves" that represents a continuous change in electrical activity—more accurately, a continuous change in voltage—over a period of time. Typically, the time frame of an evoked response—a momentary perturbation of the EEG caused by a discrete stimulus—is sometimes only a fraction of a second. Researchers typically induce many evoked responses by the use of repeated stimulation with lights or tones. When many evoked responses are averaged to remove the "noise" of unsystematic fluctuations, a relatively "clean" pattern, the averaged evoked response, emerges.

The average evoked response can be used to assess the integrity of brain mechanisms that underlie sensory information processing. Depending on where in time an abnormality appears in the averaged evoked response—immediately after the stimulus or a fraction of a second later—the investigator can estimate at what stage in sensory information processing a defect exists, anywhere from the unconscious registration of a stimulus in sensory neurons to its transformation into a conscious and memorable perception by association cortex.

We can now describe an interesting method for investigating the widely held view that schizophrenia involves a defect in the ability to *gate,* or filter, sensory information. In this research, an *auditory* evoked potential is elicited by each of two clicks, the second click occurring 500 milliseconds after the first. Normally, the evoked response to the second click is smaller—it has a lower amplitude as indicated by a smaller deflection of the EEG pens—than the evoked response to the first click. This suggests that, normally, the auditory part of the brain takes more than half a second to "recover" from the first click.

Schizophrenics typically do not show this pattern of reduced second-click response; their response to the second click is almost as strong as the response to the first click. The difference between normals and schizophrenics is illustrated in Figure 11.11. Note that the downward ("positive") deflection at about 50 milliseconds after the second click (P-50) is greater for the schizophrenic (Adler, Waldo, & Freedman, 1985; Siegel et al., 1984).

Siegel et al. (1984) also found that many schizophrenics with this EEG abnormality have the eye-tracking abnormality as well. Curiously, while the normal parents of the schizophrenics also tended to have elevated overall rates of these abnormalities, both abnormalities were unlikely to co-occur in the same parent. The results suggest that a person with both abnormalities, each one perhaps inherited from a different parent, has a greater chance of being pushed over the threshold for developing schizophrenic disorder. A single liability factor may not be sufficient to exceed the schizophrenic threshold.

The abnormal P-50 pattern also occurs in some nonschizophrenic patients, but disappears when they recover. In contrast, the abnormality occurs more frequently in schizophrenics whether they are disturbed or in remission, and also in their well relatives. It is possible that the P-50 abnormality is part of the *liability* to schizophrenia, even though it is common during the acute phase of many other disorders.

Action Monitoring

Research on attention deficit in schizophrenia typically assumes that there is something wrong with the "input" side of information processing, with the way that schizophrenics perceive and think about external events. Another

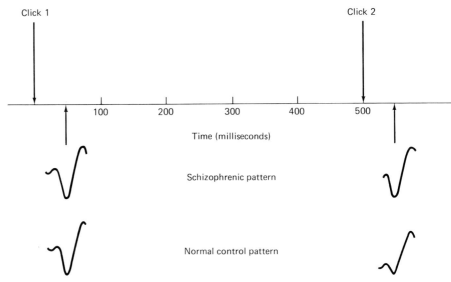

FIGURE 11.11 Averaged evoked EEG patterns in response to successive clicks. The positive (downward) component about 50 milliseconds after the second click—the so-called P-50 component—is abnormally prominent in the schizophrenic's response, given the normal control pattern. (From Siegel et al., 1984)

possibility is that the problem involves the "output" side. According to Frith and Done (1988), schizophrenics are dysfunctional in monitoring spontaneous, or self-initiated, actions, and in distinguishing these from their reactions to external stimuli. For example, hearing voices, or believing that one's thoughts are being "inserted" by an external source, could be explained as a failure to recognize self-initiated inner speech or thought.

Scientific tests of the action-monitoring deficit hypothesis are now being carried out. For example, in normal subjects, there is a large difference in the evoked EEG response to self-produced tones (small response) and to externally produced tones (large response). The action-monitoring deficit hypothesis predicts that schizophrenics will display large responses under both conditions, and there is preliminary evidence consistent with this prediction (Frith & Done, 1988). It is still too early to assess the validity and importance of the action-monitoring deficit hypothesis for schizophrenia, but it seems potentially capable of explaining many of the positive symptoms that characterize the disorder.

Affect, Motivation, and Schizophrenic Deficit

Many schizophrenics are chronically undermotivated, and they display this clinically in the form of negative symptoms. On laboratory tasks, too, they perform better only when artificially motivated by physiologically significant stimuli, such as shocks, or verbally significant stimuli, such as harsh criticism. Compared with normals, schizophrenics are differentially affected by different stimuli in the following manner, according to Buss (1966):

Verbal reward (praise):	No effect
Urging:	Little effect
Verbal punishment (censure):	Effect as great as for normals
Physiologically significant punishment (shock, noise):	Strong effect and greater than that for normals

What is the significance of schizophrenic undermotivation? Is it a cause or an effect of cognitive deficit, or is it an independently co-occurring factor that interacts with cognitive deficit to make a bad situation even worse? Schizophrenic undermotivation might be a *cause* of cognitive deficit, although no one has shown how. On the other hand, schizophrenics undermotivation might be an *effect* of cognitive deficit; that is, it might express hopelessness in the face of unremitting and glaring inadequacies in managing one's life.

A third view is that undermotivation and cognitive deficits are *co-occurring* primary factors. Neither causes the other, but each interacts with the other in the same person to produce an all-encompassing psychological "rootlessness" that sets thought adrift and prevents the secure development of normal feelings and attachments. This third view reflects the Kraepelin/Bleuler tradition that holds that schizophrenia is, fundamentally, as much a disorder of motivation as of cognition.

Problems with the Psychological Approach

General Problems   There are various problems with research on the psychological deficit(s) of schizophrenia. These include failure to replicate findings, deficiency of theoretical understanding, and failure to utilize proper control groups in experimental studies. Failures to replicate findings in schizophrenia research may reflect differences in samples or measurement or, more importantly, failure to control for the influence of factors such as psychosis, hospitalization, or local conditions that are not specific to schizophrenia.

Theoretical progress in schizophrenia is limited by theoretical progress in general psychology. To the extent that we are uncertain about terms like attention, it will remain difficult to develop useful theories of attentional deficits that do anything more than merely summarize our observations. For example, the results of performance on span of apprehension, continuous performance, and other tests of attention show smaller intercorrelations than we would expect, assuming that a single common underlying process is present.

Specificity of Schizophrenic Deficit   Inadequacy of controls is a serious problem. For example, much of the research involves comparisons between schizophrenics and nonpsychiatric, or normal, controls. The IQ distribution of schizophrenics is typically somewhat lower than that of controls. This difference means that any or all of the important findings in the cognitive area—the effects of masking or distraction, for example—could reflect differences in intelligence rather than differences in psychopathology. Therefore, in order to study schizophrenics and nonschizophrenics of equal intelligence, one is forced to study either a nonrepresentative sample of brighter than average schizophrenics or an equally nonrepresentative sample of duller than average normals. The latter has been the preferred method.

However, without a *set* of control groups, differences have minimal theoretical or practical usefulness. Is an interesting finding specific to schizophrenia or does it reflect psychosis (or organicity) more generally? To determine whether the observed behavior is specific to schizophrenia, the investigator requires manic-depressive psychotics and other psychiatric controls. Do obtained differences reflect the quality and duration of hospitalization? To find our, the researcher would need nonschizophrenic patients with either psychiatric disorders, such as depression, or medical disorders, such as chronic heart conditions, who are subject to somewhat similar hospital experiences. Do differences reflect a liability to schizophrenia or merely a schizophrenic psychosis? The answer would require data on premorbid and postmorbid conditions and on the relatives of schizophrenics. In short, we need good control groups to determine if, and in what way, a psychological deficit is specifically schizophrenic (Lewine, 1984).

Variability of Schizophrenic Behavior   Variability within a single subject is a frequently observed feature of schizophrenia: deficits within one person may come and go from day to day, year to year, and even test to test within a single session. Schizophrenic behavior, by its very nature, seems to include episodic or periodic deficits superimposed on a more chronic cognitive disorder. This variability raises an important question about cognitive deficit: is it also variable, and if so, why? If the underlying cognitive deficit is chronic, how do we explain the behavioral variability so typical of schizophrenia? If the cumulative effect of cognitive deficit is the degradation of intellectual and social competence, how do we explain social and intellectual recoveries of chronic schizophrenics? And if cognitive deficit is merely another aspect of schizophrenia, if it does not provide the theoretical mechanism to explain the clinical phenomena of schizophrenia, what does?

SUMMARY

A schizophrenic disorder, as currently defined by the behavioral criteria of *DSM-III-R*, is typically characterized by hallucinations, delusions, thought disorder, and autistic egocentricity. Its motivational features include social withdrawal, affective flatness, and apathy. Its adverse impact on self, family, and society makes it one of the costliest of human problems.

Within recent history, diagnostic fashion has emphasized either the *process* aspect of the disorder, reflecting Emil Kraepelin's focus on the developmental features of insidious onset, chronic course, and debilitating outcome, or its *syndromal* aspect, reflecting Eugen Bleuler's focus on fundamental symptoms such as mental fragmentation and autistic withdrawal. *DSM-III-R* includes criteria that take both aspects into consideration.

Evolving from the Bleulerian tradition of investigating abnormal psychological mechanisms, modern laboratory research on attention has yielded important clues about schizophrenic deficits. The prime suspect appears to be a malfunction of one or more components of the active memory mechanism that retains and processes sensory information free from the disorganizing effects of irrelevant information. Markers for the hypothetical defect(s) of attention include (1) abnormal reaction time, (2) deficiency on continuous performance tasks, (3) susceptibility to the effects of stimulus degradation, (4) sensory flooding, and (5) correlated abnormalities in the way the eye tracks smoothly moving visual stimuli.

The evidence suggests that an attentional dysfunction underlies the clinically more familiar peculiarities of thinking and language of schizophrenics. Equally important, similar abnormalities observed in the nonschizophrenic first-degree relatives of schizophrenic patients suggest that mild versions of schizophrenic deficit may be markers of a liability to the disorder. Evidence in the next chapter suggests that the deficit is *neuro*psychopathological.

There are problems with the research methodology used to investigate schizophrenia. For example, the *specificity* of the so-called schizophrenic deficit depends on its occurring only in schizophrenics and persons at risk for schizophrenia, that is, schizophrenics in remission, people who later become overtly schizophrenic, and relatives of schizophrenics. However, many studies, especially the older ones, merely compared schizophrenic patients with normals without controlling for psychosis per se (for example, comparing actively psychotic schizophrenics with schizophrenics in remission), or for type of psychotic disorder (schizophrenia versus manic-depression, for example), or for medication, confinement, intelligence, and other factors. Therefore, we are not sure that the so-called schizophrenic deficit is really specific to schizophrenia.

Schizophrenia: 2. Biopsychological Origins

In the last chapter we described some of the major psychological characteristics of schizophrenia that appear both in the laboratory and in everyday life; namely, poor reality testing, thought disorder, and delusions. We then reviewed evidence that the thought disorder of schizophrenia may reflect defects in the mechanisms of attention that are responsible for integrating perceptions and memories. Now we turn to the evidence that heredity and brain abnormalities underlie these psychological abnormalities.

DEVELOPMENTAL DEFICITS

The onset of a schizophrenic disorder typically occurs during late adolescence or early adulthood. Behavioral abnormalities may, however, show up during childhood and even as early as infancy. Let us therefore take a closer look at research suggesting a developmental connection between certain abnormal behavior patterns of childhood and the schizophrenic disorder of adulthood.

Personal and Social Deficits

Early behavioral signs that predict schizophrenia can be revealed either by retrospective or prospective studies (Watt et al., 1984). The *retrospective* strategy reconstructs *pre*schizophrenic patterns of behavior from the childhood records of adult schizophrenics. The *prospective* strategy (Mednick & Schulsinger, 1968) follows the development of children of schizophrenics, the high-risk group, and compares this with the development of the children of normals, the low-risk group. Roughly 10 percent of the high-risk children will eventually become schizophrenic, and others will show at least mildly schizophrenic behavior.

A practical problem with the prospective strategy is that a large number of high-risk children must be tracked because evidence suggests that only 10 percent of them will become frankly schizophrenic, although others may have different behavioral problems. Also, since most schizophrenics do *not* have a schizophrenic parent, some of the results obtained from the prospective study of high-risk subjects may apply only to those schizophrenics who have a schizophrenic parent. To simplify our summary, we will combine the results of both retrospective and prospective studies of *preschizophrenic* behavior patterns during infancy and childhood.

Preschizophrenics have been found to be excessively distractable and to have disorganized and peculiar associations on many laboratory measures (Asarnow et al., 1978; Mednick & Schulsinger, 1968). Preschizophrenics often strike others as ''odd'' because of their peculiar ideas and emotional flatness, and also as ''egocentric'' because of their self-preoccupation, their insensitivity to others, and their apparent lack of insight about their peculiarities. Compared to children who never develop schizophrenia, preschizophrenic children are psychologically immature (Mednick & Schulsinger, 1968). In males, this immaturity is manifested by antisocial patterns of aggressive, unstable, abrasive, defiant, and cheerless behavior, while in females, immaturity is manifested more by introversion and social isolation (Mednick et al., 1984; Watt & Lubensky, 1976; Watt, Grubb, & Erlenmeyer-Kimling, 1982).

If a single expression can capture the essence of a pattern of results so complex as the one for the schizophrenics, it is emotional immaturity. . . . There were frequent references to "crying with slight provocation," "being overshadowed by older siblings," "insensitivity to the feelings of others," "late development in physical and scholastic skills," "temper outbursts," and "self-consciousness." The introversion of the girls and the extreme alienation of the boys, especially in later childhood, seemed like a natural outgrowth of a history of retarded emotional development (Watt et al., 1979, p. 268).

Neurointegrative Deficit

Certain traits observed in high-risk subjects suggest that a subtle but general form of organic abnormality may underlie schizophrenia (Fish, 1977; Meehl, 1962). These traits do *not* clearly indicate brain damage the way an abnormal CT scan, a grossly deviant EEG, or a loss of reflexes does. Rather, they are "soft signs," that is, relatively ambiguous nonspecific indicators of presumed neurological dysfunction. Soft signs include deficiencies in fine motor coordination, abnormal quiescence, poor muscle tone, clumsiness or awkwardness, and variation, or "scatter," in test performance, with subjects sometimes failing easy tests but passing difficult tests (Fish, 1977, 1984; Hanson, Gottesman, & Heston, 1976).

Research on the physical growth and psychological development of high-risk infants has consistently yielded two basic observations (Fish, 1984; Marcus et al., 1984). First, certain abnormalities can be observed during infancy, especially in a *subgroup* of 40 to 50 percent of the high-risk children. These abnormalities include (a) postural-motor deficits—for example, retarded development of the ability to sit or stand unaided; (b) visual-motor deficits—for example, in orienting to, or reaching for, an object, or continuing to search for one that is now hidden from view; (c) auditory-motor deficits—for example, in searching for a noisy object hidden from view; and (d) bimanual deficits—for example, in manipulating an object with right and left hand or in transferring an object from one hand to the other at the midline. Collectively, these abnormalities are called *pandysmaturational* to underscore an apparently abnormal maturation of many interrelated neuropsychological functions (Fish, 1984).

Second, these kinds of abnormalities are *correlated* with three things: birth complications, low birth weight, and psychiatric symptoms of the schizoid, schizotypal, and/or paranoid variety that appear during childhood and beyond (see Table 12.1). In a nutshell, a *developmental* syndrome of physical, sensorimotor, and psychiatric abnormalities frequently found for a subgroup of high-risk children strongly suggests a biologically based vulnerability to schizophrenia. It is worth noting, however, that in some cases there is little or no detectable evidence of pandysmaturation prior to the adolescent or adult onset of schizophrenia. This absence may be an artifact of insensitive methodology, or it may express a relatively mild liability, or a dormant liability that

TABLE 12.1   PERCENTAGE OF CHILDREN WHO "HIT" ON THE PRESCHIZOPHRENIA
BEHAVIORAL INDICATORS

Indicator(s)	Children of parents who are			
	Schizophrenic ($N = 30$)	Other psychiatric patients ($N = 30$)	Normals, matched ($N = 29$)	Normals, not matched ($N = 27$)
Poor motor skills	30%	10%	21%	7%
Large within-person test score variance	53%	30%	28%	19%
"Schizoid" behavior at 4 and 7 years	27%	3%	10%	0%
Hits on all three indicators	17%	0%	0%	0%

Source: Hanson, Gottesman, and Heston, 1976, p. 148.

becomes operative only after a long period of normality, like in Huntington's or Alzheimer's disease.

In sum, the developmental studies using retrospective and prospective techniques indicate that childhood behavior patterns most characteristic of the preschizophenic include: (1) antisocial or asocial (schizoid) personality, (2) cognitive or attentional deficits, and (3) "soft" neurological signs (Erlenmeyer-Kimling et al., 1984; Friedman, Erlenmeyer-Kimling, & Vaughn, 1984; Marcus et al., 1984; Neuchterlein, 1984). Collectively, these neuropsychological and neurological signs suggest a *neurointegrative deficit,* a disorder of the timing and integration of neurological development (Fish, 1984, p. 427). Unfortunately, we do not yet know just what the neurointegrative deficit of schizophrenia might be.

NEUROPSYCHOLOGICAL ABNORMALITIES

In light of the developmental data, it is not surprising that adult schizophrenics show evidence of neurological abnormalities as reflected in neuroanatomy, neurometabolism, electrophysiology, and psychomotor behavior (Heinrichs & Buchanan, 1988; Seidman, 1983). CT scans suggest that some schizophrenics have abnormally enlarged cerebral ventricles and cortical atrophy, while PET scans suggest abnormalities in the rate and distribution of cerebral metabolism—for example, abnormally low metabolic rates in the frontal cortex. Investigations using microscopic techniques have yielded evidence of excesses, deficiencies, and even misalignment of neurons in various areas of the brains of schizophrenics (Benes et al., 1987; Colter et al., 1987; Conrad & Scheibel, 1987). Abnormally fast, slow, and "choppy" EEG patterns, sometimes all in the same record, also suggest that brain abnormality accompanies schizophrenic disorder. An example of this is recently reported evidence of abnormal auditory-evoked EEGs in schizophrenics with auditory hallucinations (Lindstrom et al., 1987). EEG abnormalities of this type suggest a dysfunction in the brain stem, a vital subcortical component of the sensory information processing mechanism.

Some of the evidence regarding brain abnormality in schizophrenia is more indirect, coming in the form of behavioral "soft signs" of neuropathology, including poor coordination and less-than-normal eye wobbling, or nystagmus, in response to deliberate rotation of the head. Additionally, schizophrenics also have an elevated rate of minor physical anomalies (MPAs)—for example, curved fingers or low-seated ears (Guy et al., 1983). These bodily signs of developmental abnormality may reflect a prenatal insult that could adversely affect brain development as well, thereby explaining why elevated rates of MPAs seem to be related to the severity of the disorder. Severity is sometimes defined in terms of *early onset* because early onset often predicts greater disorganization and chronic course. Green et al. (1987) reported that three or more MPAs were detectible in 50 percent of early-onset (younger than 19 years) compared to about 7 percent of later-onset schizophrenics. This finding is consistent with the view that the more severe the schizophrenic disorder, the more apparent the underlying pathophysiology (Green et al., 1989).

As we look at the following small subset of the research, keep a few things in mind. First, the percentage of schizophrenics showing one or more signs of brain abnormality varies across studies and methods. Second, those rare studies that measure more than one of these signs find that they correlate poorly, making it hard to argue for a single general defect. Third, although chronic schizophrenics are much more likely than less severely affected schizophrenics to show evidence of neurological dysfunction, this does not tell us whether the neurological defect is a *primary cause* of schizophrenia or a co-occurring nonspecific factor that makes a bad situation even worse. And finally, we still have little idea how these organic indicators might relate to other biological abnormalities—for example, the neurotransmitter abnormality suggested by the dopamine hypothesis (discussed below).

Frontal Lobes

Since the days of Kraepelin, experts have suspected that schizophrenia involves a pathology of the frontal lobes. A frontal deficit could produce negative symptoms by diminishing the schizophrenic's capacity to sustain positive involvement with the external world and to maintain a stable self-concept. A frontal deficit could also produce positive symptoms by failing to exercise its normal inhibitory influence on other areas of the brain (Franzen & Ingvar, 1974). Research over the past fifteen years has tended to supported the frontal deficit hypothesis, though not always (Weinberger & Berman, 1988).

With the help of rCBF, CT, and PET techniques, investigators frequently find evidence of neuronally less dense and metabolically less active frontal lobes in schizophrenics (Wolkin et al., 1988). For example, one study used the rCBF technique to track brain function in schizophrenic and control subjects during a psychological test designed to engage frontal lobe function (Weinberger, Berman, & Zec, 1986). Unlike the controls, the schizophrenics failed to show an expected increase in frontal metabolic activity while taking the test. One cannot be sure whether this result indicates a causal role for the frontal lobes or whether it merely reflects the extent to which the schizophrenics are *unengaged* in taking the test, but the results do point to underlying metabolic differences between the patients and controls.

Left Hemisphere

Some neuropsychological research on schizophrenia specifically suggests a left-hemisphere abnormality (Flor-Henry, 1976). First, anatomic, metabolic, and EEG anomalies of the left-hemisphere EEG are more frequently observed in schizophrenics than in schizoaffectives or manic-depressives (Flor-Henry, 1976; Losonczy et al., 1986). Second, schizophrenics are more likely than other psychiatric patients to perform poorly on tests of language, auditory memory, attention, and naming that tap left-hemisphere function (Taylor, Greenspan, & Abrams, 1979). For example, schizophrenics have relatively slow reaction times to visual stimuli processed by the left hemisphere in comparison to stimuli processed by the right hemisphere (Posner, Early, Reimer et al., 1988).

Finally, schizophrenics tend to show peculiarities of laterality: nonright-handedness, left-eyedness, left-footedness, or inconsistent lateral preference (Piran, Bigler, & Cohen, 1982). For example, many schizophrenics show left-handedness and right-footedness, or right-handedness but left-eyedness. This inconsistency among these measures of laterality suggests that a left-hemisphere dysfunction, perhaps arising during early development, may have induced a shift toward an abnormal dominance by the right hemisphere.

Ventricles

CT scan studies have revealed cortical atrophy—a shriveling up of the brain's cortex due to cell loss—and enlarged cerebral ventricles in many schizophrenics (Johnstone et al., 1978; Seidman, 1983). Ventricular enlargement, observable even in acute, never-medicated schizophrenics, is sometimes more pronounced on the left side of the brain (Losonczy et al., 1986). Nevertheless, two observations make ambiguous the causal significance of enlarged ventricles. First, for schizophrenic patients, there is a low-to-zero correlation between ventricle size and symptom pattern; in other words, ventricle size is not strongly related to the pattern of negative versus positive symptoms. Second, only modest association exists between enlarged ventricles and schizophrenia; in fact, some schizophrenics have normal or even small ventricles.

Actually, some progress has been made in explaining the modest connection between enlarged ventricles and schizophrenia. One study of seven pairs of identical (MZ) twins *discordant* for schizophrenia found larger ventricles in the schizophrenic twin six out of seven times (Reveley et al., 1982; Reveley, Reveley, & Murray, 1983). Identical twins have the same genotype; so if the affected co-twin tends to have the larger ventricles, perhaps adverse environmental factors producing large ventricles can push the person with a genetic liability to schizophrenia over the threshold for expressing the disorder.

The evidence on acquired neurological abnormality suggests that nongenetic factors—prenatal oxygen deprivation or infectious disease, for example—can produce brain abnormalities that potentiate schizophrenia; however, those individuals with a strong genetic disposition to schizophrenia as indicated by positive family history may not require such severe environmental insults to become schizophrenic (Lewis & Murray, 1987).

In sum, current research is yielding increasing evidence that for both genetic and nongenetic reasons, the brains of schizophrenics are abnormal. Nevertheless, uncertainty remains about the exact nature of the abnormality and its possible connection to schizophrenic symptoms.

BIOCHEMICAL ABNORMALITIES

Developmental research suggests that schizophrenic behavior is one manifestation of an evolving brain abnormality whose earliest behavioral expression may, in some cases, be detectible as far back as the first year. Neuropsychological research suggests an association between observed symptoms and anatomical or functional abnormalities in the brain. The biochemical approach suggests that schizophrenic behavior may be explained in terms of abnormalities at the synaptic level, where neurotransmitters and neuronal receptors interact.

Many biochemical hypotheses for schizophrenia have attracted research attention ever since antipsychotic drugs were introduced in the 1950s, but most have come up empty-handed (Meltzer, 1979). One hypothesis holds that some metabolic error can change a neurotransmitter into a "false transmitter" or even a toxic substance that has pathological effects. Other hypothetical factors have been proposed, including psychoactivating proteins, vitamin and mineral deficiencies, "slow viruses" that produce neural deterioration over time, and excesses or deficiencies of certain hormones. Each of these hypothetical factors was at one time or another considered a "breakthrough" discovery, and each continues to spark some interest even now, yet none commands the attention currently devoted to the dopamine hypothesis.

The Dopamine Hypothesis

In brief, the dopamine hypothesis holds that psychotic behavior is caused by the receptor hypersensitivity of certain dopamine (DA) neurons in the limbic forebrain. As a result, even a normal level of DA causes excessive and disorganized responding by these neurons (Gruzelier, 1978; Meltzer, 1979). Presumably this neural abnormality underlies the uninhibited and disorganized cognitive behavior of schizophrenic psychosis. Unfortunately, we cannot characterize with any precision the neurotransmitter-psychological correspondence or say exactly how the one causes the other. (At this point, you may want to reread the material on synaptic mechanisms in Chapter 8, pp. 216–220.)

Why do we suspect that an abnormality of dopamine (DA) neurons underlies schizophrenia? The best evidence comes from the effects of psychoactive drugs and antipsychotic medication. First, the extended use of DA-stimulating drugs such as amphetamine and cocaine produces thought disorder and delusions like those seen in manic and paranoid psychoses. Second, these drug-induced psychotic symptoms are reduced by antipsychotic drugs, or *neuroleptics*. These major tranquilizers block postsynaptic DA receptors—in particular, the so-called type 2 DA receptors (D_2) that are concentrated in subcortical regions of the brain, such as the basal ganglia (see Figure 8.1, Chapter 8, p. 202). Furthermore, the greater a drug's ability to block those D_2 receptors, the more powerful its antipsychotic effect, and consequently the smaller the dose required (Snyder, 1984). In sum, psychotic symptoms can be elicited or reduced by using drugs like amphetamine that stimulate DA neurotransmission, or drugs like chlorpromazine that inhibit DA neurons.

Why does it take as much as two weeks or more for the *abrupt* drug-induced blockade of D_2 receptors to produce only a *gradual* decrease of psychotic symptoms? Current speculation envisions a two-stage process to explain the time-course of drug effects. At first, the drug molecules "compete" with dopamine molecules by quickly occupying many of the postsynaptic D_2 receptor sites. This postsynaptic blockade induces a compensatory increase in the dopamine output of presynaptic neurons. At least initially, this compensatory activity prevents the kinds of changes in postsynaptic firing that would otherwise produce corresponding changes in symptoms. In time, however, the compensatory overactivity of the presynaptic neurons gradually subsides and the balance shifts in favor of the drug. The net effect is less dopamine and more drug at the postsynaptic site, and consequently diminished neurotransmission and less psychotic behavior (Pickar et al., 1984; White & Wang, 1983).

Controversies and Questions

The dopamine hypothesis is currently our best guess about the biochemical basis of thought disorder, but it is not clear whether there exists a unique dopamine deficit *specific to schizophrenia* (Alpert & Friedhoff, 1980;

Donaldson et al., 1983; Haracz, 1982; Van Kammen et al., 1982). Consider the following two claims that raise questions about the specificity assumption. First, cocaine and similar dopamine-*enhancing* drugs produce a psychotic condition, but typically not the full schizophrenic syndrome with its negative as well as positive symptoms. Second, these drugs are said to have little effect on the negative symptoms of schizophrenia. These two claims about the effect of dopamine-enhancing drugs would seem to argue against the hypothesis that schizophrenia involves a specific dysfunction only of dopamine mechanisms.

There is, however, other evidence that the dopamine-*blocking* neuroleptic drugs can be effective against the negative, as well as positive, symptoms of schizophrenia (Goldberg, 1985). Clearly, such evidence is at last consistent with the dopamine hypothesis (Crow, 1985). To complicate matters, certain negative symptoms—feelings of unreality, emptiness, and artificiality, for example—may actually intensify while other types of symptoms, including negative, positive, and deficit types, are receding in response to antipsychotic medication (Bernheim & Lewine, 1979). In sum, there is evidence on both sides of the argument about a specific dopamine deficit in schizophrenia, as well as observations that don't fit neatly into any hypothesis.

Seemingly incompatible observations about drugs inevitably stimulate controversies about the definition and classification of positive, negative, and deficit symptoms, and raise questions about whether some of these symptoms are fundamental while others are merely secondary, and about which ones do or do not respond to neuroleptic medication (Crow, 1985). Clearly, the fate of the dopamine hypothesis is linked to the ultimate resolution of these and other controversies and questions. For example, it is possible that two factors operate in schizophrenia: one that initiates the disorder and another that intensifies it, with a dopamine dysfunction underlying at least the second factor. Or it may be that there are two types of schizophrenia—one dominated by positive, the other by negative, symptoms—and only the positive type involves the dopamine dysfunction (Meltzer, 1979; Crow, 1980).

> In view of the myriad schizophrenics who continue to deteriorate despite neuroleptic treatment and all efforts for social rehabilitation . . . it is apparent that we have not come close to identifying the cause of the disorder in these patients. For these individuals, slow virus infections, genetically determined enzymatic deficiencies, or loss of regulatory mechanisms may be responsible. For those patients who have only acute schizophreniform episodes, and who are not misdiagnosed as having affective psychoses, it is not impossible that increased dopaminergic activity is the major biological factor in the pathogenesis of this disorder. If this is so, then this last decade has seen a historic development in schizophrenia research, for it would represent the first identification of a major subgroup of the schizophrenic syndrome for whom pathogenesis has been partially identified (Meltzer, 1979, p. 114).

This view of positive- versus negative-symptom schizophrenia draws heavily on evidence that psychosis-inducing drugs cause, and antipsychotic drugs block, positive symptoms, and that negative symptoms are relatively unaffected either way. The other view—that schizophrenia is a unitary syndrome—takes seriously the evidence that neuroleptics also reduce some negative and deficit symptoms. It remains to be seen which of these two views of schizophrenia—the dual or the unified concept—will prove to be more valid.

The dopamine hypothesis, whether applied to schizophrenia or any psychotic disorder, not only points to a biochemical abnormality, but also to certain locations in the brain where abnormalities exist. For example, Won et al. (1986) reported evidence that the brains of schizophrenics—specifically, the basal ganglia—have an elevated number of D_2 receptors. Unfortunately, a study by Farde et al. (1987) failed to confirm the Wong et al. finding, but as yet for unknown reasons. (The two studies differed in many ways, including patient characterisitics, methodology, and regions of the basal ganglia studied.) Even if the Wong et al. findings were eventually sustained, it would not be clear how (or if) an elevation of D_2 receptors explains schizophrenic symptoms (Kleinman, Casanova, & Jaskiw, 1988).

It is important to appreciate how little we know about abnormal neural mechanisms and how they might explain behavioral and mental abnormalities. The dopamine hypothesis of schizophrenia is no exception. For one thing, a defect in neural mechanisms that use the dopamine neurotransmitter might be a small though important component of a larger mechanism that involves nondopamine components as well. In addition, this larger mechanism might be controlled by still other unknown mechanisms that are ''upstream.'' Finally, while a model of dopamine dysfunction may tell us something about the neural mechanisms of thought disorder, it may not explain the ultimate cause of schizophrenia or other psychotic disorders.

In sum, although no one neurological or neurobiochemical factor has emerged as *the* key to schizophrenia, the evidence from behavioral, pharmacological, and brain research continues to support the hypothesis of an underlying organicity. Just what the organic abnormality might be and where it comes from is still unclear, but evidence that schizophrenia is heritable suggests one possible source. We now describe research showing that the risk of developing schizophrenia is determined, in part, by genetic factors.

GENETIC ETIOLOGY

The lifetime risk for at least one schizophrenic episode is usually estimated at 0.85 percent for the general population but between 2 and more than 10 percent for relatives of schizophrenics. As Table 12.2 makes clear, the difference in risk depends on the closeness of genetic relationship. The lower rate of schizophrenia in the parents of schizophrenics in comparison to other first-degree relatives is probably the result of a sampling artifact. Schizophrenics generally have lower rates of reproduction. Consequently, severely disturbed schizophrenics are unlikely to reproduce and the sample of parents who do reproduce will be late-onset schizophrenics or will be less likely to manifest schizophrenia even if they carry the schizophrenic liability. Nevertheless,

TABLE 12.2 RISKS OF SCHIZOPHRENIA FOR RELATIVES OF SCHIZOPHRENICS

Relationship	Number of studies	Morbid risk, %
First degree		
Parents	14	5.6
Siblings	13	10.1
Children	7	12.8
Children of two schizophrenics	5	46.3
Second degree		
Half siblings	5	4.2
Uncles/aunts	3	2.4
Nephews/nieces	6	3.0
Grandchildren	5	3.7
Third degree		
First cousins	3	2.4

Source: Gottesman & Shields, 1982, p. 85 (*Schizophrenia: The Epigenetic Puzzle.* Adapted with permission from Cambridge University Press).

since genetic and social closeness are correlated, how do we evaluate the relative importance of each in the overall set of data? Behavior genetic studies of twins and adoptees can help answer this question.

Twin Studies

Rationale In principle, increased risk for schizophrenia could reflect the influence of schizophrenic genes, schizophrenia-causing environments, or some combination of the two. Twin studies attempt to separate these potential causes by studying MZ and DZ twins. Recall that each MZ twin pair is identical genetically, while each DZ twin pair overlaps genetically about 50 percent. Because MZ genotypes are identical, any difference, or discordance, between the two members of an MZ pair must reflect environmental differences, while differences between the two members of a DZ pair can reflect environmental and/or genetic differences because there is only a 50 percent genetic overlap.

TABLE 12.3 PAIRWISE CONCORDANCE RATES IN OLDER AND MORE RECENT STUDIES OF SCHIZOPHRENIA

Set of studies	MZ pairs		DZ pairs*	
	N	Concordant, %	*N*	Concordant, %
Old	348	64	467	14
New	309	38	466	14

*Same-sex pairs only.
Sources: Gottesman & Shields, 1982; Kendler & Robinette, 1983.

Concordance Rates   Table 12.3 shows the concordance rates for MZ and DZ twins that have been reported in studies published before 1960 ("old") and after 1960 ("new"). The table shows that recent estimates of MZ concordance are lower than older estimates, though DZ concordances are the same. The reason for the higher concordance rates in the "old" studies probably reflects less systematic effort to obtain *all* schizophrenics who were twins, as well as a tendency to select only the most severely schizophrenic for study. But the *difference* between MZ and DZ concordance in the newer studies is still striking and consistent with a strong genetic effect.

Naturally, concordance rates will vary *among* studies, partly because of the breadth or narrowness of diagnostic criteria, but this does not much affect the MZ-DZ comparisons *within* studies. *Breadth* of criteria refers to the kinds of behaviors in the co-twin that are accepted as equivalents of the disorder in the index, or target, twin. If an investigator requires that the co-twin display *the same* disorder (a narrow criterion), concordance rates will be lower than if the investigator requires only that the co-twin display *some* psychiatric disturbance (broad criterion)— for example, eccentric, paranoid, or nervous behavior. Concordance rates for *both* MZ and DZ twins are lower for narrowly defined categories, and higher for more broadly defined categories. Nevertheless, the striking *difference* in concordance rates between MZ and DZ twins is always observed, and this difference, as well as absolute levels of concordance, points to heritability.

Another major influence on concordance rates is the *severity* of disorder in the index twin, the patient with whom the investigation starts. The more severely affected index cases are more likely to have a schizophrenic co-twin. For example, Gottesman and Shields (1966) reported a 75 percent concordance rate for MZ pairs when the index twin was severely disturbed, but only a 17 percent rate for MZ pairs when the index twin was mildly disturbed. This implies that the more severe the schizophrenia, the greater the genetic influence. There is further evidence for this conclusion about the greater heritability of severer forms of schizophrenia if we assume that the more severe the schizophrenia, the more the disorder will be dominated by negative symptoms.

A reanalysis of twin data by Dworkin and Lenzenweger (1984) shows how twin studies using diagnostic criteria that emphasize negative symptoms yield higher heritability estimates than studies using criteria that emphasize positive symptoms. Specifically, four of five recent twin studies obtained substantially greater MZ than DZ concordance for schizophrenia when the index twin displayed more negative symptoms, regardless of the number of positive symptoms. This finding is consistent with the hypothesis that there are two types of schizophrenia (Crow, 1985), one expressed primarily in negative symptoms and the other in positive symptoms, with only the former showing high heritability (McGuffin et al., 1984).

A distinction between positive and negative symptomatology is consistent with the view that process schizophrenia is dominated by negative symptoms while reactive and schizoaffective disorders are dominated by positive symptoms (see Table 12.4). It is also consistent with two other observations: the

TABLE 12.4 CLASSICAL (KRAEPELINIAN) VS. NONCLASSICAL SCHIZOPHRENIA

Characteristic	Classical	Nonclassical
Clinical symptoms	Negative	Positive
Diagnostic labels	Process	Reactive
	Simple	Schizoaffective
	Chronic	Acute
Prognosis	Chronic	Uncertain
Response to antipsychotics	Poor	Relatively good
Possible dopamine abnormality	Underactive	Overactive
Neuroanatomical abnormalities	Often seen	Rarely seen
Familial pathology	Schizophrenia	Schizoaffective
Heritability	High	?

relative uselessness of positive symptoms for differentiating between schizophrenic, schizoaffective, and affective disorders (see pages 283–284 in Chapter 10) and the relevance of the dopamine theory for positive rather than negative symptoms. And we should keep in mind that the evidence we will now describe for the heritability of schizophrenia is based largely on studies of chronic schizophrenics with prominent negative as well as positive symptoms.

Discordant Twins and Offspring Risk   It is clear from the roughly 50 percent MZ *dis*cordance that nongenetic factors are certainly at work in the typical schizophrenia disorder, though the nature of those nongenetic factors is still a mystery. Surprisingly, while studies of *discordant* MZ twins provide compelling evidence for nongenetic factors in schizophrenia, they also yield some of the most impressive evidence *for* its heritability.

If the *risk* for developing schizophrenia has a strong genetic component, then the offspring of MZ twins discordant for schizophrenia should have the same elevated risk regardless of which twin parent had schizophrenia. Fischer (1971) looked at the offspring of sets of female identical twins discordant for schizophrenia; that is, where one MZ mother was schizophrenic while her co-twin was not. About 10 percent, or 3 out of 31, of the offspring of the schizophrenic twin eventually developed schizophrenic disorder. The corresponding risk for the offspring of the *nonschizophrenic* co-twin was 3 out of 23, or approximately 13 percent.

These two concordance rates are comparable, and they are remarkably close to the roughly 10 percent value expected for the offspring of one schizophrenic parent (see Table 12.2). Although we cannot identify the nongenetic factor(s) that might trigger the expression of schizophrenia in one twin or block it in the other, one thing seems clear: whatever nongenetic factors are operating, they seem to be environmental factors *other than* exposure to psychotic parental behavior.

Adoption Studies

The results of adoption studies yield further evidence of a genetic liability for schizophrenia. The rarest type of adoption data comes from occasional studies of MZ twins *reared apart,* that is, where at least one member of a pair is raised in an adoptive home. Across all studies, the overall concordance for schizophrenia of such ''MZ-apart'' pairs is 58 percent (Gottesman & Shields, l982), a figure that is roughly comparable to the overall rates across all studies for MZ twins reared together (see Table 12.3). Now, let us consider three additional sets of adoption data on *singleton* subjects implying that the genetic evidence from twin data are generally applicable to the nontwin population as well.

High-Risk Offspring in Adoptive Environments   The classic adoption study was reported by Heston (1966). Heston identified forty-seven chronic schizophrenic and fifty control mothers whose offspring had been placed in foster care within a few days of birth. The infants were comparable in terms of age, type of placement, and quality of rearing. Their eventual psychiatric status during adulthood was assessed by personal interviews and official records. Table 12.5 shows the elevated rates of schizophrenia, psychopathy, and mental retardation found in the adopted-away offspring of the schizophrenic versus the normal control mothers. The 5 in 47 (11 percent) rate of schizophrenia is again roughly that expected from population surveys of risk for schizophrenia in the offspring of schizophrenics who rear their own children (see Table 12.2). The elevated rates of psychopathy and mental retardation in the offspring of the schizophrenics, according to Heston, probably reflects traits of the men who mated with these schizophrenic women.

Two years after the Heston report, another adoption study (Rosenthal et al., 1968) confirmed his findings. Since the publication of the Rosenthal et al.

TABLE 12.5   DEMOGRAPHIC CHARACTERISTICS AND INCIDENCE OF PSYCHOPATHOLOGY IN THE ADOPTED-AWAY OFFSPRING OF SCHIZOPHRENIC AND NORMAL MOTHERS

Trait	Normal mother	Schizophrenic mother
Subjects	50	47
Males	33	30
Age (mean)	36	36
Schizophrenia	0	5
Mental deficiency	0	4
Sociopathic personality	2	9
Neurotic personality disorder	7	13
IQ (mean)	104	94
Years of school (mean)	12	12
Children, total	84	71
Divorces, total	7	6
Never married, over 30 years old	4	9

Source: Heston, 1966, p. 822.

study, new cases have been added and the results have been updated (Gottesman & Shields, 1982). Adopted offspring of sixty-nine schizophrenic parents, the high-risk adoptees, and seventy-nine control adoptees were matched in terms of sex, age, age at adoption, and socioeconomic status of the rearing environment. On the basis of psychological testing and interviews done when the adoptees had become adults, 19 percent of the high-risk adoptees versus 10 percent of the control adoptees were diagnosed as possible or definite schizophrenics.

Later, *DSM-III* criteria were applied to thirty-nine carefully matched pairs of high-risk and control adoptees from the Rosenthal et al. (1968) study. Schizotypal disorders—schizophrenia, schizotypal personality, and schizoid disorder—were found for 28 percent of high-risk versus 10 percent of control adoptees. No differences between the two adoptee groups were found for percentage of affective or borderline disorder (Lowing, Mirsky, & Pereira, 1983). In a more recent study of similar design, Tienari et al. (1985) found psychotic disorder in six of ninety-one adopted-away offspring of schizophrenic mothers but in only one of ninety-one adopted-away offspring of control mothers, thus again confirming the earlier results.

Risk in Cross-Fostered Adoptees   So far, we have considered high-risk adoptees who are reared in adoptive environments that have been selected as desirable. But what about *low*-risk adoptees reared in a less optimal environment—for example, with a schizophrenic adoptive parent? A study of this sort would permit an examination of the consequences of being reared by a disturbed parent, but without the ambiguities of a genetic connection between the disturbed parent and the child (Wender et al., 1974). A remarkable *cross-fostering* study (Wender et al., 1973) addressed this question.

Cross-fostering refers to cases of offspring of *non*schizophrenics who are reared by an adoptive parent who becomes a schizophrenic after adopting the child. A strict social learning view predicts elevated rates of schizophrenia in these cross-fostered adoptees. In contrast, if social factors associated with schizophrenic behavior are not important to etiology, there should be no elevation in the rate of schizophrenia in these cross-fostered offspring. Only offspring of schizophrenics would be predicted by genetic theory to have elevated rates despite normal adoptive rearing.

The cross-foster study of Wender et al. used a scale to rate the *degree* of schizophrenic disorganization in the adoptees. The results indicated that only the index adoptees with a schizophrenic biological parent had elevated rates of schizophrenic disorganization while the schizophrenia rates for children without a schizophrenic heredity were lower and comparable to the control rates, as predicted by genetic theory. There is thus no evidence of elevated risk for infants with nonschizophrenic heritage when raised in a "schizophrenic" environment.

Risk in Relatives of High-Risk Adoptees   The adoption studies considered thus far have used the high- and low-risk *adoptees method*. Such studies assess risk for schizophrenia in the adopted-away *offspring* of schizophrenic versus control parents. In contrast, the adoptees *family method* assesses the risk for schizophrenia in the biological and adoptive *relatives* of schizophrenic and nonschizophrenic control adoptees. For example, Kety et al. (1968) found an elevated risk for chronic schizophrenia and ''borderline schizophrenia''—what the *DSM-III-R* now calls schizoptypal personality disorder—in the biological, but not in the adoptive, relatives of chronic schizophrenic adoptees in Copenhagen.

Recently, a reanalysis of the Kety et al. (1968) study using *DSM-III* criteria has been carried out by Kendler and Gruenberg (1984). As expected, the risk for schizophrenia and schizotypal personality disorder was elevated in the biological relatives of schizophrenic adoptees (10 percent and 20 percent for the two disorders, respectively) compared to (a) the biological relatives of nonschizophrenic adoptees (0 percent for both disorders) and (b) all adoptive relatives (0 percent for both). Comparable differences were also found for a much larger sample of second-degree relatives of the schizophrenics and the controls.

The Kety et al. study has recently been replicated in a study of Danish adoptees outside the Copenhagen area (Kety, 1987). Like the Copenhagen study, this so-called provincial study found that only the biological relatives of chronic schizophrenic adopteees showed the expected elevated risk of chronic schizophrenia (about 5 percent versus less than 1 percent in controls) and schizotypal personality disorder (about 8 percent versus less than 2 percent in controls).

Until recently, the inference of a genetic basis for schizophrenia has rested on behavior-genetic research, which, however, cannot reveal the gene(s) involved. Molecular genetic research, on the other hand, can do just this. Let's take a look at current developments in this work.

Identification of a Genetic Marker

A 20-year-old Chinese-Canadian college student, hospitalized with schizophrenia, was observed to have physical anomalies—for example, widely spaced eyes and an especially prominent forehead (Bassett et al., 1988). What was so interesting about this case was the mother's report that her schizophrenic brother—the boy's uncle and the only other schizophrenic in the family—resembled the boy in many of these anomalous features. Investigators, intrigued by this cross-generational connection between schizophrenia and the physical anomalies, did chromosome analyses on all eight family members.

The investigation revealed that the boy and his uncle—the only two relatives with schizophrenia—had inherited an extra copy of chromosome 5 material attached to chromosome 1. Each of their two chromosomes 5 was normal; in other words, they were partially *trisomic* for that genetic material, with three rather than the normal two copies. The mother of the boy also had the same chromosome 5 material translocated to chromosome 1, but in her case, this material was missing from one of her chromosomes 5, leaving her with the normal complement of genetic material.

The partial trisomy of genetic material from chromosome 5 appears to be associated with the development of schizophrenia in this family. However, it is probably not a generally important factor in schizophrenia, since most schizophrenics lack trisomies of any kind. Rather, an extra copy of genetic material might alter gene regulation, for example, by increasing the quantity of a particular protein that has something to do with schizophrenia.

The Bassett et al. findings prompted other investigators to examine chromosome 5 in several pedigrees containing many schizophrenic patients (Sherrington et al., 1988). Using restriction fragment length polymorphisms (see Chapter 7, p. 196), these investigators confirmed that a region of chromosome 5 was co-inherited with schizophrenia in seven families of Icelandic and English origin. Another group of investigators, also prompted by the Bassett et al. observation, reported an *absence* of linkage to chromosome 5 in a pedigree from northern Sweden (Kennedy et al., 1988). The optimistic explanation for these conflicting results is that distinct genetic causes for schizophrenia exist in different families that are genetically isolated. However, a less optimistic explanation is that there was no real linkage in the families between schizophrenics and chromosome 5 abnormalities, since questions have been raised about the Sherrington et al. interpretation of their complex statistical analysis. Further research ought to resolve these possibilities.

ENVIRONMENT AND HEREDITY

Twin and adoption studies suggest that the liability to schizophrenia includes a strong genetic component. On the other hand, MZ discordance rates imply that the liability to schizophrenia must also include a *non*genetic component. It is reasonable to assume that certain features of the social environment are part of this nongenetic component, but the adoption data do not confirm the assumption. Rather, they suggest that the nongenetic component probably involves *non*social environmental factors.

It is true that many studies have documented statistically significant differences between the rearing environments of schizophrenic and control subjects raised by their *natural* parents, but the direction of causality is questionable, especially in light of the cross-foster study showing no elevated risk for schizophrenia in genetically low-risk adoptees raised by schizophrenic mothers. True enough, retrospective and laboratory studies have revealed statistically modest differences in the parents of schizophrenics and controls (Schofield & Balian, 1959). Also, observation of family interactions (Mischler & Waxler, 1968) and psychological testing (Singer & Wynne, 1965) reveal deviant parental behavior, including excessive or insufficient emotional expression and disjointed or peculiar verbal communication. In the light of adoption data these parental patterns might best be interpreted as *expressions* of the schizophrenic genes carried by nonschizophrenic family members, and not necessarily an indication that parental behavior causes schizophrenia in the offspring.

Moreover, abnormal parental behavior patterns may, in part, be *reactions* to the psychopathology of the child (Liem, 1974). For example, evidence that mothers of schizophrenics are psychologically more intrusive—dominant and overprotective, yet rejecting (Frank, 1965)—than mothers of nonschizophrenics may be explained as reactions to a difficult and needy child. Unfortunately, the evidence is ambiguous because studies rarely include control groups of mothers of impaired *non*schizophrenics (children with polio or asthma, for example); that is, mothers who also might appear behaviorally disturbed by the challenges of caring for a child with an abnormality.

The fact is, no one has ever shown convincingly that any specifiable social factor can *cause* schizophrenia. If exposure to schizophrenic child rearing does not necessarily increase the risk for schizophrenia, then *nonsocial* environmental causes are involved, though, again, it is not clear what they might be. Some investigators have argued that *pregnancy and birth complications* (PBCs)—premature rupture of placental membranes, placental abnormality, prolonged labor, premature delivery, or oxygen deprivation (anoxia)—could produce neural abnormalities, such as enlarged ventricles, that could enhance even further the risk for eventually developing schizophrenic disorder in those infants with schizophrenic genes (Gottesman & Shields, 1982; McNeil & Kaij, 1978). Indeed, schizophrenics often have a history of being exposed to an excess of PBCs (McNeil & Kaij, 1978), suggesting proactive ecopathology that increases the risk for schizophrenia in those already at risk for genetic reasons.

Recall from Chapter 11 that the vast majority of schizophrenic patients and nearly half of their first-degree nonschizophrenic relatives have smooth pursuit eye movement (SPEM) abnormalities. In addition, MZ twins discordant for schizophrenia are nevertheless typically concordant for eye movement abnormalities. On the basis of this and other evidence, Holzman et al. (1988) have hypothesized the existence of an autosomal dominant gene which damages brain areas responsible for eye movements and which, if the damage is sufficiently widespread, can produce the neuropathology leading to schizophrenia.

Our understanding of environmental factors on the course of schizophrenia is no less ambiguous than our understanding of its etiology. Nevertheless, environmental factors must be operating. To appreciate the importance of nongenetic factors on the course of schizophrenia, consider a unique case of identical (MZ) quadruplets concordant for schizophrenia (Rosenthal, 1963). Each of the Genain quadruplets (see Figure 12.1) was hospitalized in her early twenties with a diagnosis of schizophrenia. Despite many psychotic symptoms in common—social withdrawal, confusion, and hallucination, for example—the quads showed major differences in other symptoms, as well as differences in the course of their illness, social adjustment, biological functions, and psychological competencies (DeLisi et al., 1984; Mirsky et al., 1984). These differences, some of which are shown in Table 12.6, make clear just how varied and unpredictable the specific manifestations of the schizophrenic disease pro-

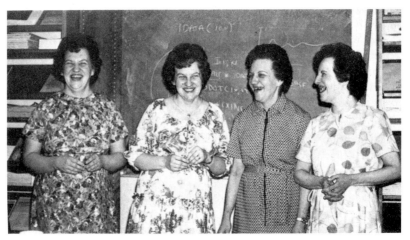

FIGURE 12.1   The Genain sisters shown here at their fifty-first birthday party.

cess are, even in genetically identical people growing up under the same roof. Clearly, nongenetic factors must influence the development of the disorder. Yet what and how important those nongenetic factors might be remains unknown.

What can we conclude about the origins and development of schizophrenia? Twin and adoption data clearly implicate a specific schizophrenic heredity while providing few clues about physical or social environmental causes. Nevertheless, MZ discordance for disorder (Fischer, 1971) and MZ differences in the behavioral expression of concordance (Genain quads) clearly implicate nongenetic factors that influence whether and how the genetic liability becomes manifest. If we look at the various liability factors that have been hypothesized for schizophrenia over the years (Table 12.7), we are struck by how little, beyond the genetic factor, is really understood about the causes of schizophrenia.

SUMMARY

Evidence continues to reinforce the idea that some abnormality of neural wiring underlies schizophrenia. At the biochemical level, overactivation of the mesolimbic dopamine system has been hypothesized, an explanation that could account for the deleterious effects of psychoactive drugs and the positive effects of antipsychotic drugs. Although this dopamine hypothesis does account for many observations, questions remain about how specific it is for schizophrenia—does it explain the *positive* symptoms of any psychotic disorder or does it reflect something basic about the *schizophrenic* disorder?

To explain schizophrenia, investigators have proposed abnormalities of brain function in general—that is, some "neurointegrative deficit"—as well as

TABLE 12.6   SAMPLE OF BEHAVIORAL DIFFERENCES IN MZ QUADRUPLETS CONCORDANT
FOR SCHIZOPHRENIA

Category	Nora	Iris	Myra	Hester
Social Adjustment				
No. of hospitalizations	8	6	4	3
Total time in the hospital (yrs)	6	16	4	16
Education level	H.S. grad	H.S. grad	Business coll. (2 yrs)	11th grade
Ever worked (sec'y/clerk)	Yes	Yes	Yes	No
Parental status:				
Married	No	No	Yes	No
No. children	None	None	two sons (foster care)	None
Friends	Ex-patients	Ex-patients	None	None
Social function	Grossly inadequate	Grossly inadequate	Fair	Grossly inadequate
Cognitive function without medication	Psychotic	Psychotic	Not psychotic	Psychotic
Biological Function				
Response to antipsychotics	Relatively good	Little/none	Adverse	Improved
Response to removal of antipsychotics	Decompensation	Improvement	Improvement	Decompensation
Dexamethasone test	Nonsuppression	Normal suppression	Normal suppression	Normal suppression
"Soft" neurological signs (number)	6.0	2.5	2.0	5.5
Cognitive Mechanisms				
Continuous performance test (CPT):				
On medication	Normal	Normal	Poor	Poor
Off medication	Very poor	Very poor	Very poor	Very poor
Reaction time (RT):				
On medication	Normal	Normal	Normal	Poor
Off medication	?	Poor	Poor	?
Smooth pursuit eye movements (SPEM)	Normal	Abnormal	Normal	Borderline

Source: Adapted from DeLisi et al., 1984; and Mirsky et al., 1984.

abnormalities in specific areas—the frontal lobes, for example. Evidence for such theorizing includes data on (1) *abnormal development* involving immature patterns of motor, personal, and social behavior; (2) *neuroanatomical abnormalities* such as large brain ventricles; (3) *neuropsychological dysfunction* such as EEG and eye tracking anomalies, and mixed laterality—left-eyedness with right-footedness, for example. That these abnormalities can precede the

TABLE 12.7   LIABILITY FACTORS RELEVANT TO THEORIES OF SCHIZOPHRENIA

Personal vulnerability*

1. Genetic sources (inherited)

  (a) Schizotypal genes (e.g., for "cognitive slippage")
  (b) Nonschizotypal genes (e.g., anxious temperament)

2. Environmental sources (acquired)

  (a) Physical environment (e.g., trauma, disease)
  (b) Psychological environment (e.g., modeling, verbal communication, reinforcement/
     punishment)

Situational factors†

1. Physical stressors (e.g., fatigue)
2. Social stressors (e.g., rejection)

  *Personal vulnerability refers to the neuropsychological wiring and programming already characteristic of the person.
  †Situational factors act on vulnerability to influence the liability to disorder.

onset of schizophrenic disorder strongly implies that some neurological abnormality does underlie the liability to schizophrenia.

Genetic studies reinforce a faulty neural wiring hypothesis for schizophrenia. Risk for schizophrenia increases in direct proportion to genetic overlap with a schizophrenic and, more important, this role is unaffected by the presence or absence of schizophrenic behavior in the rearing environment. Moreover, recent research has identified a region of chromosome 5 that, in some pedigrees, is associated with the development of schizophrenia.

Discordance for schizophrenia among MZ twins strongly implies that risk for schizophrenia includes a *non*genetic (environmental) component. Although the timing, course, and content of schizophrenic symptomatology are probably influenced by social factors, risk for initially *developing* the disorder appears to depend on genetic and nonsocial environmental factors that operate on the brain to create a neuropsychopathology.

CHAPTER 13

Affective Disorders 1: Major Syndromes

OUTLINE

At least 15 percent of the nonpsychiatric population report experiencing significant anxiety and depression (Boyd & Weissman, 1982). Regardless of cause, there is much unhappiness in the normal population. For example, a surprisingly high percentage of "normal" females in one study reported depression-related experiences such as being unpraiseworthy (46 percent), constantly anxious (25 percent), easily hurt (60 percent), and crying easily (43 percent) (Altman & Wittenborn, 1980). Recruited from women's clubs, church groups, and local industry, none of these women had a history of mental illness.

A complaint need not be a symptom of disorder (Akiskal, 1979). Depressive complaints may be part of normal reactions to stress and frustration, commonplace hazards of the home and workplace. Or they may be truly symptomatic of an affective *disorder,* the focus of this and the next chapter. We begin with the concept of affect, and then describe severe affective and related disorders, leaving to the next chapter a fuller discussion of mechanisms and etiology.

THE AFFECT CONCEPT

Affective states involve significant shifts from psychological neutrality to the "positive/happy" or "negative/sad" poles of experience. The term *affect* can refer to a variety of feelings (depression, anxiety, anger), and even the absence of feelings (apathy). Nevertheless, in the realm of abnormal behavior, the term *affective disorder* (or mood disorder, as it is called in *DSM-III-R*) conventionally refers to the sadness and/or apathy of depressive disorders, and to the euphoria and/or irritability of manic disorder. Our exclusion of anxiety and anxiety disorders (Chapter 15) from our discussion of affect and affective disorders will respect this convention.

Components of Affect

The *mood,* or feeling, component of affect refers to private experiences like joy and sadness. The *ideational,* or intellective, component represents affect in fantasy, words, and attitudes about the self and one's prospects; painful subjective feelings, for example, can be translated into the language of lowered self-esteem and deep pessimism. The *expressive,* or emotional, component includes certain qualities of movement, gesture, and vocalization (crying, for example) by which affect is outwardly expressed. The *physiological* component of affect includes changes in appetite, sleep, endocrine balance, and other bodily functions. These physiological changes are "affective" because they typically co-occur with changes in the mood, ideational, and expressive components of affect. Changes in the components of affect may occur more or less independently of external conditions, or they may be driven by external conditions, or both.

Each of the four components of affect can provoke the other. Negative thinking, for example, can amplify sad feelings while sad feelings can drive negative thinking. In severe depression, the evidence suggests that physiological events including hormone imbalances can produce negative changes in feeling, emotion, and ideation. This can be illustrated by a model of depression shown in Figure 13.1 (Ross & Rush, 1981). According to the model, physiological changes controlled by subcortical and paleocortical mechanisms are translated by the posterior right hemisphere into a nonverbal representation, an unconscious affective "idea" that can then be translated by other parts of the cortex: by the posterior left hemisphere into conscious, verbally mediated mood; by the anterior left into verbal communication; and by the anterior right into emotional expression.

This particular model was derived from research on patients with organic affective disorder, that is, affective disorder associated with lesions in different parts of the brain. Nevertheless, it can also explain the affective behavior of normal subjects studied in the EEG laboratory (Davidson et al., 1979). Apparently, then, both normal and abnormal affect can be understood as a change in one or more *components* of neuropsychological activity.

Partial Expression of Affect

We can get a better appreciation of the componential nature of affect by looking at the *partial* expression of affect in atypical affective disorders where only one component of affect is expressed in the absence of others. Consider the following examples of atypical affect displayed by brain-damaged patients (Ross & Rush, 1981). A male patient, claiming to be depressed, speaks affectlessly in a monotonous, robotlike fashion; and a female patient denies feeling depressed altogether. Yet both patients show the classic physiological signs of depression—for example, insomnia, anorexia, and endocrine abnormality. Can we interpret those signs as indicating depression in people who

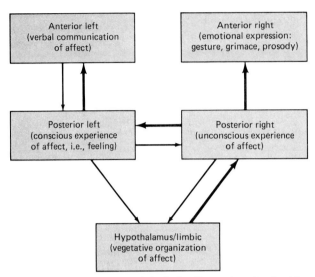

FIGURE 13.1   Diagram of major neuropsychological pathways hypothesized for affective disorder. Major affective disorder diagrammed with dark arrows, mild affective states diagrammed with light arrows. Subcortical dysfunction in major depressive disorder is translated by the posterior right hemisphere into a nonverbal apprehension that can then be (a) expressed outwardly by anterior right frontal cortex, (b) apprehended in verbal thought by posterior left cortex, and (c) communicated verbally by anterior left cortex. Selective damage can isolate emotion from feeling or emotion from words, or completely block feeling or emotion (see text). (Adapted from Ross & Rush, 1981)

otherwise—in their expressiveness or self-reports—give no evidence of being depressed?

Recall that the psychopathological meaning of physiological events depends on psychological correlates—painful feelings, weepy expressions, and pessimistic outlook, for example—that typically co-occur with the physiological events. Nevertheless, even if these psychological correlates are absent or uninterpretable, other evidence may exist to confirm (or disconfirm) the hypothesis that the observed physiological signs displayed by a patient are actually the *partial* expression of an affective disorder.

Consider the two patients we just mentioned. The classic physiological signs of depression that they display seem contradicted both by the male patient's affectively neutral style while claiming to be depressed, and by the female patient's outright denial of being depressed. Nevertheless, there are two good reasons for suspecting depressive disorder. First, the patients had either a personal or a family history of severe depression, and second, each patient had a type of brain damage which could explain the observed behavior as a partial, or incomplete, expression of depression.

The male patient had a lesion in the anterior right hemisphere, making it impossible to impart *prosody,* or rhythm and tonal variation, to his speech. The syndrome, called *aprosodia,* can prevent the appropriate expression of depressed feelings. The female patient's extensive right-hemisphere damage presumably blocked the translation of the subcortical (physiological) component of affect into cortical (ideational) representations. Right-hemisphere damage made the patient affectively "blind," although she could feel and express sadness about depressing events that had occurred *prior to* the brain damage. Apparently, affective memories that are initially laid down in both hemispheres can be retrieved by the intact left hemisphere despite its inability to appreciate *current* affective stimuli arising either from within or from the social context (Heilman, Scholes, & Watson, 1975). In sum, affect is a multicomponential state whose forms and intensity of expression depend on both normal and abnormal conditions in the brain.

While most affective disorders are "functional," with no discernible signs of organicity, some do involve hidden brain abnormalities in locations from the cerebral hemispheres to deeper parts such as the basal ganglia (Trautner et al., 1988). At this point, however, we will ignore causes, and begin with a description of the symptoms of *major,* or severe, depression. Later, we will describe mania and discuss its connection to depression. Once we have a clear picture of a severe affective disorder at both the depressive and euphoric "poles" of the positive-negative dimension of affect, we will be able to consider theoretical questions about underlying psychopathology.

MAJOR (SEVERE) DEPRESSIVE SYNDROME

Severe depressions include extreme changes in mood, motivation, cognition, and behavior, changes that are sufficiently debilitating to warrant hospitalization. These can include apathy, avolition, social withdrawal, pessimistic delusions, and suicidal impulses. The main *DSM-III-R* criteria for major depressive episode are given in Table 13.1. They include both psychological and physiological abnormalities. When depression is associated with hallucinations, thought disorder, and/or delusions, it is called *psychotic* depression.

Melancholic Aspects

The term *melancholia,* derived from the Greek for black bile, originated in the ancient humoral theories of Hippocrates and Galen (see Chapter 2). Today, the term refers to a type of depression that characterizes about 40 to 60 percent of severe episodes. *DSM-III-R* provides behavioral criteria for melancholic depression that include (a) apathy and/or anhedonia, (b) anorexia or weight loss, (c) diurnal variation in mood; that is, depression typically worse in the early morning, (d) morning insomnia characterized by early (about 4 A.M.) final awakening, with an inability to fall back to sleep despite feeling tired, and (e) psychomotor retardation—the extreme slowness of thought and movement,

TABLE 13.1 DIAGNOSTIC CRITERIA FOR MAJOR DEPRESSIVE EPISODE

A. At least five of the following symptoms have been present during the same two-week period and represent a change from previous functioning; at least one of the symptoms is either (1) depressed mood or (2) loss of interest or pleasure. (Do not include symptoms that are clearly due to a physical condition, mood-incongruent delusions or hallucinations, incoherence, or marked loosening of associations.)

    1. Depressed mood (or can be irritable mood in children and adolescents) most of the day, nearly every day, as indicated either by subjective account or observation by others

    2. Markedly diminished interest or pleasure in all, or almost all, activities most of the day, nearly every day (as indicated either by subjective account or observation by others of apathy most of the time)

    3. Significant weight loss or weight gain when not dieting (e.g., more than 5% of body weight in a month) or decrease or increase in appetite nearly every day (in children, consider failure to make expected weight gains)

    4. Insomnia or hypersomnia nearly every day

    5. Psychomotor agitation or retardation nearly every day (observable by others; not merely subjective feelings of restlessness or being slowed down)

    6. Fatigue or loss of energy nearly every day

    7. Feelings of worthlessness or excessive or inappropriate guilt (which may be delusional) nearly every day (not merely self-reproach or guilt about being sick)

    8. Diminished ability to think or concentrate, or indecisiveness, nearly every day (either by subjective account or as observed by others)

    9. Recurrent thoughts of death (not just fear of dying), recurrent suicidal ideation without a specific plan, or a suicide attempt or a specific plan for committing suicide

B. 1. It cannot be established that an organic factor initiated and maintained the disturbance.

    2. The disturbance is not a normal reaction to the death of a loved one (uncomplicated bereavement). *Note:* Morbid preoccupation with worthlessness, suicidal ideation, marked functional impairment or psychomotor retardation, or prolonged duration suggest bereavement complicated by major depression.)

C. At no time during the disturbance have there been delusions or hallucinations for as long as two weeks in the absence of prominent mood symptoms (i.e., before the mood symptoms developed or after they have remitted).

D. Not superimposed on schizophrenia, schizophreniform disorder, delusional disorder, or other psychotic disorder.

Source: American Psychiatric Association (1987), pp. 222–223. Reprinted with permission from the *Diagnostic and Statistical Manual of Mental Disorders, Third Edition, Revised.* Copyright © 1987 American Psychiatric Association.

stooped posture, heavy gait, apathy, and withdrawal—or psychomotor agitation—weeping, complaining, and restlessness (including pacing back and forth, hand wringing, and pulling on one's clothes). Patients with the melancholic form of major depression also typically show an obsessive preoccupation with guilt, failure, and inadequacy.

Temporal Aspects: Onset, Duration, and Relapse

A severe depression can develop in two to three weeks, and sometimes even faster. Typically, the patient is not hospitalized until months later, when coping is no longer possible or when the person is manifestly suicidal. The duration of the episode can vary considerably, typically from three months to about a year, depending on the person, with the duration tending to remain relatively constant from episode to episode. Significant recovery from an episode of severe depression occurs in about 70 percent of the cases, the others remaining chronically impaired with low-grade depressive symptoms that can adversely affect normal functioning and produce adverse social consequences such as isolation or stigma.

At least one relapse will be noted in half the cases followed up for many years after recovery from the initial episode (Belsher & Costello, 1988). On the average, about 20 percent of the original sample will have a postrecovery relapse by two months, and about 40 percent by twelve months. These rates are higher for the patients with (a) preexisting dysthymic disorder, (b) significant postrecovery stresses, and (c) limited social support or therapy.

In patients with multiple episodes, the latency (time) to relapse usually gets progressively shorter. Since the duration of each depressive episode is relatively constant, the decreasing latency to successive episodes reflects those briefer postepisode recovery periods. This pattern of decreasing latency from recovery from one episode to the onset of the next may explain why major depressions that first show up relatively late in life, during the 40s or 50s, often have shorter symptom free intervals. Finally, there is a progressive increase in the severity and acute onset of subsequent episodes, with a corresponding decrease in the apparent importance of preepisode stress. In other words, the more severe later episodes seem to be less dependent on the occurrence of significant life events (Gold, Goodwin, & Chrousos, 1988a).

Major depression often runs in families, and does so in a fairly systematic fashion (Bland, Newman, & Orn, 1986; Weissman et al., 1984). The age of onset and frequency of recurrence of depression in a patient predicts the risk of depressive disorder in that patient's biological relatives. More specifically, earlier onset cases have a higher number of similarly affected relatives (Figure 13.2), and patients with more recurring episodes have a higher number of similarly affected relatives. Patients with both early onset and recurrent depressions have relatives with a 17 percent risk for developing major depressive disorder (Bland, Newman, & Orn, 1986). These observations suggest that early onset-recurrent depressions reflect a more severe underlying vulnerability.

Co-morbidity

Major depressive episodes are often associated with one or more types of psychopathology; between 30 and 50 percent of patients with major depression satisfy *DSM-III-R* criteria for disorders such as anxiety disorders, somatoform disorders, impulse disorders, personality disorders, and even schizophrenia (Kocsis & Frances, 1987). The co-occurrence of major depression and other psychopathology has raised important theoretical questions. In particular, is the depression a cause or effect of the co-occurring disorder, or are the co-

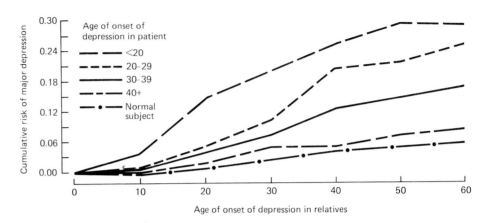

FIGURE 13.2 Cumulative risk of major depression in relatives by age of onset of depression in patients. Each curve reflects the relationship for patients with different ages of onset of depression. These curves show that risk for depression depends on the age of onset of depression in both an individual *and* the individual's biological relatives. (Weissman et al., 1984, p. 1138 *Archives of General Psychiatry*, 1984, *41*, 1136–1143. Copyright © 1984, American Medical Association)

occurring disorders actually variants of some common underlying psychopathology? For example, current evidence suggests that major depression with panic and panic disorder with depression are basically different psychopathologies even though they overlap behaviorally (Coryell et al., 1988).

COGNITIVE ASPECTS OF MAJOR DEPRESSION

Severe depression is characterized by striking changes in thinking. These can include negative biases in the interpretation and recall of events and, in the severest cases, the appearance of psychotic features, including delusions and even thought disorder.

Negative Interpretation of Experience

In some ways, the thinking of the severely depressed patient is like the thinking of the paranoid. Given a false first premise (for example, "I am stupid, ugly, and worthless"), it is logical to assume that even a trivial event (forgetting to return a book, for example) has deep personal significance ("I am selfish"). However, unlike the paranoid, who seems driven to deny feelings of inferiority, the depressive seems driven to amplify feelings of worthlessness. In the most severe cases, the depressed patient may even claim responsibility for natural disasters or global unrest.

Beck (1967) describes some basic cognitive mechanisms that produce a negative bias in the ideation of depressed patients. *Arbitrary inference* is the drawing of a negative conclusion from inadequate or contrary evidence—for example, "Those people over there must despise me because they didn't smile at me." *Selective exaggeration* raises a minor event to towering significance; a mild criticism may be perceived as vilification. *Overgeneralization* transforms a situationally specific event into one of sweeping and enduring significance, such as inferring incompetence as a mother from dirt stains on her child's shirt. Here are illustrations of these negative features:

> [A] lecturer notices that one or two people in his audience walked out of the hall while he was speaking. He arbitrarily infers that they had not enjoyed his lecture; he then overgeneralizes and thinks that no one else present liked it and that, in fact, he has always been a "loser" at public speaking; consequently, he is worthless as a person and his life has no meaning. A newly divorced woman, thinking over the history of her experiences with men, selectively abstracts the bad ones as characteristic and concludes that she will never have a satisfying relationship with a man. She may attribute her difficulties to innate and irremediable flaws in herself. This woman also magnifies the importance of certain events, such as her current boy-friend's calling to cancel a date or criticizing her for some minor fault, and minimizes positive experiences (Beck & Greenberg, 1977, p. 204).

Depressive disorders are marked by a "depressive cognitive style"—the tendency to use the types of negative thinking described by Beck (1967) and others (Abramson, Seligman, & Teasdale, 1978). Nevertheless, the *causal* significance of depressive cognitive style continues to be debated (Coyne & Gotlib, 1986). For one thing, the scores of never-depressed subjects on tests of depressive cognitive style do not seem to correlate with risk for depressive disorder—high scorers are no more likely than low scorers to develop a depressive disorder at some later point. Second, although some so-called "recovered" depressives continue to display a depressive cognitive style (Eaves & Rush, 1984), many do not (Coyne & Gotlib, 1986). Perhaps only the latter are really recovered. We discuss these two points in more detail in Chapter 14. Here we need say only that depressive cognitive style is certainly a feature of depressive disorder and even its aftermath, but its causal significance remains uncertain.

Negatively Biased Memory

The kinds of negative bias described by Beck can distort memory, self-evaluation, and judgment. A good example of negative bias comes from research on *incidental learning* during tests of recall where normal subjects are asked to pay attention to one aspect of a task, but are tested without warning for their retention of other (incidentally learned) aspects. Consider three explicit tasks requiring subjects to answer questions about adjectives. In the "structural" task the subject is required merely to indicate if each word is printed in upper- or lower-case letters. In the "semantic" task, the subject indicates if the word has the same or different meaning from a target word. In the "self-referent" task, the subject indicates if the adjective is a good self-descriptor. After completing one of these three tasks, the subject is given a surprise recall test. Recall is usually best for adjectives of the self-referent task. Derry and Kuiper (1981) wanted to understand why this effect could not be obtained with depressed subjects.

The answer seemed to lie in a basic incongruity between the positive adjectives typically used by experimenters and the negative cognitive bias of depressed subjects. These investigators instead used negative adjectives to see if the depressed subjects would do better in the self-referent task. With negative adjectives (bleak, dismal, guilty, and helpless, for example), depressed subjects had better recall in self-referent than in other tasks.

Another example of negatively biased memory comes from a recent study of incidental learning (Halberstadt et al., 1987). Depressed and nondepressed subjects were asked to imagine themselves experiencing psychologically neutral facts—for example, "I woke up and it was eight o'clock." Other segments were more "loaded," setting the occasion for subjective elaborations—in particular, depressive inferences, such as "I left the room and thought about how I did on the exam."

The following day, subjects received a surprise memory test. Depressed subjects displayed evidence of remembering things that had not actually been given in the story. Specifically, they were more likely than nondepressed controls to endorse depressively toned statements that were not objectively true about the "loaded" segments of the story—for example, "I left the room and thought I did poorly on the exam." On the other hand, there were no differences between depressed and nondepressed subjects in their recall of neutral segments, thus ruling out a general memory deficit as an explanation of the effect. Overall, the results support the thrust of Beck's (1967) cognitive approach that emphasizes how personal experience is subjectively modified with depressively toned inferences to the point where memory becomes negatively biased.

Psychodynamics

In an attempt to explain the seemingly inordinate self-deprecation displayed by severely depressed patients, Freud developed a hypothesis that major depression involves *pathological identification* with a lost object.

> If one listens patiently to the many and various self-accusations of the melancholiac, one cannot in the end avoid the impression that often the most violent of them are hardly at all applicable to the patient himself, but that with insignificant modifications they do fit someone else, some person whom the patient loves, has loved or ought to love. . . . So we get the key to the clinical picture—by perceiving that the self-reproaches are reproaches against a loved object which have been shifted on to the patient's own ego (Freud, 1917/1959, p. 158).

In other words, Freud concluded that self-abasement is actually aggression against internal representations of a person both loved and hated. An irrevocable loss of such a person, whether real or imagined, is equated unconsciously with "abandonment" and this sparks hostility toward the lost person. Consciously, abandonment provokes lowered self-esteem and heightened self-directed anger, two qualities which distinguish pathological depression—what Freud called "melancholia"—from the bereavement depression that normally occurs in reaction to the loss of a person loved unambivalently. Freud's theory of the transformation of unconscious hostility toward another into self-directed anger, though by no means universally accepted, has had a deep hold on clinical theorizing about depression.

Psychotic Features

Major depression sometimes includes psychotic features, such as delusions of personal sinfulness, global disintegration, hallucinations of bodily decay, loose associations, and idiosyncratic communications. Consider the following classic description by Kraepelin of a psychotic depression (a major depression with psychotic features).

> The patients become profoundly despondent, and indulge in all sorts of *self-accusations*. They feel that they have been great sinners, have neglected their duties and made many enemies, have never done anything right, and their whole life has been one long series of mistakes. They accuse themselves of bringing misfortune on others or of causing some great calamity. They claim that they are devoid of feeling and sympathy for others. . . . *Hypochondriacal delusions* are prominent and are usually associated with numerous false bodily sensations: their health is ruined as the result of masturbation; they are succumbing to some malignant disease, and their organs are wasting away; cloudy urine signifies profound disease of the kidneys; they can never recover, and their body and face are altered. Female patients complain of being pregnant, and often accuse themselves of immorality and masturbation (Kraepelin, 1907/1981, p. 403).

In older depressed patients, affective disorder may include symptoms of *pseudodementia*—an apparent inability to remember things or follow simple requests—that superficially resembles, and may sometimes be misdiagnosed as, real dementia (see Chapter 9, pp. 255–256).

PHYSIOLOGICAL ASPECTS OF MAJOR DEPRESSION

Major depression is marked by *physiological* abnormalities involving sleep, appetite, body temperature, energy, and hormone regulation and also by *biochemical* abnormalities involving certain neurotransmitters. We will focus on those abnormalities with the most research evidence and potential theoretical significance.

Sleep Abnormalities

Normal Sleep   To appreciate the sleep abnormalities frequently associated with episodes of major depression, one should look first at normal sleep patterns. Figure 13.3 shows a person with surface electrodes attached to the scalp, at the edge of each eye, and under the chin. The body's electric signals—tiny changes in voltage—are amplified and sent to special pens whose deflections scratch out recordings on slowly moving paper. The signal from the scalp becomes the electroencephalogram (EEG). The signal from the eyes becomes the electrooculogram (EOG). The signal from below the chin becomes the electromyogram (EMG), or muscle tension pattern.

Five major stages of sleep can be identified from the largely discrete patterns of EEG, EOG, and EMG. Four of these are typically without rapid eye movements (REMs) and so are called non-REM (NREM). These stages, from 1 through 4, include increasing amounts of low-frequency, high-voltage "delta" waves. Rapid eye movements (REMs) are typical of the REM stage of sleep when dreaming is most intense, complex, and storylike (Cohen, 1979).

The progression of sleep stages during a night of normal sleep constitutes a biorhythm of roughly ninety-minute cycles, each with an NREM and a REM component. The "architecture" of each ninety-minute NREM-REM cycle is shown in Figure 13.4. Notice the fairly predictable progression from NREM to REM, the roughly ninety-minute latency from sleep onset (stage 1) to REM sleep onset, and the progressively longer REM sleep periods till the fourth, with subsequent ones about the same or slightly shorter.

FIGURE 13.3   Electrode placement for recording sleep characteristics. The top two recordings (electro-oculogram, or EOG) show eye movements in the form of mirror-image deflections. The electromyogram (EMG) displays muscle tone recorded from the chin. Placement and recording of the electroencephalogram (EEG) is also shown. The EOG, EMG, and EEG show the onset of rapid eye movement (REM) sleep. Note the sharply decreased EMG, appearance of conjugate eye movements, and shift to low-amplitude, mixed-frequency EEG. (From Rechtschaffen & Kales, 1968)

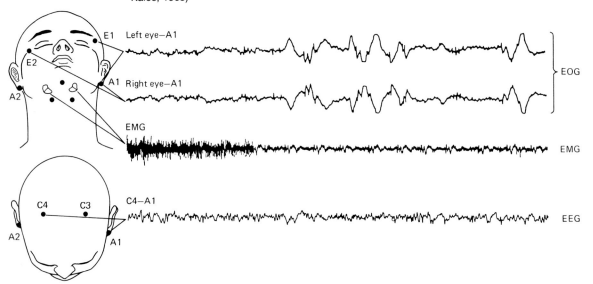

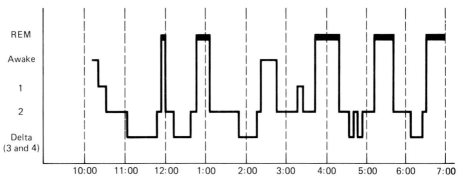

FIGURE 13.4   A typical pattern of normal sleep. Notice the progression from wakefulness to stage 1 and then on to stage 2, and finally to stages 3 and 4 (delta sleep). Notice the roughly ninety-minute latency from sleep (stage 1) onset to REM onset, the progressively longer REM periods, and the progressively shorter delta periods.

Sleep in Major Depression   Now look at the pattern of sleep in a depressed patient shown in Figure 13.5. Notice the short duration of time from sleep onset to initial REM period (less than thirty minutes); depressed patients often display such *short REM onset latencies*. Also notice that the initial REM period is *unusually long*, with subsequent REM periods either as long as the first or progressively shorter. Finally, notice the *diminished delta* sleep, frequent brief awakenings, and early final awakening (sometimes called early morning insomnia). All these are characteristic of sleep during episodes of major depression. Not shown, but frequently observed in major depression, is relatively large amounts of eye movement within REM periods (high "REM density"), especially during the first REM period of sleep.

FIGURE 13.5   A typical pattern of sleep in the depressed. Notice the long sleep onset latency, short REM onset latency, and frequent awakenings during the night. The normal increase in duration of successive REM periods is not observed. There is little delta sleep. And there is a failure to maintain sleep (early morning, or terminal, insomnia).

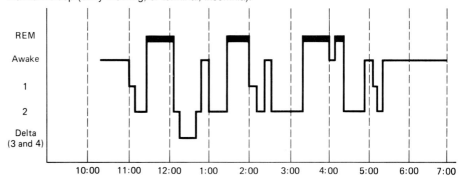

These then are the sleep abnormalities in cases of major depression where sleep duration is relatively *short,* a condition known as *hypo*somnia. Two related questions about sleep in major depression remain unanswered (Gillin & Borbely, 1985; Reynolds & Kupfer, 1987). First, what is the significance of these abnormalities to a theory of depression? Much of the theorizing about depression and sleep involves technical ideas about the neurophysiological regulation of sleep-wake and REM-NREM rhythms. Suffice it to say that much uncertainty remains about the nature and causal significance of sleep abnormalities. Nevertheless, there is one interesting finding regarding short REM-onset latency. Apparently it is associated not only with depression itself, but also with an increased risk for depression, that is, it can be observed even in nondepressed people who have had, or will later develop, major depression (Rush et al., 1986; Giles et al., 1988). In other words, short REM-onset latency may be a biological marker of a liability to depression.

Second, what is the significance of the *hypersomnic* pattern of sleep abnormalities observed in some major depressions? This pattern includes (a) normal or decreased sleep onset latency, (b) increased total sleep time with few or no arousals, yet (c) the same reduced REM-onset latency seen in the hyposomnic pattern. (While the hyposomnic pattern is typical of major *unipolar* depressions, the hypersomnic pattern is often evident in major *bipolar* depressions; differences between unipolar and bipolar depression are described shortly.) The fact is, we still do not know if the hypersomnic and hyposomnic patterns reflect different abnormalities or merely different variants of the same abnormality.

In sum, major depression is characterized by hyposomnic and hypersomnic abnormalities whose significance to theory and classification of depressive disorder is still uncertain. The same may be said for certain neuroendocrine abnormalities that are also often associated with episodes of major depression.

Neuroendocrine Abnormalities

The sleep abnormalities we have just described support the widely held view that major depression involves defective mechanisms in the deepest part of the brain—most likely including the hypothalamus and other parts of the limbic system. Also consistent with this idea is evidence that major depression is often characterized by abnormal hormone regulation in the limbic system. To get a better appreciation of this aspect of major depression, we need to understand a little more about the way that the hypothalamus controls hormone levels by controlling the *endocrine* (hormone-producing) glands.

A "smart" gas heater "knows" when to go on and off because it is equipped with a thermostat that is sensitive to room temperature. When room temperature is *fed back* to the thermostat, any difference from target set point is corrected by the *opposing action* of the thermostat. Thus, when the room temperature goes up the thermostat turns the heater off; when the room temperature goes down, the thermostat turns the heater on. The result is a narrow range of variation around a physical set point. This principle of *negative feedback* also characterizes certain physiological processes—for example, those that permit only a narrow range of variation around a biological set point for hormone levels.

Neuroendocrine Regulation by Negative Feedback The hypothalamus regulates vegetative processes like the sleep-wake cycle, glucose metabolism, and physical growth. For some of these, hypothalamic influence is indirect, operating through an endocrine "middle man" called the pituitary gland. Situated just below the hypothalamus in the center of the brain, the pituitary secretes hormones into the blood. The targets of pituitary hormones include thyroid, gonads, and adrenals (Figure 13.6). In short, the hypothalamus controls the pituitary, the pituitary controls the target endocrine glands, and, as we shall see, the hormonal output of those target glands is fed back to the hypothalamus.

One of the target glands is the adrenal, named for its location *adjacent to* the *kidneys* (ad renal). The middle (medulla) of the adrenal, under excitatory control of the autonomic nervous system, produces adrenalin which, with its excitatory effect on heart rate, is important to preparing the body for fight or flight. The outer surface (cortex) of the adrenal, under pituitary control, produces cortisol and other hormones. These have numerous effects, including facilitation of glucose metabolism and protein synthesis. Abnormalities of cortisol secretion are common in major depression.

Cortisol secretion is normally controlled by a hormone from the pituitary called *a*drenal *c*ortico*t*rophic (cortex-facilitating) *h*ormone, or ACTH, which in turn is controlled by a hypothalamic hormone called *c*ortico*t*rophin *r*eleasing *f*actor, or CRF. Secretion of CRF is in turn controlled by the inhibitory effect of cortisol levels. Thus, the *h*ypothalamus, *p*ituitary, and *a*drenal (HPA) constitute a negative feedback system, that is, the output (cortisol) at the A end of HPA is fed back to the H end as corrective input (see Figure 13.7).

HPA Defect Many patients with major depression show high levels of cortisol associated with the hypersecretion of CRF by the hypothalamus. It is not yet known, however, if CRF oversecretion reflects an abnormality of the hypothalamus alone or an abnormality of paleocortical structures that regulate the hypothalamus. Since patients with the high-cortisol pattern show *normal* cortical levels during premorbid and intermorbid periods, the abnormality should be viewed as a sign of a depressed *state* rather than as a biological marker of the liability to depression.

In normal people, the HPA system can be "fooled" by introducing a synthetic cortisol called *dexamethasone*. In a procedure called the *d*examethasone *s*uppression *t*est, or DST, dexamethasone is administered orally at 11 P.M., with plasma cortisol levels assessed the next day at 8 A.M. and 4 P.M. Just like natural cortisol, dexamethasone inhibits CRF production

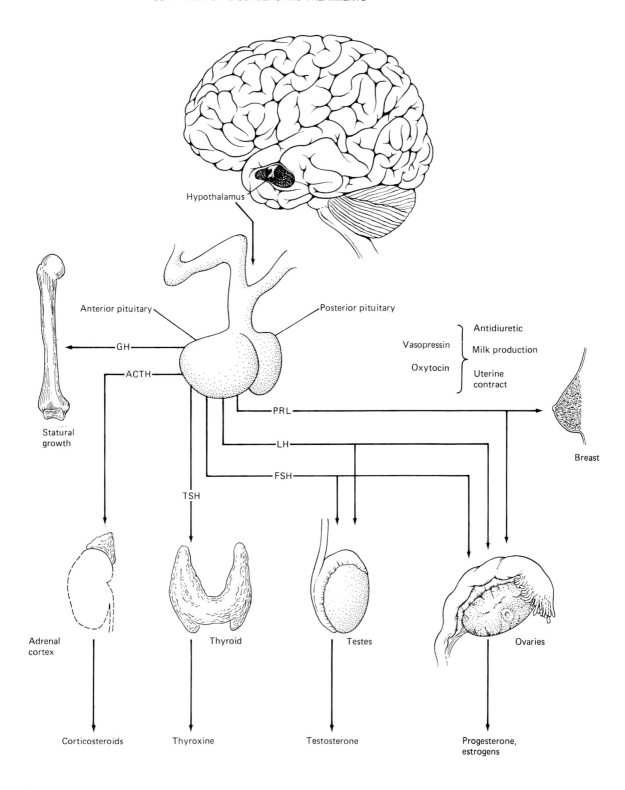

Hypothalamus

Anterior pituitary

Posterior pituitary

GH

ACTH

Vasopressin

Oxytocin

Antidiuretic

Milk production

Uterine
contract

PRL

LH

FSH

Statural
growth

TSH

Breast

Adrenal
cortex

Thyroid

Testes

Ovaries

Corticosteroids

Thyroxine

Testosterone

Progesterone,
estrogens

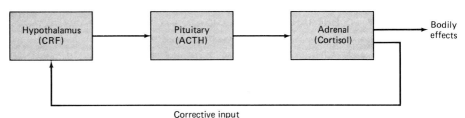

FIGURE 13.7 A negative feedback loop of particular relevance to major depression is the hypothalamus-pituitary-adrenal (HPA) loop. The hypothalamus produces CRF which activates the pituitary. The pituitary then produces ACTH, which activates the adrenal cortex. The adrenal cortex produces cortisol, which suppresses CRF production by the hypothalamus. The figure shows only one of many negative feedback loops within and among the hypothalamus, pituitary, and adrenal glands.

by the hypothalamus (see Figure 13.7). This in turn reduces ACTH, therefore indirectly reducing cortisol production.

However, about 40 to 60 percent of patients with major depression (often those with cortisol hypersecretion) show little suppression. The percentage is even higher (about 70 percent) for severe melancholic depression with psychotic symptoms. This abnormal pattern on the DST is often called "nonsuppression," even though "nonsuppression" is a misnomer because typically, a brief period of *less than normal* suppression of cortisol level is followed by a *faster than normal* return to pretest levels. Thus, when we use the conventional term "nonsuppression," we really mean "early escape from suppression."

There is one other intriguing observation about those depressed patients with the "nonsuppression" pattern on the DST. If they show a gradual normalization of DST, they generally have a good clinical outcome. However, if they continue to show "nonsuppression," they generally have a bad clinical outcome, including reoccurrence of symptoms and even suicidal behavior. In other words, failure of the "nonsuppression" pattern on the DST to normalize is a poor prognostic sign (APA Task Force, 1987).

While early escape on the DST frequently occurs in major depression, in many cases it does not; also, "nonsuppression" can occur in nondepressive disorders and in perhaps 10 percent of normals, thus raising questions about

---

FIGURE 13.6 The pituitary gland, connected to the hypothalamus at the base of the brain, has two lobes and two functions. The posterior lobe of the pituitary stores and passes on to the general circulation two hormones manufactured in the hypothalamus: vasopressin and oxytocin. The anterior lobe secretes a number of other hormones: growth hormone (GH), which promotes statural growth; adrenocorticotropic hormone (ACTH), which stimulates the cortex of the adrenal gland to secrete corticosteroids; thyroid-stimulating hormone (TSH), which stimulates secretions by the thyroid gland, and follicle-stimulating hormone (FSH), luteinizing hormone (LH) and prolactin (PRL), which in various combinations regulate lactation and the functioning of the gonads. Several of these anterior pituitary hormones are known to be controlled by releasing factors from the hypothalamus. (Guillemin & Burges, 1976, p. 134)

how specific it is to depressive disorder (Arana, Baldessarini, & Ornsteen, 1985). Our safest conclusion is that the hypothetical HPA defect suggested by "nonsuppression" on the DST is *only one of many* possible physiological abnormalities that could explain depression.

In fact there is new evidence that patients with major depression respond abnormally when their HPA and other neuroendocrine control systems are "challenged" in different ways other than by the DST. For example, many depressed patients, even some with normal DST responses, nevertheless produce abnormally low levels of ACTH in response to insulin-induced hypoglycemia (low blood sugar), perhaps indicating an insensitivity of the hypothalamus to changes in glucose (Meller et al., 1988).

In sum, major depression seems to involve a variety of physiological abnormalities in the deepest parts of the brain, including the hypothalamus. However, the significance of such abnormalities—whether they are causes, effects, or merely correlates of the psychological symptoms of major depression—is anyone's guess.

Neurochemical Abnormalities

Hypotheses about the biochemical basis of major depression have become increasingly popular ever since the early 1960s when drugs that produce or block depression were discovered. We will take a brief look at the evidence that major depression may involve abnormalities in at least two neurochemical systems, one involving neurons that use neurotransmitters norepinephrine and serotonin—classified as *bioamines* on the basis of their chemical structure—and one involving neurons that use the neurotransmitter acetylcholine.

Norepinephrine and Serotonin The original bioamine hypothesis for major depression was developed on the basis of three striking observations. The first observation was that reserpine, a drug used to treat hypertension, produced severe depression in some patients. Reserpine dissolves the vesicles which normally protect serotonin and norepinephrine molecules from being degraded by intraneuronal MAO (see Chapter 8, pp. 216–217). The depressive effect of reserpine therefore suggested that some major depressions might involve decreased levels of these important neurotransmitters.

The second observation was that drugs that block MAO—the MAO inhibitors—could counteract either natural or reserpine-induced depression; so, even if reserpine dissolved the storage vesicles, MAO inhibitors could compensate by blocking the destructive effect of MAO on the exposed neurotransmitter molecules. The net effect would be a higher level of bioamines.

The third observation was the beneficial effect of tricyclic drugs, named for their triple carbon rings. Tricyclic antidepressants block neurotransmitter reuptake, thereby maintaining higher levels of norepinephrine and serotonin in the synaptic space. The therapeutic effect of tricyclics—along with the observations of reserpine-induced depression and the antidepressive effects of MAO inhibitors—seemed consistent with the bioamine hypothesis that depression reflects deficient bioamine function.

Unfortunately, things have gotten more complex in recent years, with increasing doubts raised about the general applicability of the original bioamine hypothesis for depression (Baldessarini, 1975). For example, there is now evidence that some major depressions are associated with *elevated* levels of catecholamines, and that the therapeutic effect of antidepressive drugs, which takes two to three weeks, involves a gradual *attenuation,* or "down regulation," of catecholamine activity (Gold, Goodwin, & Chrousos, 1988a). In addition, there is increasing evidence that major depression is associated with abnormalities in other neurochemical systems, in particular, those that use the neurotransmitter acetylcholine (Davis et al., 1978; Zis & Goodwin, 1982).

Acetylcholine The relevance of an acetylcholine mechanism is suggested by abnormalities of REM sleep that were discussed earlier. You will recall that the latency, duration, density, and nightly distribution of REM periods is often abnormal in depression; some or all of these characteristics are believed to be controlled by acetylcholine mechanisms. For example, acetylcholine-enhancing drugs can shorten the latency to the onset of REM sleep, especially in depressed patients who already have abnormally short REM onset latencies (Berger et al., 1989; Sitaram et al., 1982). This suggests that an abnormally sensitive acetylcholine mechanism characterizes depressive disorder (Janowsky et al., 1972). Moreover, REM sleep is inhibited by antidepressant drugs that also inhibit cholinergic function. Perhaps this explains why REM deprivation produced by waking the depressed patient at the onset of each REM period can improve mood, although it is an impractical and short-lived treatment. This antidepressant effect takes about two weeks, and it works with the same patients who are responsive to the antidepressant drugs. In short, the evidence points to abnormalities in at least two interacting neurochemical systems, a bioamine and an acetylcholine system (McCarley, 1982; Vogel et al., 1980).

Recent research on the biochemistry of depression suggests still other abnormalities. Recall that major depression is often associated with endocrine abnormalities such as excess production by the hypothalamus of the stress hormone releaser, CRF. Some investigators have pointed out that there are many behavioral and biochemical parallels between major depression and reactions to life-threatening events. In their view, abnormalities of catecholamine, acetylcholine, and hormone function make sense if we think of major depression as stress reaction gone awry (Gold, Goodwin, & Chrousos, 1988b).

UNIPOLAR AND BIPOLAR DEPRESSIVE DISORDERS

Diagnostic Distinctions

So far we have ignored the fact that in some cases, major depression is associated with mania either in the patient or in a close relative. Such cases are called *bipolar* depression. When a depressive disorder is diagnosed as bipolar on the basis of manic behavior *in the relatives* rather than in the patient, the clinician is making an inference about the patient's underlying psychopathology. One could argue, therefore, that a major depression is truly unipolar only if there is no manic element in the patient or relatives.

We will use the term *major* depression for *any* severe depression, unipolar or bipolar. In this way, we can keep separate two independent features of affective disorders: (1) their *polarity* (bipolar versus unipolar depressions) and (2) their *severity* (major versus minor depression). Here we will continue our discussion of major (severe) depression with a special focus on polarity, the association or lack of association of depression with mania. In the next chapter we will turn to the question of why both unipolar and bipolar depressions vary in severity.

What Is Unipolar Depression? Our understanding of depressive disorder depends on behavioral and physiological information, the history of the problem, drug responsiveness, and the familial context of the disorder. Clearly, then, without good information in these areas, a diagnosis of unipolar disorder based on strictly behavioral criteria may be somewhat ambiguous because in some cases a so-called unipolar depression might turn out to be a unipolar *expression* of a bipolar disorder. For example, a patient diagnosed as unipolar depressive might develop manic behavior in response to antidepressive medication, or more spontaneously over time. Even when we can rule out bipolar disorder, a unipolar diagnosis may still be ambiguous because there is undoubtedly more than one cause of unipolar depression.

In short, the *heterogeneity* of the unipolar category makes ambiguous any comparisons of behaviorally defined bipolar and unipolar depression. Nevertheless, some insights may be gained by such comparisons, and we give some below. But before proceeding, we need to say something more about manic behavior.

What Is Unipolar Mania? The depressive and manic episodes of a bipolar disorder may be widely separated by periods of relative normalcy. Other times one follows rapidly upon the heels of the other. Sometimes, switches back and forth between the two states can occur many times within a single day. "The *switch process* in bipolar illness is one of the most dramatic events in psychiatry. . . . A bipolar depressed woman, withdrawn, taciturn, appearing like a wizened old lady, may suddenly blossom into an energetic, joking, seductive young woman after switching into mania. Though less common, the switch from mania to depression may be equally sudden and dramatic" (Mendelson, Gillin, & Wyatt, 1977, p. 167).

What does manic behavior look like clinically, and how should it be understood: as a distinctly separate *unipolar disorder* (manic type) or as an incomplete expression of a *bipolar disorder*? To get an answer, we will briefly consider the unipolar manic disorder.

DSM-III-R criteria for manic episodes are given in Table 13.2. Unipolar mania occurs in patients who never suffer from major depressive episodes, but

TABLE 13.2   DIAGNOSTIC CRITERIA FOR MANIC EPISODE*

A. A distinct period of abnormally and persistently elevated, expansive, or irritable mood

B. During the period of mood disturbance, at least three of the following symptoms have persisted (four if the mood is only irritable) and have been present to a significant degree:
1. Inflated self-esteem or grandiosity
2. Decreased need for sleep; e.g., feels rested after only three hours of sleep
3. More talkative than usual or pressure to keep talking
4. Flight of ideas or subjective experience that thoughts are racing
5. Distractibility; i.e., attention too easily drawn to unimportant or irrelevant external stimuli
6. Increase in goal-directed activity (either socially, at work or school, or sexually) or psychomotor agitation
7. Excessive involvement in pleasurable activities that have a high potential for painful consequences; e.g., the person engages in unrestrained buying sprees, sexual indiscretions, or foolish business investments

C. Mood disturbance severe enough to cause marked impairment in occupational functioning or in usual social activities or relationships with others, or to necessitate hospitalization to prevent harm to self or others

D. At no time during the disturbance have there been delusions or hallucinations for as long as two weeks in the absence of prominent mood symptoms; i.e., before the mood symptoms developed or after they have remitted

E. Not superimposed on schizophrenia, schizophreniform disorder, delusional disorder, or other psychotic disorder

F. It cannot be established that an organic factor initiated and maintained the disturbance. (*Note:* Somatic antidepressant treatment—e.g., drugs, ECT—that apparently precipitates a mood disturbance should not be considered an etiologic organic factor.)

*A manic syndrome is defined as including criteria A, B, and C above. A hypomanic syndrome is defined as including criteria A and B, but not C; i.e., no marked impairment.
Source: American Psychiatric Association, 1987, p. 217. Reprinted with permission from the *Diagnostic and Statistical Manual of Mental Disorders, Third Edition, Revised.* Copyright © 1987 American Psychiatric Association.

this is relatively rare, with a lifetime risk of roughly 2 per 1000. In the milder or *hypo*manic state, the behavior is playful, festive, and uninhibited, and can have an infectious influence on the mood of others. In the full-blown state, manics can be irritable, abrasive, and inconsiderate. Manic states may sometimes include strong feelings of depression as well as anxiety and anger. Such "dysphoric manias" seem to reflect a particularly severe form of affective disorder in that they are associated with relatively frequent prior hospitalizations for affective disorder and relatively poor responsiveness to lithium treatment (Post et al., 1989).

Upon first admission to the hospital, manics can be as thought-disordered as schizophrenics (Harrow et al., 1982). Occasionally, the manic state can be intense and delirious, with the patient suddenly becoming disoriented, assaultive, hallucinated, delusional, and even tearful, the condition appearing and disappearing rather mysteriously in only a few chaotic days (Bond, 1980).

Typically, the exuberant and extraverted *premorbid* behavior of manics gives the superficial impression of normalcy, or even mental health. However, in many cases, histrionics, abrasiveness, mood shifts, and alcohol abuse indicate character disorder. In still other cases, both healthy and defective qualities co-exist, with admirable traits like ambition, sociability, imagination, and even true creative genius sometimes "spoiled" by offensive traits like irritability, belligerence, and egocentricity. The association between mania and creativity has often been noted and is the subject of increasing research interest. For example, creative writers appear to be at greater risk for manic and depressive mood shifts (Andreasen, 1980).

Many manics develop mild or marked depressive features when administered *lithium carbonate,* the treatment of choice for bipolar depression. More important, the relatives of unipolar manics have increased risk for bipolar and other depressive disorders. Therefore, unipolar mania is probably a *rare variant* of bipolar disorder.

We now return to our focus on major depression with a more detailed description of the unipolar and bipolar types of depressive disorder. An outline of the discussion is given in Table 13.3. While the episodes of bipolar and unipolar disorders can be severe or mild (see Chapter 14), we now focus on the major versions.

Epidemiology

Lifetime Risk The bipolar syndrome has a lifetime risk of about 0.5 percent compared with roughly 5 percent for the unipolar syndrome (Robins, Helzer, Weissman et al., 1984). For the relatives of affected individuals, the lifetime risk for either syndrome is increased roughly by a factor of 10, though figures vary considerably from study to study. More specific estimates of the risk can be made from information on the age of the affected relative and the age of onset of the illness in the patient (Figure 13.2 above).

Sex and Age The female/male ratio is 2 to 1 or greater in unipolar disorder but close to 1 to 1 in bipolar disorder. It is unclear how much of this difference

TABLE 13.3 COMPARISON OF UNIPOLAR AND BIPOLAR DISORDER

Characteristics	Unipolar (UP)	Bipolar (BP)
Base rate (population)	Approx. 5%	Approx. 0.5%
Sex ratio (F:M)	Greater than 2:1	Less than 2:1
Socioeconomic status (SES)	Average	Upper class overrepresented
Age of initial onset	35–45	Late 20s
Episode duration (mos.)	Approx. 6–9	Approx. 3–6
Episode frequency	1–2 (usual)	3+ (usual)
	4–6 (maximum)	7–9 (maximum)
Family liability for first-degree relatives	UP: 8%	UP:10%
	BP: 1%	BP: 6%

in sex ratios reflects sex differences in physiology, defensiveness, reporting bias, and social expectations (Nolen-Hoeksema, 1987).

The initial episode tends to occur during the late 30s to early 40s in unipolar disorders as compared with the late 20s to early 30s in bipolar disorders. The onset of bipolar disorder during adolescence, a rare occurrence, carries an especially high risk of suicide for both men and women.

Social Class   The prevalence of affective complaints (not disorder) varies with social class (Boyd & Weissman, 1982). A greater frequency of depressive complaints is observed in the lower social classes, probably because of greater dissatisfaction at work and home, less opportunity, fewer luxuries, and lower levels of coping ability. On the other hand, the rate of unipolar disorder does not vary by social class. Perhaps the evenly distributed rate of unipolar disorder across socioeconomic classes reflects a more equitable distribution of one or more endogenous liabilities.

Surprisingly, the higher social classes have an excess of *bipolar disorder*. Why should upper-class status be associated with relatively more of what appears to be the severest type of affective disorder, a pattern just the opposite to the one we noted in schizophrenia? If social class is considered an *effect* rather than a cause, the excess rate makes good sense. Temperamental qualities of drive, sociability, and imaginativeness that are characteristic of the mildest symptoms of bipolar patients could translate otherwise unremarkable competence into extraordinary achievement. Thus, while bipolar *disorder* is a disadvantage, bipolar *traits,* or mild bipolar *symptoms,* may actually confer a distinct advantage.

Clinical Features

Many of the clinical features of major depressive episodes that we described earlier (Table 13.1) characterize both unipolar and bipolar depression. Manic and severe depressive episodes may also include psychotic features.

Psychotic Aspects   The thought disorder associated with mania—derailed, tangential, goalless—is in many ways similar to that of schizophrenia, though it tends to be more pressured and distractible, and less impoverished (Andreasen & Grove, 1986; Harrow et al., 1982). For example, about 15 percent of both manics and schizophrenics have incoherent speech. Compare the responses of a schizophrenic and a manic patient to a question about the energy crisis of the mid 1970s. (Can you tell who the manic is?)

> They're destroying too many cattle and oil just to make soap. If we need soap when you can jump into a pool of water, and then when you go to buy your gasoline, my folks always thought they should get pop but the best thing to get is motor oil and money. May many as well go there and trade in some pop caps and uh tires and tractors to gra . . . car garages, so they can pull cars away from wrecks, is what I believed in. So I didn't go there to get no more pop when my folks said it. I just went

there to get an ice cream cone, and some pop in cans, or we can go over there to get a cigarette (Andreasen & Grove, 1979, p. 381).

Well it's just one of those things, if you will spend all your energy . . . cooking and heating milk and destroying the vitamins in it, and if you will do these things you will have problems. And if you will not breed enough horses so that in good weather there's no reason why people when they go shopping couldn't take a cart and spend a day or two and camp in the summertime and bring home groceries, instead of um using up all the gas there's so many things that they could do these things if they want to. They just, they want to fool around and usually it's another issue than what they say too. It's usually somebody with a lot of pull and with a lot of lead in his pantry or something that will come out and intimidate somebody in Congress or that they won't do the things they need to do it would have to be (Andreason & Grove, 1979, pp. 382–383).

The presence of psychosis in affective disorder (as in the second example above) often complicates both diagnosis and classification. Until recently, a diagnosis of affective disorder required the *absence* of psychotic symptoms. However, psychotic and nonpsychotic patients with major affective disorder have the same responsiveness to lithium and the same proportion of relatives with affective disorder. In short, the presence of psychotic disturbances, including thought disorder, delusions, and hallucinations, has relatively little value for deciding if a psychotic patient has schizophrenia or affective disorder (Pope & Lipinski, 1978). Only a careful evaluation of other aspects—the nature of the thought disorder, the presence of mood shifts, the number of negative symptoms, development of the psychosis, family history, drug response—will yield a more confident diagnosis.

Temporal Aspects   Unipolar and bipolar episodes differ in duration and frequency, though there is much overlap (Angst, Felder, & Frey, 1979). The duration of a unipolar episode is typically six to nine months compared with three to six months for a typical bipolar episode. The number of unipolar episodes over a lifetime is typically one or two but may be as high as six. This compares with a typical frequency of more than three with a maximum of seven to nine for bipolar episodes.

Both disorders increase in frequency with age. In bipolar disorder, it is the depressive more than the manic episodes which increase in frequency with age. Both disorders carry a higher risk for relapse within twenty-four months of initial episode in older than in younger patients.

Seasonal Aspects   In *seasonal affective disorder,* or SAD, recurrent episodes of major depression have their onsets typically during the winter months—hence the term "winter depression"—followed by a shift toward normalcy from mid-February to mid-April. There is some question about the presence and severity of manic symptoms during the spring and summer months following recovery from such winter depressions; consequently there is u ncertainty about the connection between SAD and bipolar disorder (Blehar &

Rosenthal, 1989). The depressive episodes of SAD are characterized by atypical vegetative symptoms such as excessive fatigue, hypersomnia, hyperphagia (excessive eating), and cravings for carbohydrates such as crackers, donuts, and chocolate. These cravings are often normalized by antidepressive drugs that boost serotonin, but the implication of this effect for a neurochemical theory of SAD remains uncertain (Wurtman & Wurtman, 1989).

That SAD is controlled by lighting conditions is suggested by its spontaneous occurrence during winter months especially in northern latitudes where long nights are the rule, and by its responsiveness to phototherapy: exposure to very strong light for up to two hours a day (Lewy et al., 1980, 1987; Wurtman & Wurtman, 1989). Unfortunately, there is still much controversy over hypotheses that explain SAD as the effect of an interaction between light and specific neurochemical and circadian abnormalities (Blehar & Rosenthal, 1989).

Mortality   The lifetime risk for suicide in the depressed is probably ten to twenty times the population risk. In bipolar depression, suicide is rare during manic episodes, but rather tends to occur *during a shift* into or out of deep depression, especially in young males. The elevated risk for suicide during the period of shift may have something to do with the patient's energy level. When severely depressed, the energy level may be too low to support the effort of attempting suicide; when in the process of shifting from one pole to the other, energy levels are not so severely compromised as to make the suicidal effort seem impossible.

Biological Treatments

Response to Medication   Tricyclic antidepressants not only alleviate depression; they also can prevent or delay subsequent episodes. Occasionally, tricyclics will induce hypomanic attacks or rapid cycling between depression and mania in a seemingly "unipolar" patient. When this occurs, the clinician should suspect a latent bipolar disease.

Lithium carbonate is highly effective in the treatment of bipolar disorder, and there are remarkably few serious side effects if it is used correctly (Schou, 1988). In about 80 percent of cases, lithium carbonate can ameliorate depressive as well as manic episodes; its use during periods of remission can delay, or even prevent, the onset of new episodes (Coppen, Metcalfe, & Wood, 1982). It takes about two weeks for lithium to reduce the euphoria, aggressiveness, and grandiosity of manic episodes; the treatment has relatively little effect on hyperactivity and psychotic thinking (Sheard, 1980; Zis & Goodwin, 1982). For these reasons, lithium treatment of mania is often supplemented with antipsychotic drugs like chlorpromazine. While the antipsychotic effects of major tranquilizers may be due to their ability to normalize dopamine systems (see Chapter 12), the mechanism for lithium is still largely unknown. Perhaps lithium normalizes the balance between neurotransmitter systems, possibly by influencing neuronal membrane characteristics (Aldenhoff & Lux, 1981; Janowsky & Judd, 1981; Treiser et al., 1981).

Electroconvulsive Treatment (ECT) Severe depression with psychomotor retardation, vegetative abnormalities, and suicidal impulses may not respond well to drug treatment. Some of these drug-resistant cases may respond to ECT (Kiloh, 1982). A half-second current with a frequency of 120 to 150 pulses per second passed through the head produces a seizure. The number of seizures required depends on the patient, but six to twelve spaced forty-eight to seventy-two hours apart is typical (see Chapter 22).

Heterogeneity of Unipolar Depression

Recall that, compared with the symptoms of bipolar depression, the symptoms of unipolar depression are more variable and unpredictable across patients. This heterogeneity implies corresponding diversity of causality:

1 Relatively mild versions of bipolar disorder disease
2 Expressions of a unipolar depressive psychopathology *other than* that of bipolar disorder
3 By-products of personality disorder or medical disease
4 Any one of the above aggravated by adverse external conditions
5 Situation-specific reactions to depressing events in an otherwise normal individual

In the next chapter, we examine evidence that bears on all of these distinctions.

SUMMARY

Affective disorder is expressed by clinically significant changes in any of four broad psychological components of affect: (1) *vegetative* (for example, insomnia, anorexia, apathy), (2) *subjective* (for example, anhedonia, dysphoria), (3) *expressive,* or emotional (for example, crying, withdrawal, inaction), and (4) *ideational* (for example, poor self-concept, pessimistic ideas). Each of these psychological components is controlled by a different part of the brain, for example, the vegetative component is controlled by brain stem and paleocortical structures of the "limbic system." Some severe affective disorders include thought disorder and/or delusions, in which case they may be described as *psychotic.*

Four commonly observed aspects of major depression can be described, including (1) *negative cognitive bias* such as irrational expectations of failure, (2) *neuroendocrine dysfunction* (in particular, the excess production of the adrenal hormone, cortisol, apparently because of hypothalamic dysfunction), (3) *sleep/wake abnormalities,* such as early morning insomnia, and (4) possible *biochemical abnormalities,* such as the hypothetical cholinergic/catecholamine imbalance.

One view of affective disorder assumes that abnormal hypothalamic mechanisms adversely influence the right-hemisphere mechanisms of unconscious thought and the left-hemisphere mechanisms of conscious thought; the more severe the disorder, the more important are endogenous (internal) hypothalamically induced changes in motivation. This view is consistent with evidence on abnormalities in the regulation of sleep, hormones, and neurotransmitters. However, the exact nature and causal significance of these abnormalities remain uncertain.

Two major affective disorders—bipolar and unipolar—can be diagnosed from observing the patient's behavior and from information about psychopathology in the patient's relatives. An association between depression and episodes of manic euphoria and excitement distinguish the bipolar from the unipolar type, but there are other differences—for example, the bipolar type has earlier onset and more episodes, each of shorter duration. These and other observations suggest that the bipolar type is a severer affective disorder than most unipolar types.

In the next chapter, we review evidence that bipolar and *some* unipolar disorders reflect a highly heritable *manic-depressive disease* that can be distinguished from other causes of affective disorder.

Affective Disorders 2. Etiology

The etiology of affective disorders can be boiled down to a few broadly defined causal factors involving heredity, medical disease, psychopathology, cognition, and adverse events. Presumably, the balance of these factors will determine the pattern of symptoms by which a conventional classification system like *DSM-III-R* distinguishes different affective disorders. We begin with evidence that at least one of these—namely, the manic-depressive (bipolar) type—is highly heritable.

GENETIC FACTORS AND MANIC DEPRESSIVE DISEASE

The clearest evidence of a genetic factor in affective disorders, especially the bipolar kind, comes from twin and adoption studies of people displaying major episodes ("full syndrome") and less severe episodes ("subsyndromes") of affective disorder. Since studies of full-syndrome affective disorders are most prevalent, we start with these.

Full-Syndrome (Major) Disorders

We will address two related questions: Does twin research on concordance for the presence and polarity of affective disorder suggest an inherited diathesis, and is this inference sustained by adoption research on the effect of rearing conditions?

Polarity Concordance in Twins Consider the study by Bertelsen et al. (1977) involving fifty-five MZ and fifty-two DZ twin pairs having at least one twin member diagnosed with major affective disorder. MZ twins were consistently more concordant for affective disorder than DZ twins. MZ concordance was much higher for *bipolar* disorder (74 percent) than for unipolar disorder (43 percent). DZ concordance was 17 percent for bipolar and 19 percent for unipolar disorder.

These twin data (see also Bertelsen, 1979) are remarkably consistent with many other twin studies of affective disorder carried out in different countries during the last sixty years (Allen, 1976; Slater & Cowie, 1971). Collectively, these studies show comparatively lower MZ concordance rates for unipolar disorder (40 percent versus 11 percent for DZs) than for bipolar disorder (72 percent versus 14 percent for DZs). These numbers support the hypothesis that bipolar disorder is even more highly heritable than unipolar disorder. This hypothesis is also consistent with family studies that typically find markedly elevated rates of *both* unipolar and bipolar disorder in the relatives of bipolars, but markedly elevated rates of *only* unipolar disorder in the relatives of unipolars (for example, Gershon et al., 1982).

Diathesis versus Rearing   Recall that Fischer (1973) found comparably elevated rates of schizophrenia (about 10 percent) in the offspring of either the normal or the schizophrenic member of MZ pairs discordant for schizophrenia (Chapter 12, p. 330). Likewise, Bertelsen (1985) has reported comparably elevated rates of bipolar disorder for the offspring of MZ mothers discordant for the disorder. Specifically, the rate of bipolar disorder was 10.5 percent for the offspring of the disturbed twins and 9.3 percent for the offspring of the clinically normal co-twins. The bottom line: elevated risk for bipolar disorder appears to be determined by the *genetic* rather than the social connection to a person with bipolar disorder.

Adoption Research   The results of the first adoption study of bipolar disorder (Mendlewicz & Rainer, 1977; Mendlewicz, 1981) are roughly consistent with those of family and twin studies. The investigators looked at the rates of bipolar and unipolar affective disorder in the biological and adoptive parents of bipolars, the biological and adoptive parents of normals, and the biological parents of polio victims. (The polio group was used to assess the rate of affective disorder associated with rearing a problematic child.) Table 14.1 shows that the risk for affective disorder is greater for the biological parents of bipolars than for any of the control groups.

In a more recent adoption study, Wender et al. (1986) found markedly higher rates of unipolar disorder, alcoholism, and suicide in the biological rel-

TABLE 14.1   AFFECTIVE DISORDER IN PARENTS OF BIPOLAR ADOPTEES VERSUS CONTROLS

	Bipolar adoptees		Bipolar nonadoptees	Normal adoptees		Polio nonadoptees
	Biol par. (N = 57)	Adopt par. (N = 57)	Biol par. (N = 61)	Biol par. (N = 43)	Adopt par. (N = 42)	Biol par. (N = 40)
Parents with affective disorder, %*	28	12	21	2	7	10

*Figures are percentages rounded off to the nearest whole number.
Source: Abridged from Mendlewicz & Rainer, 1977. (Reprinted by permission from *Nature,* Vol. 268, pp. 327–329. Copyright © 1977 Macmillan Magazines Ltd.)

atives of adoptees with major affective disorder than in the biological relatives of nonpsychiatric control adoptees. The rates of unipolar disorder, alcoholism, and suicide in the *adoptive* relatives of the two groups of adoptees were low and comparable to each other.

Genetic Markers for Bipolar Disorder   Behavior-genetic evidence thus far discussed tells us only that a genetic factor probably exists for some affective disorders. Recent groundbreaking research has dramatically increased our ability to be more precise about the location of genetic abnormalities in affective disorder. In some families genes for bipolar disorder and genes for other traits seem to exist close together on the same chromosome. This genetic linkage can be inferred from a nonrandom association between the disorder and an established genetic trait such as color blindness or some other genetic marker. To appreciate this, we need to understand that genes that are physically close to each other on a chromosome tend to be inherited together. Let us spell this out more clearly for families with numerous instances of bipolar disorder and another genetic trait.

Two types of nonrandom relationship between the traits can exist: an associative or a dissociative type. In families in which the *associative* relationship is evident, the two abnormal traits reliably co-occur or both absent —for example, the bipolar relatives in these families tend to be the ones with color blindness while the psychiatrically normal relatives tend not to have color blindness. In families in which the *dissociative* relationship is evident, the abnormal traits reliably do not co-occur; that is, an individual displaying one typically does not display the other. In our example, then, the bipolars of these families tend not to have color blindness, while the psychiatrically normal relatives do tend to have color blindness.

The essential point is that we can infer genetic linkage if relatives who are alike for one trait (two bipolars, for example) are also predictably alike on the other trait (both have, or do not have, color blindness). Of course, the close proximity of genes along a chromosome suggesting a linkage implies nothing necessarily about a causal relationship between the respective traits. Rather, linkage studies are important in developing a better model of the genetics of bipolar disorder.

Consider two research findings suggesting genetic linkage between manic depression and either of two traits, depending on the family. The first comes from a study of bipolar disorder in families of Israeli Jews of non-European descent (Baron et al., 1987). The study of pairs of family members revealed a genetic linkage between the presence or absence of bipolar disorder and the presence or absence of color blindness, an abnormality caused by a gene on the X chromosome. This linkage is illustrated by the pedigree shown in Figure 7.6*d* (see p. 183).

A second study, in this case of family members of the Old Amish community, isolated an unusual genetic fragment on chromosome 11, using restriction fragment length polymorphisms (see Chapter 7, pp. 195–196). The investigators showed a linkage between the presence or absence of the fragment and the presence or absence of bipolar disorder (Egeland et al., 1987).

The inferred genetic abnormalities on chromosome 11 and on the X chromosome are completely independent of each other, implying at least two genetic sources of bipolar disorder. It is possible that both abnormalities will be found to affect different steps along the same biochemical pathway, or that each abnormality affects a different biochemical pathway. In any case, not all bipolar disorders can be explained by linkage with a color blindness gene on the X chromosome and a specific DNA sequence on chromosome 11 (Hodgkinson et al., 1987; Detera-Wadleigh et al., 1987). This means that the search for other genetic and nongenetic causes for bipolar disorder must continue while investigators pursue the question of how the two identified genetic locations produce their results.

One hopes that it soon will be possible to close in on the specific biological processes that are altered by these genes. For example, it is probably significant that the defective gene on chromosome 11 is very near or identical to a gene that codes for tyrosine hydroxylase, an enzyme that is important in the synthesis of dopamine and norepinephrine. These neurotransmitters already figure prominently in theorizing about the biochemistry of schizophrenia (the dopamine hypothesis—see Chapter 12) and major depression (the bioamine hypothesis—see Chapter 13).

From follow-ups of Amish with the genetic defect on chromosome 11, we know that only about 63 percent will actually express a bipolar disorder. This means that other genetic or environmental factors also contribute to its expression. It will be important to identify these other factors in future work, as they may contribute significantly to prevention and treatment.

The behavior-genetic evidence on full-syndrome affective disorder strongly supports the age-old hypothesis of a highly heritable manic-depressive disease that can manifest itself in bipolar and even unipolar syndromes. Moreover, there is increasing evidence that certain less severe "subsyndromes" are alternative expressions of the manic-depressive disease.

Manic-Depressive Subsyndromes

Subsyndromes are, in some ways, behaviorally milder versions of full-syndrome manic or depressive episodes. Three affective subsyndromes have been identified: the *dysthymic* (depressive), the *hypomanic*, and the *cyclothymic* (bipolar). To illustrate, consider the following cyclothymic pattern.

A 29-year-old car salesman . . . was reluctant to admit that he might be a "moody" person. According to him, since the age of 14 he has experienced repeated alternating cycles that he terms "good times and bad times." During a "bad" period, usually lasting four to seven days, he oversleeps 10–14 hours daily, lacks energy, confidence, and motivation—"just vegetating," as he puts it. Often he abruptly shifts, characteristically upon waking up in the morning, to a three-to-four-day stretch of overconfidence, heightened social awareness, promiscuity, and sharpened think-ing—"things would flash in my mind." At such times he indulges in alcohol to en-hance the experience, but also to help him sleep. Occasionally the "good" periods last seven to ten days, but culminate in irritable and hostile outbursts, which often herald the transition back to another period of "bad" days. He admits to frequent use of marijuana, which he claims helps him "adjust" to daily routines. In school, A's and B's alternated with C's and D's, with the result that the patient was con-sidered a bright student whose performance was mediocre overall because of "un-stable motivation." As a car salesman his performance has also been uneven, with "good days" canceling out the "bad days"; yet even during his "good days" he is sometimes perilously argumentative with customers and loses sales that appeared sure. Although considered a charming man in many social circles, he alienates friends when he is hostile and irritable. He typically accumulates social obligations during the "bad" days and takes care of them all at once on the first day of a "good" period (Spitzer et al., 1981, pp. 31–32).

In terms of number of symptoms, subsyndromes may seem less severe than full syndromes; however, in other ways—including chronicity and co-occurring personality disorder—subsyndromes may be at least as severe as full-syndrome disorders (Kocsis & Frances, 1987). Dysthymic disorder, for ex-ample, usually involves low energy, poor self-esteem, work inefficiency, inap-propriate guilt, pessimism, and other dysfunctional qualities. Moreover, like other subsyndromes, dysthymic disorder is frequently associated with one or more Axis I or II disorders, and the combination may constitute an especially severe problem.

Consider, for example, "double depression": a major depression arising out of chronic dysthymic disorder. Compared with patients with major depression, patients with double depression are typically more severely depressed, more often melancholic, and more suicidal; in addition, they have more personality disorder, are subject to more social stress (including isolation and conflict), have a poorer prognosis, and have more relatives with unipolar and bipolar disorders severe enough to warrant hospitalization (Klein, Taylor, Harding, & Dickstein, 1988). These observations suggest that at least some dysthymic dis-orders—especially early onset, chronic dysthymic disorder with episodes of major (full-syndrome) depression—are expressions of a severe affective disor-der, often the manic-depressive type.

There is increasing evidence that cyclothymic and hypomanic, like some dysthymic, disorders are expressions of manic-depressive disease (Akiskal et al., 1977; Akiskal et al., 1985; Klein, Depue, & Slater, 1985). This evidence can be boiled down to the following six points.

1 The behavioral qualities of subsyndromal disorders like cyclothymia (Table 14.2) are similar to those of full syndromes.

2 A shift from normal to hypomanic or manic states (Figure 14.1) can be elicited in cyclothymics by drugs used in the treatment of bipolar depression.

3 Cyclothymics have increased risk for eventually developing a full-syndrome bipolar disorder.

TABLE 14.2 DIAGNOSTIC CRITERIA FOR CYCLOTHYMIA

A. For at least two years (one year for children and adolescents), presence of numerous hypomanic episodes [all of the criteria for a manic episode (see Table 13.2, p. 359), except criterion C, that indicate marked impairment] and numerous periods with depressed mood or loss of interest or pleasure that did not meet criterion A of a major depressive episode.

B. During a two-year period (one year in children and adolescents) of the disturbance, never without hypomanic or depressive symptoms for more than two months at a time.

C. No clear evidence of a major depressive episode or manic episode during the first two years of the disturbance (or one year in children and adolescents).

D. Not superimposed on a chronic psychotic disorder, such as schizophrenia or delusional disorder.

E. No organic factor, such as repeated intoxication from drugs or alcohol, known to have initiated and maintained the disturbance.

Source: Abridged from American Psychiatric Association, 1987, pp. 227–228. Reprinted with permission from the *Diagnostic and Statistical Manual of Mental Disorders, Third Edition, Revised.* Copyright © 1987 American Psychiatric Association.

4 A cyclothymic parent sometimes provides the only genetic "link" between a bipolar grandparent and a bipolar child, as can be seen in Figure 14.2.

5 The relatives of full-syndrome patients have increased risk for subsyndromal disorder, while relatives of subsyndromal disorder have increased risk for full-syndrome disorder.

6 The risk for full-syndrome bipolar disorder may be as elevated in the relatives of cyclothymics as in the relatives of full-syndrome bipolars.

Just as the rates of bipolar depression and the cyclothymic subsyndrome are elevated in the offspring of bipolar patients, the rates for unipolar major depression and the dysthymic subsyndrome are elevated in the offspring of patients with unipolar major depression (Klein, Clark, Dansky, & Margolis, 1988). Together with the twin and adoption data described earlier, this evidence points to the heritability of affective psychopathology, whether expressed in major or subsyndromal form. Nevertheless, patients with affective

FIGURE 14.1 Affective shifts in a hypothetical individual subject to bipolar disorder (Adapted from Depue et al., 1981, p. 386. Copyright 1981 by the American Psychological Assocation. Reprinted by permission.)

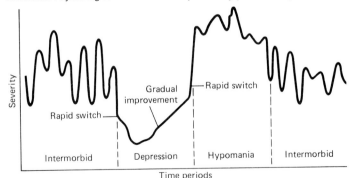

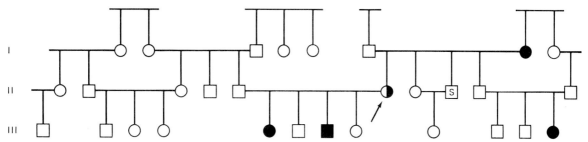

FIGURE 14.2   The cyclothymic patient indicated by the arrow appears to be a "genetic link" in this three-generational pedigree reflecting manic-depressive illness. The Roman numerals to the left indicate generations; black squares and black circles equal manic-depressive male and female relatives, respectively; white squares and white circles equal unaffected relatives; S equals completed suicide (male); and half white and half black circle equals cyclothymic index case. (Akiskal et al., 1977, p. 1231. *American Journal of Psychiatry, 134,* 1227–1233. Copyright © 1977, The American Psychiatric Association. Reprinted by permission.)

disorder often report being adversely influenced by recent negative events, especially during the month immediately prior to the onset of an episode of major depression (Bebbington, Brugha, MacCarthy et al., 1988). This suggests that even highly heritable depressions may not occur "out of the blue." Often they seem to be "reactive"; that is, precipitated by adverse, or even relatively innocuous, external events. In short, a reactive depression can involve any of the psychopathological and ecopathological factors discussed in this chapter.

MEDICAL AND PSYCHOPATHOLOGICAL FACTORS

We have seen that some depressions involve a specific affective pathology; the clearest example is manic-depresssive disease. Others, which we discuss next, appear to be by-products of medical disease or psychological disorders not conventionally classified as "affective." Still others, discussed later in the chapter, may be the by-products of cognitive traits—low self-confidence, for example—that, while not necessarily psychopathological, can interact with adversity to produce pathological depression.

Depressions Associated with Medical Disease or Other Physiological Factors

Major depressive disorders can occur in the context of neurological and somatic diseases, and also with the natural process of aging. We will briefly give a small sample of illustrative examples.

Neurological Disease   Damage to certain areas of the brain can produce affective symptoms and, in some cases, a syndrome that meets *DSM-III-R* criteria for major depression (or even mania). For example, left-hemisphere damage, especially toward the frontmost part (anterior pole), can produce a severe depression (Lipsey et al., 1983). Subcortical damage can also produce affective disorder; for example, damage to the basal ganglia can produce either depression or mania, the latter especially in people at risk by virtue of having relatives with affective disorder (Robinson et al., 1988).

Exactly how and why specifiable brain damage produces affective disorder is uncertain, although at least two possibilities have been raised. One possibility is that the neural mechanisms of affect are more easily activated, perhaps because they are "released" by damage to inhibitory mechanisms. In other words, the brain damage has made the person more sensitive and emotionally reactive. Another possibility is that the spared parts of the brain may enable the patient to recognize the loss of a subjectively important function. For example, patients with Broca's aphasia (anterior left damage) are more likely to develop severe depression than patients with Wernicke's aphasia (posterior left damage). Perhaps this difference lies in the fact that in Broca's aphasia, the posterior temporal and parietal cortex responsible for comprehension is spared; this sparing enables the patient to appreciate the sudden loss of subjectively important left frontal functions such as those related to a coherent and enduring sense of self, or personal identity (Dimond, 1980).

In sum, depressions associated with brain damage may express a damaged affective mechanism per se, while others may represent a normal depressive mechanism mobilized in an objectively depressing situation involving the sudden loss of subjectively important functions.

Endocrine Disorder   Affective disorders also may be by-products of endocrine abnormalities. In Cushing's syndrome, for example, hypersecretion of adrenal corticotrophic hormone (ACTH) by a *dysfunctional pituitary* gland causes hypersecretion of cortisol by the adrenal gland. [This contrasts with bipolar and unipolar depressions, where hypersecretion of cortisol results from the hypersecretion of corticotropin-releasing hormone (CRH) by a *dysfunctional hypothalamus*—see Chapter 13.] Cushing's syndrome is associated with weight gain, rounding of the face ("moon face"), acne, and loss of menstruation. In addition, the syndrome often includes depressions of varying severity in up to 40 percent of the patients (Jefferson & Marshall, 1981). These depressions are in many ways similar to major depressions—depressed mood, fatigue, impaired memory, decreased libido—although there are some differences, such as feeling better in the morning than later in the day (Starkman, 1988). Cushing's syndrome is a good example of a medical disease that can produce psychological symptoms that are in some ways indistinguishable from those of so-called functional disorders.

Depressive syndromes are associated with the premenstrual phase of the menstrual cycle in up to 30 percent of women (Dan, 1980; Golub, 1980; Jefferson & Marshall, 1981). The most common symptoms include pain, water retention, inability to concentrate, depression, anxiety, and irritability. An increase in various appetites including food, drink, sex, and sleep may also occur, making the syndrome "atypical" because, as we saw in Chapter 13, typical unipolar depressions are usually associated with decreases in these appetites. Figure 14.3 shows depression ratings that illustrate a correlation between menstrual and depression cycles (Halbreich, Endicott, & Nee, 1983).

A few points are worth noting about depressions associated with the menstrual syndrome. First, in *rare* instances, menstrual cycle–dependent depressions may be severe enough to include psychotic disorganization. Second, the cause of the depression probably involves a shift in the estrogen/progesterone balance and possibly other endocrine factors. One bit of evidence for this is that when the cyclic release of ovarian hormones is blocked by hormonal drug treatment, both the psychological and physical symptoms of the syndrome disappear (Muse et al., 1984). Third, researchers are currently exploring the possibility that similar hormonal factors explain postpartum depression, that is, depression in women who have just given birth (Susman & Katz, 1988). Interestingly, women with a liability to major affective disorder may be especially prone either to premenstrual syndrome or to postpartum depression (McClure, Reich, & Wetzel, 1971).

Aging Depression is frequently associated with aging (Eisdorfer, Cohen, & Kechich, 1981). Depression in the elderly could represent any of the following complex changes: (a) a lowered threshold for expressing a preexisting depressive liability, (b) diminished endocrine, metabolic, and/or brain functions that interfere with the capacity for pleasure (secondary depression), (c) the effect of prescribed medications (that is, physician-caused, or *iatrogenic* depression), and (d) a conscious reaction to diminished capacities with a consequent reduction in self-esteem (situational depression). Depression in the aged is

FIGURE 14.3 Self-ratings of depression recorded in the morning (continuous line) and evening (dashed line) by a woman with menstrually related mood disorder. (From Rubinow et al., 1984, Figure 1. *American Journal of Psychiatry, 141,* 684–686. Copyright © 1984, The American Psychiatric Association. Reprinted by permission.)

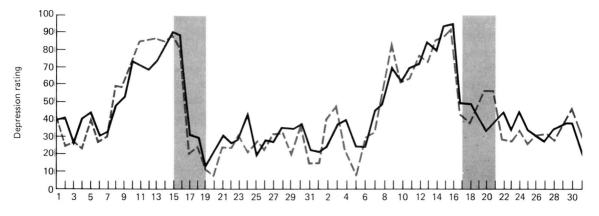

thus a good example of the many possible, and possibly interacting, causes of depression.

Depressions Secondary to Psychopathology

Depression is frequently associated with anxiety, hysterical, and personality disorders (Pilkonis & Frank, 1988). Such depressions are usually subsyndromal and nonpsychotic; the classical physiological symptoms of major depression as described in Chapter 13 tend not to occur, or they occur in an atypical form: the patient feels worse in the evening rather than in the morning and tends to overeat rather than lose appetite.

Depression and Personality Disorders Depression frequently accompanies those personality disorders that display what many clinicians call "neurotic" traits: anxiety, dependency, defensiveness, immaturity, sensitivity, and emotional instability (Gunderson & Elliot, 1985; von Zerssen, 1982). The following vignette illustrates the mixture of personality and emotional disturbances in a depression marked by anxiety and irritability.

> Ernest F. was a thirty-year-old married bus driver, the father of two small children. Chief among his complaints were the following. He felt tired, discouraged and unfit for work all the time. He slept badly and spent part of each night roaming around the house downstairs. His legs and ankles ached. He had backaches, especially at work. His head ached and his eyes smarted; sometimes while driving the bus everything would blur. He had no appetite, he was constipated, sex desire was infrequent, and part of the time he was impotent. He took no pleasure in anything any more.
>
> What worried Ernest most was his incompetence on the job. He had always been a dependable, steady worker who prided himself on leaving and coming back from each bus trip on the dot. Now he was having difficulty in remembering the schedules. Whenever he was shifted to a different route he would skip some of the stops. Once, to the passengers' consternation, he went the wrong way. He was now growing irritable with passengers and with vehicles that blocked his way. He made angry jerking stops and starts. To the passengers' protests he gave angry retorts. They reported him to the company. At home Ernest felt lonely, irritable and aloof. He lost his temper with his children and quarreled with his wife. Each time this happened he hated himself for it and called himself all kinds of humiliating things. He was a no-good, run-down bum, he said, and a failure in life. (From Norman Cameron, *Personality Development and Psychopathology: A Dynamic Approach*, pp. 419–420. Copyright © 1963 by Houghton Mifflin Company. Used with permission.)

The clinical picture of any depression depends on preexisting personality patterns. For example, depressions associated with histrionic and borderline personality patterns have a flamboyant and self-destructive quality. A particularly severe example is sometimes called *hysteroid dysphoria* (Liebowitz & Klein, 1979). Its central features are extreme intolerance of rejection coupled with depression expressed in overeating, craving sweets, oversleeping, and self-destructive behavior including threats and even half-hearted attempts to commit suicide, all designed to express anger and elicit attention and gain support. Patients with this reactive disorder—the term reactive indicating an excessive and hair-trigger, rather than normal, response to an adverse condition—are attention junkies who pursue romantic attachments with reckless abandon. They become intoxicated with affection, provoke rejection, and react with a depressive crash before streaking ahead toward fresh engagements.

Depressions associated with inhibited, overconscientious, and overcontrolled personality patterns are quite different, tending to be relatively mild and persistent. Nevertheless, these unobtrusive depressions can deepen with age until they reach major (full syndromal) proportions. Both clinical impression (Chodoff, 1974) and empirical evidence (von Zerssen, 1982) suggest that late-onset unipolar depression in females, the so-called involutional melancholia of menopause, often arises out of the quiet desperation of the inhibited personality style. To understand what "arise out of" means, let us consider some follow-up data on the kinds of depressions we have just discussed

What Is a Neurotic Depression?   The label neurotic has traditionally been applied to relatively minor, nonpsychotic, highly reactive depressions that are associated with anxiety, sensitivity, and inner conflict and with inhibited or socially disruptive behaviors like those we described earlier (Gersh & Fowles, 1979). Akiskal et al. (1978) followed up 100 such patients over a three- to four-year period. At follow-up, 40 percent of them had developed a major affective disorder, 18 percent bipolar and 22 percent unipolar. The investigators therefore concluded that the term neurotic depression will be misleading to the extent that it misidentifies people as neurotic when they have either an affective subsyndrome or are at an early neurotic stage in a developing major affective disorder.

The neurotic behavior of neurotic depression can be thought of as a cause or an effect. First, consider it as a *cause*. The neurotic behavior of a sensitive and emotional person increases the liability to depression. For example, reactive depressions often occur when such a person becomes acutely aware of the self-destructive and socially disruptive consequences of his maladaptive behavior. Moreover, the repetition of such experiences may lead to a decline in self-esteem, an increase in negative expectations about prospects, and consequently an even further increase in liability to depression.

Neurotic behavior can also be an *effect*—in particular, a defense against the liability to depression. For example, compulsive, hypochondriacal, or seductive behavior can deflect attention from depressing thoughts or depressed mood, perhaps delaying the onset of even a genetically influenced affective disorder. The depression that finally occurs could represent, among other things, a breakdown of defensive coping.

COGNITIVE AND SITUATIONAL FACTORS

Our discussion of the causes of major affective disorder has focused on clearly pathophysiological and psychopathological factors such as (1) manic-depressive heritability, (2) medical disease, and (3) psychological disorders. We now shift our focus to two broad classes of factors which figure importantly in many theories of depression: (1) adverse external conditions involving loss or failure and (2) cognitive factors, or negative patterns of thinking regarding, for example, one's guilt, incompetence, or unfortunate prospects. Before proceeding, however, we should point out a couple of things about such cognitive and situational factors.

First, while cognitive factors are clearly important features of depression, there is some debate as to their causal significance. For example, is negative self-concept a cause rather than an effect of depression, and if such negative patterns of thinking are causal, how do they develop? Second, while it is normal for truly depressing events such as personal loss to cause depression—indeed, it would be abnormal for depression *not* to occur—do such external factors play a role in *pathological* depressions as well? For example, could the *cumulative learning effect* on personality development of depressing experiences with maternal loss, rejection, or personal failure produce a depressive psychopathology? This could explain depressive reactions to minor or even innocuous events. To get a better idea about the role of cognition and situations, we will explore the depressions associated with separation and helplessness.

Separation, Psychopathology, and Depression

Maternal Loss   Maternal loss or separation, especially during infancy, can produce similar depressive reactions in infant animals and humans (McKinney & Bunney, 1969; Mineka & Suomi, 1978; Spitz, 1945). The reaction is typically biphasic, with the initial "protest" phase including anxious vocalization, and the later "despair" phase including self-clinging and huddling (Bowlby, 1969; Bowlby, 1980). These situation-specific reactions are normally often reversible with the reappearance of the primary caretaker, but the ambivalent and hostile behaviors that are sometimes directed at the caretaker may not dissipate for weeks or even months.

We should consider three basic questions about acute separation reactions in infancy. First, do they constitute a good *behavioral model* of adult depression? The protest phase does resemble some aspects of agitated depression, and the despair phase does resemble certain features of retarded depression. Also, antidepressive medication is effective in treating or preventing separation depression in infant monkeys (Suomi et al., 1981). If the infant's reaction is behaviorally similar to the adult's reaction, then environmental factors that are known to cause the former can more confidently be hypothesized for the latter. If, in the case of adult depressions, careful observation fails to disclose such events in the current external environment, we may suspect cognitive and/or physiological factors. The cognitive factor might be a disposition to magnify or even invent a depressing scenario; that is, a tendency of certain personality disorders to make depressing "mountains" out of situational "molehills." The physiological factor, on the other hand, might be some sort of neurological abnormality—a manic-depressive mechanism, perhaps—which, quite apart from cognitive style, activates instinctive mechanisms of depressive behavior even in the absence of significant external provocation.

Second, do *individual differences* in the infant's response to maternal separation reflect differences in preexisting vulnerability? Research has indicated that some species of monkey are especially reactive—for example, rhesus and pigtail macaques—while other species seem relatively invulnerable—for example, bonnet macaques (McKinney & Moran, 1982). Likewise, only a small percentage (less than 15 percent) of human infants have been observed to display major depressive reactions to maternal separation (Spitz, 1945). Many investigators believe that age, sex, and social support or disruption interact in a complex fashion with individual differences in resiliency or vulnerability (Rutter & Garmezy, 1983). But where do these individual differences come from—inheritance, prior conditioning, or both—and how important are they in explaining the risk for and severity of the reactions? We still do not know.

Finally, what are the *lasting effects* of early maternal separation? Lasting effects of early maternal loss have typically been investigated by comparing psychiatric and control samples. For example, one study found relatively higher rates of maternal loss prior to age 11 in a community sample of depressed women compared with matched nondepressive controls; maternal loss after age 11 was not associated with depression (Brown, Harris, & Copeland, 1977). One interpretation of the data is that early maternal loss adversely affects the development of self-esteem in particular, thereby increasing the vulnerability to adult reactive depressions (Brown, 1979). If there is any truth to this speculation, it probably describes only a minority of patients, because most of the research finds, overall, a weak or zero correlation between early parental loss and depressive disorder (Crook & Eliot, 1980; Roy, 1985; Tennant et al., 1981).

The reason for this weak overall correlation is that long-term effects of maternal separation may be minimal, negative, or even positive depending on how separation is defined and the social context within which it occurs (Tennant, 1988). Maternal loss from nonsuicidal death seems generally unrelated to the child's risk for depression in adulthood, undoubtedly because adequate substitute caretaking and continuity of other positive social arrangements are generally the rule (Rutter & Garmezy, 1983). On the other hand, maternal loss due to physical separations and/or maternal psychopathology, family discord, or divorce can have negative or positive long-term effects. The effects may be negative—for example, persistently neglectful and abusive childhood environments are often reported by patients with "neurotic depressions" (McKinney, Suomi, & Harlow, 1971). However, the long-term effects may be positive if postloss social arrangements become more loving and supportive (Tennant, 1988).

It is important to understand that the long-term effects we have been discussing are inferred mostly from correlational evidence. However, the causal significance of a correlation is often ambiguous, and this is true for correlations between measures of childhood maternal loss and adult-offspring psychopathology. Such correlations may indeed reflect the social influence of a parent's behavior on the offspring's development. On the other hand, they may reflect the largely *independent expression* of a possibly common psychopathology in parent and offspring. For example, maternal loss due to death by suicide may be correlated with adult offspring depression because both mother and offspring share a heritable affective disorder; likewise, maternal absence due to parental conflict may be correlated with depression and personality disorder in the adult offspring because of a shared underlying psychopathology.

Adoption studies could yield estimates of the degree to which parent-offspring correlations represent parent-to-child causality or the independent expression of underlying psychopathology. Unfortunately we typically have only group-comparison studies—of the childhood experiences of depressives versus nondepressives, for example—and these studies yield correlations whose causal significance remains theoretically ambiguous.

Bereavement (Mourning)   Situational depression in adulthood is common following a personal loss (Clayton, 1982). Clinical observation suggests that bereavement often evolves through two general phases. The initial phase of psychological "numbness" is marked by dazed and automatic behavior suggesting a partial interruption of attention and consciousness. After days or weeks, a "recoil" phase begins, and may last weeks or months before dissolving. Recoil is a mixture of protest, yearning, and despair. The *protest* component of recoil includes irritability, restlessness, and sometimes panic. The *yearning* component involves painful preoccupations sometimes even to the point of hallucinating the loved one's face or voice. The *despair* component of recoil includes aimless, disorganized, and apathetic behavior. Although protest and yearning are more akin to anxiety, despair seems a purer form of depression. While protest and yearning represent the *struggle against helplessness,* despair represents acceptance of helplessness, a resignation to defeat and an affective giving up (hopelessness.)

Normally, bereavement rarely lasts for over a year, and rarely includes the psychomotor retardation, suicidal behavior, morbid guilt, and physiological abnormalities that are typical of pathological depression. Only 2 to 3 percent of bereaved persons require hospitalization, and these patients often show evidence of pathological vulnerability: prior depressive disorder, family history of depressive disorder, chronic low self-esteem, poor social supports (estrangement from relatives, for example), and excessive demands at home or at work. Thus, in abnormal grief reactions, personal loss seems to interact with affective vulnerability or other psychopathology.

Speculation about Separation Depression   We are affectively attached to individuals and groups, in part because these attachments provide experiences that reinforce our sense of well-being. Personal loss represents disruption of these relationships. That depression is an instinctive reaction to separation from people is most clearly evident in the reactions of individuals with the deepest attachments—infants and highly dependent adults, for example—who have the most to lose and therefore are at greatest risk.

Normally, self-esteem and mood are influenced by the quality and reliability of supportive connections to people—parents, offspring, friends, and colleagues, for example—and to ideas—about cultural norms, resources, opportunities, and reciprocal obligations, to name a few (Osterweis, Solomon, & Green, 1984). Separation depression represents a disruption of such vitally important relationships. It may have an *instrumental* aspect involving an instinctive cry for help that can enlist aid and comfort (Becker, 1973). This instrumental aspect may have neurotic overtones in cases where the cry for help is used to manipulate others—for example, to gain attention and favors. Separation depression may also have an *aggressive* aspect, permitting the depressed person to express anger at the lost love object (Bowlby, 1980). In short, the instrumental and aggressive aspects of separation depression represent a kind of coping, an emotional struggle against slipping from a state of uncertainty regarding interpersonal attachments—from which recovery is at least psychologically possible—to a state of hopelessness—from which recovery seems impossible.

Helplessness, Psychopathology, and Depression

The sense of well-being is sustained by the recognition, not only that one is loved, but also that one is capable of mastering the environment (White, 1963). The prolonged frustration of *competence* motivation can produce a chronic sense of not being in control that, in turn, can produce disinterest, withdrawal, and inactivity. We will now turn our attention to depression reactions in situations that frustrate competence motivation.

Uncontrollable Events   Depressed people complain of hopelessness, of being unable to control emotionally significant facts of life. A "learned helplessness" theory was originally developed to explain how exposure to uncontrollable adversity can explain some types of exogenous depression (Seligman, 1975). The theory evolved from experimental research on dogs utilizing a "triadic design" with three groups of animals. One group—the *escapable* (or controllable) group—is exposed to electric shocks which can be escaped by learning an effective response. Another group—the *inescapable* (uncontrollable) group—is yoked to the first group in the sense that it receives the same duration and number of shocks but has no way to escape them; in other words, there is no relationship between the yoked animal's behavior and the presence or absence of shock. A third, or *base-line control,* group is exposed to the same environment, but without shocks.

Compared with escapable and base-line control groups, the inescapable group typically shows a wide variety of abnormalities that resemble some of the symptoms of depression in humans. For example, after an initial period of agitation, many of the animals develop a motivational deficit; they become passive, withdrawn, less aggressive, and even lose their appetite for food and sex. More remarkably, they develop a cognitive deficit; they are unable to learn to avoid the shock even when conditions are changed so as to make shock-avoidance learning possible—even easy.

The triadic design has also been used in research with humans (Hiroto, 1974). A mild version of the helplessness manipulation exposes subjects to uncontrollable events such as aversive noise in a task that, unbeknownst to the subject, cannot be solved. Like rats and dogs, human subjects exposed to such conditions typically come to display a variety of performance deficits in the original, and even subsequent, tasks. These include deficits in learning to escape aversive but controllable stimulation (cognitive deficit), passivity and withdrawal (motivational deficit), and dysphoria or disinterest (affective deficit). In contrast, subjects in controllable or base-line conditions typically do not display these reactions.

These initial findings provided a basis for Seligman's theory of learned helplessness depression, or LHD. According to LHD theory (Seligman, 1975), expectations that one's actions no longer exert any control over events in one's life can produce a "helplessness depression" with the characteristics just described. Four problems with the application of LHD to humans were noted by Abramson et al. (1978). First, it didn't readily explain why a helplessness depression is short-lived or enduring. Second, it didn't explain why a helplessness depression might be cross-situational rather than situation-specific. Third, the theory was silent with respect to low self-esteem, a hallmark of depression. And finally, the theory didn't explain why in some cases, depression *doesn't* occur in situations involving uncontrollability. To accommodate these problems, Abramson et al. offered a revision of LHD which gave special emphasis to certain kinds of cognitions.

Revised Learned Helplessness Theory   According to the revised theory, helplessness depressions are the products of three kinds of *attributions,* or interpretations, of stressful events. An *internal* attribution locates the cause of the events within the self ("It's my fault") with the effect of lowering self-esteem; in contrast, an external attribution ("This task is unfair") would protect self-esteem so that depression might be less likely. A *stable* attribution ("Failure has happened to me before and is likely to recur") represents the element of hopelessness that explains the persistence of a depressive reaction; in contrast, an unstable attribution ("I was in a bad mood") would tend to shorten the duration of any depression. Finally, a *global* attribution ("This kind of failure seems to occur in many situations") would explain why a depression might generalize to other situations that are objectively different from one another; in contrast, a specific attribution ("I do poorly in math") would tend to make any depression situation-specific.

Critics of LHD theory have raised many interesting questions about the revised LHD theory (Costello, 1978; Snyder et al., 1981; Weiss et al., 1979). It is clear, for example, that depressed persons engage in the kinds of negative attributions described by revised LHD and other cognitive theories of depression (Beck, 1967; Raps et al., 1982; Sweeney, Anderson, & Bailey, 1986). After all, it is natural to seek or even invent explanations for deep feelings. LHD assumes, however, that the attributions we described earlier are more than just cognitive features, they are *causes* of depression. More precisely, they are assumed to be exaggerations of a premorbid cognitive style that increases the chance that depressing events will cause a depressive disorder. To date, critics of LHD argue, the evidence for this causal assumption is questionable.

Some of this evidence comes from prospective studies showing that measures of attributional style predict the onset and maintenance of depressive *mood* in response to subsequent negative life events (Metalsky et al., 1982; Metalsky et al., 1987). But, according to the critics, no study has yet shown convincingly that cognitive style predicts later depressive *disorder* (Brewin, 1985; Coyne & Gotlib, 1983). And even if a predictive relationship were established, it would not be conclusive evidence of causality because such a relationship is merely a correlation—specifically, a correlation between a measure of cognitive style at time 1 and a measure of clinical disorder at time 2.

Further evidence for the hypothesis that traitlike cognitions play a causal role in major depressions comes from studies that compare the cognitive style of former (so-called recovered) depressed patients and never-depressed controls. Some studies (Eaves & Rush, 1984) support the cognitive model—more helplessness attribution and negatively biased thinking in the former depressed patients suggesting a predisposition, or causally significant trait. Nevertheless, some studies find no such differences (Gotlib & Cane, 1987), suggesting that depressive cognition during remission is merely a residual symptom, in other words, that the person, though diagnostically in remission, is not yet fully recovered.

To appreciate this better, consider a frightening auto or plane accident. A posttraumatic reaction may occur with anxiety, vegetative changes (for example, disturbed sleep), and fearful thoughts. Even after the reaction subsides (remission), there is a good chance that, for a while at least, the person will tend to exaggerate the risk of accidents and the probability of being harmed. Yet this negative cognitive bias, clearly the *effect* of the experience, may have no causal significance in explaining the original reaction. Therefore, like posttraumatic reactions, remitted depressions may involve negative cognitive patterns that represent the lingering components or effects of a bad experience; but, in many cases, they need not signify predisposition. Of course, they may indeed indicate a predisposition in some cases and merely an effect in other cases. Unfortunately, available evidence allows no confident conclusions (Coyne & Gotlib, 1986).

In sum, causal assumptions of the cognitive model of depression are still being debated because they rest on evidence that is either supportive but somewhat indirect—predicted changes found for the mood of *nonpatients* rather than depressive disorders of patients—or direct but unreliable—former patients and controls sometimes do, but sometimes do not, differ in the predicted direction. On the other hand, it does seem safe to conclude that depressed mood has a profound effect on cognition.

First of all, negative cognitions, including helplessness attributions, are more evident as depressive mood deepens; the darker the mood, the more obsessional and delusional the cognitive symptoms. This is clearly evident in the highly heritable bipolar depressions where mood appears to be driving the cognitions rather than vice versa. In the second place, recovery from depressive disorder is associated with a corresponding decrease in depressive cognitions, often to normal levels, even when cognitive change is not the explicit goal of therapeutic efforts (Simons, Garfield, & Murphy, 1984). So, while cognition and affect can influence one another, and while cognitive symptoms are associated with affective disorder, the hypothesis that the cognitive traits specified by LDH can *produce* affective disorder remains an open question (Barnett & Gotlib, 1988).

Summary Comment

It would appear that the consequences of the loss of loved ones (separation) or the loss of control (helplessness) depend on personal strengths and weaknesses. Involuntary separations or uncontrollable calamities can make even normal individuals at least temporarily depressed. At the other extreme, highly dependent or sensitive individuals require little in the way of separation or failure, whether perceived or real, to become depressed.

What is the causal significance of adverse life events? First, their effect on depressive symptoms is generally small; perhaps 9 percent of the variation in symptom intensity is explainable by variation between normal and stressful life conditions (Grant et al., 1982). We suspect that this small overall relationship represents a negligible depressing influence of adverse events on most people and a relatively large influence of such events on a few others. Second, the impact of adverse events often depends on prior reactivity, suggesting that the events *release* the symptoms of a preexisting depressive vulnerability. As Winokur (1979) says about adverse events: "It is not that they are unimportant to the individual, but they are omnipresent and seem to be found in all kinds of depressions. . . . They should be evaluated on the basis of a lifelong propensity to respond, i.e., a reactive personality" (p. 145).

Consistent with this point about vulnerability is the third observation, namely, that most stresses turn out to be rather *mundane* (recall that broken shoelace example in Chapter 5, p. 134). And, as Paykel suggests, "it seems probable that in most cases these events are negotiated without illness so that some other factors must contribute to the development of depression" (Paykel, 1979, p. 257).

At the beginning of the last chapter we distinguished between highly prevalent depressive symptoms and less prevalent depressive disorders. Some depressions, perhaps insufficiently severe to warrant a *DSM* diagnosis, can nevertheless motivate people to seek help. These personally distressing experiences may reflect the joint effect of personal and environmental characteristics, *none of which alone* can be thought of as pathological. In other words, many mild depressions are neither psychopathological nor ecopathological but rather problems of living caused by person-environment conflicts.

For example, a woman with five children and a self-preoccupied husband may develop a depression; with two children and a supportive husband she might never have been troubled. A modestly competent man promoted to a position requiring much personal responsibility develops depression; in a less demanding job he too might never have been troubled. In both cases, we observe a *mismatch* between personal needs or competencies and environmental demands. It would seem that regardless of its validity for major depression, helplessness and other cognitive models apply nicely to the relatively mild depressions arising from such frustrating person-situation mismatches. In sum, many depressions are the products, not of affective disorder or traumatic events, but rather of mundane and often unpredictable circumstances interacting with relatively normal human vulnerabilities and need for support.

SUICIDE

As we will see, the data on suicide reinforce common sense that depression is a major causal factor. Many suicides occur in association with a diagnosable depressive disorder. Conversely, depressive disorder increases the risk of suicide. Therefore, liability to suicide is a major consideration in any discussion of affective disorder (Sainsbury, 1968; Juel-Nelson, 1979).

Epidemiology

Overview of Suicide versus Suicide Attempt   The annual incidence of suicide per 100,000 is roughly fifteen in the United States and United Kingdom, and ranges from twenty-five in Czechoslovakia to two in Mexico. Given a life expectancy of 75 years, assuming that young children do not commit suicide, the *lifetime risk* is roughly $15 \times 65 = 975$ per 100,000, or about one per 100 in the United States.

Suicide should be distinguished from suicide attempts and suicide threats. For example the male/female ratio for suicide attempts is roughly 1 to 3 but 2–3 to 1 for actual suicides. Also, the ratio of suicide attempts to actual suicide is roughly between 100 and 200 to 1 in high school populations, 10 to 1 in college populations, and 1 to 1 for those over 55 (Hendin, 1982). The difference appears to be a function of two things that develop with age: first, the older person is more committed to the act for its own sake than as a means of manipulating others, and second, the older person is more competent to plan and execute the act. Finally, the more lethal the attempt—the more likely death would have occurred had it not been for some fortunate accident like being discovered in time—the more likely a subsequent suicide will occur.

Major risk-enhancing factors for suicide are summarized in Table 14.3. The highest rates for the nonpsychiatric population are for elderly white males (see Figure 14.4), especially when divorced or widowed, or disabled by disease. The highest rates in the psychiatric population are for those with a personal or family history of depressive disorder, followed by those with alcoholism. There is less agreement about the significance of other psychiatric disorders, including schizophrenia, anxiety, and antisocial personality (Miles, 1977, as against Robins, 1981). Also, there is evidence that young adults between 15 and 24 have had, in recent years, the highest *increase* in rates of suicide (Shneidman, 1985) as well as remarkably high rates—between 5 and 10 percent—of self-reported suicide attempts (Schwartz & Wirtz, 1988).

Psychiatric Disorder The 1 percent figure for lifetime risk of suicide in the general population is a conservative estimate because many suicides are unintentionally misidentified or intentionally mislabeled, for example, as accidents. Nevertheless, the estimate can be compared with the 16 percent rate for patients with major depressive disorder (Sainsbury, 1968). This estimate is, in all

TABLE 14.3   RISK-ENHANCING FACTORS IN PREDICTING SUICIDE

Risk-enhancing factor	Description
Sex	Male rates are always higher. On the average, the M:F ratio is roughly 2:1, reduced from 4:1 about thirty years ago, and compared to a 1:3 ratio of suicide *attempts*.
Race	Whites have a higher rate than blacks, though the rate for blacks has doubled in recent years.
Age	The elderly have the highest rates, with male rates climbing throughout the life cycle vs. female rates which peak between 40 and 60 years and then decline (see Figure 14.4).
Living conditions	Family strife increases the risk.
Physical condition	Physical infirmity or disability increases the risk.
Personal loss or failure	In males, loss of a job or any significant downward mobility in socioeconomic status is paramount. In females, loss of, or failure to attain, a personally significant relationship with a lover, spouse, or friend is of greater significance.
Bereavement or isolation	Divorced or separated males have an especially high rate (roughly 69 per 100,000); the rate for females is much lower (about 18). Lack of community affiliation (church or social groups) or interests (hobbies) increases the risk even further.
Time of year	Risks are greatest during the springtime, especially in April.
Behavioral factors	History of alcohol abuse, previous suicide attempts, or a note or other communication of intent is a significant risk-enhancing factor.
Psychiatric diagnosis	Personal or family history of depressive disorder or suicide is a major indicator. Alcoholism is another major risk factor.

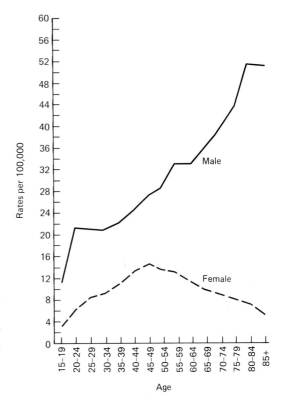

FIGURE 14.4 Male and female suicide rate per 100,000 in the U.S. white population, by sex, 1970 to 1974. (Source: National Center for Health Statistics, 1976) Nonwhite rates were similar to white female rates, except for an earlier peak (ages 25 to 34).

likelihood, also conservative because many people suffering with major depressive disorder will kill themselves before ever having been psychiatrically diagnosed. The results of a major study of 134 suicides reported in the St. Louis area (Robins, 1981) are summarized in Table 14.4. The study suggests that most suicides are associated with depression and alcoholism, but some may occur because of other disorders such as schizophrenia, or for rational reasons, such as a terminal illness.

Why do depression, alcoholism, and other psychiatric disorders increase the risk for suicide? One likely reason is that they, and especially depression, are associated with an enhanced sense of hopelessness about one's self and one's prospects. Consistent with this is evidence that measures of hopelessness are even better predictors of suicide than measures of depression. For example, Beck, Steer, Kovacs et al. (1985) obtained questionnaire estimates of depression, hopelessness, and suicidal thoughts for each of 207 people hospitalized because of an expressed desire to commit suicide. During the follow-up period of at least five years, fourteen subjects (7 percent) committed suicide. Compared with the nonsuicides, the fourteen suicides had earlier scored significantly higher only on the hopelessness scale, although their depression

TABLE 14.4 CHARACTERISTICS OF DEPRESSION-RELATED VS. ALCOHOLISM-RELATED SUICIDE

Characteristic	Depression-related	Alcoholism-related
Percentage of total sample of 134 suicides	47%	25%
Male:female ratio	Less than 3:1	Approx. 6:1
Mean age at suicide	Mid-50s	Mid-40s
Notes of intent	40%	60%
Interpersonal/social complications (loss of affectional relationships, or work, family, or legal problems)	Less frequent	More frequent
Intrapersonal problems (e.g., guilt, hopelessness)	More frequent	Less frequent
Physical problems (e.g., gastritis, nausea)	Less frequent	More frequent

Source: Adapted from Robins, 1981.

scores were somethat higher as well. These results suggest that the hopelessness component of depression, alcoholism, and other disorders is a major psychological reason for elevated risk of suicide.

Genetic Influence The liability to suicide appears to have a genetic basis (Schulsinger et al., 1979; Wender et al., 1986). Specifically, a markedly elevated risk for suicide occurs in the biological, but not adoptive, relatives of suicides and patients with affective disorder. Additional evidence suggests that the apparent heritability of suicide is, to a large extent, a function of the association between suicide and highly heritable depressive disorders. Earlier, we described evidence from research on Amish families that a genetic abnormality on chromosome 11 can account for some bipolar depressions (Egeland et al., 1987). These researchers have also provided evidence of a close association between depression and suicide.

The study considered *all* of the twenty-six documented suicides in the Old Amish community during the past 100 years (Egeland & Sussex, 1985). This traditional community is renowned for supportive, cohesive, and nonviolent qualities. Not surprisingly, the overall suicide rates are relatively low. However, 73 percent of all the suicides that did occur in this community came from just four extended families representing 16 percent of the total population, a finding clearly consistent with the evidence that genetic factors operate in suicide (see Figure 14.5). For more than 90 percent of the suicides, a diagnosis of psychopathology, mainly affective disorder, could be established.

Although psychopathology and heredity can explain why specific people commit suicide, these individual difference factors can be ameliorated or potentiated by general social factors related to migration, war, and economic conditions.

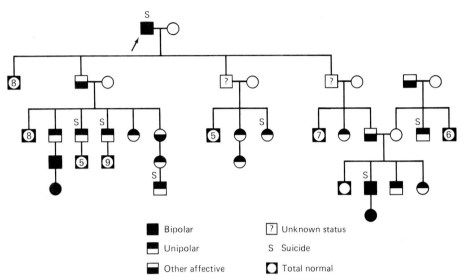

FIGURE 14.5 A pedigree illustrating the marked familiality of suicide in the Old Amish community. (Egeland & Sussex, 1985, p. 916. *Archives of General Psychiatry,* 1985, *254,* 915–918. Copyright © 1985, American Medical Association)

Migration and War Suicide rates of immigrants are two to four times greater than rates of those who remain behind. However, the rates of a particular group of immigrants can be predicted from the overall rates in the *original* country, and *not* from the overall rates in the new country (see Table 14.5). For example, Austrians have a higher rate than Mexicans, and Austrian immigrants have a higher rate than Mexican immigrants.

While migration is associated with increased risk for suicide, war is associated with decreased risk. During World War II, there was a greater percentage decrease for male suicide in belligerent countries than in neutral countries (Sainsbury, 1968). Perhaps the difference is related to an increased sense of community and purpose, less boredom, and more employment opportunities. War seems to strengthen attachments to love and work, an effect that is incompatible with suicide. Sainsbury suggested "that if psychiatrists do not know how to prevent . . . suicides . . . at least sociologists do; even if their remedy is to go to war" (1968, p. 5).

Durkheim About 100 years ago the sociologist Émile Durkheim (1858–1917) developed an ecopathological theory of suicide. It explained suicide as a function of migration, economic collapse, and other factors that undermine social supports and constraints that he believed are necessary for mental health. The result is deregulation and disorientation, a normless condition Durkheim called *anomie.* By anomie, he meant the liberation of impulsive tendencies from normal social controls.

TABLE 14.5 SUICIDE RATES IN 1959 OF FOREIGN-BORN U.S. CITIZENS FROM SELECTED COUNTRIES RELATED TO THE SUICIDE RATES OF THEIR COUNTRIES OF BIRTH

Country	*A* Suicide rate/ 100,000 of foreign-born in U.S. (1959)	*B* Suicide rate/ 100,000 of country of origin (1959)	Rank order of *A*	Rank order of *B*
Sweden	34	18	1	4
Austria	33	25	2	2
Czechoslovakia	32	25	3	1
Germany, Fed. Rep.	26	19	4	3
Poland	25	8	5	6
Norway	24	8	6	7
England and Wales	19	12	7	5
Italy	18	6	8	9
Canada	18	7	9	8
Ireland	10	3	10	10
Mexico	8	2	11	11

Source: Sainsbury, 1968, p. 2.

Appetites, not being controlled by a public opinion become disoriented, no longer recognize the limits proper to them. . . . With increased prosperity desires increase. At the very moment when traditional rules have lost their authority, the richer prize offered these appetites stimulates them. . . . The state of deregulation or anomie is thus further heightened by passions being less disciplined, precisely when they need more disciplining. Above all, since this race for an unattainable goal can give no other pleasure but that of the race itself . . . once it is interrupted the participants are left empty-handed. . . . How could the desire to live not be weakened under such conditions (Durkheim, 1897/1955, p. 390)?

Durkheim contrasted *anomic* suicide with *egoistic* suicide. Egoistic suicide represents the failure of society to enforce commitments to social activities. When individuals are prevented from joining social groups or contributing to social projects, they fail to develop psychological attachments to society. Egoistic suicide reflects a basic deficiency rather than a loss of social influence over people.

According to Durkheim, both loss (anomie) and deficiency (egoism) are rooted in *exogenous* social and economic circumstances. However, the rarity of suicide in the presence of high frequencies of social and economic stress and its strong association with familial depression suggest that Durkheim's sociological theory can account for only one aspect of suicide, namely, ecopathological conditions which interact with psychopathology. In short, a strictly sociological theory cannot account for the rarity and heritability of suicide. Rather, it seems to suggest that there are social and economic events which might lower the threshold to the suicidal expression of depressive as well as other types of psychopathology.

Psychology

Behavior and Motivation   Building on Durkheim's writings and clinical observations, Shneidman (1972) has described three types of suicide. *Dyadic* suicide involves the frustration of intense needs for contact with others. It is a mixture of disappointment, hostility, longing, and despair, the typical pattern of dependent, immature, and sensitive people. The psychoanalytic theory of depression as anger toward a lost love turned toward the self suggests that a dyadic suicide is "murder in the 180th degree" (Shneidman, 1985, p. 34).

> Most suicide notes are dyadic in their nature. Suicide notes, usually prefaced by the word, "Dear," are typically addressed to a specific person, an ambivalently loved love-one. (A prototypical example: "Dear Mary: I hate you. Love, George."). . . . The victim's best eggs are in the other person's flawed basket (Shneidman, 1972, p. 17).

In contrast, *egotic* suicide is essentially intrapsychic, the outcome of a highly intellectual process arrived at through an inner debate uninfluenced by situational events. In psychotic individuals, for example, egotic suicide can have delusional, nihilistic, and irrational qualities.

The final type, called *agenerative,* refers to suicide primarily in older persons who gradually become disaffected and detached from society and self. It is a social psychological failure resulting from a diminution of social supports and inner resources.

> Ageneratic suicides are those in which the self-inflicted death relates primarily to the individual's "falling out" of the procession of generations; his losing (or abrogating) his sense of membership in the march of generations and, in this sense, in the human race itself. . . . This kind of suicide grows out of a sense of alienation, disengagement, familial ennui, aridity, and emptiness of the individual in the "family of man" (Shneidman, 1972, pp. 18–19).

According to Shneidman (1985), all true suicides are *intentional*: directly arranged conscious acts with little possibility of rescue, or risky acts likely to cause death—for example, armed provocation of the police, or playing Russian roulette. Intentional self-destruction may reflect the belief that one's identity continues after physical annihilation, and by romantic notions about reuniting with loved ones or uniting with God. But the driving force is usually an intolerable need state which dramatically alters the way a person thinks about himself and the world. Four components of this state of mind include (1) painful agitation, (2) self-devaluation, which may include self-directed hatred, (3) constricted thinking focused on helplessness-hopelessness, which reduces problem-solving capacity or the ability to see viable alternatives, and (4) termination of pain as the only meaningful solution (Shneidman, 1985).

Arguments against Suicide   What keeps people from suicide even when depressed? A self-report study (Linehan et al., 1983) yielded a small number of fundamental reasons including (a) a sense that life is meaningful, pleasurable, and manageable, (b) a sense of responsibility to family and children, (c) moral and religious objections to suicide, and (d) fear of the physical and existential consequences of the suicidal act. Clearly, choosing to live instead of committing suicide must involve the capacity to experience love and work as meaningful balanced against the fear of social censure and existential unknowns.

SUMMARY

This chapter discusses the many biological, psychological, and situational causes of affective disorder. These causes can be divided into a few broad categories: (a) genetic factors interpretable as a heritable liability to bipolar disorder (manic-depressive disease); (b) neurological disease (for example, involving the anterior pole of the left hemisphere) and somatic diseases (for example, involving hormonal abnormalities) that alter brain physiology; (c) diagnosable psychopathology (for example, personality disorders involving dependency, emotional reactivity, and sensitivity to signs of separation or rejection), and other psychological factors—in particular, negative cognitive traits—all of which can interact with adverse circumstances to increase the risk, and influence the content, of affective disorders.

Clues about the psychology of depression come from situational depressions that are caused by two kinds of *loss*: (1) loss or rejection by loved ones and (2) loss of competence capacity—for example, because of the loss of an arm or the loss of employment. Loss, or "helplessness," depressions are characterized by anxiety, grief, longing, and crying. In the rarer and severer depressions, there seems to be a shift to a "defeat" or "hopelessness" type of depression characterized by apathy, inactivity, and unresponsiveness even to a positive change that normally would lighten mood.

Some depressions are the products of manic-depressive or medical diseases that have a largely biological etiology. In these largely biologically based depressions, social environmental factors may have minor causal significance, or they may be causally significant because of the sensitivity and reactivity of the person (producing a "reactive" depressive pattern). Other depressions appear to be the products of negative thinking—for example, an irrational tendency to blame oneself—that is characteristic of personality disorder or that is programmed by adverse social conditions. That social ecopathology—abuse, rejection, separation, loss, and the like—can trigger some depressions is hardly debatable. More uncertain is the role of social ecopathology in the development of negative patterns of cognition, and the etiological significance of those negative cognitive patterns—in other words, the degree to which they are depressogenic.

Suicide is associated with psychiatric disorder, especially depression or alcoholism, with social infirmity and aging, especially in white males, and with the psychodynamics of self-hatred, getting even, and hopelessness—in other words, when options for escaping unbearable psychological pain are no longer perceived. Some suicides seem to have a genetic basis—the biological relatives of suicides have a significantly higher risk for suicide than the adoptive relatives or the general population.

CHAPTER **15**

Anxiety Disorders

GENERAL ASPECTS OF ANXIETY

In the last five chapters we have focused on disorders associated with psychotic symptomatology. In this and subsequent chapters we shift our focus to neurotic, antisocial, addictive, and sexual disorders where psychotic symptoms are minor or absent. We begin here with anxiety disorders.

Anxiety is a familiar experience and a surprisingly prevalent complaint. Three components of anxiety are generally recognized. The *somatic* component includes racing heart, rapid breathing, and shakiness, physiological changes usually experienced as distressing. The *cognitive* component, sometimes called psychic anxiety, refers to changes in perception, thinking, and memory, such as thought-blocking, distraction, and fearful preoccupations with anticipated danger. The *behavioral* component includes phobic avoidance, compulsive rituals, and other actions to defend against real or imagined danger.

Somatic Aspects

A major hallmark of anxiety is the complex set of bodily changes mediated by the *autonomic nervous system,* or ANS (Figure 15.1). The *sympathetic,* or arousal, component of the ANS is automatically activated when massive energy expenditure is required—for example, in preparing physiologically for fight or flight. In the full-blown anxiety state, sympathetic arousal produces breathlessness, light-headedness, shakiness, nausea, blurred vision, immobility, urinary urgency, increased heart rate, sweating, and pupillary dilation. While anxiety typically involves sympathetic arousal, the opposite, or *para*-sympathetic arousal, can also occur. For example, phobic stimuli involving blood or injury elicit sharply *reduced* heart rate, *lower* blood supply to the brain, and fainting (Connolly, Hallam, & Marks, 1976; Marks, 1988).

Large and reliable individual differences exist in the *pattern* of somatic symptoms (Martin & Sroufe, 1970). For one individual, changes in heart rate may predominate, while for another, it is sweating (Lacey, Bateman, & VanLean, 1953). Anxiety can sabotage basic "vegetative" processes, reducing appetite, inhibiting sexual arousability, and disrupting sleep. All of these effects can cause dysphoric mood, lowered self-esteem, and more anxiety (Hall, 1980b; Lader, 1978).

Cognitive and Behavioral Aspects

High anxiety levels impair intellectual capability (Martin & Sroufe, 1970). Attention narrows, becoming erratic like a thin beam of light shifting willy-nilly in a darkened room. The result is a set of intense but discontinuous experiences. Derealization, depersonalization, apprehensions about dying or going crazy, and even hallucinations can give full-blown anxiety states a psychotic quality. Anxiety is also associated with an *attentional bias* toward threatening information. That is, anxious people are especially prone to detect and focus on stimuli which are congruent with their anxious feelings and fearful fantasies (MacLeod, Mathews, & Tata, 1986).

Tendencies to faint, freeze, flee, or fight are aspects of an instinctive fear reaction. In humans, these defense mechanisms are transformed by imagination and judgment into complex, sometimes symbolic, expression. In psychopathological form they emerge as phobic avoidance, persistent and uncontrollable thoughts, and compulsive rituals where certain behaviors are carried out in a highly specific fashion and in a highly predictable sequence. Some of these defensive behaviors are *pseudo*instrumental "solutions"; that is, they provide only the illusion of control without actually changing the cause of, or liability to, the anxiety. Nevertheless, the illusion of control is deeply comforting and, therefore, other things being equal, resistant to change.

Some behavioral aspects of anxiety can actually worsen the condition. Overbreathing, or *hyperventilation,* produces chemical changes in the blood that can intensify anxiety and even cause panic attacks. People with anxiety brought on by overbreathing can be taught to breathe through the nose rather

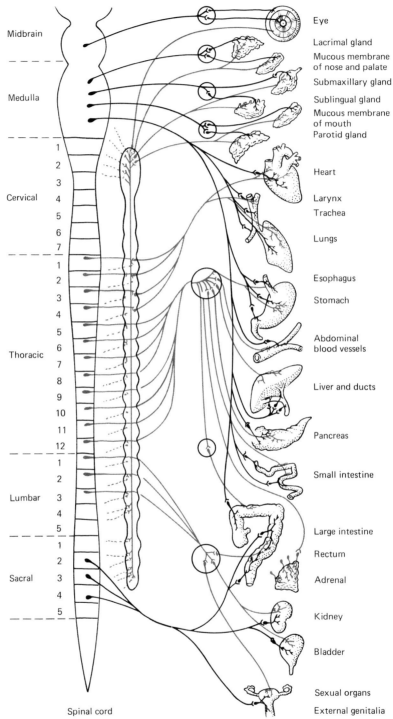

Midbrain

Medulla

Cervical
1
2
3
4
5
6
7

Thoracic
1
2
3
4
5
6
7
8
9
10
11
12

Lumbar
1
2
3
4
5

Sacral
1
2
3
4
5

Spinal cord

Eye
Lacrimal gland
Mucous membrane
of nose and palate
Submaxillary gland
Sublingual gland
Mucous membrane
of mouth
Parotid gland

Heart

Larynx
Trachea

Lungs

Esophagus

Stomach

Abdominal
blood vessels

Liver and ducts

Pancreas

Small intestine

Large intestine

Rectum

Adrenal

Kidney

Bladder

Sexual organs
External genitalia

FIGURE 15.1 The autonomic (peripheral) nervous system (Funkenstein, 1966, p. 72): *parasympathetic* branches (in black) devoted to increasing energy—e.g., by promoting relaxation and digestion; *sympathetic* branches (in gray) devoted to energy expenditure—e.g., in tension and action. Anxiety reaction to danger typically includes both parasympathetic (e.g., urinary urgency) and sympathetic (e.g., increased heart rate) components.

than the mouth so that the number and intensity of anxiety attacks are diminished (Bonn, Readhead, & Timmons, 1984; Lum, 1981).

Dissociative Aspects

Each of the three objective components of anxiety—somatic, cognitive, and behavioral—can intensify somewhat independently of the others, and the person may not be conscious of such changes. That an unconscious *dissociation* of a more active component from other, less active components can occur suggests that anxiety should be thought of as a set of loosely coupled components rather than as a lump (Lang, 1968; Lang, 1978; Hodgson & Rachman, 1974; Rachman & Hodgson, 1974; Rachman & Hodgson, 1980).

Some anxiety disorders are marked by somatic arousal—including increased heart rate, sweating, tension, and the like—but with little or no behavioral avoidance of something that is feared. Other anxiety disorders are marked by cognitive anxiety—apprehensive thoughts or fear of certain things—in the absence of marked somatic arousal. If anxiety disorders, like normal anxiety (Fenz & Epstein, 1967), are somewhat componential, then therapy may be directed at just one of the components.

There are, for example, two kinds of drug that reduce two kinds of "nervousness." One reduces somatic anxiety by blocking feedback from the autonomic to the central nervous system while the other reduces cognitive anxiety by directly altering neural firing in the brain. Also, behavioral treatments can be targeted specifically for either cognitive anxiety or behavioral avoidance without having much impact on the nontargeted behavior (Steketee, Foa, & Grayson, 1982). Certain techniques that effectively extinguish avoidance behavior in obsessive-compulsives do not necessarily reduce anxious preoccupation with feared stimuli such as dirt; conversely, the reduction of anxious preoccupation with a stimulus does not automatically reduce behavioral avoidance of that stimulus (Steketee, Foa, & Grayson, 1982). In sum, the dissociative aspect of anxiety suggests that it is made up of components that may sometimes be only loosely coupled (Lang, 1968; Lang, 1978).

Subjective Aspects

What determines the intensity of the subjective experience of anxiety? According to an early view promoted independently by William James and Carl Lange, we feel scared because we act scared, and the intensity of fear is proportional to the intensity of fearful activity. In other words, we are afraid when we become conscious of our physiological arousal and motor activity. The same objective threat occurring in the absence of rapid breathing or running away, for example, would be experienced as less frightening.

The James-Lange hypothesis implies that somatic feedback—bodily information fed back to the central nervous system—should influence affective life, and there is evidence that it does. For example, the higher the spinal cord damage in a neurological patient, the less the feedback from the autonomic nervous system, and the less intense the experienced affect (Hohmann, 1966). Also, drugs that reduce autonomic arousal can relieve the psychic anxiety symptoms of some patients with anxiety disorders, though not of others. It seems safe to say that somatic arousal can enhance anxious feelings just as anxious feelings can enhance somatic arousal. Perhaps the James-Lange theory is most applicable to people who are especially sensitive to autonomic feedback (Fehr & Stern, 1970; Reisenzein, 1983).

GENERAL ASPECTS OF ANXIETY DISORDERS

Anxiety is symptomatic of an anxiety *disorder* when it is abnormally intense, persistent, and debilitating, and/or when it is irrational, that is to say, elicited by essentially innocuous stimuli. We now give a preliminary overview of some of the general aspects of anxiety disorders, beginning with basic information on their prevalence, development, and co-occurrence with other disorders. To facilitate our introductory discussion, Table 15.1 gives brief summaries of the relevant anxiety disorders.

Prevalence

Population estimates of the lifetime prevalence of anxiety disorders listed in Table 15.1 vary across studies and locations, and change with revisions of diagnostic criteria. Currently, the estimates range from about 1.5 percent for panic disorder (and at least 5 percent for panic disorder with agoraphobia), to 2 to 3 percent for obsessive-compulsive disorder, to at least 3 to 4 percent for generalized anxiety disorder, to at least 10 percent for all phobic disorders (including agoraphobic, social, and simple types). Over a lifetime, a person may receive more than one diagnosis, and the lifetime prevalence of people with any anxiety disorder is estimated to be about 15 percent (Barlow, 1988; Robins, Helzer, Weissman, et al., 1984). Where sex ratios have been established, some disorders show marked female predominance—in agoraphobia, for example—while others show no sex difference—in obsessive-compulsive disorder, for example—or a slight male predominance, as in social phobia.

Anxiety disorders tend to run in families (Carey & Gottesman, 1981; Marks, 1987). The first-degree relatives of patients with various anxiety disorders have about a 15 percent risk for similar disorders. Risk of anxiety disorder for siblings of anxiety patients increases with the number of parents also affected with anxiety disorder, from about 5 percent when neither parent is affected to about 30 percent when one is affected, and 40 percent when both parents are affected. Also, concordance for a severe anxiety disorder varies from 30 to 60 percent for MZ twins as compared with 4 to 13 percent for DZ twins (Marks, 1987).

TABLE 15.1   MAJOR FEATURES OF ANXIETY DISORDERS

Category	Major features	Impairment	Sex ratio
Simple phobia	Avoidance of objects (e.g., animals) or specific situations (e.g., enclosed or high places)	Depends on circumstances	F > M
Social phobia	Painful self-consciousness and anxiety about social scrutiny. Avoidance of public places, self-disclosure, or self-exposure	Inconvenience is more typical than psychological impairment	M > F
Agoraphobia	Anxiety about being alone or in public places, especially about future panic attacks in such situations. Secondary depression and increased dependency. Agoraphobia is a frequent secondary feature of panic disorder (see below)	Significant	F > M
Panic disorder	Intense psychophysiological arousal, dread, disorganized thinking, behavioral paralysis, or flight. Reactive anxiety and depression are common. Agoraphobia (see above) is a frequent secondary complication of panic disorder	Demoralizing and potentially incapacitating	F = M
Generalized anxiety disorder	Chronic tension, nervousness, apprehension, psychophysiological arousal, vigilance, and mild depression	Mild to moderate	?
Obsessive-compulsive disorder	Generalized anxiety plus obsessions and compulsions, often with secondary depression	Moderate to severe	M = F
Posttraumatic stress disorder	A mix of anxiety and depression: vigilance and detachment; arousal and apathy. Painful and recurrent recollections and/or flashbacks about the trauma. Irritability and aggressive outbursts not uncommon (discussed in Chapter 5)	Mild to severe	?

Co-morbidity and Cross-morbidity

Symptoms of different anxiety disorders and also of depressive disorders often *co-occur in the same person,* something called *co-morbidity* (Barlow, 1985). For example, agoraphobic patients often display generalized anxiety, depression, and obsession (Buglass et al., 1977; Charney, 1982). Unfortunately, it is usually difficult to tell which if any of the co-occurring disorders is primary.

Relatives of patients with certain anxiety disorders have elevated rates of other disorders, a relationship called *cross-morbidity.* For example, the relatives of anxiety patients have elevated rates of major depression and alcohol abuse. More specific examples of cross-morbidity for specific anxiety disorders will be described below. Unfortunately, the data on cross-morbidity are limited (Fuller & Thompson, 1978; Marks, 1987; Munjack & Moss, 1981). Therefore, we can only speculate about underlying biological and psychological commonalities between any one particular anxiety disorder and other, behaviorally different but correlated disorders.

Temporal Aspects

Onset and Course   The onset of most anxiety disorders affecting adults occurs between the ages of 15 and 30. Follow-up studies of anxiety patients suggest some spontaneous remission of symptoms five years or more after initial contact with a professional. Fifty percent or more of these people are well or only mildly affected, but 15 percent continue to have persistently debilitating symptoms. Some disorders show recurrent cycles of intensification and remission. Relatively poor outcome is associated with poor premorbid adjustment and with symptoms sometimes sufficiently intense to require hospitalization (Goodwin & Guze, 1979).

Developmental Aspects   Different kinds of anxiety tend to predominate at different ages (Rutter, 1972). Animal and situational fears of the dark, for example, predominate during the preschool years. School phobias are more typical in the primary grades than later. Obsessive-compulsive rituals are more likely to emerge between the ages of 7 and 10, while anxious self-deprecation and depression predominate around puberty. But what is the developmental connection between childhood and adult anxiety disorders?

Children with phobic and obsessional disorders are at higher risk than controls for developing adult neurotic disorders (Cox, 1976), but not always the same disorder; a school phobia in childhood, for example, might precede an obsessive-compulsive disorder in adulthood. Nevertheless, in most cases the childhood disorder will disappear, and in some cases all that continues into adulthood is excessive sensitivity, insecurity, and dependency. When we start with adults with anxiety disorders and look back at their childhood, a similar picture emerges; although anxiety patients are more likely than normals to have had neurotic problems as children, most of them show no such history (Cox, 1976). In short, most anxiety symptoms and disorders show developmental *dis*continuity between childhood and adulthood. A possible exception is childhood obsessive-compulsive disorder, which tends to continue into adulthood (Swedo et al., 1989).

Generalized Anxiety Disorder

Sometimes a chronic pattern of anxiety occurs without phobia, panic, or obsessive-compulsive symptoms. This pattern, called *generalized anxiety,* usually includes five characteristics: (1) vague feelings of foreboding, (2) inappropriate worry and rumination about two or more "problems," (3) edginess, vigilance, and distractibility—a sense of being keyed up and subject to extreme startle reactions, (4) sympathetic arousal (for example, palpitation, sweating), and (5) fidgeting, twitching, trembling (Akiskal, 1985). These symptoms commonly precede or co-occur in many psychiatric disorders. For example, they are commonly associated with *DSM-III-R* personality disorders as well as numerous symptom disorders (Axis I), including anxiety, somatoform, addictive, sexual, and affective disorders. Nevertheless, current convention says that a diagnosis of *generalized anxiety disorder* is warranted only when inappropriate anxiety symptoms for two or more life circumstances (family finances, a child's progress at school, and the like) persist in cases where panic, phobia, obsessive-compulsive, or posttraumatic stress disorder cannot be diagnosed. In other words, the term generalized anxiety disorder is a "residual" category that is used to diagnose pathological anxiety that cannot be characterized as any other type of anxiety disorder. Here is a patient with generalized anxiety disorder.

> *Bob*: It's been an awful month. I can't seem to do anything. I don't know whether I'm coming or going. I'm afraid I'm going crazy or something.
> *Doctor*: What makes you think that?
> *Bob*: I can't concentrate. My boss tells me to do something and I start to do it, but before I've even taken five steps I don't know what I started out to do. I get dizzy and I can feel my heart beating and everything looks like it's shimmering or far away from me or something—it's unbelievable.
> *Doctor*: What thoughts come to mind when you're feeling like this?
> *Bob*: I just think, "Oh, Christ, my heart is really beating, my head is swimming, my ears are ringing—I'm either going to die or go crazy" (Spitzer et al., 1983, p. 11).

Relatively little is known about the causes of generalized anxiety disorder. Therefore, we will deal with it in the context of subsequent discussions of better-researched anxiety disorders, and also in a later section on pharmacological aspects of anxiety.

We have described the symptoms of anxiety and some general aspects of anxiety disorders, their prevalence, variety, and development. We now turn our attention to more detailed discussion of three major categories—phobic, panic, and obsessive-compulsive disorders—for which there is a good deal of research and theorizing.

PHOBIA

Phobic anxiety is crystallized around a specifiable threat—for example, animals, heights, or having a heart atttack. Phobic disorders are classified by *DSM-III-R* into three categories, depending on the type of threat that elicits fearful reactions.

Categories of Phobic Disorder

Simple Phobia   A simple phobia involves certain narrowly defined specifiable threats—for example, animals, heights, or confined spaces. The conventional term simple is, we think, unfortunate because it implies that some phobias are simple while others are complex without specifying what such a distinction means psychologically or etiologically. In fact, analyses of even simple phobias suggest that they are as complex as other psychological phenomena, as we will shortly see.

Many simple phobias involve animals. Though quite prevalent, animal phobias are not frequently seen in clinical practice because they rarely cause severe disability; typically, they do not involve reactive anxiety, depression, or the abuse of drugs that stems from attempts at self-medication. Animal phobias of childhood have a roughly equal sex ratio. In contrast, animal phobias which persist into, or begin in, adulthood are almost always reported by females, one estimate being 95 percent (Marks, 1969). Animal phobias may occur in the context of a traumatic incident (a dog bite, for example) or they may seem to develop spontaneously, "out of the blue."

Social Phobia   Social phobia revolves around the dread of being critically evaluated by observers in social situations involving eating, drinking, or speaking in public (Trower & Turland, 1984).

> For fear of shaking, blushing, sweating or looking ridiculous patients will not sit facing another passenger in a bus or train, nor walk past a queue of people. They are terrified of attracting attention by behaving awkwardly or fainting. Some may only leave their house when it is so dark or foggy that they cannot easily be seen. They will avoid talking to superiors, and stage fright will prevent them from appearing in front of an audience. They may cease swimming as it involves exposing their bodies to the gaze of strangers (Marks, 1969, p. 153).

Social phobia has a relatively chronic course and carries an especially elevated risk for depression. In contrast to other phobias, social phobia has a relatively early onset, often in adolescence, and a more equal distribution of males and females, with slightly more males affected. Also, the anxiety attacks of social phobia are predictable, being elicited by specifiable social events. Finally, social phobics do not develop panic attacks when given certain drugs that can cause panic in agoraphobics (described shortly). This unresponsiveness suggests that the anxiety of social phobia is different from that of agoraphobia (Liebowitz et al., 1985).

Agoraphobia Recognized since antiquity, agoraphobia was first described formally in 1871 by the German psychiatrist Westphal (Thorpe & Burns, 1983). It is a dread of being out in the open, in crowds, or in enclosed or other areas where impending catastrophe seems imminent but help or escape is unlikely. The agoraphobic may avoid certain places or situations, become entirely homebound, or, in extremely severe cases, become confined to a single room.

The avoidance behavior of agoraphobics is ameliorated by *safety signals* such as supportive people and familiar surroundings (Rachman, 1984). Interestingly, about one in three agoraphobic patients finds relief at night, or with dark glasses, or by keeping the curtains closed (Marks, 1969). Since light itself is arousing, perhaps darkness reduces somatic arousal that, according to the James-Lange theory, can amplify conscious anxiety and therefore the risk, or just the anticipation, of panic.

Agoraphobia, occurring for unknown reasons mostly in women, usually starts during late adolescence or young adulthood. The disorder almost always develops in response to some traumatic inner experience, such as the feeling of having a heart attack or a panic attack or of otherwise losing control. Once started, the disorder typically has a chronic course unless treated (Tearnan, Telch, & Keefe, 1984).

Evidence for Categorical Distinctions Research tends to support a categorical approach that distinguishes among types of phobia. For example, Torgerson (1979) used self-report data to estimate the degree to which phobic fears do or do not co-occur in the same person. Statistical analysis yielded five categories of phobic concern that largely support *DSM-III-R* distinctions among "simple" phobias, social phobias, and agoraphobia (see Table 15.2). Furthermore, Torgerson could estimate the heritability of each of these categories because his subjects were twins. The results are consistent with the idea that there may be partly heritable tendencies to develop certain types of phobias but not others.

Some of the categorical distinctions found by Torgerson are supported by other research—for example, on psychological differences between phobics

TABLE 15.2 CLASSIFICATION OF PHOBIAS

Category	Example	Relevant *DSM-III* category
Separation	Journeys; open spaces; being alone	Agoraphobia
Animals	Mice; rats; frogs	Simple phobia
Nature	Sharp objects; enclosed or high places	Simple phobia
Social	Eating with strangers; being watched	Social phobia
Mutilation	Hospitals; wounds; injections	Simple phobia

Source: Torgerson, 1979.

who fear animals and phobics who fear certain situations. According to a study by Seif and Atkins (1979), situational phobics (including agoraphobics) tend to perceive the world more subjectively and express their ideas more diffusely and ambiguously; the severity and content of their symptoms often depend on convenience and social context. A person with a height phobia, for example, might not be troubled by living on the top floor of an apartment house.

In contrast, animal phobics perceive the world more objectively and analytically, express their ideas more clearly, and seem relatively unaffected by context factors.

> Animal phobics appear to be consistently hypervigilant in terms of the phobic object. . . . A person who is phobic of spiders, for example, discovers spiders with alarming frequency on walls and ceilings, in corners and shadows, and in other places where nonphobics would almost never notice spiders. . . . This person separates the spider percept from the background of his or her field with remarkable ability. It appears to "pop" out of its context into focused awareness (Seif & Atkins, 1979, pp. 43–44).

Perhaps differences in cognitive style can partly explain differences in the symptomatic expression of phobic anxiety: an analytical style biasing anxiety toward "obsessional" detail-oriented behavior, and an impressionistic style biasing anxiety toward "hysteroid" globally oriented behavior (see Table 15.3). Perhaps cognitive style is part of the genetic factor suggested by the Torgerson study. Only further research will tell if this speculation has any merit.

Learning Theory of Phobic Anxiety

We began our discussion of phobia by describing what phobics fear. Now we can ask: What do phobics *really* fear? The question is especially pertinent because so many phobias seem to be about conventional things that don't scare most people. A straightforward answer is offered by Klein:

TABLE 15.3   OBSESSOID-HYSTEROID TRAITS

Hysteroid	Obsessoid
1. Excessive display of emotion	Scarcely any display of emotion
2. Vivid daydreams	Inability to indulge in fanciful thinking
3. Frequent mood changes	Constant mood
4. Underconscientious	Overconscientious
5. Given to precipitate action	Slow and undecided owing to weighing of pros and cons
6. Overdependent	Obstinately independent
7. Careless and inaccurate	Stickler for precision
8. Shallow emotionally	Feels things deeply
9. Desire to impress and gain attention	Self-effacing

Source: Foulds, 1965 (*Personality and personal illness.* Reprinted by permission from Tavistock Publications).

It bears repeating that specific phobic objects and situations are not in themselves dangerous but almost always afford an opportunity for grave danger. Phobics are not afraid of water—they are afraid of drowning; they are not afraid of cats or dogs—they are afraid of being clawed and bitten; they are not afraid of heights—they are afraid of falling; they are not afraid of public speaking—they are afraid of social humiliation; they are not afraid of enclosures—they are afraid of suffocation (Klein, 1981, p. 252).

But why does the patient develop the fear? The classical psychoanalytic view is that phobias are really about losing *self*-control due to the imminent eruption of dangerous infantile libidinal and aggressive impulses to act out. Many experts, however, doubt the usefulness of the idea that phobias are symbolic transformations of inner conflict originating in early childhood.

Even where symbolism can be shown satisfactorily, this does not prove its causative role. . . . Phobic patients, especially agoraphobics, often produce psychopathological material of great interest, richness and feeling. The temptation is then strong to link this symbol-rich material to the origin of the phobia. The temptation is even more powerful when disclosure of this material is accompanied by abreaction and temporary relief for a week or two. . . . We are all familiar with patients emerging from retarded depression who "come alive" and talk freely as they improve. The same applies to patients in remission from severe agoraphobia. Such patients talk because they are better—they are not better because they have talked (Marks, 1969, pp. 98).

In striking contrast to psychoanalytic theories, learning theories of phobia give special explanatory weight to environmental causes rather than to erotic or aggressive impulses. Accordingly, phobias are acquired through ordinary learning mechanisms that forge an association between a stimulus—an object or situation—and the painful experiences it signals. Since both the warning stimuli and the adverse events which cause pain are often imposed on the individual from external sources, learning theories typically require no special inner factors—ambiguous genetic tendencies or mysterious symbolic mechanisms—to explain either common or idiosyncratic fears.

Learning theories of phobia reinforce the idea that some phobias are indeed "simple," that is, have straightforward explanations as learned behaviors. These theories are therefore justifiably popular, given their face validity and experimental support. Nevertheless, a growing number of researchers (Emmelkamp, 1982; Marks, 1969), even those identified with learning theory (Gray, 1981; Rachman, 1978), have begun to raise questions about the application of learning theory to phobic disorders. What are the basic mechanisms suggested by learning theory and what is the evidence?

Basic Mechanisms   Learning theories of anxiety usually include at least two key mechanisms: traumatic conditioning and observational learning of fearful behavior (see Chapter 5, pp. 126–130). You will recall that the *conditioning mechanism* involves formerly innocuous stimuli that reliably elicit anxiety after they have become predictably associated with a traumatic event such as parental loss, physical abuse, panic attack, or any deeply threatening experience. Anxiety is elicited by initially innocuous but now-conditioned warning stimuli that, along with the anxiety, motivate avoidance behaviors which are reinforced by safety signals, including anxiety reduction. Through stimulus generalization, any stimulus that is physically or semantically similar to the conditioned stimuli can also elicit anxiety and avoidance. Given the richness and unpredictability of experience, a conditioning theory can, without recourse to genetic or symbolic mechanisms, account for even the most idiosyncratic phobias.

The *observational learning* mechanism is nicely illustrated in studies by Mineka et al. (1984) and Cook et al. (1985). Adolescent rhesus monkeys reared in the laboratory normally show no fear when exposed to a snake. However, they do develop fear of snakes after observing a born-in-the-wild adult monkey displaying strong fear reactions to snake and snakelike stimuli. The observer's acquired fear is persistent and its intensity is highly correlated with the intensity of the model's fearfulness. The results are fully consistent with the assumption that emotionally provocative *vicarious* learning, that is, learning by observing a fearful model, can produce phobic behavior.

Ironically, one of the most interesting things about the learning model of psychopathology is the controversy it has provoked regarding its explanation of certain observations about phobia. We will briefly describe five controversies, starting with the question: Is there a biological disposition to learn certain types of phobias rather than others?

Biologically Prepared Stimuli   Clearly, it is adapative to be able to respond fearfully to objectively dangerous events, even at the risk of temporary disruptions of other behaviors. Beck and Emery remind us of the adage that "evolution favors anxious genes"; on the average, making a false positive—seeing a "threat" where none exists—is better than making a false negative—being insensitive to a real threat. "One false negative—and you are eliminated from the gene pool. Thus, the cost of survival of the lineage may be a lifetime of discomfort" (Beck & Emery, 1985, p. 4).

Nevertheless, too much energy wasted on false positives can be maladaptive. In fact, neurotic behavior often seems to be just that sort of thing: apprehensive attention to, and avoidance of, things not objectively dangerous. This is the case of the irrational fears we call phobias. But more specifically, why are certain phobias more prevalent than one would expect given the infrequency of unpleasant experiences or potential danger involved (to elevators, for example)? Also, why are other phobias rare even though they involve real dangers (to electric outlets, for example)?

Biologically oriented learning theorists are impressed by the apparent evolutionary significance of most phobias. Separation from others, being gazed at, open spaces, enclosed, narrow or high places, and certain animals might represent evolutionary dangers *common to a species*. Has evolution built into the human nervous system a readiness to acquire fearful reactions to such *species-relevant* events (Ohman et al., 1976)? In other words, are we—and also our phylogenetically "close relatives," the apes and monkeys—*biologically prepared* (regardless of personal experience) to develop certain phobias—for example, to snakes rather than electrical outlets (Seligman, 1970)? The Mineka et al. (1984) study is consistent with this speculation, as is evidence that shock-induced conditioned reactions are more persistent if they are signaled by "prepared" CSs such as a snake rather than an unprepared CS such as a flower (Ohman, 1979). The speculation about the special conditionability of certain stimuli remains complex and controversial, however (McNally, 1987; Mineka, 1985).

There is one other intriguing question we can ask. Are some people, for unique genetic reasons, especially responsive to such species-relevant (or even *idiosyncratic*) stimuli? Sensitivity to specific potential threats would be analogous to other types of individual sensitivities—for example, to the specific colors, textures, or bodily sensations that might underlie idiosyncratic tastes and preferences. In short, people may be *biased* by heredity as well as by personal experience to react to special stimuli, thereby increasing their risk for some phobias. This idea is consistent with the results of the Torgerson study discussed earlier; nevertheless, in the absence of adoption research, it remains highly speculative.

Nontraumatic Etiology Learning theories of phobia have traditionally favored a traumatc factor to explain the intensity and persistence of phobias. Clinical and experimental evidence clearly supports the view that some syndromes—posttraumatic stress disorder, multiple personality, and certain animal phobias, for example—originate in traumatic experience. And yet, in many other cases, neither patients nor their therapists are able to discover a trauma even after exhaustive investigation (Marks, 1981).

Furthermore, attempts to produce phobias through traumatic conditioning of neutral stimuli like lights or sounds have often met with little success (Watson & Rayner, 1920). Short-term aversions to conditioned stimuli produced through repetitive pairings of neutral and noxious events often do not resemble the symptoms of anxiety disorder (Costello, 1970). Likewise, traumatic experiences with aerial bombing, life-threatening disease, or even aversion therapies have rarely produced anything resembling a phobia (Emmelkamp, 1982; Marks, 1969). In other words, even if many phobias started with traumatic experience, most traumatic experiences seem *not* to produce phobia, thus suggesting the importance of certain vulnerability factors.

The readiness to develop certain phobias may involve the readiness to *imagine* dangers even in situations that most people would feel competent to handle (Beck & Emery, 1985). Entirely normal learning mechanisms might, in vulnerable people, forge an association between anxiety-provoking fantasies and related external events.

Delayed Onset Sometimes a traumatic event can be established as *the* antecedent factor in phobia. But why does the onset of such phobias sometimes occur weeks or even months after the traumatic event? We do not yet have a generally accepted explanation. Perhaps some sort of phobic conditioning produced by noxious experiences can be suppressed temporarily by defense mechanisms such as repression or by coping skills—for example, diverting attention to safe and satisfying activities. Later, the phobia could erupt when such compensatory mechanisms are weakened, perhaps by current adversity or trauma that activates the relevant memories. This is analogous to the case of brain damage-induced behavioral deficits that disappear, only to reappear perhaps years later when neurological compensatory mechanisms weaken with aging (discussed in Chapter 9, pp. 262–263).

Persistence and Intensification Conditioning theory says that "neutral" stimuli reliably associated with trauma or adversity acquire the power to elicit anxiety; they become negative CSs. The persistence and even intensification of anxiety reactions could be explained by assuming that the negative CS is periodically reconditioned by subsequent trauma, even one that is different from the original trauma (Mineka, 1985). But why do phobic fears persist, or even intensify, when there is no evidence of periodic reconditioning (Eysenck, 1976; Bolles, 1979)? Perhaps the problem is with the evidence; undetected reconditioning may often occur either unconsciously or consciously but without recall. Another possibility is that *uncertainty* about potential threat is sometimes sufficient to sustain phobic preoccupations even in the absence of further conditioning.

Clearly, all organisms are distressed when stimulus conditions relevant to self-preservation are ambiguous (Weiss, 1977). Under conditions that threaten self-preservation, ambiguous conditioned stimuli—for example, a very brief or weak version of a stimulus that was initially associated with trauma—can elicit *even stronger* emotional distress than that produced by the initially traumatizing unconditioned stimulus (Eysenck, 1979). Are there human parallels? Nameless dread may be more distressing than objective danger. Perhaps uncertainty and ambiguity about the "real" nature of the threat prevents the extinction of phobic behavior. This would explain why behavior therapy of phobia works—it helps the person to clarify and gain control over conditions associated with threat.

Absence of Models Studies on observation learning in monkeys clearly support the idea that modeled anxiety *can* produce anxiety through observational learning (Mineka et al., 1984). But if modeling is a factor, why do most parents, siblings, and children of patients *not* have anxiety disorders? It would appear that although modeling may be *sufficient* to produce anxiety, it is not *necessary*, and may not be typical for anxiety disorders.

But consider this: learning can *immunize* as well as sensitize. Prior experiences of coping successfully with noxious events can prevent the development of depression during subsequent exposure to helplessness conditions (Seligman, 1975). Likewise, positive experiences with potentially dangerous things—growing up with pets, for example—can immunize against animal phobia. Immunization can occur through observation of others. For example, prior exposure to a model interacting *nonfearfully* with a snake can effectively prevent later conditioning of a phobic reaction to snakes (Mineka & Cook, 1986). Thus, the presence of a fearless parent could explain the immunity of a child exposed to the other parent's phobia.

In sum, we still cannot be sure how well laboratory experiments model phobic behavior, or how well learning theories explain the development of phobic disorders.

PANIC DISORDER

A *panic* experience, or "attack," involves discrete episodes of intense somatic anxiety with severe apprehension, terror, and a sense of impending doom. At least initially, these experiences are unexpected in the sense that there is no obvious explanation such as a phobic object, social scrutiny, or impending threat.

Panic Attacks and Panic Disorder

Panic Attacks According to *DSM-III-R,* a panic attack should include at least four of the following symptoms: (a) shortness of breath or smothering sensations; (b) dizziness, unsteadiness, or faintness; (c) palpitations or accelerated heart rate; (d) trembling or shaking; (e) sweating; (f) choking; (g) nausea or abdominal distress; (h) depersonalization or derealization; (i) numbness or tingling sensations (paraesthesias); (j) flushes (hot flashes) or chills; (k) chest pain or discomfort; (l) fears of dying, going crazy, or doing something uncontrolled. Typically, such panic attacks last ten to fifteen minutes but sometimes more than an hour.

> Ten minutes after they began shopping, Dennis suddenly felt very sick. His hands began to tremble uncontrollably, his vision became blurred, and his body felt weak all over. He experienced a tremendous pressure on his chest and began to gasp for breath, sensing that he was about to smother. These dramatic physical symptoms were accompanied by an overwhelming sensation of apprehension. He was terrified but did not know why. Without saying anything to Elaine, he whirled and dashed from the store, seeking refuge in their car, which was parked outside. Once there, he rolled down the windows to let in more air, laid (sic) down on the back seat, and closed his eyes. He continued to feel dizzy and short of breath for about 10 minutes more (Neale, Oltmanns, & Davison, 1982, p. 17).

The onset of a panic attack is usually sudden, seemingly "out of the blue." However, closer examination reveals that it often develops within the context of (a) chronic tension or conflict typically arising from frustrating family life or employment, or (b) special situations—for example, while in a shop, in a crowd, or on a public conveyance, while using a drug like marijuana or cocaine, or when threatened by separation from a loved one (Mathews, Gelder, & Johnston, 1981).

Panic attacks are experienced by people in the nonpsychiatric population; from 10 to 30 percent report having experienced at least one (Telch, Lucas, & Nelson, 1989). Panic attacks also occur in patients with various psychological disorders—for example, in phobic patients in the presence of a phobic stimulus, and also in patients with depressive, somatoform, or personality disorders.

Panic Disorder A diagnosis of panic *disorder* requires at least four attacks within a four-week period or at least one attack followed by a period of at least one month of persistent apprehension of having another. The disorder has a comparatively high prevalence in the population, about 2 to 5 percent, with a roughly equal sex ratio unless agoraphobia (discussed below) is prominent, in which case females outnumber males at least 2 to 1. Panic disorder first appears most typically during the late 20s and is generally persistent in the absence of treatment.

Panic disorder can be quite debilitating. Not only is it frequently associated with chronic nervousness, depression, sexual difficulties, and hypochondriacal preoccupations (Breier, Charney, & Heninger, 1984), but it also may be associated with an elevated rate of cardiovascular abnormalities, in particular, anatomical abnormalities of the heart (Margraf, Ehlers, & Roth, 1986). For these reasons, panic patients frequently seek medical advice and assurance for problems that are both real and imagined (Chambless, 1982).

Physiological and Cognitive Aspects

There are two general views on the role of physiological versus cognitive processes in panic disorder. The physiological view assumes that panic is an extreme activation of physiological events, a "discharge" of the autonomic nervous system. The primary cause of the discharge is presumed to be physiological—for example, a metabolic or neurological dysfunction. In short, the conscious thoughts and subjective experiences we call "panic" are secondary to the physiological "discharge," an instinctive behavioral pattern that is normally set off in the presence of life-threatening events. This physiological view of panic disorder as an endogenous pathology was given credibility early on by evidence that panic attacks could be produced in panic patients simply by using physiological provocations like injections of sodium lactate or inhalation of CO_2, and also by having patients hyperventilate.

An opposing view is that threat appraisals are critical both in the description and the explanation of panic attacks. In cognitive models (see Beck & Emery, 1985), panic may occur if external events are judged to be extremely dangerous—for example, when animal phobics panic in the presence of the phobic stimulus. Likewise, panic patients have panic attacks when they judge a stimulus to be extremely dangerous. The difference is that unlike the phobic patient, the panic patient typically reacts to stimuli that are both internal and innocuous—for example, a change in heartbeat or a feeling of dizziness. If such a stimulus is interpreted to mean "I'm having a heart attack" which means "I am dying," the chance of having a panic attack is increased. The individual is either uninformed—that is, naive about the insignificance of the stimulus—or misinformed through erroneous prior learning. Another possibility is that the panic sufferer has a *catastrophizing* cognitive style, that is, a general tendency to experience even innocuous events as ego- or life-threatening. In short, a critical causal factor in panic disorder is the cognitive one of threat appraisal.

The cognitive view is supported by evidence that panic attacks can be prevented by providing accurate information (internal events are not "dangerous" and panic attacks are not heart attacks and thus not dangerous). By learning effective coping skills, patients can anticipate the attacks, control or prevent them (for example, with relaxation techniques), and even turn them on at will!

The debate on the primacy of physiology versus cognition is too complex to develop fully here. It is likely that physiological and cognitive components both exist, but in different measure, depending on the case. Thus, the physiological model may be more valid for panics in which physiological factors predominate, while the cognitive model may be more valid for panics in which cognitive factors predominate. Nevertheless, both types of panic disorder could respond to cognitive therapy if we assume that cognitive therapy can increase the sense of efficacy, security, and self-control even in a basically physiological disorder. At present it is too early to be sure of the relative merits of the physiological and cognitive models, or whether each is best applied to a different type of panic disorder.

Agoraphobic Aspects

For at least a century, clinicians have noted that agoraphobia is a common complication of panic disorder (Foa, Steketee, & Young, 1984). In an early paper on obsessions and phobias, for example, Freud observed that "in the case of agoraphobia . . . , we often find the recollection of a state of *panic*; and what the patient really fears is a repetition of such an attack under those special conditions in which he believes he cannot escape it" (Freud, 1895/1959, p. 136).

It is true that most patients with agoraphobia have a history of panic attacks, but many—perhaps most—patients with panic do not develop agoraphobia (Noyes et al., 1986). Why some panic disorders evolve into agoraphobic syndromes remains uncertain, although there are many hypotheses (Tearnan, Telch, & Keefe, 1984). For example, an important cognitive factor may be low self-efficacy, in this case, the belief that one will not be able to cope with anticipated panics and therefore that catastrophic consequences are likely to occur (Telch et al., 1989). In addition, the insecurity typical of agoraphobic patients has prompted speculations about the causal significance of early events such as maternal loss or other separation experience that could promote a disposition to develop agoraphobia in the face of panic (Gittelman & Klein, 1985; Thorpe & Burns, 1983).

Another possibility is that certain cognitive and personality factors are involved (Breier et al., 1986). These could include (a) poor insight and the sense that "things just happen," (b) the tendency to catastrophize, (c) strong belief in the efficacy of avoiding situations where panics occur, and, perhaps most important, (d) a sense that the personal benefits of avoidance outweigh the personal costs. The benefits may include more than mere successful avoidance of panic; other possible advantages include escape from unpleasant adult responsibilities and gaining attention from, and even emotional control over, other people. These can be powerful incentives in the development of an agoraphobic pattern out of a panic disorder.

Whatever its origin, the agoraphobic "solution" is costly in terms of diminished freedom of movement and increased need for support from others. Nevertheless, it seems to be highly reinforcing by reducing the subjective probability of further panics. No wonder then, that in the absence of drug or behavior therapy, it tends to be a chronic disorder.

Panic Disorder versus Generalized Anxiety

Generalized anxiety and panic attacks often co-occur in the same person; for example, generalized anxiety occurs sometimes prior to, but more often subsequent to, the development of panic disorder (Breier et al., 1986). Evidence of such co-morbidity has raised two questions about *DSM-III-R* categorical distinctions between generalized anxiety and panic.

First, is the generalized anxiety "disorder" category valid? Does it represent a truly distinct psychopathology or is it merely a "residual" form of distress that is otherwise not diagnosable? Second, if it is indeed a true disorder, does generalized anxiety represent a fundamentally different type of psychopathology, or is it merely a different expression of the same underlying psychopathology? Perhaps the only important difference is that generalized anxiety represents a less severe form of anxiety psychopathology. The relatively scanty and somewhat inconclusive evidence on these two questions continues to spark debate.

The argument in favor of a categorical distinction can be boiled down to a few points. First, both the panic and generalized anxiety disorders are familial, with each disorder tending to run in different families (Noyes et al., 1987). Thus, the relatives of panic patients have a markedly elevated risk for panic disorder but not for generalized anxiety disorder—25 versus 2 percent, respectively, according to one study (Crowe et al., 1983); on the other hand, the relatives of patients with generalized anxiety disorder have a markedly elevated risk for generalized anxiety disorder but not for panic disorder. Furthermore, there is evidence that MZ concordance is higher than DZ concordance for panic disorder, but not for generalized anxiety disorder (Torgerson, 1983).

This observation suggests a genetic factor for panic disorder but not for generalized anxiety disorder.

Consistent with these familial distinctions is the idea that generalized anxiety and panic disorders represent different neuropsychological mechanisms, each designed by evolution to cope with a different kind of survival threat (Klein, 1981). In this view, generalized anxiety disorder is a pathological expression of behavior normally mobilized to cope with *anticipated* threat, while panic disorder is a pathological expression of behavior normally mobilized to cope with *perceived* danger or pain. One way to validate this theoretical distinction between anticipatory and panic anxiety is to show that panic and generalized anxiety disorders respond therapeutically to different types of antianxiety drug—for example, panic disorder to antidepressants and generalized anxiety disorder to benzodiazepines (Klein, 1981; Sheehan, 1982). To date, however, the evidence is unclear or nonsupportive (Margraf, Ehlers, & Roth, 1986).

In sum, the theoretical distinction between panic anxiety and generalized (anticipatory) anxiety has captured the imagination of many investigators. Still, the argument for the categorical separation of panic and generalized anxiety disorders in *DSM-III-R* remains inconclusive, and even contradicted by some evidence (Margraf, Ehlers, & Roth, 1986).

OBSESSIVE-COMPULSIVE DISORDER

We turn now to obsessive-compulsive disorder, a chronic and debilitating condition usually first manifesting in adolescence or young adulthood and affecting about 1 percent of high school students, and from 2 to 3 percent of the adult population. The severity of the disorder is dramatically underscored by the fact that obsessive-compulsives, compared with patients with other anxiety disorders, are more likely to consult medical specialists—dermatologists, oncologists, and neurosurgeons, for example—to require hospitalization, and, in some cases, to receive psychosurgery when all else fails. We describe the varied and somewhat bizarre clinical features and the personal and social devastation of the disorder, and briefly note what little reliable information is known about mechanisms and origins.

Clinical Features

Anxiety   Different kinds of anxiety characterize obsessive-compulsive disorder (Insel, Zahn, & Murphy, 1985). Some patients experience what might be called "doubt anxiety" in their preoccupations with questions like: Did I leave the door unlocked, or Did I hurt someone's feelings, or Am I actually a homosexual? Other patients experience "phobic anxiety" which is typically about being contaminated by germs or having cancer or heart disease. A minority of obsessional patients seem to experience no anxiety. Rather, they have an affectless quality, or "primary obsessional slowness" (Rachman, 1974)—for example, taking an hour to brush their teeth or an excessive amount of time to decide what to order in a restaurant.

The psychoanalytic view is that obsessional anxiety or slowness is a conscious expression of an unconscious awareness of "dangerous" impulses to carry out antisocial acts (Nemiah, 1980b). An alternative view is that the obsessive-compulsive's behavior is due to extraordinarily high subjective estimates that external dangers will materialize unless action is taken to prevent them (Carr, 1974). The nature of obsessions and compulsions that dominate the disorder is consistent with both of these assumptions.

Obsessions Normally, intrusive thoughts are rare and, when they do occur, they are typically dismissable (Salkovskis & Harrison, 1984). In contrast, obsessions are irresistible, often involving morbid fantasies—for example, about doing violence to a loved one. Kraines describes a woman who

> complained of having "terrible thoughts." When she thought of her boyfriend she wished he were dead; when her mother went down the stairs, she "wished she'd fall and break her neck"; when her sister spoke of going to the beach with her infant daughter, the patient "hoped that they would both drown." These thoughts "make me hysterical. I love them; why should I wish such terrible things to happen? It drives me wild, makes me feel I'm crazy . . . " (Kraines, 1948, p. 183).

Frequently, obsessions are about acting antisocially (for example, uttering obscenities, or acting out sexually), being dirty, contaminated, or infected (with special attention to bodily wastes or secretions, or dirt or germs), being the target of vague dangers, or having forgotten to do something important like locking a door or turning off the gas (Rapoport, 1988).

Compulsions Compulsions are largely involuntary, all-consuming, often stereotyped rituals (doing or saying something in an exact, highly prescribed manner), and frequently involving grooming, cleaning, touching, ordering and/ or arranging, and checking (the lights, gas, or locks, for example). Psychoanalysts interpret the compulsive ritual as a reaction formation, a defense mechanism that controls an objectionable motive by transforming it into its opposite—for example, the impulse to be dirty into compulsive cleaning, or cruel impulses into compulsive kindness (Fenichel, 1945; Schafer, 1954). Reaction formation is illustrated by excessively considerate, even self-sacrificing, acts done for individuals about whom the patient experiences hateful fantasies.

> Extreme reliance on reaction formation against hostility generally becomes itself an indirect avenue for the expression of hostility: one can be too clean, too conscientious, too sincere, too tender or too saintly for anyone else's comfort. Ultimately, exaggerated reaction formations are relentlessly demanding, accusing, guilt-provoking, and personally and socially stultifying (Schafer, 1954, pp. 346–347).

Some learning theorists emphasize the reinforcing value rather than the symbolic meaning of compulsive behavior (Bandura, 1968; Eysenck & Rachman, 1965). Adopting a pure conditioning model, they argue that any behavior, occurring for whatever reason, can become habitual if followed immediately by a sharp reduction of anxiety or discomfort; and the sharper the reduction of anxiety/discomfort, the more stereotyped the habit (Rachman & Hodgson, 1980). In short, a compulsion may have an arbitrary rather than a symbolic connection to anxious preoccupations.

Other learning theorists do see a connection between the meaning of an obsessive preoccupation and a compulsive ritual—for example, obsessions about contamination are more likely to be associated with cleaning than checking rituals. Adopting a cognitive conditioning model, they argue that symbolic meanings make certain behaviors more likely to occur and be reinforcing, even if they provide only the illusion of safety.

In this view, symptom severity stems, in part, from profound doubts about the capacity to manage specific obsessional preoccupations that are especially threatening because they are experienced as real even though the patient knows that this is illogical. For example, a patient with fantasies about murdering her child is compelled repeatedly to call the school for assurance that the child is still alive—all this even while admitting to the therapist that she couldn't have actually hurt the child. In short, a core cognitive characteristic of obsessive-compulsive disorder seems to be magical thinking—the irrational sense that one's thoughts, especially dangerous and/or guilt-ridden fantasies, have effects on objective events.

Shortly, we will describe evidence that a specific brain abnormality underlies obsessive-compulsive disorder. How this abnormality relates to the psychological abnormalities just discussed is uncertain, however.

Other Psychological and Social Characteristics Obsessive-compulsive disorder is personally debilitating and socially disruptive, as the following vignette makes clear.

> If Gerald as a teenager had ever permitted his father to hug him, the father would have been transported with delight. But Gerald developed a presentiment that his parents would contaminate him, or he them (the two ideas were mixed together), and both father and mother were forbidden to touch him or enter his room. He staked out a special corner of the living room for himself, and the parents were not permitted to step within this magic circle. There was a shelf in the refrigerator reserved for his food, and Gerald would not eat at the same table with his parents. His clothes could not be washed in the machine with their clothes nor dried in the same dryer. We heard about the father who drove 20 miles at night to get the precise variety of soap the patient insisted upon to complete a shower which had already lasted for hours. There were the mothers who were required to cleanse themselves with ritual observances before washing the patient's clothes. The humiliations and mistreatment to which the parents subjected themselves was almost unbelievable— except that the investigators had heard them so many times already (Hoover & Insel, 1984, pp. 210–212).

Obsessive-compulsive disorder is characterized by many apparent contradictions. A hand-washing compulsion driven by dread of contamination may co-exist in a person who rarely bathes. Neatness in one area is belied by dishevelment in another—for example, a sparkling clean bathroom next to a kitchen littered with dirty dishes (Rachman & Hodgson, 1980, p. 65). Apparent contradictions are also evident in magical thinking about power: power of the self over others and power of others over the self. Hoover and Insel (1984) describe the power concept that dominated the thinking of ten severely disturbed obsessive-compulsive patients.

> Their thoughts were driven by a fearful presentiment that, if certain acts were not properly performed, someone would be seriously harmed or would die. (Disease germs, automobile accidents, intruders, contamination, ill wishes, were among the fantasied mechanisms.) The patients felt a burdensome power to injure—or protect from injury—their families, acquaintances, or even complete strangers. On the reverse side of this same rationale, others persons were considered to possess deadly threatening powers over the self, a danger that might be countered by special acts of vigilance. Emphasis often shifted back and forth between these two concepts (Hoover & Insel, 1984, p. 208).

Neurophysiological Aspects

There is preliminary evidence that obsessive-compulsive disorder is associated with two possibly related neurophysiological abnormalities, one involving the connection between basal ganglia and frontal lobes, and the other involving neural systems that utilize the neurotransmitter serotonin. The hypothesis of a basal ganglia dysfunction is supported by evidence that (a) obsessive compulsive patients have abnormally small but metabolically hyperactive basal ganglia (Luxenberg, Swedo, Flament et al., 1988); (b) obsesssive-compulsive disorder is elevated in patients with various diseases of the basal ganglia (Rapoport, 1988); (c) obsessive-compulsive disorder is associated with Gilles de la Tourette's disorder (discussed below); and (d) the compulsions of the disorder resemble species-specific fixed-action patterns such as ritually circling a sleeping area before bedding down that, in lower animals, are controlled by the basal ganglia (Rapoport, 1988).

A serotonin-related dysfunction for the disorder is suggested by evidence that drugs with different effects specifically on serotonin-neuron functioning can increase or decrease the symptoms of obsessive-compulsive patients. For example, certain antidepressive drugs (in particular, chlomipramine and fluvoxamine) are therapeutic in adults and children, even when the patients are not depressed (Flament et al., 1985). These drugs are effective presumably because they eventually inhibit the activity of serotonergic neural systems (Perse, Greist, Jefferson et al., 1987). Contrariwise, drugs that increase serotonergic functioning can enhance the symptoms of obsessive-compulsive disorder (Zohar, Mueller, Insel et al., 1987). The evidence on serotonin-specific drugs is tentative and somewhat unreliable. Consequently, the hypothesis that obsessive-compulsive disorder involves a serotonergic dysfunction must be considered speculative at this point (Barlow, 1988).

Familial and Genetic Aspects

Data on familial aspects of obsessive-compulsive disorders are sparse and only suggestive (Rachman & Hodgson, 1980). Early studies of first-degree relatives of obsessive-compulsive patients revealed elevated rates of the same disorder, or at least an elevated rate of other psychiatric problems (see Carey & Gottesman, 1981). More recently, Swedo et al. (1989) reported a 25 percent risk for the disorder in first-degree relatives of patients. In contrast, Hoover and Insel (1984) could find no diagnosable obsessive-compulsive disorders in forty first-degree relatives of ten obsessive-compulsive patients. The relatives had elevated rates of depression, alcohol abuse, and anxiety and the parents displayed idiosyncracies reminiscent of obsessive-compulsive disorder, in particular, supercleanliness and overmeticulousness.

The few existing twin studies of obsessive-compulsive disorder are consistent with a hereditary factor, yielding concordance rates of 68 percent and 15 percent for MZ and DZ twins (see Turner, Beidel, and Nathan, 1985). An additional bit of evidence on behalf of a genetic component to obsessive-compulsive disorder is its association with Gilles de la Tourette's syndrome, a hereditary disorder marked by explosive motor and vocal tics (see Chapter 9, pp. 251–252). Fifty percent of Tourette's patients have diagnosable obsessive-compulsive disorder. Moreover, the biological relatives of Tourette's patients have an elevated risk for either Tourette's disorder, chronic tics (a subsyndrome of Tourette's), or obsessive-compulsive disorder (Pauls & Leckman, 1986; Pauls et al., 1986). It is therefore conceivable that some obsessive-compulsive disorders are alternative expressions of Tourette's disorder. Nevertheless, we should keep in mind that not all studies have shown a familial or genetic component to obsessive-compulsive disorder, so our ideas about the familiality, heritability, and classification of the disorder must remain tentative.

ANTIANXIETY DRUGS AND BIOCHEMICAL MECHANISMS

Our understanding of anxiety mechanisms is likely to be advanced by increasing knowledge about the neural, as well as behavioral, effects of antianxiety drugs. At this point, however, our knowledge is rudimentary. Table 15.4 summarizes some of the major points in the discussion that follows.

Benzodiazepine Antianxiety Drugs

Benzodiazepines Over 70 million prescriptions for antianxiety drugs are written each year (Rickels, 1981). Currently, the most frequently prescribed antianxiety drugs are diazepam (Valium) and alprazolam (Xanax). Benzodiazepines reduce anxiety, especially generalized anxiety uncomplicated by panic attacks or debilitating phobias. The drugs also induce sedation and muscle relaxation, effects that may be beneficial to the anxious person. Benzodiazepines require about one to three weeks to affect the symptoms of

TABLE 15.4 ANTIANXIETY DRUGS

Type	Major locus of action	Target disorder	Side effects	Addictive potential
Benzodiazepines	CNS (limbic)	Generalized anxiety	Some	Some
Beta blockers	ANS	Somatic anxiety; social phobia	Few	Little
Tricyclics	CNS	Agoraphobia; obsessions	Many	Little
MAO inhibitors	CNS	Depression; social phobia; panic	Many	Little

generalized anxiety (see Figure 15.2). But the drugs have three drawbacks: adverse side effects (vertigo, for example), addictive potential, and relapse after discontinuance unless supplemented with behavioral treatment.

Benzodiazepine Receptors   How do the benzodiazepines work? Benzodiazepine receptors exist on the membranes of certain neurons throughout the brain (Enna, 1982). Each benzodiazepine receptor is actually part of a *receptor-complex*, which includes a benzodiazepine component and a GABA (gamma amino butyric acid) component responsive to the neurotransmitter

FIGURE 15.2   Final level of functioning depends on initial degree of psychopathology and on treatment duration. (From Rickels, 1981, p. 13. "Benzodiazepines: Use and Misuse," in D. Klein & J. Rabkin (eds.), *Anxiety: New Research and Changing Concepts,* 1981, pp. 1–24. Reprinted by permission from Raven Press, Ltd.)

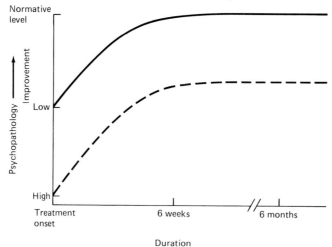

(Miller, 1981; Gray, 1985). Certain drugs that alleviate anxiety bind to the benzodiazepine receptors. These antianxiety drugs include the benzodiazepines, of course, and also alcohol.

Other chemical agents that bind to the benzodiazepine receptor complex *promote* anxiety—they are called anxio*genics*. Monkeys given an anxiogenic drug such as beta-carboline show heightened vigilance, distressed vocalization, behavioral agitation, and physiological activation. These anxietylike symptoms can be reduced by administering a benzodiazepine; moreover, the development of anxietylike symptoms can be prevented by giving benzodiazepines prior to the beta-carboline (Ninan et al., 1982; Insel et al., 1984).

No one knows exactly how antianxiety or anxiogenic chemicals work. One hypothesis is that each has a distinct effect on the benzodiazepine-GABA receptor complex and therefore on neural firing. Specifically, each chemical affects the benzodiazepine component of the receptor complex, in turn altering the GABA component's receptivity to GABA; it is this latter effect on GABA receptivity that presumably alters neural firing rates, and therefore anxiety level (Insel et al., 1984).

The competing effects of benzodiazepines and anxiogenics imply that an endogenous agent—a natural "benzodiazepine"—exists as part of the neurophysiological mechanism of normal anxiety. A biological basis for individual differences in anxiety might therefore conceivably include differences in one or more of the following: (1) level of the hypothetical endogenous benzodiazepine, (2) sensitivity of the benzodiazepine receptor, and/or (3) number of benzodiazepine receptors. In fact, there is evidence consistent with the last two possibilities. The brains of rats selectively bred for fearfulness have fewer benzodiazepine receptors than nonfearful controls (Robertson et al., 1978).

Unresolved Questions

Research on the benzodiazepine mechanism has added an important piece to the anxiety puzzle. Yet many questions remain. For example, how specific is the benezodiazepine drug effect? Some researchers used to think that benzodiazepines block generalized anxiety but not panic (Klein, 1981). However, new evidence suggests that panic can be blocked by using higher doses or newer types of benzodiazepines (Noyes et al., 1984; Sheehan, 1985). In short, while there are valid behavioral and theoretical distinctions between panic and generalized anxiety, these have not yet been clearly supported by reliable evidence of corresponding differences in pharmacological responsiveness.

There is another important question about how *non*benzodiazepine antianxiety drugs work. For example, we don't know why *antidepressants* such as imipramine can sometimes block panic anxiety (Klein, Ross, & Cohen, 1987). Assuming that they do not bind to the benzodiazepine receptor complex, does this mean that there is a distinctly different, nonbenzodiazepine mechanism in the brain, and if so, what is it (Redmond, 1985)? This is reasonable to ask because there is a nonbenzodiazepine mechanism that researchers already know about, one involving the *autonomic* nervous system. When certain neural receptors—the *beta-adrenergic* receptors—are blocked by *beta blockers* such as propranolol, some people find relief from somatic anxiety. In other words, by blocking neural feedback from the heart to the brain, beta-blockers can sometimes relieve anxiety without directly affecting benzodiazepine receptors, though the latter may be indirectly involved in the calming effects that are experienced by the person.

In sum, the benzodiazepine mechanism is only part of a complicated and still ambiguous physiological mechanism that underlies the behavior and experience of different types of anxiety. We still do not know the number and nature of the components of the mechanism, how it explains the vulnerability to different types of anxiety disorders, or how it accounts for the effects of psychological treatments that reduce anxiety.

BEHAVIORAL TREATMENT OF ANXIETY DISORDERS

Behavioral treatments are derived both from experience that tells us what works, and from theory that tells us what ought to work. In this section we focus on a select group of behavioral techniques that have been found to be effective in treating anxiety disorders, especially those associated with maladaptive avoidance behavior. We leave for Chapter 22 further discussion of such techniques, their theoretical foundations, and an empirical evaluation of their effectiveness.

Anxiety-Response Suppression (Counterconditioning)

Anxiety is only one of many possible reactions to a stimulus. It follows that strengthening a competing response to anxiety should effectively counteract, or *countercondition*, the anxiety reaction. The classic example of counterconditioning therapy is *systematic desensitization,* pioneered by Joseph Wolpe (1958). The goal of this treatment is to achieve relaxation in the face of "danger." To this end, a hierarchy of least to most feared stimuli is constructed. Then, the patient is taught how to relax various muscles of the body. The heart of the treatment involves learning how to associate relaxation initially to the least and eventually to the most anxiety provoking stimuli in the ordered set. It may take weeks or months to reach a point where the most feared stimuli are conditioned to relaxation more than to anxiety, especially when the stimuli are confronted in vivo, that is, "in the flesh."

Counterconditioning procedures have proven to be effective for some phobias (Eysenck & Rachman, 1965; Kanfer & Phillips, 1970; Marks, 1981), and may even block the otherwise anxiety-inducing effects of sodium lactate (Guttmacher & Nelles, 1984). However, counterconditioning appears to be less effective for other types of anxiety—in particular, for the anxiety of agoraphobic and obsessive-compulsive disorders (Emmelkamp, 1982). For this type of anxiety, a different technique can be effective.

Exposure

In some cases, a behavior therapist will utilize a technique that forces the patient to confront feared stimuli head-on without trying to escape. We now turn to this *exposure* technique.

If anxiety is conceptualized as largely an unconditioned reaction (UCR), then inducing repeated reactions should promote *habituation.* For example, if agoraphobic anxiety is an abnormal exaggeration of the natural tendency to be wary of potentially dangerous places, repeated forced exposure to those "dangers" should reduce fear. On the other hand, if anxiety is conceptualized as an abnormally intense conditioned reaction (CR), repeated exposure should promote *extinction,* that is, decrements in response intensity across nonreinforced stimulus presentations. Thus, whether viewed as a CR or UCR, anxiety should gradually decrease with repeated exposure to the fearful stimulus.

Exposure techniques force the phobic or obsessional patient to confront feared stimuli head-on, preferably in vivo (Marks, 1981; Stampfl & Levis, 1967). There is some controversy about the superiority of in vivo exposure over imaginal exposure. Apparently, imaginal techniques can be effective (Mathews et al., 1976), but the in vivo technique is effective more frequently (Emmelkamp, 1982). Also, therapeutic effects of exposure may in some cases be facilitated pharmacologically—for example, by combining exposure and tricyclic antidepressants to reduce anticipatory anxiety and panic in agoraphobic patients (Telch, Agras, Taylor et al., 1985).

Table 15.5 illustrates a therapeutic sequence of exposures carried out by a

TABLE 15.5 EXAMPLES OF THE SEQUENCE OF IN VIVO EXPOSURE FOR A WASHER (15 SESSIONS)

The following fear hierarchy was constructed for Steve: feces—100 subjective units of discomfort or SUDs; urine—90 SUDs; toilet seats in public bathrooms—80 SUDs; sweat—70 SUDs; newspapers—60 SUDs; doorknobs—50 SUDs. These items all have in common ability to cause disease.

During in vivo exposure treatment, the following sequence was pursued:

Session 1. Steve walked with the therapist through the building touching doorknobs, especially those of the public restrooms, holding each for a period of several minutes.

Session 2. Steve held doorknobs and newspapers.

Session 3. Steve held newspapers and doorknobs. Contact with sweat was introduced by having him place one hand under his arm and the other inside his shoe.

Session 4. Exposure began with newspapers and sweat. Toilet seats were added by having the patient sit next to the toilet and place his hand on the seat.

Session 5. Exposure began with contact with sweat and toilet seats. Urine was then introduced by having Steve hold a paper towel soaked in his own urine specimen collected that morning.

Session 6. Exposure included urine, toilet seats, and sweat with the addition of fecal matter (a piece of toilet paper lightly soiled with his own fecal matter). Homework focused on feces, urine, and toilet seats.

Sessions 7 to 15. Daily exposure to the highest three items was continued. Homework focused on the objects used during that day's treatment session. Weekend homework mirrored Friday's exposure. Periodic contact with lesser contaminants continued throughout.

Source: From Steketee & Foa, 1985.

compulsive hand-washer. Reduced anxiety occurs in many cases after repeated exposures of the sort shown in this table. Table 15.6 contains guidelines for the therapeutic technique of exposure. The procedure's effectiveness seems to depend more on exposure per se than on the intensity of the patient's reactions.

For anxiety disorders involving maladaptive avoidance behaviors, *response prevention* is an important ingredient in exposure therapy. An example is ritual prevention, widely used for treating compulsions, especially in the context of in vivo exposure. Steketee, Foa, and Grayson (1982) showed that the combination of exposure and ritual prevention was superior to either alone in reducing subjective discomfort (see Figure 15.3). The authors also showed that exposure per se tended to reduce anxiety but not the compulsion to engage in rituals, whereas response prevention tended to reduce the compulsion to engage in rituals without reducing anxiety about feared stimuli.

Cognitive-Behavioral Strategies

Cognitive-behavior therapies are highly structured, with specific agendas for problems to be explicitly confronted (Beck & Emery, 1985). One type encourages the patient to reduce irrational and self-defeating assumptions—for example, that self-assertion is "bad" (Ellis, 1962). Another type encourages patients to formulate such irrational and self-defeating beliefs in the form of specific self-statements. Gradually, these are modified so that patients acquire the ability literally to talk themselves into a healthier attitude (Meichenbaum, 1977). Table 15.7 provides examples of self-instructional statements to be acquired in four problem areas: preparing for stressors, handling stressors that actually occur, coping with anxiety, and reinforcing progress in these areas.

There is mixed evidence that one type of cognitive therapy for anxiety works better than another, or that cognitive therapies work better than alter-

---

TABLE 15.6   SUGGESTIONS FOR EXPOSURE TREATMENT

1. All designated exposure items are arranged hierarchically according to the subjective units of discomfort (SUDs) levels they evoke, and are presented in ascending order, beginning midway. That is, if the top item evokes 100 SUDs, exposure commences with items at the 50-SUD level; if the top item evokes 80 SUDs, a 40-SUD item is presented first.
2. A given item should be presented until the anxiety level provoked is reduced by half.
3. An exposure item should be repeated until it evokes no more than minimal anxiety.
4. Frequent sessions should be held, preferably three or more times per week.
5. Ideally, the intensive treatment program should be terminated when the most feared item has been confronted and provokes only mild anxiety. If substantial gains are not evident after 15 sessions, continuation of intensive treatment should be questioned.
6. Regularly scheduled follow-up sessions are recommended to consolidate treatment gains.
7. For motivated patients, detailed instructions for self-exposure may be sufficient. If the relationship between spouses or in the family is good, family members can be actively involved in the treatment program.

Source: From Steketee & Foa, 1985.

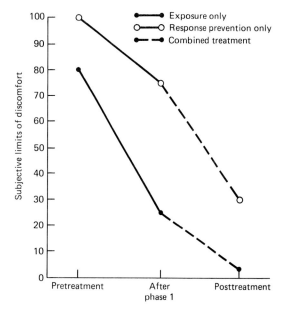

FIGURE 15.3 Mean highest subjective anxiety assessed during exposure test for different treatment conditions: (1) exposure only, (2) response prevention only, and (3) combination of both. (From Steketee, Foa, & Grayson, 1982, p. 1367. *Archives of General Psychiatry*, 1982, *39*, 1365–1371. Copyright © 1982, American Medical Association)

native types like systematic desensitization (Miller & Berman, 1983). It is likely that all the therapies we have described are effective to the extent that they promote in the patient a belief in the efficacy and relevance of the treatment (placebo or expectancy effect) and a sense of increasing personal effectiveness (self-efficacy).

SUMMARY

Anxiety is an affective state marked by somatic disturbances, apprehension, and avoidance behavior. Pathological anxiety is intense, persistent, and irrational. Its expression in the form of phobia, panic, obsession, and other disorders can be extremely debilitating.

Phobic disorders are marked by preoccupation with and avoidance of "threatening" objects such as animals, situations such as heights, or internal conditions such as panic states. Agoraphobia—typically fear behavior involved in coping with the threat of panic attacks—is qualitatively different from "simple" phobias such as fear of animals. The two traditional theoretical approaches to the origins and mechanisms of phobia are the psychoanalytic model, with its emphasis on the symbolic replay of unconscious infantile conflict, and the conditioning model, with its emphasis on trauma-induced and modeled conditioning of fear to previously neutral stimuli. Two other views are gaining increasing attention. The cognitive view emphasizes the tendency to "catastrophize" about essentially innocuous stimuli such as changes in heartbeat; the biological view emphasizes possibly heritable brain abnormali-

TABLE 15.7   EXAMPLES OF COPING SELF-STATEMENTS REHEARSED IN SELF-INSTRUCTIONAL (STRESS INOCULATION) TRAINING

Preparing for a stressor
  What is it you have to do?
  You can develop a plan to deal with it.
  Just think about what you can do about it.
  That's better than getting anxious.
  No negative self-statements: just think rationally.
  Don't worry; worry won't help anything.
  Maybe what you think is anxiety is eagerness to confront the stressor.

Confronting and handling a stressor
  Just "psych" yourself up—you can meet this challenge.
  Reason your fear away.
  One step at a time; you can handle the situation.
  Don't think about fear; just think about what you have to do. Stay relevant.
  This anxiety is what the doctor said you would feel.
  It's a reminder to use your coping exercises.
  This tenseness can be an ally; a cue to cope.
  Relax; you're in control. Take a slow deep breath.
  Ah, good.

Coping with the feeling of being overwhelmed
  When fear comes, just pause.
  Keep the focus on the present; what is it you have to do?
  Label your fear from 0 to 10 and watch it change.
  You should expect your fear to rise.
  Manageable.

Reinforcing self statements
  It worked; you did it. Wait until you tell your therapist (or group) about this.
  It wasn't as bad as you expected.
  You made more out of your fear than it was worth.
  Your damn ideas—that's the problem.
  When you control them, you control your fear.
  It's getting better each time you use the procedures.
  You can be pleased with the progress you're making.
  You did it!

Source: Reprinted with permission from D. Meichenbaum & M. Genest. "Cognitive Behavior Modification: An Integration of Cognitive and Behavioral Models," from F. H. Kanfer & A. P. Goldstein (Eds.), *Helping People Change* (2nd edition). 1980, Pergamon Press PLC.

ties that underlie panic attacks and biologically prepared predispositions to associate certain stimuli or ideas with objective or imagined threats.

Chronic (generalized) and/or acute (panic) levels of anxiety need not involve phobias. The relation between these types of anxiety disorder is uncertain, though some investigators argue that despite their behavioral overlap, panic and generalized anxiety may differ in important ways, including the amount of genetic determination and response to different drugs. Panic disorder is associated with an especially high risk for developing agoraphobia.

Generalized anxiety, like depressed feelings, is a common symptom of many neurotic and personality disorders.

Obsessive-compulsive disorder is a mixture of apprehension, obsessive pre-occupation, and repetitive or even rituallike avoidance behavior. Psychoanalytic theory holds that the disorder involves hostile impulses symbolically expressed and pathologically defended against. Learning theories argue for explanations that emphasize normal conditioning mechanisms. New evidence suggests, however, that these psychological factors are biologically predisposed by a brain abnormality, possibly involving a hyperfunction of serotonin neural systems, and probably involving the basal ganglia and frontal lobes.

Two therapeutic approaches have proven to be effective with anxiety disorders: the pharmacological and the behavioral. The former is important because antianxiety effects of specific drugs—for example, benzodiazepines for generalized anxiety, and certain tricyclic antidepressants for obsessive-compulsive disorder—imply that individual differences in vulnerability to certain kinds of anxiety are mediated by corresponding differences in types of brain abnormality. The behavioral approach is important because of its demonstrated efficacy for ameliorating anxiety, and because it suggests psychological mechanisms of anxiety regardless of possible brain dysfunction.

Somatoform Disorders

OUTLINE

The concept of hysterical neuroses has traditionally included two types of psychological disorder that simulate medical conditions. The *somatoform* type involves frequent complaints about pain, weakness, fatigue, discomfort, loss of sensation, and other symptoms suggesting bodily dysfunction. The *dissociative* type, described in Chapter 17, involves sometimes dramatic changes in consciousness, memory, and personality suggesting neurological disease. Somatoform and dissociative disorders are called *hysterical* when medical examination fails to reveal a physiological abnormality for the symptoms while psychological examination reveals stress, conflict, suggestibility, and attention-seeking. Nevertheless, there is increasing evidence that hysterical mechanisms in both somatoform and dissociative disorders often are not just mental problems but may involve abnormal brain functions (Merskey, 1986).

HISTORICAL BACKGROUND

Theories of hysteria have been recorded as far back as the second millennium B.C.E., for example, the ancient Greek view that the wandering uterus, disrupting physiological processes by displacing or compressing bodily organs, thereby causes mental changes. Hysterical disorders have played an important role in the development of modern theories of psychopathology, especially psychoanalytic theory. We will start, however, with a bit of history beginning about 100 years ago.

Anna O.

Late in 1880, Joseph Breuer was asked to examine a 21-year-old female disabled by numerous symptoms: paralysis of both legs, right arm, and neck, defects of vision, chronic coughing, and hallucinations of black snakes and "death heads." In addition, she would shift between two personality styles, one characterized by indolence and passivity, the other by agitation and rebelliousness. After first considering meningitis, Breuer settled on a diagnosis of hysteria for Anna O., as the patient has come to be known.

Hysterical symptoms often mimic physical disease yet respond to purely psychological therapy. Breuer and Anna O. developed a "talking cure" that involved what she called "chimney sweeping." This was a hypnotic exercise in free association revealing hidden memories of deep psychological significance around which symptoms seemed to have coalesced. Discovering connections between emotionally significant events and specific symptoms often proved therapeutically effective. For example, paralysis of the right arm disappeared when the patient discovered its origins in a painful dream.

The emotional basis of Anna O.'s hysterical disorder was evident in her fantastic and ever-changing symptoms, their situation specificity, and their apparent symbolism. For example, in reaction to an impending separation from Breuer, she developed the symptoms of a false pregnancy, a somatic metaphor strongly suggesting a dependency with erotic overtones. A few years later the Anna O. case would have a profound effect on the intellectual development of Sigmund Freud, a young neurologist-turned-psychiatrist who came to work with Breuer.

Some years later, the career of a remarkable young woman was beginning to take shape. A daughter of middle-class Orthodox Jewish parents, Bertha Pappenheim began her professional career as a feminist. An early accomplishment was her German translation of *A Vindication of the Rights of Women* by Mary Wollstonecraft, mother of Mary Shelley, creator of the Frankenstein story. Later, Pappenheim helped publicize the plight of poor Jewish women swindled and turned to prostitution by white slave traders. Eventually, she founded a home for wayward women and the orphaned victims of persecution and pograms. In 1936, she succumbed to cancer, and her death was widely mourned. In 1954, the German government issued a stamp to commemorate Pappenheim as its first social worker (see Figure 16.1).

At first glance, there would hardly seem to be much in common between Anna O.—a neurotically disabled child-woman who was manipulative, dependent, fractious, and shut in—and Bertha Pappenheim—that charming, moral,

FIGURE 16.1 A commemorative stamp honoring Bertha Pappenheim (Anna 0.). Courtesy of Ministry of Post, Bonn, West Germany.

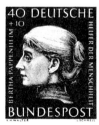

energetic individual of celebrated humanitarian and intellectual accomplishments. Nevertheless, Anna O. and Bertha Pappenheim were, in fact, the same person (Jones, 1964).

How can we explain this transformation? Was Anna O. indeed the victim of an underlying brain disorder, as Breuer first thought? Anna O.'s behavior was seemingly conflict-ridden, situation-specific, dramatically self-expressive, with psychosomatic "communications"; and all this was consistent with the diagnosis of hysteria. Yet three especially good reasons support the idea that Anna O. was, in fact, afflicted by a reversible organic mental disease, perhaps subacute limbic encephalitis (Flor-Henry, 1983). First, many of her symptoms are more typical of organic than hysterical disorder—for example, double vision, mutism, the inability to recognize familiar faces (prosopagnosia), clouded consciousness, and visual hallucinations. Second, her premorbid and postmorbid adjustment was normal—actually, quite extraordinary in the positive sense, as evident in her subsequent career—with no evidence of hysterical or other personality disorder. Third, there is growing evidence, discussed below, that many neurological patients have one or more of the classic "pseudomedical" symptoms of hysteria and that many diagnosed hysterics are rediagnosed at follow-up over months or years as having an organic disorder (Merskey, 1986).

Perhaps, after all, Anna O.'s hysterical behavior was *secondary* to a real organic disorder, but elevated to false primacy by psychoanalytically biased physicians. Unfortunately, current explanations invoking either organic disease or hysterical psychopathology seem inadequate to resolve this question. Nevertheless, the Anna O. case illustrates the nature and ambiguities of somatoform disorder—in particular, its psychological and neurological aspects. To get a better idea about these, we will first describe the behavioral symptoms of somatoform disorders. Then we will proceed to a discussion of *hysteria,* a theoretical term we use for the psychopathology that is believed to underlie at least some of the somatoform disorders (as well as dissociative disorders—see Chapter 17).

Briquet's Disorder

Occasional experiences with abdominal or chest pain, dizziness, headache, fatigue, and the like are quite prevalent, and often easily explained as normal reactions to stressful conditions involving bereavement, interpersonal conflict, or physical illness or injury (Lipowski, 1988). However, a somatoform disorder may be suspected when a persistent pattern of frequent and ever-changing somatic complaints cannot be explained simply as a matter of stress, or as symptoms of some other psychiatric disorder—major depression or anxiety disorder, for example—or medical disease.

While clinical descriptions of somatoform behavior go back to antiquity, systematic research on somatoform disorder is of much more recent vintage—in particular, research published in 1859 by Paul Briquet (pronounced brih-

KAY). Briquet studied 430 inpatient hysterics during a ten-year period (Mai & Merskey, 1980). The dominant symptoms reported by these subjects were medically inexplicable, yet classifiable into a few major categories: pain, anesthesia, paralysis, seizure, contracture, spasm, and altered sensation. The overwhelming majority of cases were female, and their first-degree relatives, especially if female, had a markedly elevated risk for the same symptoms.

Briquet concluded that a combination of genetic disposition and adverse circumstances caused hysterical disorder. The disposition was marked by emotional sensitivity and excessive impressionability, while the adverse circumstance included marital discord, death, separation, conflict, and prolonged illness. Briquet's diathesis-stress hypothesis is consistent with modern research, theory, and data on somatoform disorders.

SOMATOFORM DISORDERS AND SYMPTOMS

The category *somatoform disorder*, initially codified by *DSM-III*, includes, among other things, somatization disorder, hypochondriasis, and conversion disorder. Of these three, somatization disorder is by far the most researched.

Somatization Disorder

Diagnostic Criteria Briquet's description of what we we now call somatization disorder has stood the test of time. Currently it is represented, perhaps most closely, in the *Briquet hysteria* criteria of Perley and Guze (1962), shown in Table 16.1, and in the *somatization disorder* criteria of *DSM-III-R*, shown in Table 16.2. Differences between these two sets of criteria for somatization disorder are significant, however.

For example, dysphoric symptoms like panic or generalized anxiety and depression are considered "associated features" in *DSM III-R* but fundamental in Perley and Guze (1962). In fact, patients defined as somaticizers according to one set of criteria will sometimes not satisfy the other set (Cloninger, 1985, unpublished). More important, Perley and Guze criteria define a rarer and *severer* disorder, one that is more congruent with that described by Briquet (see Table 16.3), and one that shows clearer evidence of familial transmission. For these reasons, when we discuss data that are derived from patients diagnosed by Perley and Guze (or similar) criteria, we will use the term Briquet hysteria. Otherwise, we will use the terms Briquet hysteria and somatization disorder interchangeably.

Somatic Symptoms Briquet hysteria (somatization disorder) affects roughly 0.5 percent of the female population; it is extremely rare in males (Cloninger, 1985, unpublished). Typically, patients give vague but complicated medical histories so imprecise that the interviewer is often unable to follow the details. Past and present *polysymptomatic* complaints are described with great flair, but with insufficient specificity or distinction between essential and trivial. Consider symptom reports from some Briquet patients:

TABLE 16.1 PERLEY AND GUZE CRITERIA FOR DIAGNOSING HYSTERIA*

Group	Symptoms	Group	Symptoms
Group 1	Headaches Sickly most of life	Group 7	Dysmenorrhea Menstrual irregularity including amenorrhea for at least two months Excessive menstrual bleeding
Group 2	Blindness Paralysis Anesthesia Aphonia Fits or convulsions Unconsciousness Amnesia Deafness Hallucinations	Group 8	Sexual indifference Frigidity Dyspareunia Vomiting for all nine months of pregnancy or hospitalized for excessive vomiting in pregnancy
Group 3	Fatigue Lump in throat Fainting spells Visual blurring Weakness Dysuria	Group 9	Back pain Joint pain Extremity pain Burning pains of sexual organs, mouth, or rectum Other bodily pains
Group 4	Breathing difficulty Palpitation Anxiety attacks Chest pain Dizziness	Group 10	Nervousness Fears Depressed feelings Need to quit working or inability to carry on regular duties because of feeling sick Crying easily Feeling life was hopeless Thinking a good deal about dying Wanting to die Thinking of suicide Suicide attempts
Group 5	Anorexia Weight loss Nausea Abdominal bloating Food intolerances Diarrhea Constipation		
Group 6	Abdominal pain Vomiting		

*For strictly defined Briquet hysteria according to Perley and Guze, the person, prior to age 35, should have complained about at least 25 symptoms from nine of ten groups, with each symptom (a) interfering with the patient's life, and/or (b) associated with medication or drug taking, and/or (c) motivating the seeking of medical advice.
Source: Perley & Guze (1962). (Reprinted with permission from *The New England Journal of Medicine,* vol. 266, 421–426.)

Vomiting: I vomit every ten minutes. Sometimes it lasts for two to three weeks at a time. I can't even take liquids. I even vomit water. I can't stand the smell of food.

Food intolerance: I can't eat pastries. Always pay for it. I can't eat steak now. I throw up milk. I always throw up the skins of tomatoes.

Loss of consciousness: I passed out on the bathroom floor during my period and was still on the floor when they found me the next morning.

Weight change: I lose weight just walking down the street. I hold my breath and lose weight. I was down to 65 pounds at one time.

Dysmenorrhea: I can't work. Every month I am in bed for several days. I have

TABLE 16.2   DIAGNOSTIC CRITERIA FOR SOMATIZATION DISORDER

A. A history of many physical complaints or a belief that one is sickly, beginning before the age of 30 and persisting for several years.

B. At least 13 symptoms from the list below. To count a symptom as significant, the following criteria must be met:

1 No organic pathology or pathophysiological mechanism (e.g., a physical disorder or the effects of injury, medication, drugs, or alcohol) to account for the symptom or, when there is related organic pathology, the complaint or resulting social or occupational impairment is grossly in excess of what would be expected from the physical findings

2 Has not occurred only during a panic attack

3 Has caused the person to take medicine (other than over-the-counter pain medication), see a doctor, or alter lifestyle

Symptom list

Gastrointestinal symptoms

1 *Vomiting (other than during pregnancy)**

2 Abdominal pain (other than when menstruating)

3 Nausea (other than motion sickness)

4 Bloating (gassy)

5 Diarrhea

6 Intolerance of (gets sick from) several different foods

Pain symptoms

7 *Pain in extremities*

8 Back pain

9 Joint pain

10 Pain during urination

11 Other pain (excluding headaches)

Cardiopulmonary symptoms

12 *Shortness of breath when not exerting oneself*

13 Palpitations

14 Chest pain

15 Dizziness

Conversion or pseudoneurological symptoms

16 *Amnesia*

17 *Difficulty swallowing*

18 Loss of voice

19 Deafness

20 Double vision

21 Blurred vision

22 Blindness

23 Fainting or loss of consciousness

24 Seizure or convulsion

25 Trouble walking

26 Paralysis or muscle weakness

27 Urinary retention or difficulty urinating

Sexual symptoms for the major part of the person's life after opportunities for sexual activity

28 *Burning sensation in sexual organs or rectum (other than during intercourse)*

29 Sexual indifference

30 Pain during intercourse

31 Impotence

Female reproductive symptoms judged by the person to occur more frequently or severely than in most women

32 *Painful menstruation*

33 Irregular menstrual periods

34 Excessive menstrual bleeding

35 Vomiting throughout pregnancy

---

*The seven items in italics may be used to screen for the disorder. The presence of two or more of these items suggests a high likelihood of the disorder.

Source: American Psychiatric Association, 1987, pp. 263–264. Reprinted with permission from the *Diagnostic and Statistical Manual of Mental Disorders, Third Edition, Revised.* Copyright © 1987 American Psychiatric Association.

TABLE 16.3 ADDITIONAL STATISTICAL INFORMATION ABOUT SOMATIZATION DISORDER (BRIQUET-TYPE HYSTERIA)

Associated features	Anxiety, depression, conflict, and various types of personality disorder
Age at onset	Usually during the teen years
Course	Usually chronic with recurrence and variability of symptoms; the result is a large, weighty, and ever-growing medical record of unspecifiable "diseases"
Impairment and complications	Work inefficiency, frequent medical help-seeking, hospitalizations, and unnecessary (and therefore possibly dangerous) operations; suicide threats, attempts, and increased risk of actual suicide
Prevalence and sex ratio	About 0.5 to 1% of females and almost no males
Diagnostic pitfalls	Somatization may be secondary to organic or affective disorder, assuming that factitious disorder can be ruled out

had to have morphine hypos. There is a throbbing pain in the legs as if the blood does not circulate. Can't go to the bathroom as I faint.

Sexual indifference: Have never been interested. It's not a normal thing to me. Disgusting. I have no feelings. It's just a duty. (From Goodwin & Guze, 1979, p. 79, after Purtell, Robins, & Cohen, 1951)

Unfortunately, physicians often perform unnecessary surgical operations on these patients. By age 25 Briquet hysterics have had five times more surgery than normal controls and two and a half times more than other surgical patients (Cohen et al., 1953). Figure 16.2 gives locations and numbers of operations for hysteric and normal women. The excess is clearly in the abdominal region, where complaints are often vague but could signal something dangerously awry. This figure makes clear why the ancient Greeks named the disorder hysteria, or wandering uterus. It seems that abdominal complaints are among the most difficult to diagnose, with cautious physicians defensively suggesting operations which later prove to have been unnecessary.

Neurotic Features Briquet included impressionability and emotional reactivity in his concept of hysteria. Many clinicians have since noted the theatrical and calculating behavior of many hysterics. According to one, for example, "under the mask of comedy, caricature, clowning or trickery, there lies indeed a drama; but this drama is . . . like some law of insincerity, an organic law that falsifies his relations with other people" (Ey, 1982, p. 16).

Modern studies confirm that a large percentage of Briquet hysterics have serious emotional problems and many do have histrionic personality disorder (Kimble, Williams, & Agras, 1975). This disorder is marked by conflict-ridden tendencies to be dramatically self-expressive yet painfully self-conscious, provocative or even seductive yet rejecting, charming yet exasperating, happy-go-lucky yet prone to depression, seemingly world-wise yet naive and gullible,

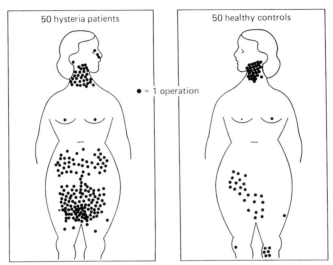

FIGURE 16.2 Comparison of number and location of major surgery procedures in fifty hysteria patients and fifty healthy control subjects. By weight, it can be calculated that the mass of organs removed in hysteria patients is more than three times that in control subjects. (Source: M. E. Cohen, E. Robins, J. J. Purtell, M. W. Altman, and D. E. Reid. Excessive surgery in hysteria. *Journal of the American Medical Association,* 1953, *151,* 977–986. Copyright © 1953, American Medical Association.)

richly imaginative yet without personal insight. (See also Chapter 3, p. 81, for additional description of this Axis II disorder.) The close connection between Briquet symptoms and histrionic traits and also the lifelong chronicity of the two suggest that somatization disorder, an Axis I category of *DSM-III-R,* might profitably be considered an Axis II personality disorder.

Hypochondriacal Features Somatization disorder may be accompanied by preoccupations with the possibility of hidden disease. There may also be an element of "doctor-shopping" as well as resistance either to negative medical findings or reassurance from the physician. In these cases where hypochondriacal features are especially prominent, the question of *hypochondriasis* versus somatization disorder may be raised (see Table 16.4).

[The hypochondriacal patient] notices various abnormal sensations, or even pains, and links these together in elaborate schemes that are incomprehensible to anyone else. He begins going from doctor to doctor presenting them with meticulously detailed descriptions of his symptoms, often accompanied by notes and diagrams. Every aspect of his treatment is followed to a ridiculous extent and he criticizes, distorts and attempts to influence doctors' opinions, becoming angry and emotional if this is resisted. Work is impossible, the patient's daily routine becomes minutely regulated, and he follows complex, self-devised regimes of medication. There is of-

TABLE 16.4   MAJOR DIFFERENCES BETWEEN BRIQUET DISORDER AND HYPOCHONDRIASIS

Characteristic	Briquet disorder	Hypochondriasis
Focus of complaint	Symptoms	Implication of symptoms, i.e., hidden disease
Style of complaint	Vague but colorful	Precise but affectless
Interaction with clinician	Attentive, seductive, grateful, trusting	Demanding, ungrateful, unreassurable
Age	20s–30s	30s–40s
Sex ratio	Usually female	Balanced or slightly more often male
Physical appearance	Often attractive	Often unattractive
Personality style	Hysteroid	Obsessive

ten a characteristic sombre, taciturn, introspective and self-centered affect, which however conceals genuine distress—and there may be considerable secondary depression (McKenna, 1984, p. 581).

Some clinicians believe that hypochondriasis involves unusual sensitivity to innocuous bodily sensations such as mild aches and pains, plus a cognitive factor that magnifies the sensitivity into morbid preoccupations and "doctor-shopping" during adulthood (Goleman, 1988a). The cognitive factor could originate from excessive parental anxiety about the child's somatic complaints. Some clinicians believe that there is a psychodynamic element as well, that many hypochondriacal patients defend against dysphoria and low self-esteem by displacing attention to bodily sensations (Ford, 1983; McKenna, 1984). These interesting speculations have yet to be verified. But the fact that anxiety and depression are freely expressed in some cases of hypochondria (Barsky, Wyshak, & Klerman, 1986) either casts doubt on the psychodynamic speculation or indicates a failure of defensive processes.

Conversion Symptoms   Somatization disorder patients sometimes display bizarre sensory and motor symptoms characterized by deficiency or excess—for example, hysterical anesthesia or convulsion, respectively (see Group 2 of the Perley and Guze system in Table 16.1). Conversion symptoms are somewhat controversial because they are both (a) *psychogenic*—they involve mental causality—and (b) *quasi-neurological*—they suggest neurological disease. Let us discuss the psychogenic quality first.

Conversion Symptoms as Psychogenic

Conversion symptoms are characterized as psychogenic when they seem to be self-serving, unconsciously motivated, and symbolically meaningful rather than caused by neurological disease. An obvious example would be a neurologically inexplicable paralysis of the legs in a soldier about to be sent to the front that disappears soon after discharge. (Conversion is a presumed mechanism in psychoanalytic theory by which unconscious conflicts are converted into a kind of body language. We need not adhere to the psychoanalytic explanation when using the term to mean psychogenic, however.)

In many cases, special tests can expose the psychogenic nature of the dysfunction. Consider the following examples.

Anesthesia-Analgesia The hysterical basis of lost bodily sensation (anesthesia) or lost pain sensation (analgesia) can be determined by evaluating certain qualities of the sensory loss. Conventional wisdom holds that, in contrast to neurological loss, hysterical loss involves an *abrupt transition* from unaffected to affected areas of the body where the sensory loss is evenly distributed within the affected area. For example, hysterical anesthesia of the hand is uniform from wrist to tip of fingers, a violation of the neurological "proximal-distal" rule which says: the further out on a limb, the greater the deficit. Thus, real sensory loss should be less at the wrist (proximal) and more toward the tips of the fingers (distal). Abrupt change from sensation above to anesthesia below the wrist indicates the influence of the patient's *idea* of hand over the normal sensory-neurological *map* of hand.

Paralysis Freud said, "Hysteria behaves in its paralyses and other manifestations as if anatomy were nonexistent, or if it had no knowledge of it" (Freud, 1893b/1959, p. 54). Like hysterical anesthesia, hysterical paralysis violates neurological rules in its uniform distribution and sharp demarcation from nonaffected areas. The hysterical basis of muscular weakness can be demonstrated by rather simple tests such as shown in Figure 16.3.

Blindness Hysterical blindness is a rare symptom that can occur bilaterally, unilaterally, or at the boundaries of the visual field, so-called tunnel vision (see Figure 16.4). Bilateral blindness is likely to be hysterical if there is evidence of a normal pupillary reaction to light and if there are jerky eye movements called nystagmus in response to a vertically striped pattern moving horizontally across the visual field.

The hysterical basis of unilateral blindness is revealed by the *lens test*. Suppose the patient complains of blindness in the right eye. A red lens is placed in front of the good (left) eye and the patient is asked to read a set of numbers, some printed in red and some in black. A patient with true unilateral blindness can read only the black numbers because the red lens in front of the good eye makes the red numbers invisible. Not knowing this, the hysteric reads all the numbers; this demonstrates that the "blind" eye is functioning normally since only it, and not the good eye, is free of the red lens.

The hysterical basis of tunnel vision (Figure 16.4) is demonstrated by what the patient reports seeing when moving toward or away from a stationary object. In real tunnel vision, the observable area of the object will vary with dis-

Elbow flexors

1. Patient is instructed to flex arm at elbow against resistance by examiner.

2. Examiner suddenly extends the arm, stretching flexor.

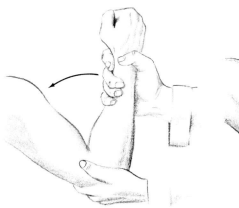
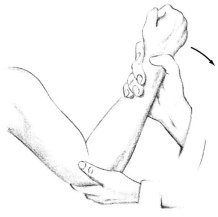

A. Response in organic paralysis

B. Response in hysterical paralysis

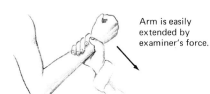

Arm is easily extended by examiner's force.

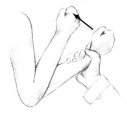

Arm extension is followed by involuntary flexion of the stretched muscle, indicating reserve strength.

Finger flexors

1. Patient grasps examiner's fingers.
2. Examiner suddenly jerks fingers back, stretching patient's flexors.

A. Response in organic paralysis

B. Response in hysterical paralysis

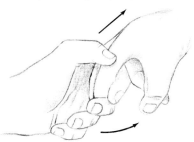
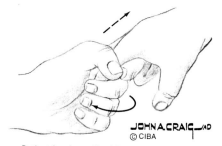

Patient's grasp is easily overpowered and examiner's fingers pull free.

Patient involuntarily tightens grasp on examiner's fingers.

FIGURE 16.3 Test for hysterical weakness in arm and hand. (Copyright © 1983. Ciba-Geigy Corporation. Reproduced with permission from *Ciba Collection of Medical Illustrations* by John Craig, M.D. All rights reserved.)

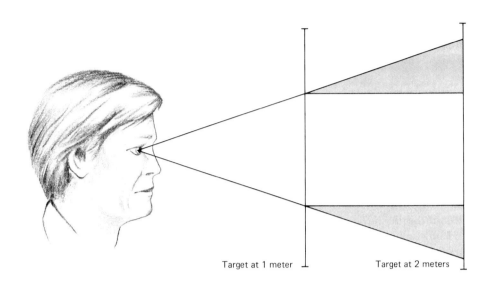

Target at 1 meter   Target at 2 meters

The normal visual field expands as a
cone of vision as the distance from
target to patient is increased.

JOHN A.CRAIG—MD
© CIBA

Normal visual field at 1 and 2 meters

2 m
1 m

Hysterical visual field at 1 and 2 meters

2 m
1 m

Normal field shows larger area at
2 meters than at 1 meter.

Hysterical fields are equal in size at
1 meter and 2 meters and may show "intertwining."

FIGURE 16.4   Test for hysterical tunnel vision. (Copyright © 1983. Ciba-Geigy Corporation. Reproduced with permission from *Ciba Collection of Medical Illustrations* by John Craig, M.D. All rights reserved.)

tance; in hysteria it will tend to remain the same. In other words, the neurological patient can see only a fraction of the *visual field* regardless of its content. In contrast, the hysterical patient can see only a fraction of some *object,* while blotting out other parts which presumably have special significance.

Deafness   An obvious test for hysterical deafness is to determine if auditory stimuli produce signs of physiological arousal during sleep. Another test involves the disruptive effect of auditory feedback. With a tape recorder and earphones, a person's speech can be fed back slightly delayed. The slight delay of feedback normally has a disruptive effect on speech unless there is profound hearing loss. Auditory feedback has been used to assess hypnotic "deafness" (Barber, 1969), and presumably could be used to test for hysterical deafness.

Convulsion   The hysterical basis of convulsive behavior can readily be inferred in many cases from certain indicators—for example, a normal EEG in the context of a "severe seizure," bodily movements and a variety of emotional expressions quite unlike the usual stereotypical convulsion, absence of "seizures" during sleep or when alone, and lack of memory impairments, confusion, or lethargy just after the episode (Fenton, 1982; Pincus, 1982). Nevertheless, hysterical convulsions are sometimes so true to form they can be misdiagnosed as epilepsy, and occasionally a true epilepsy expresses itself in such atypical forms that it is misdiagnosed as "hysteria" (Fenton, 1986). This is a good example of how difficult it is to determine if a quasi-neurological symptom is neurological (genuine though atypical) or pseudoneurological (fake).

Conversion Symptoms versus Conversion Disorder   Conversion symptoms usually are part of a syndrome like somatization disorder or depressive disorder; they rarely occur alone. They are typically stress-specific, time-limited, and nonrecurrent. When they do occur alone, they are diagnosed as conversion disorder.

Surprisingly little is known about conversion disorder or its relation to somatization disorder (American Psychiatric Association, 1980). For example, we do not know if it runs in families like Briquet disorder. We do know, however, that conversion disorder is more situation specific, arising in the context of personal crises or interpersonal conflict, and that, unlike Briquet disorder, it is *infrequently* associated with histrionic personality disorder (Chodoff & Lyons, 1958; Ljungberg, 1957; Ziegler, Imboden, & Meyer, 1960). Also, unlike Briquet disorder, conversion disorder is sometimes associated with a curious lack of concern, called *la belle indifférence*, which appears especially odd to the observer given the apparent seriousness of the claimed dysfunction. For example, a patient awakens with apparent blindness yet appears unconcerned. Finally, unlike Briquet syndrome, conversion disorder appears to involve denied or masked rather than overt depression (Katon, 1982; Matussek, Soldner,

& Nagel, 1982). Major differences between Briquet's syndrome and conversion disorder are listed in Table 16.5.

Conversion Symptoms as Quasi-neurological

The notion that somatoform disorders may reflect brain abnormality is relatively modern in comparison to the older notion that hysterical symptoms are caused by a wandering uterus. Uterine notions survived 3000 years until the seventeenth century when autopsies revealed that the uterus of hysterics is normally located (Veith, 1965). During the same century, a new hypothesis emerged about hysteria as a brain disorder. At least this hypothesis could explain male hysteria. Yet autopsies done in the late eighteenth century by Philippe Pinel suggested that the brains of hysterics were anatomically normal. Of course, the neurological methods of those days were too crude to rule out some hidden brain abnormality caused by neurological or somatic disease. Thus, even an anatomically normal-looking brain might be functioning abnormally.

Are Quasi-neurological Symptoms Fake (Pseudo) or Genuine?   As we have seen, somatoform symptoms, especially the converson type, can be called *quasi*-neurological because they suggest neurological disease, though ambiguously. Upon close inspection, quasi-neurological symptoms may turn out to be false, or *pseudo*neurological; on the other hand, they may be genuine, that is, atypical signs of neurological disorder (Merskey, 1986). Clearly, the validity of a diagnosis of somatoform disorder will depend on the *balance* of evidence.

Nevertheless, the frequent association of hysterical symptoms with real neurological disorder strongly suggests that some sort of hidden brain abnormality may indeed underlie the psychogenic symptoms of hysterical disorder.

TABLE 16.5   MAJOR DIFFERENCES BETWEEN BRIQUET AND CONVERSION DISORDER

Aspect	Briquet disorder	Conversion disorder
Typical symptom picture	Polysymptomatic	Monosymptomatic
Indifferent attitude	Rare	Relatively frequent
Situation specificity	Infrequent	Frequent
Duration	Chronic, recurring	Acute, nonrecurring
Depression	Typically manifest	Typically hidden (masked by defense mechanisms)
Histrionic personality disorder	Often concurrent	Rarely concurrent
Classification status	A syndrome	Probably not a syndrome
Theoretical status	Part of psychopathic spectrum (see Ch. 18)	Probably a symptom of any one of many disorders; e.g., depression

Let us take a closer look at research evidence bearing on this interesting diagnostic problem.

Diagnostic Ambiguities   During the past twenty-five years, researchers with increasingly sophisticated techniques have repeatedly documented a frequent association between somatoform disorders and brain abnormalities (Pincus & Tucker, 1978). Nevertheless, it is still easy to confuse conversion symptoms with underlying physiological abnormalities. This confusion stems from the fact that brain abnormalities can produce many of the classical symptoms of hysteria, including those quasi-neurological conversion symptoms that are often assumed to be pseudoneurological.

For example, Gould et al. (1986) found that most of their neurological patients displayed one or more of those classical hysterical symptoms that are supposed to rule out organicity. These included (a) conversion symptoms—for example, sharp boundaries and patchy areas on the skin separating deficient from normal sensory awareness, (b) changes in these symptoms in response to the doctor's suggestions, (c) a history of somatization and hypochondriasis, (d) la belle indifference, and (e) secondary gain, that is, using illness to avoid problems and evade responsibility.

Pincus and Tucker (1978) report experiences on a neurology ward over thirteen months. A total of 485 inpatients and outpatients were seen during that period, twelve of whom had either initially or finally received a diagnosis of conversion disorder. For these twelve the diagnosis had changed over time. Results are shown on Table 16.6.

The initial diagnosis was made by a referring physician, the final diagnosis on the neurology ward. Of the twelve, seven had an initial diagnosis of conversion disorder, but a final diagnosis of a neurological disease. Only two of these seven had a past history of psychosomatic symptoms. The five patients with an initial neurological diagnosis had a final diagnosis of conversion disorder. These five all had a previous history of psychosomatic complaints.

In short, not only are hysteric patients being reclassified as having brain abnormalities (Slater & Glithero, 1965; Whitlock, 1967; Shalev & Munitz, 1986), neurological patients with specifiable brain damage display many of the classic signs of hysteria. Incorrectly diagnosing a real neurological disease as "hysteria" could delay if not prevent treatment, and with life-threatening consequences.

A charming 45-year-old female we saw had complained of transient weakness in one arm, but repeated neurological examinations had been entirely negative; the diagnosis was conversion disorder. Her personal and professional life was satisfying and productive and there was no prior history of psychosomatic complaint. Unable to accept the diagnosis of conversion disorder, she arranged to enter a research hospital where psychological testing was entirely negative for any psychiatric disturbance. A meningioma (a tumor in the meninges lining of the brain) was subsequently discovered. Sadly, during surgery she died of hemorrhage. One cannot be sure that the operation would

TABLE 16.6 OCCURRENCE OF PSYCHOSOMATIC ILLNESS IN TWELVE PATIENTS CONSIDERED TO HAVE CONVERSION REACTIONS

Sex	Age	Chief complaint	Initial diagnosis by referring physician	Past history of psychosomatic symptoms	Final diagnosis
F	34	Generalized weakness	Conversion reaction	−	Parkinson's disease
M	40	Headache, amnesia	Conversion reaction	+	Meningitis
F	50	Seizure	Conversion reaction	+	Epilepsy
F	50	Generalized weakness, fatigue	Neuresthenia, conversion reaction	−	Cerebral metastases
F	35	Blindness	Conversion reaction	−	Uveitis-meningitis
M	50	Headache, ataxia	Conversion reaction	−	Cerebellar hemorrhage
M	32	Vertigo, ataxia	Hypochondriasis, conversion reaction	−	Ependymoma
F	21	Dyspnea	Lactose intolerance, migraine, diaphragmatic flutter	+	Conversion reaction
F	50	Hemianesthesia and paresis	Epilepsy, migraine, multiple sclerosis	+	Conversion reaction
M	40	Quadriparesis	Multiple sclerosis	+	Conversion reaction and multiple sclerosis
F	40	Seizures, paraparesis, ataxia	Epilepsy, multiple sclerosis	+	Conversion reaction
F	36	Ataxia, hemiparesis	Brain tumor	+	Conversion reaction

Source: From Pincus & Tucker, 1978, p. 266. (*Behavioral Neurology*, Oxford University Press. Reprinted with permission.)

have turned out differently had the tumor been discovered earlier. But the probability of organicity is enhanced when a psychological test battery rules out psychiatric disturbance.

If there is an association between hysteria and organicity, what can we conclude about those hysterical disorders in which, typically, brain abnormality cannot be detected (Roy, 1982)? The association does suggest that somatoform disorders may indeed be facilitated by a hidden *hysterical pathophysiology;* that is, a subtle *neurological* component of hysterical psychopathology. On the other hand, the association does *not* rule out other disposing factors such as social conditions that encourage somatization, especially in people with certain personality traits such as immaturity, suggestibility, repressiveness, and poor insight.

In short, the hysteria-organicity association takes us back full circle: behavior that initially suggests neurological disease (quasi-neurological) and then seems ''all in the head'' (pseudoneurological) may turn out to be, in part, a real neurological illness. The riddle of hysterical disorder may be especially tricky because it can involve both disease and deception, pathological play-acting in which the fakery is in some sense ''real.'' To understand this, we will need to look more closely at play acting, and then at the pathology of hysteria.

IS HYSTERIA MERELY SICK-ROLE PLAYING?

Hysterics do what normals sometimes do—exaggerate or even make up illness—but they are much more skillful and motivated. Sick-role behavior—acting like a sick person—can be mimicked by normal volunteers in laboratory studies, as we will see shortly. Outside the laboratory, sick-role behavior is a frequent feature of stress-induced reactions. It is a normal, often unconscious inclination of young children, the infirm aged, and anyone devastated by untimely disease.

As a chronic way of life, however, sick-role behavior—what is often called sick-role *playing*—is a symptom of psychopathology. It is common to all somatoform disorders, but it is often also seen in other psychiatric disorders—depression in particular—and, as we have seen, in medical disorders.

Sick-role playing provides certain "advantages": avoiding responsibility, deflecting attention from personal inadequacies or failures, attracting support, and even expressing resentment. But these advantages are costly, since they are paid for in the currency of restricted mobility, diminished self-respect, social disapproval, and decline in quality of life. In short, whether sick-role behavior is treated as normal or pathological will depend on duration, severity, and other factors.

Hysteria, Suggestibility, and Hypnosis

Normal and Hynotic Suggestibility   Nonetheless, many symptoms of medical illness can be simulated at will by normal individuals (Barber, 1969). Hypnotic induction encourages responsiveness to suggestion by dramatically reducing critical and self-conscious thinking. But hypnotic induction is not required to produce such psychological changes. Nonhypnotic methods employing highly credible suggestions can be used—for example, "This kind of thing is easy," or "You are the kind of person who can do it."

The extent to which normal individuals can be induced to simulate medical symptoms is insufficiently appreciated. Given the right conditions, attitudes, and expectations, normals can act as though suffering from anesthesia, blindness, paralysis, and other abnormalities (Barber, 1969). To illustrate, consider the cognitive changes experienced under hypnosis by Eugen Bleuler, one of the giants of psychiatry.

> Bleuler strove to cooperate with the hypnotist while keeping as much awareness as he could. He soon noticed that parts of his visual field were falling out, as it were. Finally, he could perceive only the contrast of light and shadow. He felt as though his eyes were moist and they burned slightly, but he felt relaxed. A comfortable warmth invaded his body from the head down to his legs; he felt no desire to move or to do anything, and it seemed to him that his thoughts were quite clear. He heard the hypnotist tell him to move his arms; he tried to resist the order, but failed partly. The hynotist then told him that the back of his hand was insensitive; Bleuler thought that this could not be true and that Von Speyr was joking when telling him that he was pricking it (which he was actually doing). He awoke as if from a slumber at the hypnotist's injunction (Ellenberger, 1970, p. 116).

You can now appreciate why many investigators believe that hysterics are particularly seduced by the *idea of sickness,* perhaps because they have learned that the only way they can cope with personal distress is by engaging their special ability to simulate sickness (Bliss, 1984b). This idea of sickness is often conditioned by prior personal experience with diseases such as epilepsy and bronchitis that have clear-cut symptoms (Munford & Liberman, 1982; Pincus, 1982). In fact, some patients mimic their own current medical symptoms—for example, *hysterico-epileptics* mimic their own true epileptic behavior, sometimes so skillfully that it may be difficult to distinguish the genuine from the fake!

Since the days of Liebeault, Bernheim, and the Nancy school a hundred years ago, psychiatrists have argued that hysteria is an abnormal exaggeration of the *normal* tendency to transform ideas about illness into somatic acts (Ellenberger, 1970). Ey (1982) writes of "this 'hysterical component' of the human spirit, that is to say its capacity to make use of mechanisms of expression in a dramatic or theatrical way" (p. 16). "Medical student's disease" exemplifies how the idea of disease, stimulated by textbook descriptions and exaggerated in fantasy, can magnify bodily sensations into a false disorder. Mass hysteria is another example of how the idea of disease can become exaggerated and affect many people within a group.

Mass Hysteria   One minute a single individual displays signs of real or hysterical illness. Soon thereafter, the "contagion" spreads to others. The "victims" may express any number of "symptoms" like coughing, dizziness, anxiety, crying, and even convulsion.

> Not long ago, at a high school football game in a suburb of Los Angeles, about a half-dozen persons reported feeling ill during halftime with severe symptoms of food poisoning. The examining physician ascertained that all of them had consumed soft drinks from the dispensing machine under the stands. He took into account two possibilities—one that the syrup might have been contaminated; the other that copper sulfate from the pipes leading to the dispensing units might have leaked into the beverage during the mixing process.
>
> In an effort to safeguard other spectators, the physician directed that an announcement be made requesting that no one consume soft drinks from the mixing machine. The announcement made reference to the persons who had food poisoning. The immediate result was that the entire stadium became a sea of retching and fainting persons. Hundreds rushed home and called their family physicians. Ambulances from five hospitals plied back and forth between the stadium and the emergency rooms. Some two hundred persons had to be hospitalized.
>
> Investigation yielded the information that there was nothing wrong with the soft drinks from the dispensing machine. When this word was passed along, the "ill" persons recovered as quickly and mysteriously as they had become ill (Cousins, 1984, p. 82).

Hysterical "disease" can be transmitted to receptive individuals under special situations. Initially an abnormal and unexpected event takes place, anything from psychotic behavior, distress signals, or physical events like a strange odor or bug bite (Kerckhoff, 1982). The anomalous event stimulates the idea of disease and triggers illness behavior in vulnerable individuals.

Vulnerability to mass hysteria is a function of (1) receptivity to the idea of disease, (2) empathy with others of a group, (3) personal stress, and/or (4) repressive cognitive style (Colligan, Pennebaker, & Murphy, 1982). Receptivity to the idea of disease is the prior sense that the disease has a high likelihood of occurring, whether from nuclear radiation, food poisoning, bacterial infection, or even evil spirits (Phoon, 1982). Empathy with others develops in groups that are relatively isolated psychologically or physically, as in schools, factories, or stadia. Somatic compliance with other people is a kind of togetherness (Sirois, 1982).

Stress can be an important factor in crystallizing hysterical responsiveness. Stress may be caused by monotonous conditions or information overload. It may be heightened further by the high arousal of emotional turmoil, or by ambivalence toward certain people. Another factor may be repressive cognitive style, a tendency to deny problems, that can create an "explosive potential" of pent-up frustrations interacting with the other factors (Kerckhoff, 1982). Although both sexes are susceptible, the majority of mass hysterias involve young females in schools, and older females in work settings. This sex difference in liability does not yet have a satisfactory explanation, though evidence that females are generally more suggestible than males may prove important (Eagly & Carli, 1981).

Hypnotic and nonhypnotic laboratory simulations of somatization and observations on mass hysteria suggest the following hypothesis. Hysterics are the "geniuses" of somatization: not only are they much better than normals at producing bodily symptoms, they do this more readily and more spontaneously (Bliss, 1984b).

Hysteria and Malingering

When an individual has frequent bodily complaints and behavioral symptoms of disease which cannot be substantiated medically, questions arise about *malingering,* the conscious effort to deceive. A good example is the feigning of illness or handicap in order to avoid military service.

It is often difficult to distinguish between malingering, where the motive is conscious, and hysteria, where it is unconscious. They are behaviorally and functionally similar, and they frequently co-occur; diagnosed hysterics and even medical patients sometimes invent "problems" to get more attention from a physician whom the patient suspects is insufficiently concerned. It is true that clinicians have traditionally viewed both hysteria and malingering as two kinds of deception (Ey, 1982). But the appearance of insincerity need not mean that somatoform disorders are merely forms of malingering.

Freud's great teacher, Charcot, argued forcefully that the unconscious, psychogenic psychopathology of hysterical (somatoform) disorder is different from malingering. As Freud describes it, partly because of Charcot's work,

"... gradually the sneering attitude, which the hysteric could reckon on meeting when she told her story, was given up; she was no longer a malingerer, since Charcot had thrown the whole weight of his authority on the side of the reality and objectivity of hysterical phenomena. Charcot had repeated on a small scale the act of liberation commemorated in the picture of Pinel which adorned the lecture hall of the Salpetriere" (Freud, 1893a/1959, pp. 18–19).

How can we distinguish malingering from true hysteria? First, hysterical complaints can occur despite good performance on neurological tests. In contrast, malingerers will always try to perform poorly on these tests by "faking bad." For example, a hysterically blind individual might perform perfectly on a visual detection task while continuing to claim blindness. This seemingly phony inconsistency would be avoided by the malingerer (Sackheim, Nordlie, & Gur, 1979).

Second, while sick-role behavior and even some medical symptoms such as coughing are relatively easy to simulate, as we have seen, certain somatoform symptoms are nearly impossible to simulate regardless of motivation. For example, Levy and Jankovic (1983) report that a patient who had complained about the adverse effects of her anticonvulsive medication responded to a placebo (saline) injection by lapsing into a "comatose state." During the *hysterical coma,* normally involuntary reflexes were absent: there was a loss of pupillary response to light, no optokinetic nystagmus in reaction to a moving vertical-stripe pattern, no postural reaction to pain, and no eye blink after the examiner touched her cornea. Amazingly, the absence of these primitive and normally involuntary reflexes was associated with a normal waking EEG, and, as revealed by subsequent testing, an excellent memory for all aspects of the test conditions!

How could someone lapse into an apparently comatose state where primitive involuntary reflexes disappear, yet continue to process complex information about the setting as if fully alert? The subject reported that during the deepest phase of the "coma" she hallucinated sinking into deep water and struggling to escape being caught in a net. Clearly, a reflexively nonresponsive, yet cognitively and affectively responsive, subject is not just malingering or role-playing. Role-playing theories cannot easily resolve such an extraordinary abnormality. Renaming it "skillful" role-playing is like saying that Einstein was merely a very good mathematician. In other words, whatever we call it, we need to know how it is done and why. For this reason, many investigators subscribe to the hypothesis that hysteria involves a unique type of psychology, and because of the evidence, a unique type of psycho*pathology.*

THE PSYCHOPATHOLOGY OF HYSTERIA

What kind of person displays *frequently* and *spontaneously* not only sick-role behavior that most people are capable of simulating—coughing, gagging, and bodily complaints, for example—but also rare and exotic behaviors, such as anesthesia, blindness, or paralysis? These latter symptoms might be achieved by some normals under highly suggestive conditions in the laboratory, but in the real world, they are not only difficult to produce, they are personally distressing and socially disruptive.

The question of individual differences in ability and motivation to somaticize suggests that hysteria is more than just role-playing (see Table 16.7). Rather, it is a form of psychopathology in which the normal tendency to identify somatically with disease is *exquisitely developed* and then activated under conditions of inner conflict. We will first look at the clinical and neuropsychological evidence of psychopathology in hysterics and their families, and then turn to some relevant theoretical formulations.

Concurrent and Familial Psychopathology

Clinical Evidence Hysteria has always connoted "sickness"—organic, psychopathic, demonic—depending on social or psychiatric fashions (Veith, 1965). Hysteria is a chronic condition with diverse symptoms which may change over time. According to Goodwin and Guze (1979) "twenty to thirty years of symptoms are typical, and patients who have had the illness for over forty years are not unusual" (p. 81).

Hysteria is associated with a wide variety of other kinds of psychopathology, both in patients with somatoform disorder (Shields, 1982; Slater, 1961) and in their first-degree relatives (Coryell, 1980; Ljungberg, 1957). These other kinds of psychopathology include organic, psychotic, neurotic, and psychopathic symptoms. The close association between the bodily and neurotic symptoms traditionally observed in somatization disorder is now represented explicitly in the Perley and Guze diagnostic criteria, which include anxiety and depression (Group 10).

Recent research on 859 Swedish female adoptees suggests a genetic factor (Sigvardsson et al., 1984). Analysis revealed two general types of somatization disorder: a "high frequency" type with two or more complaints per year, mostly about pain and discomfort, and a "diversiform" type marked by a much wider variety of somatic problems (Cloninger et al., 1984) (Table 16.8). Both types had elevated rates of criminality and alcohol abuse in the biological fathers (Bohman et al., 1984). These results, along with others to be discussed in Chapter 18, suggest an interesting hypothesis: some forms of somatization

TABLE 16.7   FOUR CATEGORIES OF DRAMATIC SELF-PRESENTATION*

	Normal	Pathological
Conscious	Acting	Malingering
Unconscious	Hypnosis	Hysteria

*The table suggests that hysteria represents a unique combination of unconscious and pathological factors separating it from other ways of dramatically presenting the self.

TABLE 16.8 SOMATIZATION DISORDERS

Female adoptees	Type 1 (high frequency)	Type 2 (diversiform)
Percentage of adoptee sample ($N = 859$)	4.8	12.0
Focus on headache, backache, stomach distress	More	Less
Psychiatric problems	More	Less
Sick leaves	More	Less
Diversity of problems per complaint	Less	More

Source: Adapted from Cloninger et al., 1984, and Bohman et al., 1984.

and antisocial behavior may be variants of a genetically influenced antisocial tendency (or *psychopathy*) whose behavioral expression is partly determined by sex.

Neuropsychological Evidence Riley (1984) compared neuropsychological test performance of Briquet, depressed, and normal controls selected from a large group of college students. Numerous sensory, motor, verbal, and other tests were used. Left-hemisphere function was assessed with tests of right-field sensory perception, verbal comprehension, and right-side motor skill and strength. Right-hemisphere function was assessed with tests of left-field sensory perception, visual and spatial comprehension, and left-side motor skill and strength.

The Briquet group performed relatively poorly on tests of left-hemisphere function, especially on tests of the left temporal and frontal areas. This performance deficit was particularly striking given the relatively good performance by the Briquet group on tests of right-hemisphere functioning. The Briquet group had elevated scores on many MMPI scales of neurotic and psychotic behavior. Figure 16.5 shows a remarkably similar profile both for Riley's young Briquet subjects and a group of older and more disturbed hysteric patients (Liskow et al., 1977).

There was an additional finding. For the Briquet subjects only, the *difference* between left- and right-hemisphere test scores correlated with scores on a questionnaire test of *dissociative* tendencies like absences, sleepwalking, and derealization. The greater the deficit of left relative to right hemisphere, the higher the score on the dissociation test. This correlation is consistent with the 100-year-old idea that a single brain abnormality underlies both the somatic and dissociative aspects of hysteria.

You will recall that at the turn of the twentieth century, leaders of the Salpetriere school of psychiatry in Paris were forging a neuropsychological theory of hysteria (Chapter 2, pp. 40–41). Charcot and his successor, Pierre Janet, argued that an "integrative force" of brain function normally maintains "dynamic tension" among reflexes, habits, and cognitive activities. In hyster-

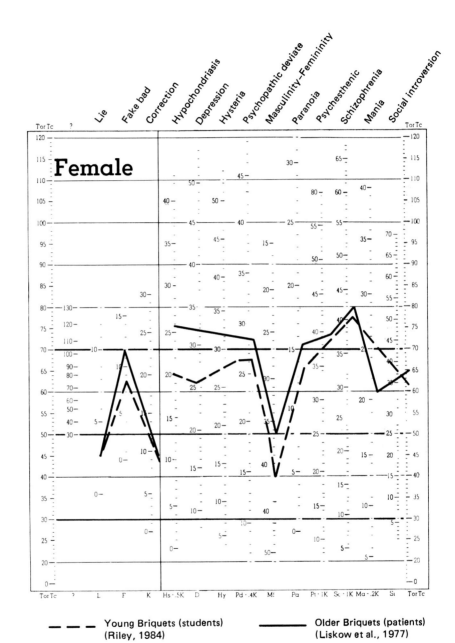

FIGURE 16.5   Average MMPI profiles for different hysterical groups. (See Chapter 4, pp. 98–99, for a description of MMPI.)

ical disorders, this integrative force is diminished for various reasons, including genetic and traumatic reasons. Under such disintegrative conditions, fragments of mental life can split off or *dissociate* from the rest. Dissociated fragments, though active and highly organized, remain unconscious. Nevertheless, under stressful conditions these fragments can gain control over cognitive, motor, and somatic behavior. This shift in control to dissociated processes is experienced by the hysteric as alien, involuntary, and inexplicable. As Janet describes it, "things happen as if an idea, a partial system of thoughts, emancipated itself, became independent, and developed itself on its own account. The result is, on the one hand, that it develops far too much, and, on the other hand, that consciousness appears no longer to control it" (Janet, 1920, p. 28).

Psychoanalytic Theory of Hysteria

Trauma and Repression   Freud differed from Janet in arguing that dissociated ideas are unconscious because they are *repressed*. They are repressed because they are associated with *traumatic* experience. Further, Freud argued that the strong affective "charge" of dissociated ideas could be *converted* into a bodily language of somatic disturbances. To this day, the term conversion implies unconscious personal *meanings*.

The concept of unconscious trauma is central to the psychoanalytic theory of hysteria. Freud (1896/1959) distinguished between two traumatic factors: an original traumatic experience that initially induces repression, and a current traumatic experience that weakens it. The original experience is traumatic because it involves (1) real danger occurring during early childhood, a time of great vulnerability; or (2) fantasied danger spontaneously arising like a nightmare. According to Freud, the original experience becomes unconscious through the active defense of repression so that the isolated, or "dissociated," experience remains affectively charged and therefore potentially disruptive. "Let no one object," he says, "that the theory of dissociation of consciousness as a solution of the enigma of hysteria is too far-fetched. . . . In fact the Middle Ages had chosen this very solution, in declaring possession by a demon to be the cause of hysterical manifestations; all that would have been required was to replace the religious terminology of those dark and superstitious times by the scientific one of today" (Freud, 1893a/1959, p. 20).

The second traumatic factor is any stressful condition in the current environment capable of diminishing repressive efficiency—for example, interpersonal conflict or a personal loss. Under conditions of weakened repression, a supplemental defense is mobilized to convert affectively charged ideas into a "language" of somatic symptoms. In short, a hysterical neurosis is the result of a traumatically induced, long-standing vulnerability interacting with a current provocation, thereby upsetting intrapsychic equilibrium and producing a "psychosomatic solution."

The meaning of a particular symptom requires analysis of mental life to discover its unique determining influences. Often, the process is effortful and time-consuming. However, under certain conditions, meanings may be revealed with little effort—for example, in a hypnotically induced crisis.

For instance, a little girl has suffered for years from attacks of general convulsions which might have been epilepsy and had in fact been taken for it. To establish a differential diagnosis she was hypnotized and was promptly seized by an attack. When asked: 'What do you see now?' she answered. 'The dog, the dog is coming!' Further inquiry revealed that the first attack of the kind had appeared after she had been chased by a mad dog. Therapeutic success later confirmed the diagnosis of a psychogenic malady (Freud, 1893b/1959, p. 37).

Sexuality Throughout its long history, hysteria has been connected in some way with sexuality, especially female sexuality. Eventually, notions about the wandering uterus gave way to hypotheses about abnormal sexual function. These hypotheses were based on observations that hysteria is often associated with sexual excess or restraint. Interestingly, Briquet concluded that, given the different rates of hysteria in nuns (low) and prostitutes (high), sexual restraint is probably not a causal factor in somatization disorders. Freud, you will recall, concluded just the opposite, at least in the case of middle-class neurotic patients.

According to Freud, the social psychological drama of oedipal conflict leaves repressed residues of affectively charged memories even in people who are sexually active or even promiscuous as adults. These residues can re-emerge in affectively charged social interactions of adulthood which are reminiscent of their earlier counterparts. You will recall that the basis of this idea was the erotic *transference,* the passionate attachment of patient to therapist which Freud considered to be the neurotic persistence of infantile patterns. For Freud, the passionate attachment of Anna O. to Breuer was a key to the great secret later revealed in the psychoanalytic theory of the oedipus complex. "The fact that a gross sexual, tender or inimical, transference occurs in every treatment of a neurosis, although this is neither desired nor induced by either party, has always seemed to me the most unshakable proof that the forces of the neuroses originate in the sexual life" (quoted by Brill, 1938, pp. 936–937).

This emphasis on sexuality created an unbreachable barrier between Freud and other psychiatric investigators. Janet, who differed with Freud on many aspects of hysteria (see Table 16.9), counteracted with numerous examples of severely hysterical women whose sexual functions were quite normal.

Evaluation Outside of psychoanalytic circles, there is little tolerance for a theory which gives so much explanatory weight to repressed memories of traumatically frustrated sexual strivings. Even those with great sympathy for psy-

TABLE 16.9 COMPARISON OF JANET AND FREUD ON HYSTERIA

Aspect	Janet	Freud
Model neurosis*	Dissociative disorder	Somatization (Briquet) disorder
Hysterical diathesis (genetic, neurological)	Important	Of varying importance
Dissociative mechanism (influence of affectively charged unconscious ideas)	Fundamental	Fundamental
Traumatic etiology	Important	Important
Repression (directed and purposeful forgetting)	Unimportant: does not explain low psychic "tension"	Fundamental: explains low psychic "tension"
Sexual motivation	Unimportant	Fundamental
Hypnoanalysis	Useful	Of little use
Dream analysis	Of some use	Essential
Psychoanalysis of somatic symbolism	Of some use	Essential

*The neurosis most often used to develop a theoretical model of hysteria.

choanalysis find monotonous the repetitive "discovery" of sexual solutions to any and all complex symptoms. And there is another problem, one having to do with any theory whose validity depends so heavily on the symbolic interpretation of behavior. According to Slater (1982), "the trouble is that with a little thought and imagination one can always find a 'symbolic' meaning for any symptom whatever—even, say, for an absent knee-jerk; and there is no objective way of proving oneself right or wrong in any interpretation one fancies. . . . Motives, like meanings, can always be supposed and can never be disproved; for, in classical depth psychology, both the patient's acceptance and his denial of a motivation are equally taken to confirm it" (p. 37).

Nevertheless, at least one aspect of the psychoanalytic theory is supported in research and, ironically, by one of Freud's severest critics. Eysenck (1982) reports questionnaire data showing that students with high scores on a test of hysterical disposition are especially conflicted over sexuality. His inference is that hysteria-prone individuals are "overwhelmingly sex-oriented, with an almost unbearable degree of tension and sexual excitement induced through a very strong libido" (p. 76). Briquet-prone individuals seem to be unhappy, guilt-ridden, and hostile with regard to sex partners. Eysenck concludes that sexual and inhibitory forces within personality are unstably balanced and in a high state of tension.

Assuming that these inferences apply to hysteric patients with various somatoform disorders, they are roughly consistent with psychoanalytic views about intrapsychic conflict over sexuality. However, they say nothing about the origins of the problem, whether erotic, traumatic, frustrative, or repressive. On these questions, the scientific literature is largely incomplete.

The singular emphasis on sexuality was modified in subsequent versions of psychoanalytic theory. Aggressive motivation was recognized as another fundamental type of pleasure striving along with the libidinal one. If the frustration of aggressive as well as sexual motivation can promote somatization, why not the frustration of fundamental motives involving security, affiliation, curiosity, mastery, etc.? There is simply no way to decide on scientific grounds what motivation is being converted, *if any*.

> Why does the patient have to resort to bodily language? Does the symptom communicate a single meaning, express a single thwarted impulse, or does it convey so many meanings that we could call overdetermined, literally choked with meanings? Why is it so stubborn, so resistant to therapy? Because it somehow "binds anxiety" and serves as a kind of bodily scapegoat to carry away guilt? Because it justifies nonfeasance, and enlists sympathy and pity from those who surround the patient? Because it bars a course of action demanded by impulses that are taboo (aggressions, cowardice, lust)? Because it is a way of getting even, of expressing hatred and of settling old scores, of defeating a stubborn mother who has insisted upon a hateful course of action? Because it is a roundabout way of preserving a dependent status, of finding security, of being excused from military service, of avoiding marriage or a career (Cole, 1970, pp. 294–295)?

Despite centuries of speculation and scientific research, the psychopathological concept of hysteria remains largely uncertain. We may profitably argue that it is not merely role-playing, malingering, or hypnosis, but we are on less sure ground when attempting to explain exactly what it is. And as we will see in the next chapter, our uncertainty is multiplied with respect to the even more mysterious dissociative type of hysterical disorders. The irony is that hysteria, seemingly the most psychogenic of disorders, also seems most refractory to satisfactory psychological explanation.

PSYCHOLOGICAL TREATMENT

Currently there are no controlled studies of psychological treatment of somatization disorder. Most such patients drop out of psychological therapies, often preferring medical treatment. The remainder represent a select group of patients unusually receptive to psychotherapeutic efforts (Ochitill, 1982).

General Strategies

In general, psychological therapies employ two general strategies. One focuses on hypothetical vulnerabilities arising out of personality development which somatization presumably reflects. This is the strategy of the talking therapies like psychoanalysis. The other strategy focuses on the eliciting and reinforcing events which sustain abnormal behavior whatever its causes. This is the strategy of behavioral therapies.

Because the problem of somatization is "in the head," therapists may be tempted to use placebo treatments that suggest "strong medicine"—for example, saline injection, sugar pill, or some hocus-pocus manipulation. However, the use of placebos is questionable on ethical grounds—it involves deception while conveying the idea that self-exploration and personal responsibility are of little importance—and also on pragmatic grounds to the extent that it reinforces sick-role behavior (Morrison, 1978). Nevertheless, the absence of systematic evaluation of the placebo treatment of hysteria makes the question difficult to resolve.

Like placebos, drugs may sometimes seem preferable to the more laborious process of uncovering psychological meanings and mechanisms.

> The physician should brace himself for some pretty unpleasant feelings of his own. Conditioned as doctors are to the concept of cure, they have trouble tolerating the patient who never improves. Week after week of continuing complaints which fail to yield to his best therapeutic efforts inevitably raises feelings of inadequacy and guilt in the most competent and conscientious physician. Uncertainty as to the next therapeutic step adds to his anger, and his instinctive reaction will be to excise the patient from his practice (Morrison, 1978, p. 458).

But like placebos, drugs carry potentially unacceptable costs. With drugs there is usually a possibility of addictive potential and unpleasant side effects.

Specific Techniques

Rewards and Punishments Whatever the etiology, specific behaviors are subject to the controlling influence of eliciting and reinforcing stimuli which can be altered or blocked for therapeutic purposes. For example, the chronic hysterical cough of a 17-year-old girl was treated successfully by having family members ignore the coughing while solicitously attending to and otherwise rewarding normal behaviors (Munford & Liberman, 1982). Without a payoff for the "illness," an important reason for coughing was removed.

Rewards and punishments can be used in the *shaping* of gradually better approximations to behavioral normality. For example, hysterical tremor was treated successfully by requiring the patient to place a stylus into successively smaller holes to avoid shocks (Liversedge & Sylvester, 1955). The following illustrates the gradual shaping of normal speech in an hysterically mute female.

> The mutism was treated by means of a reinforcement strategy called shaping; that is, rewarding the patient with weekend home visits for successive steps toward normal speech. Since she maintained rigid shoulder, head, and neck muscles and wrote that she could not control jaw and lip movements, the first behaviours to be shaped were those requiring control of these muscles. She was instructed to perform progressively ordered exercises that resulted in her accomplishing neck rolls, tongue extensions, lip pursing, grinning, and parting her teeth. Her next task was to increase control of inhalation and exhalation. After this, sound production began with plosives, then moving to consonant and vowel combinations. The final behaviours were the pronunciation of words, followed by phrases and sentences. Initially, Jennifer's speech consisted of single-word utterances at a barely audible level. How-

ever, 6 weeks later she was discharged from the hospital speaking fluently and appropriately (Munford & Liberman, 1982, p. 291).

Systematic Desensitization   The anxiety of somatization disorder may coalesce around specific situations or behaviors. In such cases it may be possible to achieve therapeutic goals by utilizing systematic desensitization. The sick-role behavior of somaticizing patients may serve the purpose of avoiding social interactions or social responsibilities. One strategy would be to get the patient to approach the feared behaviors in successive steps, either in imagination or in vivo. With the right amount of encouragement and praise at each step this treatment can be effective (Munford & Liberman, 1982).

Assertiveness Training   Many somaticizing patients are profoundly *neurasthenic,* that is, passive, weak-willed, and anergic. This debilitating style can sometimes be overcome by encouraging personal and interpersonal assertiveness. For example, a neurasthenic woman with hysterical pain was trained to be more assertive at work—saying no to requests for overtime work, for example—and at home—making requests of her husband for help with housework. In addition, she was required to keep a diary to document increasing assertiveness skills and decreasing pain. Within two weeks, hysterical symptoms had subsided and work efficiency had improved (Munford & Liberman, 1982).

Moral Support   All therapies, whether psychoanalytic, behavioral, or pharmacological, involve a certain amount of moral support for the patient as a person. Engaging the therapeutic efforts of the family is particularly important because so much of the problem is interpersonal and often domestic.

> In working with the family, keep in mind the enormous frustrations relatives face. Living with someone who must be hauled around from doctor to doctor, who takes 15 to 20 pills a day, who cannot care for herself let alone the house or the children, and who requires frequent trips to the emergency room for overdoses and suicide gestures is enough to try the patience of a saint. The complete physician should therefore be ready to support the family in moments of crisis and to retain his perspective when relatives behave less than therapeutically (Morrison, 1978, p. 458).

SUMMARY

Somatization disorder, first codified by Paul Briquet during the nineteenth century, refers to polysymptomatic bodily complaints about pain, sensorimotor deficits, gastrointestinal discomfort, altered consciousness, and dysphoria. The psychogenic and character-neurotic nature of the disorder is strongly suggested by its hypochondriacal and pseudomedical qualities, supporting the idea that severe somatization is both a symptom and a personality disorder, just as Paul Briquet suggested more than a century ago.

Modern research has repeatedly found a frequent association between hysterical symptoms and clear-cut brain disorder. Research also suggests a subtler neuropsychological abnormality of left-hemisphere function in somatization disorder even where hard signs of brain abnormality are lacking. Concomitant affective, psychopathic, and addictive symptomatology in hysteric patients and their biological relatives further reinforces the idea that somatization disorder is one expression of a distinct psychopathological spectrum of disorders. If a specific biological liability factor does exist for hysteria, it is still unclear to what extent it is sufficient to produce somatization disorder. Also, we still do not know how important environmental factors are in themselves or as potentiators of the biological liability.

In many ways somatoform and dissociative disorders seem to be the most psychogenic of the psychopathologies, yet they have defied psychological theorizing. Questionnaire data support at least the idea that somaticizing patients are highly conflicted over sexuality and are emotionally ambivalent in their interpersonal relationships. Research on mass hysteria and hypnotic simulation of illness supports the argument that individual differences in suggestibility, inner conflict, and personal identification with illness are important factors. The occasional appearance of spectacular pseudoneurological behaviors—for example, hysterical coma—that are nearly impossible to simulate even under deep hypnosis suggest abnormal "abilities," perhaps reflecting an abnormal combination of the exaggerated tendencies of normal people to somaticize when distressed or when exposed to conditions that reward sick-role behavior.

The idea that somatization disorder reflects psychopathology has a long history. Turn-of-the-century investigators like Charcot and Janet hypothesized a "weak nervous system" subject to *dissociation*; that is, the splitting of mental life into separate, poorly coordinated, mutually competitive parts that cause abnormalities of bodily experience, altered states of consciousness, and conflict-ridden behavior. The most ambitious psychological explanation was the Freudian view that the dissociative mechanism of hysteria is caused by trauma-induced repression of oedipal frustrations. What this influential theory offers in complexity and ingenuity is often offset by nontestability or disconfirmation.

CHAPTER 17

Dissociative Disorders

OUTLINE

INTRODUCTION

Early in the 1950s a 25-year-old woman was referred to Dr. Corbett Thigpen for treatment of severe headaches. Eve White, a modest and restrained person, was obviously disturbed about her headaches and depressed about an unhappy marriage. During one session she admitted hearing voices and feared she might be going insane. While the therapist grappled with this revelation, a dramatic event began to unfold.

> As if seized by a sudden pain she put both hands to her head. After a tense moment of silence, her hands dropped. There was a quick, reckless smile and, in a bright voice that sparkled, she said, "Hi there, Doc!"
>
> The demure and constrained posture of Eve White had melted into buoyant repose. With a soft and surprisingly intimate syllable of laughter, she crossed her legs. Disconcerted as he was by unassimilated surprise, the therapist noted from the corner of his awareness something distinctly attractive about them, and also that this was the first time he had received such an impression. There is little point in attempting here to give in detail the differences between this novel feminine apparition and the vanished Eve White. Instead of that retiring and gently conventional figure, there was in the newcomer a childishly daredevil air, an erotically mischievous glance, a face marvelously free from the habitual signs of care, seriousness, and underlying distress, so long familiar in her predecessor. This new and apparently carefree girl spoke casually of Eve White and her problems, always using *she* or *her* in every reference, always respecting the strict bounds of a separate identity. When asked her own name she immediately replied, "Oh, I'm Eve Black" (Thigpen & Cleckley, 1954, p. 137).

The new personality was a vain, self-indulgent, provocative "travesty of a woman" and markedly different from the other. In some ways she seemed healthier than Eve White, yet in other ways almost "defective." For example, while exuberant, resourceful, and self-reliant, she was curiously detached, "apparently almost as free of hatefulness or of mercy, or of compassion, as a bright-feathered parakeet who chirps undisturbed while watching a child strangle to death" (Thigpen & Checkley, 1954, p. 138).

Some time later, Eva White dissolved into Jane, the hoped-for integration of Eve White and Eve Black. Unfortunately, this apparent resolution was illusory. "Eve" eventually wrote a book clarifying many things about her case, including over twenty personalities, most of whom were unknown to Dr. Thigpen (Sizemore & Pittillo, 1977). In describing the riot of personalities seemingly out of control, she asks:

> Did the others come because I could not live with my reality? But other people face these same realities. Why was I different? Others have stood and faced fear, while I ran! Why? Why? There *must* be some answers. Do all people have this potential? Or was I born lacking something or having too much of something (Sizemore & Pittillo, 1977, p. 38)?

A tentative answer to these fundamental questions requires that we consider *dissociative disorders* in which psychological functions become isolated and autonomous from the rest of personality. The result is any number of anomalous behaviors, including amnesia, personality change, and somatization, all of which defy ready explanation.

PSYCHOGENIC AMNESIA AND FUGUE

Included in the dissociative disorder category of *DSM-II-R* are psychogenic amnesia, psychogenic fugue, and multiple personality. The first two of these, discussed next, involve striking lapses of memory. Multiple personality encompasses a complex pattern of such lapses and much more, as we will see later.

Psychogenic Amnesia

> A 38-year-old woman approached a policeman in New York City, reporting that she had forgotten her name. The last thing she remembered was going out for something to eat, feeling hungry and cold. Following her admission to Bellevue Hospital, she slept the remainder of the night, awakening the next morning having spontaneously regained her memory. On inquiry, it was found that she had recently returned to her husband in New York, reluctantly terminating a love affair in Florida (Abeles & Schilder, 1935, quoted by Aalpoel & Lewis, 1984, p. 225).

Definition   Psychogenic amnesia is a sudden and selective inability to recall significant *personal* information such as one's name and family, but not general information. Collectively, the following features suggest a psychogenic rather than an organic basis. The recall failure is too extensive for ordinary forgetfulness, but too selective to suggest any obvious organic brain disorder. Also, there is a normal ability to store *new* information, something not typical of conventionally defined organic amnesias (Wickelgren, 1979). Finally, the amnesia may be *completely* dissipated by using suggestion, hypnosis, or a sedative like sodium amytal—a barbiturate that dramatically reduces anxiety. Amnesias due to brain lesions, in contrast, can be made worse by sodium amytal.

Psychogenic amnesia is self-limiting, typically lasting only a few days. While rare—the exact prevalence is unknown—it is the most frequent of the dissociative disorders. It strikes females mostly in the second or fourth decade, and, less frequently, males who are under extreme personal stress—for example, under combat conditions.

Etiology and Treatment Like other dissociative disorders, psychogenic amnesia frequently involves crises, conflicts, and frustrated needs. Sometimes the condition can be traced to extreme ambivalence, love-hate conflicts which seem impossible to resolve without total forgetfulness. There are no relevant familial, twin, or adoption studies, and consequently nothing can be inferred with confidence about etiologically significant genetic or environmental factors.

Little is known about effective treatment. Obviously, psychological support can be employed while therapist and client wait for spontaneous remission. Sometimes hypnosis or sodium amytal is used in conjunction with free association and encouragement to explore the psychodynamics of hidden memories, all in the hope of accelerating remission. In the absence of systematic research, the effectiveness of such procedures cannot be evaluated.

Psychogenic Fugue

Roughly 100 years ago, an evangelist named Ansel Bourne disappeared from his home in Providence, Rhode Island. The noted psychologist William James described the case as follows.

> This morning Mrs. Bourne, the wife of Rev. Ansel Bourne, called at police headquarters and reported that her husband had been missing since Monday last. Rev. Mr. Bourne is quite widely known as an evangelist, and during the past twenty-five years he has carried on his religious work in various parts of the United States. For some years, it is said, he has been subject to attacks of a peculiar kind, which rendered him temporarily insensible, and on some occasions he has remained in an unconscious state for many hours.
>
> On January 17, 1887, he drew 551 dollars from a bank in Providence with which to pay for a certain lot of land in Greene, paid certain bills, and got into a Pawtucket horsecar. This is the last incident which he remembers. He did not return home that day, and nothing was heard of him for two months. . . . On the morning of March 14th, however, A. J. Brown, who had rented a small shop six weeks previously, stocked it with stationery, confectionery, fruit and small articles, and carried on his quiet trade without seeming to any one unnatural or eccentric, woke up in a fright and called in the people of the house to tell him where he was shopkeeping, and that the last thing he remembered—it seemed only yesterday—was drawing the money from the bank, etc., in Providence. He would not believe that two months had elapsed (quoted by Nemiah, 1980a, p. 1544).

James had the opportunity to hypnotize Bourne, who was then able to recall in great detail his experiences as Brown but nothing of his experiences as Bourne. "He had heard of Ansel Bourne, but 'didn't know as he had ever met the man.' When confronted with Mrs. Bourne, he said that he had 'never seen the woman before'" (James, 1890, quoted in Abse, 1982, p. 173).

Definition Psychogenic fugue involves sudden flight from one's home or customary place of work, adopting a new identity, and having amnesia for prior experiences. The amnesia is selective. While there is typically no loss of general information, skills, language, and cultural mores, there is amnesia for the original self, relatives, and friends. Sometimes the person is not even aware of any loss of memory. Unlike malingerers, but like the organic patient with anosognosia, the person with psychogenic fugue seems unflustered by confrontation with such apparent absurdities (Fenton, 1982). Unlike epileptics, this person experiences no auras prior to the fugal state. Unlike the multiple personality (discussed later), the person adopts just one new identity in the new location, usually a less colorful personality than the original. Also, there is mutual amnesia across the two identities—neither knows about the other—unlike the one-way amnesia typical for multiple personalities when one personality usually has full knowledge of the others. Finally, fugue more typically involves males, while multiple personality more typically affects females.

The new identity in psychogenic fugue is typified by a narrowness of existence. Observers are impressed by the single-mindedness and restricted emotion of the individual. Do these qualities help sustain the amnesia? To answer these questions, we need to know more about memory.

Memory and Psychogenic Amnesia The reversibility of psychogenic amnesia associated with fugue makes clear that the problem is *retrieval,* not the failure to store information. Interestingly, an analysis of dream content sometimes reveals lost memories relating to the original personality and living conditions. An example is the case of the Rev. Mr. Hanna, who developed a new identity away from home. The meaning of his dreams escaped him but was transparent to his relatives when they had the opportunity to hear them. In one instance, his father mentioned a place called Marinoe which had appeared in one of Hanna's dreams. Hanna's reaction was "How can you know all this, it was only a dream" (Nemiah, 1980a, p. 1546)!

How can large chunks of personally significant events be lost? One clue is that recall is impaired when certain qualities of mental function change radically from what they were. Thus, in a waking state we have trouble recalling dream experiences; when in a happy state we have trouble recalling sad experiences; and when in a sober state we have trouble recalling drug-related experiences (Bower, 1981; Cohen, 1979; Swanson & Kinsbourne, 1979). The common factor in these examples seems to be an incongruity between the mental activity and the organization of subjective experience during these initial events and later memories of them. Radical incongruity in mental activity and psychological organization across time could underlie amnesia, even for parts of the self. This analysis is fully compatible with observations that the amnesic person appears different while displaying no loss of intellectual competence.

But how would such discontinuities occur? One possibility is an abnormal shift in neural function, perhaps stimulated by stress or a physiological instability. Clinicians have long noted similarities between epileptic and dissociative disorders—for example, both can involve complicated behaviors for which there is total amnesia. Does psychogenic amnesia represent some sort of seizurelike shift in brain function with a corresponding block of memory? Then why is the amnesia so selective, typically involving personal experiences and even one's own identity but not impersonal information?

Another possibility is that amnesia could be affected by a willful shift in the thinking of a highly motivated, neurologically normal individual who is role-playing amnesia. Consider the similarity between psychogenic and posthypnotic amnesia. How does a person comply with a suggestion made during hypnosis that newly learned material be forgotten posthypnotically, that is, after the hypnotic induction has been removed? The answer may lie in how thinking is *organized* posthypnotically, so that there is a mismatch in the subjective organization of certain information during initial experience and later during attempts to remember that experience. In other words, memory will fail if the mental rules for retrieving memories are different from the mental rules for organizing specific earlier experiences. This *mismatch* of mental rules may explain why, more generally, adults—using their ''logical'' style of thinking—have so much trouble recalling childhood experiences that are organized in memory according to ''prelogical'' rules (Wilson & Kihlstrom, 1986). Unfortunately, researchers do not know if the psychological changes underlying naturally occurring psychogenic amnesia correspond to those in experimental amnesia and what role, if any, a brain abnormality plays in the psychiatric disorder.

In sum, physiological and psychological approaches to psychogenic amnesia are two ways of explaining the same phenomenon. One focuses on brain dysfunction—for example, seizurelike abnormalities—and the other focuses on mental dysfunction caused by cognitive discontinuities. The real problem is that neither explanation, nor the relevant research on each, is developed enough to enable us to decide if one is valid and the other is false, or if they are actually two valid ways of explaining the same phenomenon, one in the language of neural mechanisms and the other in the language of mental mechanisms.

Etiology and Treatment   The etiology of psychogenic fugue is uncertain though, like psychogenic amnesia, it seems to involve crisis and conflict, with anxiety and depression occurring prior to onset of the condition. Clinical writings suggest the possibility that the high-conflict state may induce a seizurelike condition unique to dissociative disorders, but this is pure speculation. ''The dissociated personality in fugue is acting out a wish-fantasy, and consciousness is suffused with feelings of well-being; these replace the consciousness of frustration and the feelings of ill-being that preceded the fugue'' (Abse, 1982, p. 175).

Uncertainties surround the question of treating dissociative disorders. Like psychogenic amnesia, psychogenic fugue usually calls for supportive psychotherapy with adjunctive hypnosis. However, the absence of systematic research makes impossible any confident evaluation of treatment effectiveness.

MULTIPLE PERSONALITY DESCRIBED

We turn now to a disorder that has the elements of psychogenic amnesia, psychogenic fugue, and more. Multiple personality is one of the most bizarre and compelling of all the behavior disorders.

Formal Definition

Consider the following comprehensive definition of multiple personality.

> Multiple personality . . . refers to the presence of one or more alter personalities, each possessing presumably different sets of values and behaviors from one another and from the "primary" personality, and each claiming varying degrees of amnesia or disinterest from one another. The appearance of these personalities may be on a "conscious" basis (i.e., simultaneously coexist with the primary personality and aware of its thoughts and feelings) or a separate consciousness basis (i.e., alternating presence of the primary and other personalities with little or no awareness or concern for the feelings and thoughts of each other) or both (Ludwig et al., 1972, pp. 298–299).

This definition includes two general criteria, one relating to the *structure* of each personality, or alter, and the other to their *gnostic* relationships, that is, the way that each alter knows (or is agnosic regarding) any of the others (see Table 17.1). Let us take a closer look at the structual and gnostic aspects of multiple personality.

Personality Structure In many cases each alter is a distinct personality with a unique and coherent set of features reliably organized over time. Cognitive features include thinking style, attitudes, and values. Temperamental features include emotionality, sociability, tastes, energy, outlook, and sexual orientation. Behavioral features include posture, handedness, handwriting, and general bearing. Somatophysiological features include the presence or absence of specific allergies, physical health, sensitivities, or insensitivities (to foods—for example), and visual acuity (Coons, 1988). There are often sex and age differences, for example, one personality may be a 3-year-old boy while another is an older woman.

Striking discontinuities across personalities can exist, some straining credulity. For example, personality X might be allergic to cats while personalities Y and Z are not.

> The doctor was amazed. Was it possible that one personality had an allergy and the other one did not? That the body reacted chemically to nylon when one personality was out, and that the reaction ceased immediately when the other one emerged? He quickly called out Mrs. White, and while casually questioning her, he watched her

TABLE 17.1 STRUCTURAL AND GNOSTIC ASPECTS OF MULTIPLE PERSONALITY

Features	Explanation
A. Structural Aspects	What is multiple personality?
1. Complex	Personality refers to a *multiplicity* of cognitive, affective, motoric, and somatophysiological traits.
2. Coherent	Each personality consists of a unique set of traits noticeably *different* from any other(s).
3. Consistent	Each personality is unerringly reproduced time after time. In short, it is *temporally reliable.*
B. Gnostic Relationships	How does each personality know about the other?
1. Inferential	Knowledge is indirect and abstract if based solely on *inference*—for example, from certain telltale signs like unraveled knitting, strange letters, or comments from friends about uncharacteristic behavior for which one has no memory but for which there is concrete evidence.
2. Mnestic	Knowledge can be based solely on *memory.* While a personality (usually the "primary") may be entirely *amnestic* (without memory) for the other(s), it may be knowledgeable through memories of the other(s)' experiences when it "comes out."
3. Perceptual	Knowledge can be based on *sensory information* as well as memory. In this case, the knowledge is immediate, and the knowledgeable personality is called a *co-conscious.* The co-conscious personality thus has concurrent consciousness of the perceptions and thoughts of the other, even though the other is completely unconscious of the co-conscious.

attitude carefully: She never once touched the red, blotchy legs or in any way indicated any discomfort. Before the doctor's incredulous eyes, the angry red quickly receded from the now motionless legs, leaving them their usual unblemished white (Sizemore & Pittillo, 1977, p. 297).

One personality may be pain-sensitive while the other is anesthetic. One may be tired and depressed, even suicidal while the other is energetic and happy. Clara Norton Fowler, immortalized by Morton Prince (1906/1969) as "Miss Beauchamp" (pronounced BEE-chum), displayed during the early stages of her therapy the classic *neurasthenic* pattern of symptoms typical of the initially presenting personality, the one first seen by the therapist. B I, as she was called by Prince, complained of aches, pains, insomnia, fatigue, and aboulia, a "failure of will" marked by lack of energy and pervasive inactivity. In contrast, the "Sally" personality (originally called B III) was vibrant, active, and insensitive to pain.

Sally has a peculiar form of *anesthesia.* With her eyes closed she can feel nothing. The tactile, pain, thermic, and muscular senses are involved. You may stroke, prick, or burn any part of her skin and she does not feel it. You may place a limb in any posture without her being able to recognize the position which has been assumed. But let her open her eyes and look at what you are doing, let her join the visual sense with the tactile or other senses, and the lost sensations at once return (Prince, 1906/1969, pp. 147–148).

Even more exotic contrasts have been reported (Goleman, 1988b; Coons, 1988). For example, one personality may perspire noticeably in a warm room in which an alter does not; one personality may wear prescription glasses while another does not; one may suffer diabetes while another shows no diabetic symptoms; one may claim to be blue-green color blind while another is not; or one may be allergic to citrus fruit while another is not. Few of these contrasts have been validated, so it is not yet clear what is really going on—for example, if a difference across personalities in the use of prescription glasses indicates a real difference (change) in visual acuity.

Multiple personality does not always involve dramatically abrupt shifts among strikingly distinct, fully formed personalities. For one thing, some of the alters have no clear-cut sense of identity, continuity over time, or even a proper name; these alters are better thought of as personality states or behavioral tendencies (Kluft, Steinberg, & Spitzer, 1988). In addition, alters—whether personalities or personality states—may emerge gradually over minutes rather than abruptly in a second or two. Finally, alters and their interrelatedness may change with age as the frequency of switching decreases—for example, one may become more dominant.

Gnostic Relationships   Gnosis means knowledge. How does any one of a set of multiple personalities come to know another? It appears that knowledge can be acquired through inference, memory, or, more directly, through perception, as outlined in Table 17.1.

An *inferential* relationship between two personalities is the least direct because it is based on logic rather than memory or perception. Typically the initially presenting personality, often with the help of a therapist, figures out that there must be another personality; there seems to be no other reasonable explanation for the odd events—a depleted bank account, unraveled knitting, frequent ''absences'' coupled with sudden consciousness of being in a new place—and also for the uncharacteristic behavior—frivolous, reckless, or even antisocial—that the person cannot deny despite having complete anmesia for them.

A *mnestic,* or memory-based, relationship is more direct. In this case, an ''awake'' B personality knows about a ''sleeping'' A personality because B has access to A's memory traces. Typically, there are two types of mnestic relationships among the personalities: two-way amnesia and one-way amnesia. In *two-way* amnesia, neither personality A nor personality B is directly aware of the other, though, as we indicated earlier, suspicions may be stirred by hints of the other's existence. In *one-way* amnesia, the A personality—typically the initially presenting personality—has no direct knowledge of B or of others, while B and the others are aware of A.

Consider the complex relationships among the four major personalities of Miss Beauchamp: B I (Miss Beauchamp), B II (a hypnotically altered B I),

B III (Sally), and B IV ("the Idiot"). B I knew nothing of B III or B IV. B IV had only a sketchy knowledge of B I but no knowledge of B III. B III knew B I intimately, except when BI used French. (When Prince wanted to keep B III in the dark about his interactions with B I, he had B I speak in French!) B III knew only the acts but not the thoughts of B IV (Prince, 1906/1969).

Sometimes the activated B personality claims to be a *co-conscious* who is continuously aware of A's experiences. In this case, B's knowledge of A is direct and immediate, based on the same perceptions and conscious experiences that constitute A's knowledge. Thus, while A is unconscious of B, B is immediately and intimately conscious of A. For example, Sally claimed to be continuously and concurrently aware of B I's experiences while awake and even while B I was dreaming, all despite B I's complete unconsciousness of Sally's "presence" (Prince, 1906/1969).

Other Characteristics

Multiple personality typically becomes apparent around adolescence, although it probably first develops around ages 4 to 6 out of personal crises involving frustration or pain (Bliss, 1980). Table 17.2 lists some objective signs and sub-

TABLE 17.2 PROMINENT BEHAVIORS AND EXPERIENCES WHOSE DIAGNOSTIC IMPLICATION FOR MULTIPLE PERSONALITY IN CHILDHOOD IS ALMOST ALWAYS OVERLOOKED

Teacher and Parent Observations
  Dazed appearance; trancelike behavior
  Uses more than one name and shows confusion when others attempt to clarify the discrepancy
  Marked changes in personality (e.g., shy, timid to hostile, extraverted)
  Inexplicable or unnatural forgetfulness
  Variation in physical skills (e.g., handwriting, visual acuity)
  Variation in preferences (e.g., food, entertainment)
  Inconsistencies in schoolwork
  Antisocial qualities (e.g., truancy, fighting, unresponsiveness to punishment, homicidal behavior)
  Denial of wrongdoing despite strong evidence
  Masochistic or suicidal behavior (e.g., self-injury, recklessness)
  Precocious sexuality (more aggressive in boys, more seductive in girls)
  Isolated (e.g., ignored, rejected, teased)
  "Hysteria" (e.g., somatization, hypochondriasis, conversion, sleepwalking)

Subjective Experiences
  Loss of time
  Perplexity (e.g., things seem changed; people use wrong names)
  Voices
  Sense of victimization (e.g., punished for another's misdeed)
  Imaginary playmates
  Loneliness

Source: Adapted from J. Fagan & J. MacMahon, "Incipient multiple personality in children," p. 29. *Journal of Nervous and Mental Disease, 172,* 197–202. Copyright © by Williams & Wilkins, 1984.

jective experiences of children who are vulnerable to, if they don't already have, multiple personality in early childhood (Fagan & McMahon, 1984). The diagnostic significance of these indicators is often overlooked by parents, teachers, and even mental health professionals.

The course of the disorder is typically chronic, with remissions and relapses that are somewhat dependent on external events. Most of the reported cases are female. However, the exact sex ratio, like the prevalence, of multiple personality is obscured by uncertainties of ascertainment. For example, there were only 200-odd cases reported in the entire literature up through the 1970s (Boor, 1982; Greaves, 1980), but hundreds, perhaps thousands, have been reported since then. It is therefore likely that the prevalence of multiple personality has been grossly underestimated (Kluft et al., 1988). For example, subtle personality changes can be taken for differences in mood, while radical changes may occur in remote social settings unknown to friends or therapist. Eve Black hung out at night in bars, settings entirely isolated from those familiar to Eve White and completely unknown to her.

In fact, the initially presenting personality typically seeks help for what patient and therapist at first assume to be the symptoms of medical problems—for example, headache or other pain, gastrointestinal disturbances, or seizurelike movements—or psychiatric problems. In fact, close scrutiny often turns up a veritable galaxy of psychiatric symptoms (see Table 17.3) that misleadingly suggests any of a number of other erroneous diagnoses, including depression, schizophrenia, borderline personality, psychopathy, hysteria, organicity, and malingering. The multiple personality diagnosis is rarely considered early in treatment and then only when fairly strong evidence overwhelms the incredulous examiner. It has been estimated that in the average case there is a six- to seven-year interval that occurs between the initial assessment of significant psychological problems and the correct diagnosis, during which time about 3.6 erroneous diagnoses are made (Putnam et al., 1986).

In order to enhance the sensitivity of diagnostic assessment to multiple personality, investigators (Bliss, 1984a; Greaves, 1980) have suggested that clinicians pay special attention to certain telltale indicators. These are given in Table 17.4. Of particular significance are absences, headaches, inexplicable changes in behavior, hallucinated voices, and a history of childhood abuse.

IS MULTIPLE PERSONALITY MERELY ROLE-PLAYING?

Flourney, in the nineteenth century, insisted that "the weight of evidence [for any hypothesis] must be in proportion to the strangeness of the fact" (Ellenberger, 1970, p. 315). Multiple personality is surely one of the strangest of facts, but unfortunately without the proportionate weight of evidence toward a scientific explanation. If it truly is a unique form of psychopathology, it must at least be distinguished from innocent (largely unconscious) role-playing and from willfully deceptive malingering.

TABLE 17.3 PROMINENT SYMPTOMS ASSOCIATED WITH MULTIPLE PERSONALITY*

Symptoms	Females, %	Males, %
Depressions	90	78
Amnesias	85	64
Dazed states	83	50
Nightmares	83	59
Suicide attempts	81	77
Multiple phobias	75	59
Anhedonia	75	50
Rapid mood shifts	71	68
Severe anxiety or panics	69	61
Sexual abuse early	60	27
Depersonalization	54	50
Derealization	54	50
Auditory hallucinations	54	45
Elimination of severe pain	52	68
Fugue states	52	50
Pain problems	50	48
Headaches	50	36
Visual hallucinations	48	32
Physical abuse early	40	32
Body anesthesia	38	32
Paranoid delusions	35	27
Limb paralysis	33	23

*These are some of the symptoms and their frequencies reported by multiples. Controls have not been included, but controls reported very few of these symptoms (Bliss, 1984b, p. 200).

Source: E. L. Bliss, "A symptom profile of patients with multiple personalities, including MMPI results," *Journal of Nervous and Mental Disease, 172,* 25–36. Copyright © by Williams & Wilkins, 1984.

Normal Role-Playing

Arguments against the normal role-playing hypothesis are fairly straightforward. Here are a few. First, normal people *do not* role-play multiple personality unless under highly motivating and artificial settings in the laboratory or on the stage. In real life, the condition is extremely punishing. It is associated with debilitating dysfunctions, emotional suffering, social embarrassment, and severe inconvenience. "The pain, chaos, and misery they experience is unsurpassed in the literature" (Greaves, 1980, p. 580). One is tempted to add that you have to be crazy to role-play craziness of this sort.

TABLE 17.4 DIAGNOSTICALLY SIGNIFICANT SIGNS OF POTENTIAL MULTIPLE PERSONALITY

Headaches, especially with blackouts or nightmares
Absences (lost time)
Behavior change with amnesia
Voices
Environmental evidence; e.g., strange letters
Polysymptomatic somatization, including conversions
Easy emergence of new identities in hypnosis

Second, normal people probably *cannot* role-play multiple personality, even if there were convincing role models or substantial payoffs which typically is not the case. Thus, their condition could not have been a matter of normal suggestibility in the context of modeling. In many instances, affected individuals have not even heard of the disorder. Finally, the notion that some of the more exotic mnestic and somatophysiological features of multiple personality can be simulated by otherwise normal people strains belief. This is especially true when the personalities are complex, multitalented, and numerous. (The median number of personalities per case is roughly ten.) For example, Billy Milligan has more than twenty distinct personalities, each with highly developed and distinctly different technical, artistic, linguistic, and other skills, not to mention different ages and sexual orientations (Keyes, 1981).

Malingering Hypothesis

Nevertheless, on a limited basis, some of the features of multiple personality can be faked. Normal subjects, given hypnotic suggestion, can simulate many of the symptoms of multiple personality—for example, admitting the existence of a distinct "other" with its own name, personality, and goals (Spanos et al., 1986). Occasionally, a malingerer can, for antisocial reasons, simulate multiple personality so skillfully that even experienced professionals may be fooled.

The "Multiple Personality" of Malingering In 1979, Kenneth Bianchi was sentenced by a California court to eight life terms for the "Hillside rape-murders." Initially, Bianchi appeared to be a humble innocent, a befuddled victim of circumstances. However, a radically different "personality" appeared under "hypnosis," a vicious, remorseless psychopathic killer named Steve Walker. Apparently, it was Steve, not Kenneth, who was responsible for the murders.

Eventually, Martin Orne, an expert on hypnosis, was able to prove that Bianchi was faking hypnosis as well as multiple personality. For example, the "hypnotized" Bianchi did not show "trance logic"—the easy acceptance of impossible or incompatible "facts"—that is typical in hypnosis and dreaming but atypical in normal wakefulness. Also Bianchi tried too hard to please the hypnotist—in particular, overresponding to hypnotic suggestions. For example, Orne requested Bianchi to imagine seeing a person in the room. After a moment, Bianchi got out of his chair, greeted the imagined person with an air of delight, and "shook hands." Orne recognized the deception; a truly hypnotized subject would not be so effusively demonstrative and would certainly not try to shake hands with a hallucination. Bianchi was overplaying his role. In short, some aspects of multiple personality can be faked. But can all aspects be faked? Is multiple personality merely an elaborate hoax?

Validity Tests for Multiple Personality There is increasing scientific evidence on the validity of multiple personality. Of the few studies done, most report EEG differences across personalities which seem incapable of simulation by controls (Ludwig et al., 1972; Pitblado & Cohen, 1984; Herbert, 1982, but see Coons, Milstein, & Marley, 1982). The tests usually involve analysis of EEG frequency components, the latency and amplitude characteristics of evoked potentials, and the correlation of these measures across personalities. One study, for example, found lower correlations across the alters of patients than across the "personalities" simulated by normal subjects; in other words, the alters were more clearly differentiated in terms of EEG (Putnam, 1986).

One of the most ambitious studies to date (Ludwig et al., 1972) involved EEG, galvanic skin response (GSR), learning, memory, and other tests on the four major personalities of a 27-year-old low-normal IQ veteran. The complaints of the initially presenting personality included violent outbursts, severe headaches, and strange experiences for which he claimed total amnesia. As is typical, the initially presenting personality, named Jonah, is conventional, retiring, frightened, confused, shallow.

In one part of the Ludwig et al. study, each of the personalities was asked to learn a different paired-associates word list. Each list consisted of ten pairs of words. Each pair included a "stimulus" word and its word associate "response." Each personality was trained to a criterion of perfect performance on his specific paired-associates list. Then, through hypnotic induction, each personality in turn was again called forth and tested on the stimulus words initially given to him and to the other three personalities. Each of the three non-Jonah personalities knew the correct responses to his and Jonah's stimulus list but not to the others' stimulus lists. Likewise, Jonah knew his responses but was completely amnesic for the correct responses to the others' lists. These results indicated a one-way amnesia separating Jonah from his other personalities.

A similar indication was evident in the GSR, an autonomic reaction of the sweat glands to affectively charged stimuli. Each of the non-Jonah personalities responded with a strong GSR to words of great affective significance to him and also to Jonah, but not to the other non-Jonah personalities. Jonah showed an elevated GSR for his affective words, but not to the affective words of any of the others. Along with differences in the EEG, the data supported the clinical evidence of four coherent, mnestically distinct, personalities.

The Ludwig et al. (1972) study is consistent with recent research—for example, on memory (Putnam, 1986). Normally, it is difficult to keep separate in memory each of two lists of highly similar words; laboratory subjects have trouble remembering which words are in which list. However, subjects with multiple personality display better than normal recall if each list is initially learned by a separate personality, especially if that personality is amnesic for the other. In contrast, subjects who role-play multiple personality do not display better than normal recall if each list is initially learned by a simulated separate personality. These observations constitute further evidence that the psychological separateness of the components of multiple personality disorder is a genuine phenomenon.

Comment

Multiple personality seems to be an exaggeration of normal tendencies toward dramatic self-presentation through inconsistent, even contradictory, behaviors. However, neither logic nor evidence requires that we treat the disorder *merely* as the exaggeration of normal tendencies. If it is a *pathological* exaggeration—as we believe the evidence suggests—then the disorder is *qualitatively* as well as quantitatively different from the norm.

When we say: "*I* couldn't help *myself*," or "*It* just came to *me* out of the blue," we imply two things: first, that there is at least one component of ourselves, other than the one with which we usually identify, and second, that behavior often seems to have a "mind of its own." Perhaps we really mean that there are many possible components of ourself, each with action capabilities and different goals, but operating out of consciousness (Jaynes, 1976). Perhaps multiple personality involves a pathological loss of the ability to organize and inhibit *components* of personality, with a consequent exaggeration of the normal tendency toward behavioral inconsistencies plus a lack of insight about how much and how often this is so.

The tendency to engage unconsciously in inconsistent behavior appears to be rooted in normal development. Research using sodium amytal and split-brain techniques suggests that each of us, right from early childhood, consists of separate selves which arise out of situational-specific behavior (Gazanniga & LeDoux, 1978).

> Could it be that in the developing organism a constellation of mental systems (emotional, motivational, perceptual, and so on) exists, each with its own values and response probabilities? Then, as maturation continues, the behaviors that these separate systems emit are monitored by the one system we come to use more and more, namely, the verbal, natural language system. Gradually, a concept of self-control develops so that the verbal self comes to know the impulses for action that arise from the other selves, and it either tries to inhibit these impulses or free them, as the case may be. [Perhaps] the mind is not a psychological entity but a sociological entity, being composed of many submental systems. What can be done surgically and through hemisphere anesthetization are only exaggerated instances of a more general phenomenon. The uniqueness of man, in this regard, is his ability to verbalize and, in so doing, create a personal sense of conscious reality out of the multiple mental systems present (Gazzaniga & LeDoux, 1978, pp. 150–151).

Perhaps, under some very special circumstances—whether artificial (hypnotic induction) or physiological (brain abnormality)—the rare and maladaptive combination of frustration, dissociation, and repression produces a psychopathological splitting of personality whereby the componentially organized self becomes a disorganized set of full-fledged selves.

THE PSYCHOPATHOLOGY OF MULTIPLE PERSONALITY

We seem to have come full circle back to Janet's core neuropsychological concept of dissociation as the effect of weak integrative "tension" (Chapter 16, p.

448). What then is the evidence that multiple personality involves some sort of brain abnormality?

Organic Factors

The Epilepsy Question Many investigators have suspected that multiple personality is related to temporal lobe epilepsy (Benson, Miller, & Signer, 1986). For one thing, multiples have an elevated risk for seizure disorder and may experience epilepticlike symptoms such as auras, somatic sensations, changes in consciousness, and deepening of emotions (Sutcliffe & Jones, 1962). Conversely, epileptics have an elevated risk for multiple personality. In the first recorded case of an apparently epilepsy-related multiple personality, a man named Sorgel dissociated into a decent and an antisocial counterpart. On one occasion, his antisocial personality chopped up a woodcutter and drank his blood. This was a case of one-way amnestic multiple personality in which the decent personality had no knowledge of the other's bizarre doings (Taylor & Martin, 1944).

A connection between temporal lobe epilepsy and multiple personality also makes sense on purely theoretical grounds. The temporal lobe is an important part of the limbic forebrain that controls affective and physiological functions, and that plays an important role in memory. The limbic connection would explain the overlap between the two disorders in symptoms such as depersonalization, altered consciousness, intense feelings, and disturbances of memory.

New research reinforces the hypothesis of a neuropsychological link between epilepsy and multiple personality. Elevated rates of multiple personality continue to be found for patients with temporal lobe epilepsy; these rates are higher than for any other population, whether normal, psychiatric, or neurological. In addition, a close relationship may occur between seizures and the switch between personalities. In one case, medication-induced relief from seizures produced a hostile, aggressive personality; whenever the drug treatment was discontinued and seizures returned, so did the normal, loving personality (Benson, Miller, & Signer, 1986).

Mesulam (1981) reported that twelve of sixty-one temporal lobe epileptic patients had dissociative disorder. Seven of these (12 percent) had multiple personalities. One was a 19-year-old woman with attacks of "absence" since the age of 12 and an abnormal EEG over the left temporal lobe. Two of her personalities had a one-way amnestic relationship. Edna has no direct awareness of Linda while Linda is directly conscious of Edna.

> Edna and Linda have distinctly different styles of speaking. Edna has a high-pitched voice, frequently uses stereotypes and contractions, and writes with her left hand. Linda, on the other hand, speaks in a low-pitched and gutteral tone, uses precise articulation without stereotypes or contractions, and writes with her right hand. Edna projects an image of naivete and submissiveness, whereas Linda imparts a sense of authority and self-importance (Mesulam, 1981, pp. 176–177).

An additional study (Schenk & Bear, 1981) corroborates the association between temporal lobe epilepsy and multiple personality. Three out of forty epileptics were found to have multiple personality, a rate of 7.5 percent. And when only female temporal lobe epileptics were considered in the analyses, the percentage was even higher.

However, these relatively high rates of dissociative disorder in epileptics could reflect a bias in the patients seen at behavioral neurology clinics rather than psychiatric hospitals; in other words, these patients may constitute an unrepresentative sample of dissociative disorders. After all, most multiple personality patients studied so far have *normal* EEGs. Moreover, there appear to be almost no medical, psychological, behavioral, or social differences between multiple personality patients who have or do not have abnormal EEGs (Putnam, 1986). Thus, while some cases of epilepsy may involve a neurological condition that is conducive to multiple personality, it is probably best not to think of multiple personality as a form of epilepsy.

The Headache Symptom   Multiple personality is frequently associated with headache, especially prior to the emergence of new personalities (Ludwig et al., 1972; Prince, 1906/1969; Thigpen & Cleckley, 1954). In fact, headache is the most common complaint of the initially presenting personality (Putnam et al., 1986). Headache is a frequent correlate of neurological and somatic disorder (Glaser, 1975; Pincus & Tucker, 1978), and also is frequently experienced by highly conflicted repressed individuals (Frazier, 1980). The neuropsychological significance of headache to multiple personality is still uncertain, but may prove substantial.

Ecopathology

It seems unlikely that Freud would have abandoned the seduction hypothesis if, early in his career, he had specialized in dissociative disorders rather than somatization and conversion hysteria. Traumatic ecopathology is a well-documented causal factor in almost all cases of multiple personality (Bliss, 1980; Stern, 1984), including abandonment, betrayal, inconsistency, rigid repressiveness, beatings, sexual abuse, burnings, and cuttings (Table 17.5). Occasionally, these traumatic events are truly bizarre, as in this case of multiple personality.

> A favorite ritual . . . was to separate Sybil's legs with a long wooden spoon, tie her feet to the spoon with dish towels, and then string her to the end of a light bulb cord, suspended from the ceiling. The child was left to swing in space while the mother proceeded to the water faucet to wait for the water to get cold . . . she would fill the adult-sized enema bag to capacity and return it to her daughter. As the child swung in space, the mother would insert the enema tip in the child's urethra and fill the bladder with cold water. "I did it," [her mother] would scream triumphantly when her mission was completed, "I did it." The scream was followed by laughter, which went on and on (Schreiber, 1974, p. 109).

TABLE 17.5 FIRST PERSONALITY PRODUCED BY EACH OF FOURTEEN MULTIPLE PERSONALITY PATIENTS

Name of first personality	Age at first appearance	Circumstances	Purpose	Rape reported by patient	Total no. of personalities
Sally	4	Mother held her under water and "tried to drown her"	Control and feel anger and handle homicidal rage	Yes	18
Jane	5	Frightened and sick on a train	Care for her when frightened or needed help	Yes	2
Sue	4	Spanked by father for having a temper tantrum	Control anger, get angry for her, keep a smile on her face	Yes	30
Betsy	5	Lonely and frightened; parents constantly fighting	Playmate	Yes	4
Joan	4	Wanted to cry and hide; lonely and unhappy	Playmate	?	4
Debbie	4	Molested by a man	Handle that frightening episode and thereafter handle sex	Yes	17
Bill	5	Brother dies and wanted a brother	A brother to be a companion and protect her	Yes	6
Linda	5	Being taken to surgery for a tonsillectomy: she had defective legs and feared real purpose was to amputate them	Cry for her because she was punished when she cried	Yes	5
Little girl	4	Appeared when mother remarried and the patient was very unhappy	Make her happy with beautiful early memories	No	3
Judy	5	Lonely	Playmate	No	2
Sarah	5	?	?	?	?
Jill	6	Lonely	Playmate	?	3
Naomi	6	Lonely	Playmate	Yes	4
Barbara	5	Lonely	Playmate	Yes	2

Source: Bliss, 1980 (*Archives of General Psychiatry,* 1980, 37, 1388–1397. Copyright © 1980, American Medical Association).

The causal significance of early childhood trauma is suggested by the following two observations: first, the greater the frequency and variety of traumas, the greater the number of personalities and the earlier they emerge in development; and second, the more numerous the personalities, the longer it takes to arrive at a satisfactory therapeutic resolution of the problem (Putnam et al., 1986). Nevertheless, traumatic ecopathology alone is too common to explain the comparatively rare multiple personality disorder. In other words, although there is a high probability of discovering familial ecopathology in patients with the disorder, there is still a relatively low probability of discovering the disorder in people who have been subjected to such ecopathology. Something more seems to be required.

Dissociative Psychopathology

The fact that traumatic ecopathology is insufficient to produce multiple personality implies that when it does occur, it potentiates a dissociative disposition. The fact that such a rare disorder can be found running in families over two and even three successive generations (Kluft, 1984) also implies a special disposition. However, in the absence of genetic studies, we cannot estimate the degree to which the hypothetical disposition is inherited or acquired.

The Self-Hypnotic Mechanism In some cases, the disorder seems to emerge in a perversely creative, emotionally sensitive person for whom conventional outlets for dramatic self-expression are simply inadequate. Take the case of Miss Beauchamp.

> In Miss Beauchamp's heredity and childhood, then, we find ample to account for the psychopathic soil which has permitted her present condition. She was never strong, as a child, became easily tired, and suffered from headaches and nightmares. Attacks of somnambulism also occurred. On one occasion when about fourteen years of age she walked out into the street at night in her nightgown and was brought home by the policeman. For years she was in the habit, from time to time, of going into spontaneous trance-like states.... For instance, one day, an attack came on while she was crossing the Public Garden. At the moment she was headed for Park Square. When she came to herself she was walking in an opposite direction, in a different part of the Garden.
>
> As a child, then, [she] was morbidly impressionable, given to daydreaming and unduly under the influence of her emotions. She took everything intensely, lived in a land of idealism, and saw the people and the world about her not as they were but as they were colored by her imagination (Prince, 1906/1969, p. 13).

New studies reveal that multiples have a surprising facility for attaining the hypnotic state spontaneously, voluntarily, and without the help of someone else. Bliss quotes one of the multiple personalities of a patient: "She creates personalities by blocking everything from her head, mentally relaxes, concentrates very hard, and wishes" (Bliss, 1980, p. 1392). It is important to understand that this change in consciousness is a spontaneous "primitive defensive reflex," not the product of modeling and instruction (Bliss, 1984a). It is *discovered* to be effective in dealing with traumatic experiences whatever their origins. Another patient reported: "I feel as though I have always been able to hypnotize myself. I don't honestly remember a time when I couldn't. I could always get inside myself and I always thought everyone could and did" (Bliss, 1980, p. 1392).

Some investigators have suggested that this spontaneous self-hypnotic state is akin to a dream process, the difference being that the many dream characters are manifested in the waking behavior of the person rather than merely imagined during sleep (Ellenberger, 1970). Perhaps the different characters of our dreams represent the different selves which normal people are able to inhibit or sublimate without splitting, while the pathology of multiple personality is the inability to prevent multicharacter dreams from coming true.

Functional Aspects of the Personalities   Each of a set of multiple personalities can serve an important function. It may gratify repressed or irrepressible desires for sexual or aggressive pleasure. More often, the personalities seem to serve a self-defensive function through belligerent, instrumental, conservative, or even masochistic behavior (see Table 17.6).

To illustrate, consider the following example of self-defensive function from the story of Billy Milligan's twenty-four personalities. The therapist is interviewing one of them, a tough, violent Yugoslavian named Ragen who acts as "defender" in dangerous situations. The "spot" referred to in the narrative is the center stage of consciousness.

"You see, Billy knows nothing about us," Ragen said. "He has—vat you call it?—amnesia. Let me put it this way. Ven he is in school, losing so much time, he goes up to roof. He starts to jump. I remove him from spot to stop him. He is asleep ever since that day. Arthur and I keep him asleep to protect him."

"When was that?" Judy asked.

"Right after sixteenth birthday. I remember he vas depressed because his father makes him vork on his birthday."

My God," Gary whispered. "Asleep for seven years?"

"Is still asleep. He vas only for few minute avak. It vas mistake to let him on spot."

"Who's been doing things?" Gary asked. "Working? Talking to people ever since?

" . . . To answer question: Allen and Tommy are mostly on spot ven dealing vit other people."

"They just come and go as they please?" Judy asked.

TABLE 17.6   FUNCTIONAL ASPECTS OF MULTIPLE PERSONALITY

Functional aspects	What purpose does a personality serve?
1 Wish-fulfilling	Pleasure striving serves to gratify repressed or irrepressible desires; e.g., sexual, aggressive
2. Self-defensive	Protective functions can be expressed through different styles (a) *Belligerent:* tough, take-charge, aggressive style (b) *Instrumental:* intelligent and resourceful problem-solving style (c) *Conservative:* avoidant or escapist style (d) *Masochistic:* Pain-absorbant style
3. Self-punitive	A personality may torment or humiliate another as atonement for guilt or to express self-contempt
4. Self-fulfilling	Each of many personalities may express frustrated dispositions (e.g., for adventure, drama) and talents (e.g., arithmetic, musical, artistic). Hysteria as self-fulfilling is romance in the sense of self-presentational story-telling

TABLE 17.7 SOME OF BILLY'S PERSONALITIES

Name	Age	Description	Function
Arthur*	22	British intellectual, fluent in Arabic, self-taught in physics and chemistry	Determines which personality will take "the spot" in a given situation
Ragen*	23	Aggressive, violence-prone Yugoslavian, fluent in Serbo-Croatian	Defender in dangerous situations
Allen	18	Con man, drum player, artist	
Tommy	16	Antisocial; knows electronics, plays saxophone	Escape artist
David	8	Sensitive, confused	Accepts pain, suffering of other personalities
Christine*	3	Bright but dyslexic English girl	
Adalana*	19	Shy, introverted lesbian with spontaneous nystagmus (jiggling of the eyes)	
Samuel	18	Orthodox Jew, sculptor and woodcarver	Preserves religious conviction
Shawn	4	Deaf and often taken for retarded	

*See Figure 17.1 for portraits of these personalities done by the Allen personality.

"Let me put it this vay. In different circumstances, spot is ruled by me or by Arthur, depending on situation. In prison I control spot—decide who goes on, who stays off—because is dangerous place. As protector, I have full power and command. In situations vere is no danger and vere intelligence and logic are more important, then Arthur dominates spot" (Keyes, 1981, pp. 37–38).

A personality may also serve self-punitive functions in depressive and guilt-ridden moods. In fact, one alter may have homicidal impulses toward another sometimes expressed in self-mutilation, but how often these impulses result in suicide cannot be determined (Putnam et al., 1986). A personality may also serve any one of many nonpathological dispositions, aspirations, and talents that are frustrated by conventional life. Table 17.7 provides a sketch of nine of twenty-four Milligan personalities, many with significant talents, skills, and responsibilities. Figure 17.1 shows portraits of some of Milligan's personalities done by the Allen personality.

In sum, we can think of multiple personality as a set of defensive maneuvers arising out of personal frustration or traumatic distress and complicated by their own unfortunate effects (Greaves, 1980). The primary defenses, dissociation and repression, are solutions to the problem of psychic survival, of preserving life and limb in the face of unacceptable impulses, frustrated talents, and otherwise insurmountable circumstances (Bliss, 1984c). Other defenses

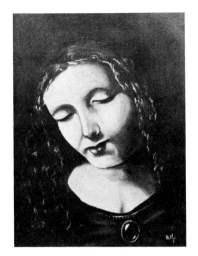

"Adalana."
Oil painting
by Allen

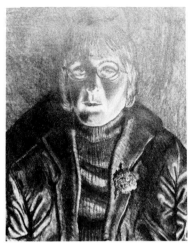

"Arthur."
Pencil sketch
by Allen

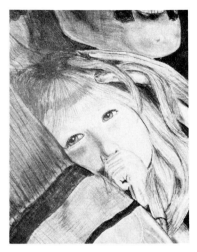

"Ragen Holding Christine."
Pencil sketch by Allen
(Christine spells her own name with an
"e"–Christene–whereas the other
personalities spell it as usual, with an "i.")

FIGURE 17.1　Artwork by Billy Milligan. (From *The Minds of Billy Milligan* by Daniel Keyes. Copyright © 1982 by Daniel Keyes. Reprinted by permission of Random House and Bantam Books.)

protect against personal difficulties caused by the comings and goings of personalities with different goals and behavioral styles.

Is Multiple Personality a Form of Hysteria?

From Janet to the present, investigators have argued over whether the theoretical category of hysteria should include multiple personality. Janet believed it should, and hypothesized a common dissociative mechanism which produces a narrowing of consciousness (Ellenberger, 1970). Other greats like Charcot, Binet, and Freud concurred.

If somatoform and dissociative disorders share a common psychopathology, certain predictions can be made. For example, Briquet hysterics and their relatives should be at greater-than-normal risk for multiple personality, while multiples and their relatives should have an elevated risk for somatoform disorder. Empirical evidence is meager on this question. What little there is (Bliss, 1980, 1984a, 1984b; Roy, 1982) supports the hypothesis that multiple personality and Briquet disorder are versions of a common spectrum (but see Greaves, 1980, for a dissenting view). For example, Bliss (1984b) reports that a large percentage of Briquet patients show evidence of multiple personality.

In Chapter 18 we will describe evidence that the first-degree relatives of Briquet patients have increased risk for antisocial disorders. Likewise, at least one of the personalities of the multiple personality disorder can usually be described as antisocial. In female multiples, antisocial behavior is expressed in childish, irresponsible acting out or pranksterism. In males, it is more aggressive and physically destructive. In both, lying, stealing, vandalism, and general deception are the rule. In short, evidence of common antisocial tendencies further links, albeit indirectly, multiple and somatoform disorders

Current evidence suggests that both Briquet (Bliss, 1984b) and multiple personality (Bliss, 1980) disorders are associated with excellent hypnotic susceptibility. In addition, Briquet and multiple personality disorders apparently share a common pattern of psychopathology. Figure 17.2 shows sets of three MMPI profiles, two for Briquet disorders we have seen before in Figure 16.8 (p. 449), and an additional one for a set of fifteen multiples (Bliss, 1984a).

The pattern similarity is evident. But more, the figure suggests a continuum of severity linking the two disorders, from mild (young Briquet students) to modest (older Briquet patients) to severe (multiples). These data support Janet's and Freud's view that the Briquet and multiple personality disorders are two forms of hysteria, the common neuropsychological link being the dissociative mechanism. Freud states that the "splitting of consciousness, which is so striking in the well-known classical cases of double conscience, exists in a rudimentary fashion in every hysteria and that the tendency to this dissociation—and therewith to the production of abnormal states of consciousness, which may be included under the term 'hypnoid'—is a fundamental manifestation of this neurosis" (Freud, 1893/1959, p. 34).

In sum, meager data tend to support the hypothesis that dissociative and somatoform disorders involve a common hysterical psychopathology, but the hypothesis remains highly speculative.

TREATMENT OF MULTIPLE PERSONALITY

Treatment typically involves psychodynamic therapy, sometimes also including drugs and videotaping. Drugs like sodium amytal promote the recall of affectively charged childhood memories by reducing anxiety. Videotaped evidence forces the patient to confront the reality of other personalities (Hall, LeCann, & Schoolar, 1978).

There are no controlled outcome studies of the treatment of multiple personality. Basic assumptions about what is therapeutic include the desirability of fusion or reintegration through therapeutic support, free association, and encouragement of remembering and *abreaction*: emotionally reliving a traumatic experience through both hypnotic and nonhypnotic suggestion. All assumptions about therapeutic goals are based on clinical lore and common sense and are subject to philosophical as well as scientific questions.

The Goal of Integration

Consider the common assumption that the major goal of therapy should be the reintegration of personality by fusing its separate, dissociated components (Combs & Ludwig, 1982; Prince, 1906/1969; Thigpen & Cleckley, 1954).

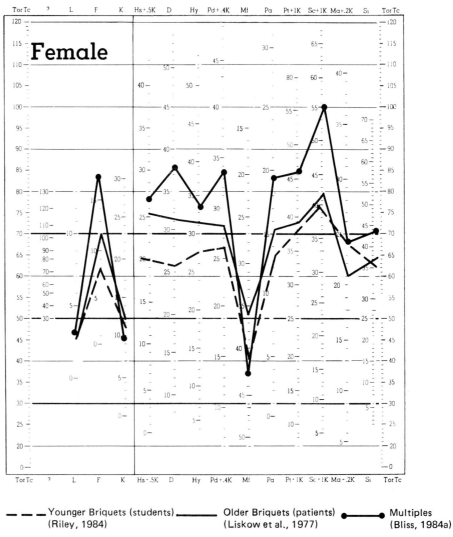

— — — Younger Briquets (students) ——— Older Briquets (patients) ●——● Multiples
      (Riley, 1984)   (Liskow et al., 1977)   (Bliss, 1984a)

FIGURE 17.2 Mean MMPI profiles of students (Riley, 1984) and patients (Liskow et al., *American Journal of Psychiatry, 134,* 1137–1139. Copyright © 1977, The American Psychiatric Association. Reprinted by permission.) with Briquet disorder, and patients with multiple personality (Bliss, 1984a).

Validity of the Assumption First, it is possible that the assumption is flawed. The separate personalities, at least some of them, might be psychologically healthier than the integrated one. Ludwig et al. (1972) reported that the apparently integrated Jonah of their study seemed sicker than the separate personalities, and suggested that "the separate functioning of the alter identities may represent a more effective way of handling anxiety than a coalescence of identities. If we remain scientifically openminded we must entertain the possibility that perhaps 'four heads are better than one''' (p. 310).

Ethics of the Assumption   A more provocative question is this: Does the therapist have the moral right to work toward personality integration when this means a kind of "euthanasia" of personalities (Sizemore & Pittillo, 1977)? Unless suicidal, each personality, like any living system, is motivated to survive.

> Sally pleaded that she had "just as much right to live" as had Miss Beauchamp; that she "enjoyed life just as much" as her other self, and complained bitterly of the dull time she has when she could not get out of her shell. Almost piteously she pleaded, "Why can't I live as well as she? I have got just as much right to live as she has." To her it was a question which should die and which should live. She never could be made to recognize the identity of the two personalities (Prince, 1906/1969, pp. 142–143).

Does the therapist have the right to work toward the annihilation of an individual self, which is psychologically comparable to physical death (Prince, 1906/1969)? And if the goal of therapy is the preservation of personality, with whom does the therapist establish the primary therapeutic alliance? Which of the personalities is the "real" one? It is not at all clear that the initially presenting personality is the "real" personality. Apparently it was not in the case of the B I personality of Miss Beauchamp, or the Eve White personality of Chris ("Eve") Costner. Was Prince morally correct to act on the assumption that "poor Miss Beauchamp, the saint, whom we knew so well, whom we had protected and cared for, would be only a dissociated personality, a somnambulist, and must no longer be allowed to live" (1906/1969, p. 240)?

Therapeutic Support

Another assumption of most therapies is the desirability of therapeutic support through patience, talk, attention, even friendship. Even such a reasonable assumption has potential pitfalls. For example, how does the therapist prevent the highly suggestible patient from engaging in further dissociations? Concern about *iatrogenic* (physician-caused) disorder is reiterated in the literature (Coombs & Ludwig, 1982; Bowers, Brecher-Marer, Newton, et al., 1971), and yet there is no simple formula for preventing such an outcome. On the other hand, does the therapist have the moral right to prevent the emergence of a personality?

It is commonly assumed that each personality should be treated with respect as an individual. Often, it is hoped that one personality may be convinced to work toward integration by supporting the interests of the others.

> At night when A is asleep her guard against you (B) will be lowered and you will be able to speak to her. Tell A everything we have discussed, especially how desirable it is that you become one person. Upon awakening A will know that she has dreamt. She will have a vivid memory of the dream and a strong wish to report its contents to me the next time we meet (Combs & Ludwig, 1982, p. 313).

Here again, many perplexing questions arise. How does the therapist prevent biases for or against a particular personality from becoming antitherapeutic prejudice? Does each personality have the right to know the others' thoughts, assuming that this knowledge would be helpful to the therapeutic work? Or does the right to privacy take precedence? Was Prince on ethically sound ground when he addressed B I in French to keep B III (Sally) from knowing what was going on? There are simply no good answers to such scientific and philosophical questions.

SUMMARY

Dissociative disorders include psychogenic amnesia, psychogenic fugue, and multiple personality. Psychogenic amnesia refers to a sudden inability to recall significant chunks of personal experience. Its psychogenic basis is readily suggested by the personal crises which typically antedate it, and by its selectivity, self-serving nature, and apparently nonorganic basis. Psychogenic fugue includes a sudden change in identity, flight to new surroundings, and adoption of a new lifestyle with amnesia for prior experience. General information and intellectual capacity are retained despite selective amnesia, affective constriction, and narrowness of interests and activities. Psychological theories of psychogenic fugue have focused on radical changes in cognitive function, driven either by heightened unconscious motivation, including massive repression and self-hypnotic mechanisms, or by a seizurelike abnormality akin to epilepsy.

Multiple personality refers to two or more distinct personalities coexisting within the same brain. Structural aspects include complex and coherent trait patterns within each personality that are consistent over time. Gnostic relationships among the personalities—the way one personality knows others—may be *inferential* (based on the logical implications of telltale signs), *mnestic* (based on shared memories), or *perceptual* (based on concurrent shared experiences, or co-consciousness).

The hypothesis of an underlying abnormality resembling epilepsy is supported by the elevated rate of multiple personality in temporal lobe epilepsy, but contradicted by the frequent absence of an epileptic EEG. The role-playing hypothesis is supported by personality qualities of suggestibility, deceptiveness, and dramatic self-expressiveness, but controverted by differences between personalities (e.g., in allergies, psychophysiology, handedness), and by extraordinary complexity and unerring consistency within each of the personalities, all of which are nearly impossible to simulate voluntarily. Also, there is increasing evidence from laboratory research on involuntary behavior and electrophysiology that the personalities are real.

Like other dissociative disorders, multiple personality frequently evolves as a massive defense against traumatic ecopathology. However, its occasionally nontraumatic origins, self-hypnotic mechanisms, and extraordinarily creative aspects suggest the operation of a unique dissociative disposition that can operate autonomously.

Antisocial Personality

OUTLINE

All personality disorders appear to have their origins early in life. Rigid and maladaptively responding to stress, adults with personality disorders generally are egocentric and disabled in love and work, viewing others as threats or objects for exploitation. Because they do not see their own maladaptive traits as ego-alien or undesirable, they often fail to understand why others are distressed by their actions. Their motivation for change is as low as their resistance to treatment is high. Consequently, any psychological treatment will usually be marked by intense ambivalence toward the therapist and by self-destructive acting out. If anxiety erupts, they tend to flee rather than try to discover the cause. These patients are almost always "treatment failures." As Vaillant and Perry (1980) put it:

> [Personality disorder patients] demonstrate to mental health professionals the limits of their expertise, yet no group of emotional disorders is more often encountered in psychiatric practice. Those with personality disorders crowd the rosters of clinic dropouts, treatment failures and referrals to other agencies. . . . Those with personality disorders are functionally more disabled than the neurotics (p. 1562).

Personality disorders are characterized by adaptive inflexibility, vicious cycles, and tenuous stability (Millon, 1981). *Adaptive inflexibility* means that coping resources are few, stereotyped, and often ill-suited to situational demands. The person knows only a few tunes and plays them regardless of their appropriateness. *Vicious cycles* imply that the person's habitual attempts to cope intensify rather than resolve preexisting difficulties. *Tenuous stability* is the person's lack of resilience in the context of stress. Episodic deterioration from, and recovery to, marginal levels of adjustment is the rule for these basically fragile people.

Clinical descriptions of personality disorders have a protean quality and clear distinctions are hard to pin down. Generally, the personality disorders are clustered into three categories on Axis II in the *DSM-III-R*. The first cluster includes the paranoid, schizoid, and schizotypal; these people are said to be odd, eccentric, or remote. The second cluster includes the histrionic, narcissistic, antisocial, and borderline; people with these personality disorders are described as overly dramatic, emotional, or erratic. The third cluster includes avoidant, dependent, compulsive, and passive-aggressive personality disorders, with pervasive anxiety or fearfulness the common thread apparently tying this cluster together. For a more comprehensive description of all the personality disorders see Chapter 3, pp. 80–83. In addition, the psychology of personality disorder—in particular, ego deficit and compensatory defense mechanisms—are discussed in Chapter 6, pp. 167–169 and the symptoms of personality disorder as expressions of both a vulnerability to, and defense against, anxiety and depression are discussed in Chapter 14, pp. 376–377.

Although the eleven personality disorders are conventionally accepted diagnostic entities, research on their classification and validity is only beginning to indicate that reliable distinctions among some of them can be made (Loranger et al., 1987). However, antisocial personality, one of the disorders in Cluster 2, is fairly reliable diagnostically and has been the target of much important research. Therefore, it will be the focus of this chapter.

CATEGORIES OF ANTISOCIALITY

Clinical descriptions of antisocial personality tend to include a variety of behavioral signs and personality traits. One thoughtful description of the antisocial personality refers to:

> . . . those non-psychotic and non-retarded adults who have multiple difficulties in many life areas, difficulties broadly characterized as a failure to conform to social norms. While no one behaviour is diagnostic, it is hard to imagine applying that label to anyone who is described by his boss as a good worker or who is law-abiding. Typically, we refer to someone who fails to maintain close personal relationships with anyone else, performs poorly on the job, who is involved in illegal behaviours (whether or not apprehended), who fails to support himself and his dependents without outside aid, and who is given to sudden changes of plan and loss of temper in response to what appears to others as minor frustrations. These characteristics must be chronic and more or less typical of the whole life history up to the point of diagnosis. A sudden appearance of antisocial behaviour in a previously conforming adult suggests mania, paranoid schizophrenia, drug intoxication, organic brain disease, even new political allegiances, but not antisocial personality (Robins, 1978, pp. 255–256).

The diagnosis of antisocial personality disorder conventionally requires a childhood or adolescent history of conduct problems in addition to chronic failures to conform to adult social norms. Common features of the disorder include a history of truancy, running away, fighting, cruelty to people and animals, forced sexual activity, destroying property, setting fires, stealing, and lying. As adults, these people have trouble remaining employed, commit illegal acts, and are often reckless and irresponsible both as citizens and as parents. Antisocial personality disorder is much more frequent in males. Using diagnostic criteria similar to the *DSM-III*, about 4.6 percent of adult males and 0.8 percent of adult females in the general population receive that diagnosis (Robins et al., 1984).

In line with the belief that the disorder is manifested primarily in social misbehavior, the term *sociopathy* is often used interchangeably with antisocial personality (Birnbaum, 1914). The sociopathy perspective emphasizes disturbances in social relations, implying that such individuals would behave normally if isolated on a deserted island.

The more influential explanation for antisocial personality has used the concept of *psychopathy* (Cleckley, 1950). This concept implies that some sort of psychopathology, perhaps with a biological basis, underlies antisocial behavior. Although we often use psychopathy interchangeably with the *DSM-III-R* diagnosis of antisocial personality disorder, Cleckley's criteria are much broader. The *DSM-III-R* criteria, although including the absence of remorse, focus mainly on behavioral signs of criminality and delinquency, ignoring exploitive, Machiavellian, and disloyal qualities that would not necessarily involve legal difficulties. Cleckley's more personality-oriented criteria include noncriminal aspects such as superficial charm, absence of anxiety, pathological egocentricity, poverty of emotional reactions, lack of insight, and vulnerability to alcohol (see Table 18.1).

Recent work has further clarified differences between *DSM-III-R* diagnostic criteria for antisocial personality disorder and Cleckley's criteria for psychopathology (Harpur, Hare, & Hakistan, 1989). A Psychopathology Checklist was completed for more than 1000 male prison inmates on the basis of interviews and examination of official files. Statistical analysis revealed two correlated factors described as: (1) ''selfishness, callousness, and remorseless use of others''; and (2) ''chronically unstable and antisocial life style; social deviance.'' The first—a ''Cleckley'' factor—was captured by such items as superficial charm, deceit, lack of emotional depth, and a grandiose sense of self-worth. The second—a ''*DSM-III-R*'' factor—was captured by items such as low frustration tolerance, childhood conduct problems, impulsivity (e.g., often quiting jobs without good reason, or moving to different cities on whim), and being a poor parole risk.

It will be important in future studies to verify the reliability and validity of these factors in nonincarcerated populations, as well as in females. It is quite possible that inconsistent results across studies on antisocial personality arise because different diagnostic criteria have been used to select subjects.

Childhood Patterns

A scheme for classifying adult antisocial behavior grows out of the *DSM-III-R* classification for types of conduct disorder, childhood versions of antisocial per-

TABLE 18.1 CLECKLEY'S (1950) CRITERIA FOR PSYCHOPATHY

1. Superficial charm and good intelligence
2. Absence of delusions and other signs of irrational thinking
3. Absence of nervousness
4. Unreliability
5. Untruthfulness and insincerity
6. Lack of remorse or shame
7. Inadequately motivated antisocial behavior
8. Poor judgment and failure to learn by experience
9. Pathological egocentricity; incapacity for love
10. General poverty in major affective reactions
11. Specific loss of insight
12. Unresponsiveness to general interpersonal relations
13. Fantastic and uninviting behavior with drink and sometimes without
14. Suicide rarely carried out
15. Sex life impersonal, trivial, and poorly integrated
16. Failure to follow any life plan

sonality disorder. The *DSM-III-R* has three categories of antisocial behavior in childhood: group type, solitary aggressive type, and undifferentiated type. The *group type* can establish affectionate bonds with others, although they may behave callously toward "outsiders." Their conduct disorder may involve stealing and vandalism, but usually with companions and without direct confrontation of the victim. The *solitary aggressive type* displays a pattern of repetitively aggressive interactions toward others, often without any group support. The *undifferentiated type* displays a mixture of the group and solitary aggressive types and thus cannot be classified into either of the other two types.

Adult Patterns

Socialized Antisocials   As adults, socialized antisocials can form close personal attachments, at least to a select few. They are able to empathize and feel guilt about their misbehaviors. Included in the socialized category are those who were regarded as *subcultural delinquents* in their youth. Reared in delinquent and/or lower class environments, subcultural antisocials form normal allegiances to those in their "in group," yet display callousness toward those outside it. Presumably, their antisociality arises from environmental forces that promote delinquent behavior and egocentric attitudes. One gets the impression that these people are shaped by their immediate society to behave this way. If this is true, the term sociopathy might be most applicable to them. Many of these people desist in their antisocial behavior in adulthood as they become acculturated to the larger society.

Also included in the socialized antisocial category are the antisocial neurotics, or *secondary psychopaths*. Their antisocial behavior is believed to reflect underlying neurotic conflicts that are often anxiety-laden, guilt-producing, ego-alien, symbolically expressed, and inexplicable even to the person engaging in the behavior. They are best thought of not as real psychopaths but as otherwise disturbed people whose problems are manifested in antisocial activities.

Undersocialized Antisocials   Undersocialized antisocials, or *primary psychopaths*, report little worry or anxiety, form no close personal attachments, callously disregard the norms of social conduct, lack empathy, exploit others, and seem motivated only by cheap thrills (Karpman, 1955). Primary psychopaths have been the target of much psychological research because their behavior seems so inexplicably harmful both to themselves and to others and cannot readily be explained by reference to obvious organic, psychotic, or environmental conditions. In general, undersocialized antisocials are more likely than socialized types to persist in their antisocial behavior (Henn, Bardwell, & Jenkins, 1980).

Another group of antisocials does not fall neatly into either the socialized or undersocialized category. Individuals of this group often have EEG bursts of paroxysmal brain wave activity consistent with the episodically explosive and violent behavior occasionally observed in them. Others have a high proportion of waking EEG theta wave (4 to 7 Hertz) activity rarely found in the EEG records of normal people over 10 years of age, and suggestive of cortical immaturity (Monroe, 1978). Although their behavior is often violently antisocial, during "good periods" their behavior may be nearly normal.

Given our summary of the many different patterns of antisociality, superficially similar antisocial behaviors turn out, upon close inspection, to be psychologically different and to have different origins. Consider a group of belligerent activists agitating for a "cause." Among them is the thrill-seeking psychopath motivated by selfish pleasure, the psychotic motivated by delusional fantasies of grandiosity and personal destiny, the neurotic symbolically acting out against authority, and the healthy person motivated by genuine idealism.

Institutionalized versus Community Psychopaths

Much of what we know about the personality and behavior of primary psychopaths derives from studies of imprisoned criminals. But an obvious question is whether such results can be generalized to the nonincarcerated population. One study suggests that they can. The investigator placed this clever ad in a Boston underground newspaper:

> Wanted charming, aggressive, carefree people who are impulsively irresponsible but are good at handling people and at looking after number one. Send name, address... (Widom, 1978, p. 72).

The idea was to identify noninstitutionalized psychopaths by providing a personality description which many psychopathic types, as defined by prisoner studies, would find socially desirable. The respondents were interviewed and given a variety of personality tests. Like many incarcerated prisoners, the respondents obtained their highest scores on the Psychopathic deviate (Pd) and Hypomania (Ma) scales of the Minnesota Multiphasic Personality Inventory (MMPI). These results thus indicate that the psychopathic personality profile does not depend on having been in prison. Indeed, many individuals with this profile are never incarcerated.

DEVELOPMENTAL ASPECTS

Many psychologists believe that primary psychopathy is present in very early childhood, perhaps even before school begins (Yochelson & Samenow, 1976). If it is true that such pre-antisocials are already insufficiently sensitive to social influences, parental threats of loss of love or punishment do not persuade them to redirect their behavior into more appropriate channels. Often, such children have rejected their parents before the parents have rejected them. Here is one history of early onset antisocial behavior.

C was involved in just about everything from an early age. The stealing pattern began at 4, when he took toys that weren't his, and then he began taking nickels and
dimes from his grandmother's purse. When he was 8, the breaking and entering began. This continued for some time, with stealing money and major items, such as
cameras, jewelry, radios, and so forth. From this time on, he was breaking into au-
tomobiles. Around age 8, he decided to hang another youngster by putting a noose
around his neck. He threw the end of the noose over a stick and kicked the can out
from under the child, but the stick broke and the child fell to the ground. About 9
years of age, C was becoming pretty convinced that crime was the best way of life.
At age 11, he organized and headed a protection racket with 9 other boys. They
managed to get 450 students in the school to contribute a dollar a week. At age 12,
he was fencing stolen goods. Also at about this time, he became a member of a gang
and soon became one of its leaders. At ages 16 and 17, he was very much involved
in the gang fighting and had his own gun. C was a war council chief, directing other
members of the gang in their fights with zip guns, chains, and knives (Yochelson &
Samenow, 1976, p. 18).

This boy's undersocialized antisocial behavior began in early childhood, becoming more sophisticated and dangerous with age. Although this history of a
budding psychopath is more violent than most, prospective and retrospective
longitudinal histories of psychopaths yield much the same picture.

Longitudinal Studies

Substantial longitudinal continuity exists between childhood and adolescent or
adult antisocial behavior. In summarizing the results of many predictive studies of antisocial behavior in youngsters, Loeber (1982) concluded as follows:

1 The higher the rate of early antisocial behavior, the more likely it is to
continue.
2 The more settings in which antisocial behavior occurs (at home and at
school), the more likely it is to continue.
3 The greater the variety of antisocial behavior (for example, lying, theft,
vandalism, *and* aggression), the greater the risk for later antisocial behavior.
4 The earlier the onset of antisocial behavior, the more likely it is to persist.

Only a fraction of all delinquents are psychopaths, but among persistent delinquents, the percentage of psychopaths is higher. Although most preadoles-
cent and adolescent delinquents do not become adult antisocials (Cloninger &
Gottesman, 1987), most antisocial adults will have had a childhood and adolescent history of antisocial behavior.

Robins (1966, 1978) obtained clinical records of 524 children first seen in the
1920s and early 1930s. Thirty years later she interviewed these subjects and
examined official records. She rated childhood antisocial behavior, using a
checklist of twenty-six symptoms, including incorrigibility, physical aggression, marked impulsivity, truancy, vandalism, running away, pathological lying, difficulties in getting along with peers, lack of guilt about antisocial acts,
and thefts. It turned out that the sheer number of childhood symptoms was

strongly related to the eventual diagnosis of adult psychopathy. Although 43 percent with ten or more of the symptoms were so diagnosed in adulthood, only 4 percent with fewer than four eventually became diagnosed psychopaths.

Table 18.2 gives the percentage of these psychopaths who had symptoms on the checklist as children and who have the symptoms as adults. The fact that no one childhood symptom was invariably associated with an adult diagnosis of psychopathy indicated that a single cardinal antisocial behavior could not be used to diagnose prepsychopaths in childhood. Thievery, the most frequent antisocial symptom, found in 83 percent of the adult psychopaths, occurred in only 31 percent of the prepsychopathic children.

Other longitudinal studies of delinquents coincide with those of Robins. A comprehensive study by West and Farrington (1973, 1977) followed up 411 lower-class boys until they were 21. At various intervals these boys were interviewed, rated by teachers, and given psychological tests. By the age of 21, fifty had been convicted both as juveniles and as adults, that is, they were recidivists. Comparisons with the 269 nondelinquents revealed differences on a host of social, behavioral, and possibly genetic variables (see Table 18.3). The delinquents came from larger families with lower incomes, received inadequate supervision, and had parents with criminal records. As early as 8 years of age, the eventual delinquents were clumsier, had lower nonverbal IQs (verbal IQs were not measured), and had been held back in school more fre-

TABLE 18.2 CHILDHOOD SYMPTOMS PREDICTIVE OF ANTISOCIAL PERSONALITY

Symptom	Percentage of adult antisocials who had symptom	Percentage of children with symptom who became antisocial
Theft	83	31
Incorrigibility	80	30
Truancy	66	34
Running away	65	33
Bad companions	56	30
Staying out late	54	30
Physical aggression	45	32
Poor employment record	44	32
Impulsivity	38	35
Reckless, irresponsible	35	29
Slovenly appearance	32	34
Enuresis	32	29
Lack of guilt	32	38
Premarital intercourse	28	31
Pathological lying	26	39
Sexual perversion	18	37

Source: Data from L. N. Robins, *Deviant Children Grown Up: A Sociological and Psychiatric Study of Sociopathic Personality.* Williams & Wilkins, Baltimore, 1966 (in Vaillant & Perry, 1980).

TABLE 18.3 THE RELATION BETWEEN ADULT DELINQUENCY AND EARLY BACKGROUND CHARACTERISTICS

Background characteristic	Age when assessed	269 nondelinquents, %	50 convicted as both adult and juvenile, %
Poor parental behavior	8–9	19.0	42.6*
Low nonverbal IQ	8 and 10	20.1	40.0*
Low nonverbal IQ	14–15	17.9	38.0*
Criminal parents	10	15.2	54.0*
Acting out	8–9	14.1	40.0*
Troublesome at school	8 and 10	13.8	58.0*
Low family income	8–9	17.8	42.0*
Broken home for reasons other than death	15	8.9	24.0*
Nervous-withdrawn	8–9	27.8	17.8
Psychomotor clumsiness	8 and 10	21.9	38.0*
Poor school achievement	11	24.2	52.0*
Teachers' rating aggressive	12–13	16.9	36.2*
Teachers' rating aggressive	14–15	13.3	55.3*
High score on self-reported delinquency (tests at two ages combined)	14 and 16	10.4	60.0*
High score on self-reported aggression (tests at two ages combined)	14 and 16	11.9	52.0*

*Comparing the percentage shown with the percentage among 269 nondelinquents, the difference is statistically significant.
Source: After D. J. West and D. P. Farrington, *The delinquent way of life.* London: Heinemann, 1977, pp. 142–143.

quently. Throughout adolescence they were more aggressive, according to self-report and teachers.

On only one item did the controls tend to exceed the recidivists; they were rated as more nervous and withdrawn at ages 8 and 9. One hypothesis, to which we will return, is that anxiety reduces the likelihood of delinquency. Presumably, the contemplation of aggressive or antisocial actions by nondelinquents would more easily arouse anxiety and this would inhibit further antisocial ideation.

Predicting Delinquency

How can the tangled web of variables, such as inadequate child rearing, criminal parentage, and low social class, in the West and Farrington study be interpreted? The investigators later tested whether each key factor, independent of the others, contributed to delinquency (Farrington & West, 1981). For example, they matched delinquents and nondelinquents for the presence of criminal parents. After matching, they found that early separation of the child from his parents made no independent contribution to delinquency.

Matching analyses revealed only three personal and four background factors that independently predicted delinquency. The personal factors were (1) primary school teachers' ratings of troublesomeness, (2) daring, and (3) low IQ. The background factors were (1) poorer families, (2) larger families, (3) criminal parentage, and (4) poorer parental child-rearing behavior. When

Farrington and West combined all the risk factors into a single predictive formula, they found that only about 50 percent of the recidivists could have been identified in advance. The teachers' ratings of troublesomeness well would have predicted the outcome about as well.

Many anticipated bad outcomes do not materialize. Consider again the "troublesome at school" item in Table 18.3. Although only 13.8 percent of the 269 good-outcome children had been rated as troublesome in elementary school versus 58 percent of the 50 recidivists, more good-outcome than poor-outcome children had been troublesome (37 as against 29). Of all the children rated as troublesome, only 44 percent (29 out of 66) became recidivists. This story puts the challenge of successfully predicting infrequent events in a nutshell. Without a perfect test, many good-outcome people will be predicted to have bad outcomes, and many of those with eventual bad outcomes will have been missed (see also Loeber & Dishion, 1983).

It is more than an academic matter to identify the most violent and potentially recidivistic antisocials early. They account for the majority of violent crimes among juveniles. Although they do eventually get caught, they are often incarcerated only briefly. Chronic juvenile offenders—those who commit five or more offenses—account for 52 percent of all delinquent acts, although they represent only 6 percent of the total population of delinquents (Wolfgang, Figlio, & Sellin, 1972).

SOCIAL, BIOLOGICAL, AND BEHAVIORAL ASPECTS

The complexity of antisocial behavior calls for an analysis of each of its many-faceted aspects. Let us now briefly review some possible social and biological causes of antisocial behavior.

Family Environment

The family environments of antisocials are likely to be more undesirable than those of normals. Parental caretaking and discipline are often harsh, lax, inadequate, or all of these (West & Farrington, 1977). Observations of antisocial children and their interactions within the family reveal that faulty parental management techniques can cause a spiraling increase in undesirable interactions between parents and children (Patterson, 1986). For example, relatively trivial misbehaviors such as whining, teasing, and yelling can elicit from parents explosively aggressive punishment if the children fail to comply to parental demands. It is as if the parents of these children have few effective methods of discipline short of violence. To be sure, some children have temperaments that make them difficult to handle, and well-meaning parents can be repeatedly frustrated by their unsuccessful efforts at less harsh discipline.

The parents, particularly the fathers, of antisocial boys tend to be aggressive themselves, a behavior that might facilitate the same kinds of behavior in their children (Bandura & Walters, 1959). Parental influence of this sort cannot be too potent, however, because most siblings of antisocials are not themselves antisocial, and there are explanations for parent-child correlations other than parental misbehavior causing psychopathology in their children (Chapter 5). For example, because of failure to obey, antisocial children can elicit punitive behavior even from mothers of normal children who have never met them before (Anderson, Lytton, & Romney, 1986).

Physiological Aspects

Antisocials are relatively more aggressive and daring even as children, and threats of punishment do not effectively deter their antisocial behavior. Because anticipation of punishment arouses anxiety in normal people, a central question is whether antisocials differ from others in anxiety responsiveness. There is evidence that delinquents are more likely to have lower levels of adrenaline than controls, which does suggest lower autonomic arousal (Magnusson, 1987; Levander, Mattsson, Schalling, & Dalteg, 1987). If experienced anxiety is lower in antisocials, then it cannot serve so well to deter their misbehavior. The question of low anxiety has been investigated in many behavioral studies of psychopathic and nonpsychopathic prisoners

Electrodermal Aspects of Anxiety   If a calm subject is made anxious, sweat gland secretions act as an electrolyte that increases the conductance of an electrical current between two points on the skin. Some laboratory studies of skin conductance have suggested lower anxiety in psychopathic prisoners.

Hare (1965) sequentially presented the numbers 1 to 12 to psychopathic and nonpsychopathic prisoners who had been told that on number 8 they would receive an intense shock. The nonpsychopaths showed increased skin conductance early in the number sequence and an intense response to the shock. The psychopaths, however, showed relatively low skin conductance when the first few numbers were presented, and a slightly less intense response to the actual shock. This pattern of results suggesting comparatively little anticipatory anxiety mirrors the picture seen in the real world. Psychopaths often do not anticipate early enough the consequences of their actions and, if apprehended, appear less threatened by the prospect of punishment (Lykken, 1957).

Differences in skin conductance between psychopathic and nonpsychopathic subjects are especially large in the context of extremely aversive stimuli. When Hare (1978) presented tones varying in intensity from loud to very loud—the latter about the loudness of a nearby jackhammer—the two prisoner groups differed significantly only for the loudest noise, the psychopathic prisoners reacting less intensely to the deafening stimulus than the nonpsychopathic prisoners (see Figure 18.1).

Do these findings suggest that hyporesponsiveness to threat accounts for the inability to learn from punishment? Perhaps psychopaths are less able to directly experience anxiety in anticipation of their actions or vicariously experience the anxiety that their actions arouse in others. In the same way that the

FIGURE 18.1   Mean skin conductance responses of psychopathic (Low Socialization) and nonpsychopathic (High Socialization) prisoners to tones ranging in intensity from 80 to 120 decibels. Note that the two groups of prisoners differed only slightly in skin conductance when the intensity of the tone was fairly modest, but the High Socialization prisoners showed a much more intense increase in skin conductance than the Low Socialization prisoners when it became extremely loud (From R. D. Hare and D. Schalling, Eds., *Psychopathic behaviour: Approaches to research.* Copyright © 1978, John Wiley and Sons, Ltd.)

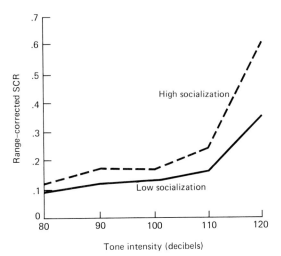

sightless cannot appreciate the beauty of a sunset, the "anxietyless" may not fully comprehend the consequences of their antisocial behavior, the personal danger, the harm to others, and the like.

Heart Rate   If skin conductance data suggest low anxiety among psychopaths, heart-rate data suggest something different. When beat-to-beat changes are continuously recorded in subjects who anticipate a noxious loud sound, psychopathic prisoners show *accelerating* heart rates while nonpsychopaths show surprisingly little change.

Figure 18.2 shows heart rates for psychopathic and nonpsychopathic prisoners in anticipation of the noxious event separately for the first and second trials. On trial 1, subjects had not yet experienced the noise, but there is already some evidence that the heart rates of the psychopaths are accelerating. On trial 2 the difference between the two groups of prisoners is accentuated. Actually, heart-rate acceleration and low skin conductance observed in other studies of psychopaths are not necessarily contradictory signs of a common underlying process. Hare argues that heart-rate acceleration, especially in the context of negligible changes in skin conductance, indicates successful "tuning out" of aversive stimuli (Lacey, 1967; Lacey & Lacey, 1974). But why the acceleration in the first place? Perhaps it is part of a preparation for action that is so typical of the psychopath. If psychopaths have an action, rather than a reflective, orientation, they might be more prone to think about escaping, not because of intense anxiety but rather because they are simply aware of danger, like someone reacting quickly to avert an automobile accident before experiencing the anxiety. In short, an action orientation diminishes sensitivity to incoming information (acceleration in heart rate) and reduces anxiety (little change in skin conductance).

Physique

Not surprisingly, antisocials, especially the aggressive types, are more *meso-morphic,* that is, they are more muscular and have a large bone mass. This observation emerged from a study of 500 delinquents and their matched nondelinquent controls (Glueck & Glueck, 1956). Sixty percent of the delin-quents had a predominantly mesomorphic physique compared with only 31 percent of the controls. Furthermore, only 14 percent of the delinquents were *ectomorphic*—that is, skinny and angular—compared with 40 percent of the controls. Among those who were *endomorphic*—that is, fleshy and rotund—no differences in frequency between delinquents and nondelinquents appeared. Physique is strongly heritable, but it seems improbable that genes for physique would also be directly responsible for antisocial behavior. Rather, stronger people—that is to say, mesomorphs—are more likely to be rewarded for being physically aggressive.

But how can we explain antisocial ectomorphs? Because they are more fragile, they should more often receive punishment for aggressive antisocial behavior. Perhaps their antisocial behavior takes the form of covert activities involving "sneakiness" in which aggressive confrontation is less likely. Un-fortunately, we don't know whether there are differences in the types of anti-social behavior displayed by mesomorphs and ectomorphs. One other possi-

FIGURE 18.2 Changes in heart rate shown by psychopathic (P) and nonpsychopathic (NP) inmates during the twelve-second period prior to an anticipated 120-decibel tone (From R. D. Hare and D. Schalling, Eds., *Psychopathic behaviour: Approaches to research.* Copyright © 1978, John Wiley and Sons, Ltd.) In contrast to Figure 18.1, it is the psychopathic prisoners who now show greater reactivity.

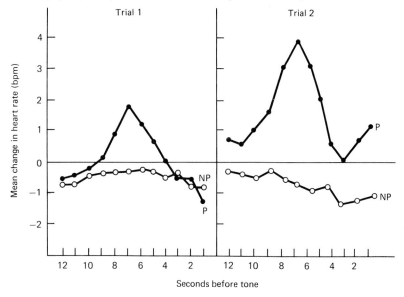

bility, however, is that at least some ectomorphic delinquents can't help themselves; they are driven to their delinquency because of hyperactivity. Table 18.4 gives the percentage of delinquents and controls who were "extremely restless in early childhood." Almost twice as many delinquents as nondelinquents had been hyperactive, but by far the most hyperactive were the ectomorphic delinquents. Eighty-two percent of them had been hyperactive, as compared with only 34 percent of the ectomorphic controls.

Hyperactivity, a possible indication of neurological abnormality, can increase the risk for delinquency (Satterfield, Hoppe, & Schell, 1982) and adult criminality (Magnusson, 1987). In the presence of a sturdy body build, the distinctive role of hyperactivity is less apparent, but hyperactivity may be almost an essential condition for delinquency in ectomorphs.

Intelligence

Delinquents tend to have lower IQs than nondelinquents, even after parental socioeconomic status and race are statistically controlled (Hirschi & Hindelang, 1977). This means that for a given socioeconomic status or racial group, lower IQ people are at greater risk for delinquency. Furthermore, chronic delinquent offenders have lower IQs than one-time offenders (Wolfgang, Figlio, & Sellin, 1972). Some have argued that the negative relationship between higher IQ and lower rates of delinquency arises because higher IQ delinquents are better able to escape detection. But this argument appears doubtful because low IQ also relates to the number of *self-reported* delinquent acts, and the low IQ-delinquency association is independent of whether the acts have been detected or not (Moffitt & Silva, 1988).

Closer examination of the components of IQ suggests that delinquents and adult antisocials are especially impaired in verbal, as opposed to nonverbal, thinking (Glueck & Glueck, 1956; Yeudall et al., 1982). As early as 4 years of age, but certainly by age 7, children who will be diagnosed with conduct disorder in adolescence already show signs of low verbal IQ (Schonfeld, Shaffer, O'Connor, & Portnoy, 1988). Moreover, reading and spelling disabilities also are more frequent in psychopaths than in controls matched for IQ (Henning &

TABLE 18.4 RATES OF EXTREME RESTLESSNESS IN DELINQUENTS AND NONDELINQUENTS IN EARLY CHILDHOOD AS A FUNCTION OF PHYSIQUE TYPE

Physique types	Delinquents (*N*-60) %	Nondelinquents (*N*-30) %
Mesomorph	52	27
Endomorph	59	32
Ectomorph	82	34
Balanced	68	26

Source: Physique and Delinquency by S. Glueck and E. Glueck. Copyright © 1956 S. and E. Glueck. Reprinted with permission of Harper & Row, Publishers, Inc.

Levy, 1967), and serious delinquents have often been regarded as especially deficient in expressive language (see Brickman et al., 1984, for example). Deficiencies in verbal functions could make it more difficult to act reflectively and anticipate the long-term consequences of one's actions. Moreover, they could produce an impairment in verbalizing and experiencing feelings. These verbal deficiencies in delinquents and psychopaths have suggested to many experts a neuropsychological deficit in the left hemisphere.

Consider a letter received by Vaillant (1975) from a distressed schoolteacher about her psychopathic son: "He is inarticulate and quarrels quickly and finds fault. He writes like a child and misspells words" (p. 179). There is a good possibility that inarticulateness, handwriting difficulties, and misspellings, especially in a person from an educated household, are signs of lefthemisphere damage. Quay (1986a) argues, however, that signs of a verbal or left-hemisphere deficit are characteristic only of undersocialized antisocials. These, of course, will be the ones most likely to be classified as psychopaths.

Learning

Studies of primary psychopaths have shown that they learn less from physical punishment than do secondary psychopaths, the anxious antisocials (Lykken, 1957; Schmauk, 1970). In these experiments, prisoners were asked to learn a maze with four levers at each step. Pressing the correct lever allowed subjects to advance to the next step, but pressing a particular one of the three incorrect levers resulted in an intense shock. The explicit task — the one clearly explained to the subjects—was to learn the maze in the fewest number of trials, but the incidental task—the one that the subjects had to discover for themselves — was to avoid the shock lever when making errors. The hypothesis was that if primary psychopaths, in contrast to controls, do not easily condition to punishment because of a deficient anxiety response, they would not learn especially to avoid the shock lever at each step of the maze.

All groups learned the explicit task in the same number of trials, demonstrating that primary psychopaths are not generally deficient in learning ability. In comparison with anxious antisocials or normal controls, however, primary psychopaths made a greater proportion of shocked errors, confirming the expectation that primary psychopaths are less easily conditioned by physical punishment. Perhaps the poor performance of primary psychopaths on the shocked levers was an artifact of their inability to realize a connection between a particular incorrect response and the shock it produced.

Indeed, this failure to realize a connection between a particular response and shock seems very important. Newman and Kosson (1986), for example, found that psychopathic prisoners made more errors on a subtle "incidental" aspect of a task even when errors resulted only in the loss of money, but that psychopathic and nonpsychopathic prisoners did not differ in performance on an explicit aspect of a task. Collectively, the research suggests that psychopaths are as able as others to respond appropriately to conspicuous rewards or punishments, but not to subtle or incidental aspects of their experience. Once fixated on a particular approach, psychopaths seem less able than others to consider alternative courses of action.

A focus on only low anxiety about physical punishment as a cause of psychopathy may have been misplaced; the psychopathic deficit may be broader, encompassing a more general cognitive deficiency involving the inability to integrate rationally both the positive and negative consequences of a particular choice of action, especially when one or the other of the consequences is not obvious.

Organic Brain Deficit

Can organic brain dysfunctions explain psychopathy? Like anxiety, depression, and other symptoms, certain psychopathic qualities can be simulated by experimentally produced lesions in the midline frontal lobe region or in closely related structures (Gorenstein & Newman, 1980). Lesions in these areas produce impulsive animals who profit little from punishment and have trouble inhibiting previously rewarded responses even though such responses are now punished. These animals are also hyperactive and easily distracted.

Frontal-Lobe Dysfunction The behavior of psychopaths and of those with known frontal lesions is often quite similar; both display lack of foresight, insight, or conscience (remember Phineas Gage discussed on page 223), along with fearlessness, aggressiveness, and self-defeating behavior (Elliot, 1978). For example, some studies find that psychopaths and frontally damaged patients show behavioral perseveration on tests requiring mental flexibility. That is, they persist in responding in a certain way, unable to shift to a new response when the original is no longer appropriate (Newman, Patterson, & Kosson, 1987).

These inflexible people are also overly influenced by the immediate stimulus environment, seeming to forget or ignore even recent experiences. In one experiment psychopathic subjects, patients with frontal-lobe damage, and normal controls were presented cards on which there was either a plus or minus sign. The subjects' first task was to indicate whether a plus or minus had appeared on the card previous to the one they were currently looking at, and on this task the groups did not differ; both psychopaths and frontal patients did just as well as controls. However, when asked to report the symbol *two cards back*, the performance of psychopaths and frontal patients was grossly inferior to that of controls (Gorenstein, 1982). Not all psychopaths display this pattern (e.g., Hare, 1984; Sutker & Allain, 1987), but the resemblance to frontal patients is often striking.

We do not know why some psychopaths and not others display behavioral abnormalities akin to patients with frontal damage. There is a slight tendency for studies yielding positive results to contain younger subjects and it is possible that as subjects grow older, their ''frontal'' behavior diminishes. Another possibility is that drug abuse, a frequent concomitant of psychopathy, is responsible for the abnormality. It also has been suggested that psychopaths with a history of attentional deficit hyperactivity disorder are most likely to display frontal impairments (Moffitt, in press). Indeed, a childhood history of hyperactivity is common in psychopaths, and it would be useful to differentiate psychopaths according to this factor.

Frontal impairment, however caused, might explain the elevated heart rate in some primary psychopaths in response to threat. Luria (1973) writes of frontally damaged patients presented with a problem who, "with their distinctive impulsiveness, never start with a preliminary analysis of the task's conditions but immediately attempt to solve" (p. 15). Like the patient with frontal damage, the psychopath is notorious for his impulsivity. Yochelson and Samenow (1976) describe the psychopath as always ready for action, always thinking of ways to rob, steal, or deceive. One consequence of preparing for action rather than reflecting on its implications is an elevated heart rate (McGuinness & Pribram, 1980), which might explain why Hare (1978) found accelerating heart rates in psychopaths about to be exposed to a loud noise.

Figure 18.3 illustrates regions of the frontal lobe, and the left side of Table 18.5 provides a summary of the major symptoms of frontal damage and their anatomical locations (Kolb & Whishaw, 1980). The right side of the table provides evidence that the performance of psychopaths resembles the performance of patients with established frontal damage. Parallels are inexact because relatively recent frontal damage in a previously normal person differs

FIGURE 18.3   A simplified picture of some regions of the frontal cortex that may be relevant to psychopathy. Much of our knowledge about these regions comes from patients with tumors and traumatic injuries that produce damage often not confined to a circumscribed region of the frontal lobe. (From Kolb & Whishaw, 1980)

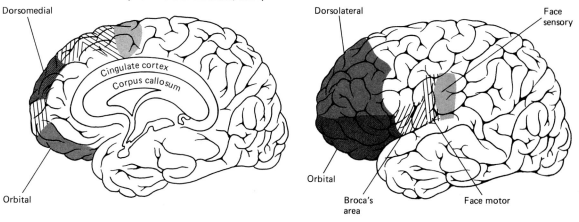

Dorsomedial

Cingulate cortex

Corpus callosum

Orbital

Midsagittal View

(a)

Dorsolateral

Face sensory

Orbital

Broca's area

Face motor

Lateral View

(b)

TABLE 18.5 A COMPARISON OF BEHAVIORAL SYMPTOMS OF PATIENTS WITH KNOWN FRONTAL-LOBE
DAMAGE AND PSYCHOPATHS OR PERSISTENT DELINQUENTS

Frontal-lobe symptoms	Anatomic location	Psychopathic symptoms
Aphasia	Broca's area	Low verbal IQ (Yeudall et al., 1982)
Impaired response inhibition	Dorsolateral and dorsomedial	Impulsivity (Cleckley, 1950)
Impairments in visual gaze (cannot efficiently search a complex field to locate an object)	Dorsolateral and dorsomedial	?
Poor recency memory	Dorsolateral	Captured by the immediate stimulus, cannot use information from recent past (Gorenstein, 1982)
Impaired corollary discharge*	Dorsolateral	?
Poor movement programming	Dorsolateral	Clumsiness (West & Farrington, 1977)
Impaired spatial orientation	Dorsolateral	?
Impaired social behavior	Orbital	Callousness (Cleckley, 1950)
Altered sexual behavior	Orbital	Casual sexuality, inability to form enduring attachments (Cleckley, 1950)
Reduced behavioral spontaneity	Orbital	Perseveration (Newman et al., 1987)
Impaired phonetic discrimination	Face	?
Poor spelling	Face	Academic learning deficits (Yeudall et al., 1982)

*Normally, if the eyeball is pressed, the world seems to move; if the eye moves voluntarily, the world remains still. This is explained by neurons firing in a corollary fashion only if the eye moves voluntarily. A deficit in corollary discharge occurs with damage to dorsolateral frontal cortex.
Source: Left side of table after Kolb & Whishaw, 1980.

from an impairment arising early in life. For example, nonpsychopathic adults who undergo surgery to remove portions of the frontal cortex do not become psychopathic.

Nevertheless, striking correspondences between established frontal-lobe symptoms and psychopathic symptoms do appear. Only four of the frontal damage symptoms in Table 18.5 have not been assessed in psychopaths. Evidence for them would add weight to the frontal-lobe hypothesis about psychopathy. One would, however, have to ascribe to psychopaths unrealistically massive structural lesions to account for all the parallels. A more likely hypothesis is a subtle but pervasive anomaly of frontal-lobe maturation.

Maturational Lag   Normally, the frontal lobes mature later than the other lobes (Yakovlev & Lecours, 1967), a fact that perhaps explains the egocentricity and impulsivity of early childhood. Frontal lobe myelination occurs in two spurts: (1) between 2 and 4 years of age and (2) during adolescence and beyond (Pontius, 1974). Peterson et al. (1982) have shown in a longitudinal study that youths who eventually engaged in repeated thievery show more signs of EEG immaturity even *before* the youngsters commit crimes; the EEGs of prethieves yielded a pattern suggesting brain activity more characteristic of younger children.

The cause of the immature EEG patterns is unknown, but such patterns are consistent with a maturational-lag hypothesis. Delayed maturation could explain both typical psychopathic behavior and the observation that some psychopaths "burn out," that is, they become less impulsively aggressive and more law-abiding in their 40s (Hare, McPherson, & Forth, 1988). Thus, the burnout phenomenon may be a consequence of neural maturation that could be influenced by genetic as well as environmental factors.

GENETIC ASPECTS

Many investigators have observed that criminality tends to run in families. Unfortunately, psychopathy is imperfectly related to criminality, so genetic investigations of criminality shed a somewhat indirect light on the causes of psychopathy. In fact, no adequately sized twin study of psychopathy per se has ever been conducted. Nonetheless, behavior genetic studies of criminality do provide information that can be used in understanding the genetics of antisocial behavior.

Twin Studies

Twin concordances for criminality vary with the age of the twins (see Cloninger & Gottesman, 1987). The average MZ and DZ concordance rates for *juvenile delinquency* are about 87 percent and 72 percent. Such high DZ rates differing so little from MZ rates indicate that shared environmental factors potentiate juvenile delinquency, and remind us that faulty parental management techniques may figure importantly in antisocial behavior during childhood and adolescence (Patterson, 1986). Nevertheless, MZ and DZ concordance rates for *adult criminality,* averaging about 61 percent and 18 percent, support a genetic hypothesis. It would appear then that juvenile delinquency arises in most cases for largely environmental reasons, but some juvenile delinquents go on to become adult criminals partly for genetic reasons.

Adoption Studies

Two types of methodology have been employed in adoption studies of psychopathy and criminality. In one, investigators first identify antisocial adoptees and then examine their biological and adoptive relatives for evidence of antisocial behavior. In the other, investigators start with antisocial people who have given up a child for adoption and then examine their adopted-away offspring for signs of antisocial behavior.

Using the first method, Schulsinger (1972) started with a nationwide Danish register of adoptees. He searched the criminal and psychiatric records to identify 57 adult adoptees (forty males, seventeen females) who met his criteria for psychopathy. These criteria were: (1) a consistent pattern beyond adolescence of impulse-ridden or acting-out behavior, and (2) emotionality judged by the

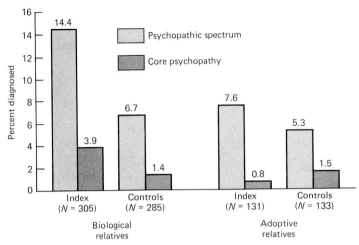

FIGURE 18.4 Psychopathic disorders in the biological and adoptive relatives of psychopaths and control adoptees. (After Schulsinger, 1972)

clinician to be more intense than warranted by the provocation. Neurotics and psychotics were excluded. Control adoptees were closely matched to the index adoptees for sex, age, age at first transfer to the adoptive family, and social class of the adoptive family. The biological and adoptive relatives of both groups of adoptees were then evaluated for evidence of psychopathy without knowledge of the group to which the relatives belonged.

The results appear in Figure 18.4. These are divided by whether the relatives were diagnosed by narrow criteria that are closer to *DSM-III* descriptions or by broad criteria which allowed for the diagnosis even if the person could only be described as an alcohol abuser. There is a significant excess of psychopathy in the biological relatives of the psychopaths regardless of whether narrow or broad criteria are employed. Interestingly the adoptive relatives of either type of adoptee did not differ in the frequency of psychopathy, suggesting that it is unnecessary to have an adoptive parent with an antisocial diagnosis to increase the risk for having the disorder in the offspring.

Using the second method, Crowe (1974) assessed the adopted-away offspring of incarcerated female felons in Iowa. Each of the forty-six index adoptees was matched to a control adoptee for age, sex, race, and age at adoption. For estimates of antisocial behavior, Crowe used arrest records and follow-up psychiatric interviews. Results indicated that the criminal mothers had produced an excess of antisocial offspring, the antisocial behavior involving mostly an excess of misdemeanors rather than violent offenses. Interviews showed about 13 percent of the index offspring, but none of the control adoptees, met the criteria for antisocial personality disorder.

Additional evidence of a genetic factor comes from the largest adoptees' families study of criminality, one based on the criminal records of more than

14,000 Danish adoptees and their biological and adoptive parents (Mednick, Gabrielli, & Hutchings, 1984). The criminal convictions could not be characterized in great detail except for noting whether the adoptees' crimes were violent or offenses against property. While criminality in the adoptive parents was unrelated to adoptee criminality, criminality in the biological parents was correlated with the rate of property crimes in their adopted-away children. Moreover, the greater the recidivism in the biological parent, the greater the likelihood that the adopted-away offspring would eventually have a criminal conviction. As you can see in Figure 18.5, the adoptee conviction rate increases fairly regularly as a function of convictions in biological parents. Biological parent recidivism has a marked effect on property offenses among their offspring, but is not significant for violent offenses, suggesting, like the Crowe (1974) study, that the propensity for petty criminality as opposed to violent criminality is more likely to be genetically transmitted.

A retrospective study using MMPI profiles of mothers who had released their children for adoption revealed that the mothers of seemingly antisocial offspring had MMPI profiles suggestive of antisocial personality (Willerman, Loehlin, & Horn, unpublished). All these mothers had been administered the MMPI during their pregnancies about seventeen years earlier. Figure 18.6 compares the MMPI profiles of the biological mothers of antisocial and control children. In comparison to the mothers of the well-behaved adoptees, the biological mothers of the antisocial adoptees were elevated on several of the MMPI scales indicative of psychopathology, the statistically largest difference between the two groups of mothers being on the Psychopathic deviate scale of the MMPI.

In sum, there is evidence for the genetic transmission of criminal behavior

FIGURE 18.5 Percentage of adoptees convicted of violent and property offenses as a function of criminal convictions in the biological parents (From S. A. Mednick, W. F. Gabrielli, Jr., & B. Hutchings, Genetic influences in criminal convictions: Evidence from an adoption cohort. *Science, 224,* 891–894. Copyright © 1984 by the AAAS.)

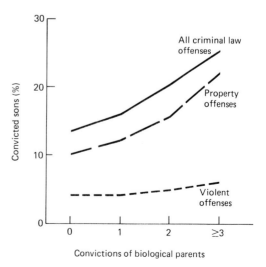

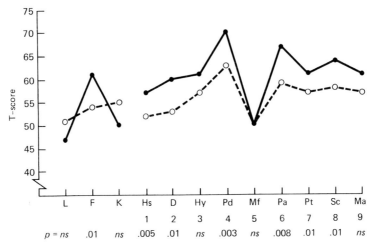

FIGURE 18.6 MMPI profiles of birth mothers of antisocial (solid line) ($N = 20$) and well-behaved (dashed line) ($N = 48$) adoptees. Significance levels at the bottom refer to MMPI scale differences between the birth mothers of the two groups of adoptees. (From Willerman, Loehlin, & Horn, in preparation)

probably to the extent that antisocial personality is a factor. But equating criminality with either the *DSM-III-R* diagnosis of antisocial personality disorder or Cleckley's diagnosis of psychopathy is not entirely warranted. Only about half of adult incarcerated criminals meet *DSM-III* diagnostic criteria for antisocial personality disorder or Cleckley's criteria for psychopathy (Hare, 1983). Obviously, not all criminals are antisocial personalities and not all antisocial personalities do time in prison.

BRIQUET-ANTISOCIAL PERSONALITY CONNECTION

Antisocial personality in males and females and Briquet in females not only run in the same families (Cloninger et al., 1975; Guze et al., 1986), but also can coexist within the same person. Indeed, one study showed that 26 percent of female felons were diagnosed as having antisocial personality *and* Briquet's syndrome (Cloninger & Guze, 1970).

A recent family study of Briquet's and antisocial personality confirms earlier reports of their connection. Table 18.6 presents results from interviews of the first-degree relatives of Briquet females and the relatives of control psychiatric patients (Guze et al., 1986). The first-degree relatives of the Briquet patients not only have substantially elevated rates of Briquet's but also elevated rates of antisocial personality, suggesting that the two disorders have something in common.

The hypothesized commonality is especially significant because there is no obvious overlap in the diagnostic criteria for each disorder. This result sug-

TABLE 18.6   RATES OF BRIQUET'S SYNDROME AND ANTISOCIAL PERSONALITY IN THE FIRST-DEGREE RELATIVES OF PSYCHIATRIC PATIENTS WITH EITHER BRIQUET'S SYNDROME OR SOME OTHER PSYCHIATRIC CONDITION

Patient's diagnosis	Female relatives' diagnosis of Briquet, %	Male relatives' diagnosis of antisocial personality, %
Briquet	6.6	18.7
Not Briquet	2.4	10.5

Source: From Guze, Cloninger, Martin, & Clayton, *British Journal of Psychiatry,* 1986, p. 20.

gests a common etiology, but expression of the abnormality may be affected by sex-specific biological and cultural factors (Warner, 1978). One cultural factor could be stereotypic biases of how men and women are expected and encouraged to behave. For example, males with antisocial personality are said to have "impersonal" sexual relations while female Briquets are said to have "promiscuous" sex, but it would seem that these different terms only represent culturally loaded interpretations of the same behavior.

A recent adoption study that bears on the issue of sex-specific expression showed a connection between many somatic complaints in women adopted early in life and elevated rates of either alcoholism or criminality in their biological fathers (Sigvardsson et al., 1984; Cloninger et al., 1984; Bohman et al., 1984). No psychiatric diagnoses were made, and the number of women who specifically had Briquet's syndrome is uncertain. Nevertheless, the important idea is that a lifelong history of multiple somatic complaints of one kind or another in daughters is associated with alcoholism or criminality in biological fathers.

The antisocial personality-Briquet hysteria connection is too close to be accidental (Cloninger, 1978). Perhaps a common thread tying them together is an inability to reflect before taking action. As noted in the previous chapter, females with Briquet's syndrome are not psychologically minded; the same obviously holds for those with antisocial personality. Not being introspective, people with Briquet's syndrome or antisocial personality attribute unlabeled or dysphoric feelings to more obvious sources—for example, physical symptoms, faults of others, bad friends. This introspective deficiency is exemplified by observations that antisocial personalities are more likely to report symptoms of somatic anxiety and tension such as unexplained restlessness, sweating, and severe headaches, than they are to report symptoms of psychic anxiety such as worry (Schalling, 1978).

TREATMENT

Yochelson and Samenow (1976) believe that psychopathy is characterized by erroneous thinking habits that are inimical to good conduct. When simply entering a store, for example, psychopaths immediately "case the joint," locating the cash register and developing an escape plan. Yochelson and Samenow do not believe that uncovering early childhood roots of this behavior is helpful to treatment. Only by drastically altering antisocial thinking habits is there any hope for therapeutic change. Their treatment approach includes relentless scrutiny of the psychopathic pattern: manipulativeness, maliciousness, and mendacity. Even nonarrestable misbehaviors, such as buying a car without enough money to maintain payments, are harshly criticized.

Although there is little reason for optimism in the treatment of adult antisocial personality disorder, occasional "successes" in treating its childhood version—conduct disorder—provide reason for cautious optimism. One study used a treatment approach called "cognitive-behavioral problem-solving skills training" (PSST), comparing it both with another form of therapy called "nondirective relationship therapy" and with an essentially untreated control group (Kazdin et al., 1987). On average, the results indicated a substantial advantage of PSST over the other two "treatments." An especially informative analysis asked about the proportion of children who were "normal" one year later. Only 23 percent of the PSST children were indistinguishable from normal children in comparison to 9 and 10 percent in the two other groups. Thus, a relatively successful treatment may not result in complete remission of symptoms for even a majority of children. However, decreasing deviance indicates modest success of the program, even if it falls short of complete normalization of function for the majority of children.

The treatment of antisocial adults is more complicated because parents usually cannot expose the person to treatment as they can with their young children. Often motivated only by a court order for treatment, antisocial adults are noncompliant and only superficially engaged, and leave therapy at the first opportunity. Thus, one of the biggest challenges to therapy with antisocial adults is to motivate them in treatment for a sufficient period of time (Offord & Reitsma-Street, 1983).

One pharmacological approach classifies antisocials by their distinctive problems—for example, are they aggressive, do they have deficits in avoidance learning or deficits in impulse control, and do they have EEG abnormalities (Cloninger, 1983)? A given patient may be normal for some of these qualities and abnormal for others. Cloninger prescribes lithium for impulsively aggressive individuals and anticonvulsant medication for those with seizurelike EEG abnormalities. Predatory bullies who are chronically but not impulsively aggressive may require a different chemical approach. Not many data are available on the success of these pharmacological treatments, but one study has confirmed the efficacy of lithium carbonate in explosively aggressive children (Campbell et al., 1984), and several other studies have suggested the utility of lithium for people with explosively antisocial behavior (see Shader, Scharfman, & Dreyfuss, 1986).

SUMMARY

Personality disorders are characterized by stereotyped patterns of coping marked by episodic eruptions of impulsive and ill-planned actions. These disturbances are difficult to treat because the symptoms do not seem alien to the patient and therefore produce little motivation to change. For that reason, the bulk of the chapter concerns antisocial personality disorder. The chapter focuses on the most reliably diagnosed personality disorder; namely, antisocial personality disorder.

Antisocial personality, a diagnosis made only in adults, has its origins in early development. Antisocial children, who often receive a childhood diagnosis of conduct disorder, display recklessness, hyperactivity, aggression, daring, and a general failure to conform to rules. Poor school performance continues in adolescence when these children often come to the attention of the law because of delinquency. Psychological tests reveal a pattern of relatively poorer verbal than nonverbal skills, suggesting an action-oriented rather than a verbally self-reflective approach to life. Experimental measures in adults with antisocial personality suggest a possible physiological mechanism which attenuates both conscious anxiety and responsiveness to threats of punishment. Neurological tests indicate EEG signs of immaturity and other aberrations suggestive of a neurodevelopmental lag that may have its primary effects on the frontal lobes and closely related structures.

The families of antisocials are characterized by poor child-rearing practices. However, the causal ecopathological status of these practices is rendered ambiguous because adoptees eventually diagnosed as psychopathic or criminal also have biological parents marked by antisocial behavior. Daughters of such parents have an excess of multiple somatic complaints, warranting a diagnosis of Briquet's syndrome. The two different diagnoses probably reflect sex differences in the expression of a common underlying biological vulnerability. An effective treatment for adults with antisocial personality disorder is unavailable, although behavioral and pharmacological treatments have attained some successes with children.

CHAPTER 19

Addictive Behaviors

OUTLINE

THE ADDICTION CONCEPT

Addictions are compulsive preoccupations with and dependencies on certain drugs. Addicts think only of the drug to the exclusion of other things, and when the drug is inaccessible, they are often frantic. These passionate attachments can result in personal, physiological, and occupational debilitation. Personal adjustment is sabotaged because involvement in obtaining and using drugs limits interpersonal relationships to fellow users or, even more narrowly, to total self-absorption. Physical health is compromised by toxic effects, nutritional deficiencies, or unsanitary practices associated with drug use, and occupational debilitation is expressed in unstable job performance.

Many people use addictive substances, but curiously, only a fraction become addicted. For example, only 8 to 12 percent of regular drinkers are addicted to alcohol and only about 25 percent of heroin users are addicts (Jaffe, 1980). Why some people become addicted while others do not is a central question we will try to answer in this chapter.

Although addictions usually involve substances such as alcohol and opiates, it is worth keeping in mind that addictions can develop even in the absence of a substance. For example, pathological gamblers display virtually all the features of addictive behavior. They are compulsively preoccupied with the excitement of gambling to the point where their personal and occupational functioning becomes impaired; they must continually increase the stakes in order to sustain excitement just as the addict must increase the drug dose in order to produce the same effect achieved earlier; and when prevented from gambling, they may experience psychological withdrawal symptoms such as agitation and depression.

Aspects of addictive functioning may also occur in those in the grip of infatuation. It produces a total preoccupation with the loved one, lovesickness if the partner is inaccessible, and eventually the loved one becomes a less thrilling stimulus. Since infatuation is a common experience, it is not regarded as deviant or pathological, yet when unrequited, it may call for a mental health professional. These examples point out the universality of addictive potential and the fact that addicts are not necessarily a ''breed apart.''

The diagnosis and severity of addiction are usually assessed on the basis of the seriousness of four clinical features: (1) *preoccupation* with the drug; (2) *tolerance* such that a larger dose is now required to produce effects achieved earlier with a smaller dose; (3) *dependency,* that is, whether psychological withdrawal symptoms such as agitation and depression, or physiological symptoms like seizures or cramps, occur after abrupt cessation of the drug's use;

and (4) *debilitation* of social and physiological function. While these four criteria of severity can readily be applied to current users, they are unsatisfactory for the so-called recovered addict who must resist temptations to relapse. It is the sustained absence of urges in widely different settings rather than the ability to resist the urges that really signifies the recovered addict. After all, the odds are good that persistent cravings, even those resisted hundreds of times, will eventually win out.

Not all relapses are associated with immediately succumbing to cravings, however. Some alcoholics, for example, plan their next binge weeks in advance as others plan vacations, suggesting that even the anticipation of eventually satisifying a craving can reduce the immediate necessity for using the drug (Mello & Mendelson, 1978).

Relapse is much more likely to occur if the person remains in, or returns to, the environment in which the original addiction was acquired. Relapse rates for detoxified U.S. Vietnam veterans and detoxified young civilian addicts treated in federal hospitals are shown in Figure 19.1 (Robins, Helzer, & Davis,

FIGURE 19.1 A comparison of narcotic use after leaving Vietnam and after release from federal detoxification hospitals. From Robins, L. N., Helzer, J. E., & Davis, D. H. (1975). Narcotic use in Southeast Asia and afterward. *Archives of General Psychiatry, 41,* 955–961. Copyright © 1975, American Medical Association.

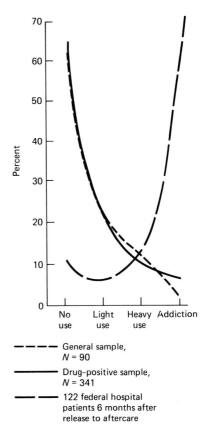

General sample, *N* = 90

Drug-positive sample, *N* = 341

122 federal hospital patients 6 months after release to aftercare

1975). While 70 percent of former opiate addicts treated in federal hospitals resumed their addiction within six months of release, less than 10 percent of the addicted veterans relapsed after discharge. Obviously, a result such as this means that addictions cannot be explained solely by the pharmacological properties of addictive drugs. Environmental factors, perhaps associated with ecopathology, peer influence, or conditioning, must figure in at least some kinds of addictive behavior. And, of course, access to an addictive substance is necessary for the eventual development of an addiction or a relapse.

The importance of accessibility as a prerequisite for addiction is shown even among those who are generally most knowledgeable about the adverse effects of addictive substances. For example, 15 percent of all opiate addicts in England are physicians and nurses (Jaffe, 1965). Social and cultural factors that increase the accessibility of addictive substances also influence the probability of addiction. In France wine is integral to social life and alcoholism is rampant. By contrast, some Middle Eastern countries do not permit alcohol. As a consequence, alcoholism is rare by comparison.

CAUSES OF ADDICTION

Theories about addiction typically focus on one or more basic causal factors such as the specific physiological properties of addictive drugs, personality traits that promote addiction, and newly acquired motivations after exposure to the drug. No one theory has yet been able to account for all the observations, however, suggesting that different theories may be applicable to different aspects of addictive behavior.

Theories which emphasize the distinctive physiological properties of addictive drugs argue that these drugs produce intense pleasurable experiences or alter physiology in ways that require more of the drug merely to feel normal. For example, rats forced to drink alcohol develop cell membranes that are less permeable than normal, presumably impairing their metabolism. Only by drinking more alcohol can the rats cause the membranes to return to normal permeability (Rottenberg, Waring, & Rubin, 1981). It would not be surprising if adverse membrane changes can be transformed into the experience of malaise which can then prompt drinking to produce relief.

Psychological theories argue that addictions arise because they fulfill a psychological need that cannot be easily satisfied in other ways. Presumably, preexisting psychopathology causes distress which is alleviated temporarily by the addictive drug. Since the drug does not eliminate the underlying problem, however, the person must repeatedly use the drug. Other theories emphasize the role of learning and conditioning in addictive behavior, especially the role of conditioned cues that elicit noxious withdrawal symptoms and cravings. For example, seeing someone take a drink may elicit conditioned withdrawal symptoms even in an abstinent alcoholic.

Addictive Potential of Specific Drugs

Drugs such as aspirin, antidepressants, and neuroleptics can reduce stress and make someone feel better, yet they are not abused. Then what are the distinctive properties of addictive drugs? A key observation is that drugs that produce addictions in humans also produce addictions in animals (Schuster, Renault, & Blaine, 1979). This indicates that the higher cognitive processes characteristic of humans are not necessary for an addiction to develop, although it is premature to say that addictions in animals are identical to addictions in humans.

One of the most important properties of drugs with addictive potential is that they are liked by the user; that is, they produce powerfully pleasurable effects regardless of their capacity to reduce pain or distress. Indeed, how well a substance is liked even after only one exposure is a good predictor of its addictive potential. Consider liking scores for six commonly used drugs in Figure 19.2. Except for Librium, a popular benzodiazepine tranquilizer, some dosage of each drug produces a higher liking score than its placebo control (Jasinski, Johnson, & Henningfield, 1984). The drug in the figure showing the highest correlation between dosage level and the degree of liking is morphine, confirming its powerful abuse potential.

The role of liking in addiction is concisely shown in the following dialogue from Cohen (1972):

FIGURE 19.2   Mean scores on the "liking" scale of the Single Dose Questionnaire. The responses are peak responses which occurred after the drug had been given. P is placebo. From Jasinski, D. R, Johnson, R. E. & Henningfield J. E. (1984). Abuse liability assessment in human subjects. *Trends in Pharmacological Sciences, 5,* 196–200. Copyright © 1984 Elsevier Science Publishing Co., Inc.

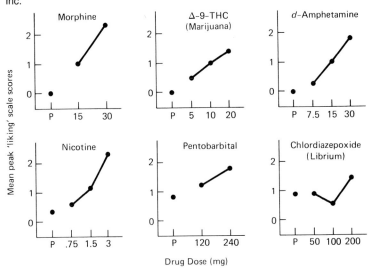

Interviewer: Why do you use drugs?
User: Why not?
Interviewer: How could someone convince you to stop?
User: Show me something better.

Distinctive anatomical substrates exist for pleasurable experiences. To illustrate, rats will compulsively press a bar in order to self-administer cocaine directly into the medial frontal cortex, but they will not do so if the drug goes to another brain area (Goeders & Smith, 1983). Indeed, animals trained to self-administer addictive substances directly into certain brain areas may even ignore their nutritional needs and die for the pleasures obtained (Falk, Dews, & Schuster, 1983).

Liking is not the whole story, however, because first experiences with many addictive substances are often decisively negative. For example, many heavy smokers remember their first cigarette as distinctly unpleasurable. In addition to the pleasurable effects of drugs, the capacity of drugs to elicit withdrawal symptoms after abstynence must also be considered. Heroin withdrawal, for example, produces cramps and chills, which can be relieved promptly only by more of the drug. On the other hand, withdrawal from cocaine produces negligible physical symptoms. Cocaine produces a psychological dependence in the absence of a physiological dependence, and probably has more to do with the pleasure obtained than with the postponement of withdrawal symptoms.

In sum, drugs may induce and maintain addiction through different mechanisms. Some drugs will mainly be pleasurable and sustain an addiction because of their desirable properties. Other pleasurable drugs will also produce severe withdrawal symptoms following abstinence, which then motivates repeated use to alleviate the symptoms.

Addiction-Prone Personality Traits

Studies of undercontrolled, hyperactive, and rebellious children reveal that they are at high risk for becoming alcoholics and drug abusers in adulthood (Jones, 1968). They are likely to have been school truants and alienated from their surroundings (Wilsnack & Wilsnack, 1979). Boys with such conduct problems are three times more likely than those without to become severe alcoholics. However, many alcoholics begin drinking in their 30s and 40s and have no prior history of misbehavior (Blane, 1979). Therefore, explanations of their addiction will not be found in personality traits associated with a history of recklessness. These late-onset cases appear to be anxious and dependent people who begin to abuse alcohol in order to relieve their current distress, and have persistent guilt feelings about their drinking (Cloninger, 1987). These alcoholics are different from the rebellious early-onset types who have little guilt over their frequent drinking.

Acquired Motivation

People who initially try a potentially addictive drug do not intend to become addicted. Instead, they are motivated by expectancies about its pleasurable properties or peer pressure. After an initial positive experience, however, the user becomes increasingly preoccupied with obtaining the drug. If the preoccupation becomes all-consuming, we say that the person is addicted. What causes a rather unremarkable and seemingly commonplace initial motive for drug use to be transformed into an all-consuming preoccupation? One popular theory of how this intense motivation is acquired is called the *opponent-process* theory (Solomon, 1977; Solomon & Corbit, 1974).

The first proposition of the theory simply says that a drug capable of producing an addiction elicits a pleasurable experience called the primary reaction. The next proposition is that this primary reaction is automatically countered by an opposite secondary reaction "wired-in" to the nervous system as a homeostatic mechanism. The secondary reaction has a distinctively different time course for buildup and decay, and would be experienced as displeasure were it to occur alone. Whereas the primary reaction occurs within a few minutes and decays rapidly as the addictive stimulus is cleared from the body, the secondary reaction has a much slower buildup and a much slower rate of decay. According to the theory, primary and secondary reactions sum algebraically to produce the overall affective state at any one point in time. In short, a positive affective state means that the pleasurable primary reaction dominates; a negative affective state means that the displeasurable secondary reaction dominates and the person is experiencing withdrawal symptoms.

Because the secondary reaction has a slower decay time, it can cumulate over repeated exposures to the addictive stimulus, becoming more and more negative if intervals between exposures to the addictive stimulus are relatively short. Upon initial exposure to an addictive drug, the secondary reaction is much less intense than the primary reaction, and the person experiences the drug as distinctly pleasurable. With repeated exposures to the drug, however, the secondary reaction gets increasingly intense and may be all that remains after the active properties of the drug have disappeared from the body. Tolerance develops to an addictive drug because the secondary reaction counters the primary reaction to the point that even the physiologically positive aspects of an addictive stimulus are no longer evident unless the drug dose is increased. Indeed, for some chronic heroin users, there is virtually no "high" from the drug anymore. The net effect of the buildup of the secondary reaction is unpleasant withdrawal symptoms and cravings, with the addict motivated solely to avoid withdrawal symptoms.

Although initially the secondary reaction is innate, it can be conditioned to various external or cognitive stimuli. In other words, *conditioned* secondary reactions can develop so that merely the sight or taste of something normally associated with a secondary reaction (the CS) can produce it, even in the absence of the drug (the UCS). This can be seen when a placebo is given to social drinkers who believe they are drinking an alcoholic beverage (Newlin, 1985). After drinking the placebo they show a reduced heart rate, quite the opposite of that produced directly by alcohol ingestion. Presumably, this conditioned secondary reaction, seen clearly in the absence of the active drug, serves normally to attenuate the positive primary reaction, and probably figures in the normal development of tolerance.

Conditioning factors typically come into play when environmental cues elicit powerful secondary reactions in the absence of the drug.

> Just as salivation and increased appetite or hunger can be evoked by the sight of food, a conditioned withdrawal syndrome with associated craving may result whenever the alcoholic passes the bar, sees other people drinking, or encounters cues relevant to previous drinking practices. Also, since anxiety, nervousness, jitteriness, and other types of emotional dysphoria may produce such physiological responses as increased heart rate and respiration, tremulousness, autonomic liability, increased sweating, insomnia, all of which represent changes associated with the alcohol withdrawal syndrome, we should anticipate that these states, induced either by arguments with spouses, employment difficulties or loneliness, may likewise evoke craving (Ludwig, Wikler, & Stark, 1974, pp. 539–540).

Conditioned secondary reactions prompt the addict to seek ways to reduce the dysphoria. The most efficient way to eliminate the negative reaction, of course, is to take more of the drug, which is exactly what is meant by a conditioned addictive cycle. The potential for a conditioned secondary reaction often remains for life, the consequence of which can be relapse years after the person has begun to abstain. This is precisely why it is so difficult to be certain that an addict is ever completely cured.

Why people try drugs in the first place is a different question, but the answer presumably includes novelty seeking, desire to seem mature and peer pressure. When initial exposure to a drug produces dysphoria, as it does so often, novelty seeking probably becomes less important, although peer pressure and continued striving for maturity still play an influential role. For example, the first cigarette usually produces dizziness, nausea, and coughing. Were these reactions alone decisive, no one would smoke again. However, because these symptoms also serve as a rite of passage or are awarded by peer approval, the user persists. Those for whom these motives are unimportant or who experience extremely negative psychophysiological reactions should be deterred after the initial dysphoric experience.

The opponent-process theory has some limitations, and recent advances which make more precise distinctions between the physiological substrates of pleasure and withdrawal symptoms may soon supplant the theory. The opponent-process theory does not specifically address addictions to drugs such as cocaine that produce psychological withdrawal symptoms like depression and fatigue rather than noxious physical symptoms like cramps and seizures (Baker, Morse, & Sherman, 1987). Indeed, these stimulants have little or no effect on the brain areas associated with dysphoric physical withdrawal symptoms. Urges arising from physical withdrawal symptoms could produce relapse if the person is addicted to opiates, but not if addicted to stimulants. Relapse among stimulant addicts is more likely to be associated with the revival of memories of their pleasurable effects.

Distinct Substrates for Positive and Negative Subjective Experiences

There are distinct physiological substrates for the euphoric versus the distress-relieving experiences associated with use or withdrawal of addictive drugs (Wise, 1988). Addictive drugs stimulate certain pathways within the *median forebrain bundle*, a component of the limbic system, producing intense pleasure by increasing the quantity of synaptic dopamine in that region. The anatomical substrate for relief of physical withdrawal symptoms, however, is associated with a different neuroanatomical substrate called the *periaqueductal gray*, an area surrounding the canal connecting the third and fourth ventricles in the brain stem. The periaqueductal gray region is also known to be involved in the mediation of physical pain through the endorphin system, which will be described at the end of this chapter. Opiates like heroin and morphine have powerful effects in the periaqueductal gray (distress relief) as well as in the median forebrain bundle (pleasure), whereas stimulants such as amphetamine and cocaine affect only the median forebrain bundle.

The factors that cause and maintain addiction might differ as a function of the brain areas that are affected by a specific drug. If only the median forebrain bundle is stimulated, euphoria is produced, but withdrawal symptoms will not develop if the drug is discontinued (Gawin & Ellinwood, 1988). Abstinence from opiates results in physical withdrawal symptoms arising from the periaqueductal gray, and relief comes only by taking the same or a substitute drug, keeping the opiate user in an addictive cycle to relieve the withdrawal symptoms. Elimination of the physical withdrawal symptoms is possible, but then one has still to deal with memories of the euphoria-producing effects of the opiate arising from past stimulation in the median forebrain bundle. The specific brain areas excited by alcohol are not entirely clear, but injections of alcohol increase synaptic dopamine levels in the limbic system in the same way as injections of cocaine or amphetamine (DiChiara & Imperato, 1988). We should keep in mind, however, that drugs have effects not only in the specific areas under investigation, but also in other areas. The behavioral architecture of responses distinctive to each drug probably depends on the specific pattern of influence of the drug on other regions of the brain.

Drugs that stimulate the median forebrain bundle do so more effectively than any "normal" forms of pleasure such as good food, sex, or the beauty of nature. Memories of past pleasures associated with previous use of the drug can continue to motivate a habit despite obvious self-destructive consequences. Wise (1988) points out that drugs of abuse are too pleasurable for our own good. Psychoactive drugs that affect the median forebrain bundle can surpass normal forms of pleasure, which is why it is so difficult to cure addiction, even when physiological withdrawal symptoms have long since disappeared.

Moreover, pharmacological treatments directed only at the unpleasant symptoms of opiate withdrawal neglect the importance of pleasurable memories in maintaining a drug addiction. If effective treatments for addiction are to be found, they will have to deal with the different roles played by the positive and negative affects arising from anatomically distinct sites.

ALCOHOLISM: DESCRIPTIVE ASPECTS

Alcohol is the most widely abused substance known and for that reason is the main focus of this chapter. Estimated to affect 10 million Americans, alcoholism costs billions in lost productivity, is a prominent source of marital discord and divorce, figures in about half the vehicular fatalities and homicides, and is associated with almost half of the more than 5 million arrests annually (Chafetz, 1975).

Behavioral Effects of Alcohol

Alcohol is a central nervous system depressant, as are sedative hypnotics such as barbiturates that produce relaxation effects at low doses and sleep at high doses. For unknown reasons, depressant drugs block inhibitory neurons more effectively than excitatory neurons. The consequence of small doses is a reduction of anxiety and discomforting self-consciousness, a pleasurable loss of inhibitory control, and an enhanced sense of efficacy. Larger amounts, however, produce dysphoria and the symptoms of intoxication: incoordination, slurred speech, and uninhibited behavior. With respect to sexuality, though alcohol "provokes the desire, it takes away the performance." Curiously, alcohol-induced delayed orgasm may sometimes be perceived as enhancing sexuality because it prolongs the sex act.

Overdoses of alcohol depress excitatory neurons as well, so that a person becomes extremely drowsy or comatose. Were barbiturates taken in the same social circumstances and doses in which alcohol is typically imbibed, they would produce symptoms virtually identical to those of alcohol. (This explains why barbiturates are not considered separately in this chapter despite their distinctively different chemical structure.)

Most states in the United States define intoxication as a blood alcohol level of 0.10 percent. For a 150-pound man, this level is achieved by loading an empty stomach with four or five cans of beer or four or five ounces of whiskey in an hour. Females, because of relatively more body fat, which does not absorb alcohol, achieve these levels with a smaller dose. A rough idea of the correlation between blood alcohol levels and behavior is given by Ray (1972).

At less than .03 percent, the individual is dull and dignified.
At .05 percent, he is dashing and debonair.
At .10 percent, he may become dangerous and devilish.
At .20 percent, he is likely to be dizzy and disturbing.
At .25 percent, he may be disgusting and disheveled.

At .30 percent, he is delirious and disoriented and surely drunk.
At .35 percent, he is dead drunk.
At .60 percent, the chances are that he is dead.

Ethnic Differences

Alcoholism rates vary among ethnic groups. Whether residing in their native lands or elsewhere, Asians have a low rate of alcoholism (less that 1 percent). One explanation is that there is something different about their physiology. Indeed, it does appear that Asians are hypersensitive to small amounts of alcohol.

Physiological Differences   Small doses of alcohol produce strikingly different reactions in Caucasians and Asians (Wolff, 1972). Only 3 percent of Caucasoids flush, in comparison to 80 percent of Asians. The racial groups also differ in subjective symptoms. Only 3 percent of Caucasoids, but 43 percent of Asians, report rapid heartbeat (tachycardia) after drinking. Asians also have higher rates of palpitations, muscle weakness, dizziness, and sleepiness.

There appears to be a good genetic explanation for these ethnic differences. A liver enzyme called aldehyde dehydrogenase (ALDH) is responsible for the breakdown of acetaldehyde, a metabolite of alcohol. ALDH actually has two forms, I and II; ALDH-I is missing in many Asians, resulting in the slower breakdown of acetaldehyde (Stoil, 1987/1988). Since acetaldehyde accumulation accounts for alcohol's unpleasant and toxic symptoms, it seems likely that many Asians drink less because alcohol is more noxious to them.

Japanese alcoholics tend not to have an ALDH-I deficiency, while nonalcoholic Japanese are often deficient in that enzyme. Table 19.1 gives rates of ALDH-I deficiency in various groups of Japanese, including normals, schizophrenics, alcoholics, and persons addicted to drugs other than alcohol. It is clear that ALDH-I deficiency is common in all groups of Japanese, except the alcoholics, suggesting that ALDH-I deficiency protects against the development of alcoholism in the Japanese. It is, however, worth noting that many of the controls have no deficiency of ALDH-I, yet do not become alcoholic, so that the deficiency alone cannot explain low rates of alcoholism in Japan. But

TABLE 19.1   FREQUENCY OF ALDH-I DEFICIENCY IN ALCOHOLICS, NONALCOHOLICS, AND NORMAL CONTROLS FROM JAPAN

Subjects	No.	% with deficiency
Normal controls	105	41.0
Alcoholics	175	2.3
Schizophrenics	86	41.9
Drug dependents	47	48.9

Source: From Harada et al., *The Lancet* II, No. 8302, p. 827.

the Japanese results should alert us to the possibility that unknown enzymatic factors in other populations could make drinking strongly unpleasant and therefore protect against developing alcoholism. Since ALDH-I deficiency does not occur in Caucasians, their alcoholism must have another explanation. But as many as 10 percent of Caucasians have unpleasant symptoms following alcohol ingestion, suggesting the possibility of other enzymatic factors operating to discourage drinking in Western groups.

Social and Cultural Factors   Noxious symptoms arising from alcohol ingestion may discourage excess intake, but are probably not sufficient in certain environments to prevent alcoholism. For example, American Indians also respond adversely to alcohol, in keeping with their Asian genetic heritage, yet they have among the highest rates of alcoholism in the world (Hanna, 1976).

Wolff (1973) suggested that visible flushing and other alcohol-related symptoms serve as cues of getting high and are more likely to be encouraged rather than censured in Indian social settings. Where drinking itself is not laden with positive emotional and personal significance—as an indication of virility or maturity, for example—the noxious symptoms alone should be a sufficient deterrent to continued drinking.

In sum, cultural factors can override physiological dispositions, and genetically related variations in alcohol metabolism can interact with the socially defined meaning of the symptoms to determine the likelihood of alcohol abuse. In one context the symptoms promote further drinking; in another they act as a deterrent.

Alcoholism rates also depend on how alcohol consumption is regulated in the family. Prohibitions are less effective in controlling drinking than are prescriptions for how, when, and where it is to be used (Vaillant, 1983a). Summarizing a report by the National Institutes of Health, Sarason (1972) says that the likelihood of alcoholism is minimized when

1 Children are exposed to alcohol early in life, but in diluted amounts, and usually within the context of some family or religious ritual
2 The beverages usually ingested have a low percentage of alcohol
3 The beverage is considered mainly as food and is usually taken with meals
4 Parents drink only moderately
5 No moral importance is attached to drinking
6 Drinking is not considered proof of virility or adulthood
7 Abstinence is socially acceptable
8 Excessive drinking is socially unacceptable, and
9 The culture group agrees on the point at which drinking has gone too far and should be stopped

These prescriptions have the effect of reducing the probability of overexposure to alcohol. As a consequence the person is unlikely to enter an addictive cycle.

Diagnosis and Classification

There are different ways to diagnose alcoholism. Some classifications empha-size physical symptoms while others emphasize the social debilitation arising from its abuse. But it seems reasonably clear that different methods of diag-nosis agree well with each other (Vaillant, Gale, & Milofsky, 1982). The diag-nosis of alcoholism can be established on the basis of physical symptoms such as tremulousness and morning drinking to stave off withdrawal symptoms or on the basis of social and occupational impairments including job loss and friends' complaints about drinking too much.

Abuse versus Dependence   The *DSM-III-R* disregards the differences among various drugs, placing all addictions into one category called either Psychoactive Substance Dependence or Psychoactive Substance Abuse. To earn a diagnosis of dependence, the patient must meet only some of the crite-ria. The abuse diagnosis is a residual category for those who fail to meet a suf-ficient proportion of the criteria for dependence. The nine original criteria for dependence can be reduced to five: (1) the development of tolerance (although cirrhotic liver damage in chronic alcoholism can actually cause tolerance to decrease), (2) failure to control excessive intake, (3) preoccupation with get-ting the drug, (4) narrowing of interests, and (5) withdrawal symptoms.

Withdrawal symptoms following either abstinence or a reduction in the usual amount of alcohol intake can be quite dramatic.

> Tremulousness, which appears within a few hours after the last drink, is often ac-companied by nausea, weakness, anxiety, and sweating. Purposive behavior di-rected toward obtaining alcohol or a suitable substitute is prominent. There may be cramps and vomiting. Hyperreflexia is prominent. Tremors may be mild or so marked that the patient may be unable to lift a glass. The subject may begin to "see things," at first only when the eyes are closed but later even while the eyes are open. Insight is at first retained, and the subject remains oriented. The syndrome at this point is often referred to as acute alcoholic hallucinosis. . . . Grand mal seizures can occur, but they are less common in alcohol withdrawal than in barbiturate with-drawal.
>
> The tremulous state reaches peak intensity within 24 to 48 hours, and seizures are most likely to occur within the first 24 hours after cessation of drinking. If the syn-drome progresses further, insight is lost; the subject becomes weaker, more con-fused, disoriented, and agitated. He may be terrified by his persecutory hallucina-tions. They are often so vivid that the subject, even after recovery, sometimes doubts their unreality. At this stage, which appears around the third day of with-drawal, the picture is that of the tremulous delirium (Jaffe, 1980, p. 553).

Table 19.2 gives the frequency of various problems and complaints associ-ated with alcohol dependence in a group of men followed from teenage until age 47 (Vaillant, Gale, & Milofsky, 1982). In comparison to social drinkers— men who drink mainly on social occasions—the dependent had many more alcohol-related problems; 90 percent of them had trouble controlling their drinking and 93 percent had friends or relatives who had complained. Only 56

TABLE 19.2   THE SYMPTOMS OF PROBLEM DRINKING THAT MOST EFFECTIVELY
DEFINED ALCOHOLISM

	Symptom frequency, %	
Symptoms of problem drinking	Alcohol-dependent (N = 68)	Social drinker (N = 240)
Symptomatic drinking	96	4
Admits problem controlling alcohol use	90	1
Family or friends complain	93	8
Morning drinking	76	1
Problems with health	78	1
Problems with job	67	0
Blackouts	80	3
Going on the wagon	79	5
Ever diagnosed alcoholic	56	0
Marital problems	71	2
More than 3 alcohol-related arrests	61	0
One hospital, clinic, or AA visit	59	0
Financial problems	49	0
Employer's complaint	50	0

Source: After Vaillant, Gale, & Milofsky, *Journal of Studies on Alcohol,* 1982, *43,* p. 225. Reprinted with permission from *Journal of Studies on Alcohol,* vol. 43, pp. 216–312, 1982. Copyright © by Journal of Studies on Alcohol, Inc., Rutgers Center of Alcohol Studies, New Brunswick, NJ 08903.

percent had been formally diagnosed as alcoholic, suggesting the existence of a large proportion of undiagnosed alcoholics in the general population.

Primary versus Secondary Alcoholism   Another distinction made by experts is that between primary and secondary alcoholism: primary when no other diagnosable disorder is thought to cause the alcoholism or secondary if the alcoholism arises as a consequence of a basically different disorder like psychopathy or depression. The primary-secondary distinction has important theoretical and practical implications. For example, many people with antisocial personality disorder are also alcoholic, but the family backgrounds of secondary alcoholics with antisocial personality disorder and primary alcoholics without antisocial personality disorder differ greatly. Indeed, children from nonalcoholic but socially troubled families have only one-quarter the risk of becoming alcoholic compared with children of alcoholic fathers from well-functioning families (Vaillant, 1983b).

WHY DO PEOPLE BECOME ALCOHOLIC?

Given that the dangers of alcohol are generally known, it is not entirely clear why people enter an addictive cycle in the first place. Since many alcoholics could easily have anticipated the negative consequences by seeing relatives affected, the familiality of alcoholism is especially surprising. To be sure, positive expectancies about the ''good'' things to be achieved by drinking, such as a loss of inhibition, increased conviviality, and illusions of increased sexual prowess can be powerful motivators that cause neglect of the possible negative consequences.

Three prominent hypotheses to explain the origins of alcoholism—(1) pleasure, (2) tension reduction, and (3) heredity—are considered here. The first hypothesis refers mainly to positive reinforcing effects of alcohol and was discussed earlier in the context of other drugs. The second hypothesis refers to the distress-relieving effects of alcohol. The third hypothesis refers to the genetic basis of high initial alcohol tolerance or more rapid metabolism of alcohol so that it produces fewer debilitating effects. These hypothetical mechanisms are not mutually incompatible; indeed, they may be operating simultaneously. Later, when the destructive results of alcoholism are perfectly clear to the user, the distinctive physiological properties of addictive substances may maintain addictive behavior, and conditioning factors may be operating to cause abstainers to relapse.

Tension Reduction

The tension reduction hypothesis says that some people drink in order to reduce anxiety, distress, or discomforting self-consciousness (Hull, 1981). The tension-reducing effects of alcohol can be seen in a study of young men given either a high or low dose of alcohol before being made apprehensive about interacting with a female confederate. The men had previously been divided into two groups according to whether they had a high or low tolerance for alcohol based on a test dose of the drug. Not surprisingly, the larger the alcohol dose the more stress-relieving its effects. But a larger dose in the highly tolerant seemed to be less effective in relieving anxiety than a smaller dose in the less tolerant (Figure 19.3).

These results reveal that alcohol can relieve tension and that the effects also depend on the drinker's prior level of alcohol tolerance. The main question is whether the low- or the high-tolerance people are more prone to become alcohol abusers. In our view it is the highly tolerant, because they must imbibe more alcohol to achieve the desired tension-relieving effects, and the overdrinking makes them more liable to withdrawal symptoms later. People with low tolerance for alcohol could achieve similar behavioral effects with smaller doses that do not importantly alter physiology; thus, low-tolerance individuals would not find it necessary to drink much alcohol even with the same degree of initial distress.

What empirical evidence is there to support the hypothesis that the tolerant are more likely to become alcoholic? Perhaps the clearest evidence comes from a study of moderate-drinking young men who were either at high risk for developing alcoholism because they had an alcoholic first-degree relative or were at low risk because they had no alcoholic relative. The men were administered alcohol and their body sway responses were recorded while standing

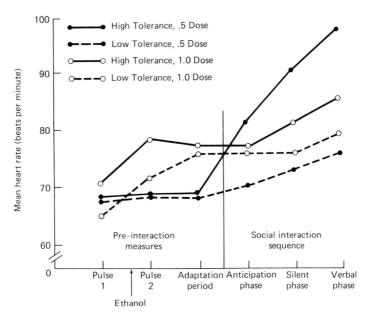

FIGURE 19.3   Mean pulse rate in beats per minute throughout the experiment. Doses indicate amount of alcohol given in grams of absolute alcohol per kilogram of body weight. From Lipscomb, T. R., Nathan, P. E., Wilson, T., and Abrams, D. B. (1980). Effects of tolerance on the anxiety-reducing function of alcohol. *Archives of General Psychiatry, 37,* 577–582. Copyright © 1980, American Medical Association.

with eyes closed (high body sway after a test dose of alcohol is used as an indication of low tolerance). The results of the body sway test for the high- and low-risk subjects are shown in Figure 19.4. Clearly, the high-risk subjects show much less body sway to alcohol, confirming the idea that highly tolerant people are more likely to come from families with a history of alcoholism. Moreover, these results support the idea that high tolerance is a risk factor for alcoholism. If high tolerance is coupled with few initial negative side effects, it would seem that there is fertile ground for developing alcoholism once drinking begins. However, one should not expect all the high-risk offspring to show elevated tolerance, even if a genetic theory is entirely correct. If just one genetic factor were important for alcoholism, only half the children of an alcoholic parent would be expected to have the deviant gene; the other offspring would be expected to be indistinguishable from controls without a family history of alcoholism.

Alcohol relieves tension by its depressant effects on the brain. It produces slow, high-amplitude, well-organized EEG waves (Figure 19.5) with correlated feelings of relaxation (Propping, 1978). One interesting idea is that prealcoholics have EEG peculiarities that are associated with higher levels of arousal and tension. The alcohol tends to "normalize" the EEG, with the cor-

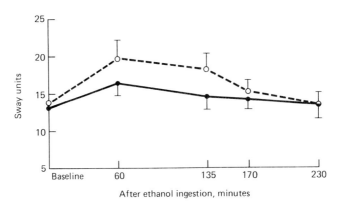

FIGURE 19.4 Mean total body sway counts following ingestion of 0.75 milliliters per kilogram for thirty four matched pairs of young men with either a positive (solid line) or negative (broken line) family history of alcoholism. From Schuckit, M. A. (1985a). Ethanol-induced changes in body sway in men at high alcoholism risk. *Archives of General Psychiatry, 42*, pp. 375–379. Copyright © 1985, American Medical Association.

related behavioral consequence of increasing feelings of well-being. If prealcoholics have especially deviant EEGs, they are more likely to benefit from the normalizing effects of alcohol. Consistent with this idea is the observation that the preteen sons of alcoholics show more EEG disorganization than preteen controls do (Gabrielli et al., 1982). Also, primary alcoholics report more hyperactivity and distractibility as children (Jones, 1968; Tarter et al., 1977), conditions often associated with aberrant EEGs. All these observations support the widely held view that some alcoholics use alcohol as self-

FIGURE 19.5 Male MZ twins with relatively poorly expressed EEG alpha waves at rest. But 120 minutes after drinking 1.2 grams per kilogram of alcohol, alpha waves have become much more pronounced. From Propping, P. (1977. *Human Genetics, 35,* 309–334.

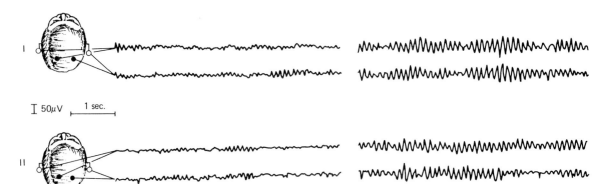

medication to relieve their dysphoria, but these studies were not designed to address the possible genetic basis of these problems, an issue to which we will now turn.

Genetic Propensity

At least 31 percent of alcoholics have an alcoholic parent, the vast majority being the father (Cotton, 1979; Harford, Haack, & Spiegler, 1987/1988). The rate is about six times that of the relatives of normal controls, and about 2.5 times that of the relatives of nonalcoholic psychiatric patients. Observations such as these raise the question of whether alcoholism or, more precisely, a liability to alcoholism can be genetically transmitted (Searles, 1988). And if the answer is affirmative, what is inherited?

Much of what we know about the genetic, physiological, and behavioral effects of alcohol derives from studies of lower animals. Mice can be bred for alcohol preference and tolerance. Consistent with what we have inferred from the data on humans, highly tolerant mice show the greatest preference for alcohol when given a choice (Fuller, Church, & Dann, 1976; Le & Kiianma, 1988). In short, evidence from animal studies indicates that alcohol preference has some genetic determination and that higher tolerance is associated with more drinking.

Although there is little doubt of familial influences on alcoholism, family studies alone cannot untangle genetic and environmental factors. Some twin research (Kaij, 1960) suggests that a hereditary factor exists for alcoholism, but more recent twin studies have not been confirmatory (see Gurling, Grant, & Dangl, 1985). While adoption studies have been somewhat more consistent in demonstrating the genetic transmission of alcoholism, the results have depended on the sex of the adoptee, with males showing more evidence of genetic transmission.

A Danish study supported a simple genetic hypothesis for the transmission of *alcoholism,* but not of heavy drinking short of alcoholism, in adopted-away sons of alcoholics (Goodwin et al., 1973). High-risk adoptees were almost four times more likely to become alcoholic than control male adoptees. An unexplained puzzle, however, was that heavy drinking and problem drinking were not in excess among the high-risk adoptees. This lack of continuity is troublesome for any hypothesis that posits multiple genetic factors for alcoholic propensity, although the existence of a single gene for alcoholism remains a possibility. Indeed, a reanalysis of the Kaij (1960) twin study on alcoholism showed extremely high heritabilities only for the most severe degree of alcoholism, chronic alcoholism for ten or more years, suggesting that milder forms might be less heritable (Gottesman & Carey, 1983).

A virtually identical Danish study of female adoptees found no evidence for genetic transmission of alcoholic propensity (Goodwin et al., 1977). Other adoption studies have also found that the sex of the adoptee must be taken into account. For example, a Swedish adoption study found clear evidence for genetic transmission of alcohol abuse in adopted-away sons, but only alcohol abuse (and not alcoholism) in the biological mother predicted of alcohol abuse in the adopted-away daughters (Cloninger, Bohman, & Sigvardsson, 1981)—and alcohol abuse in the biological father did not predict alcoholism in the adopted-away daughters. (The Swedish studies could not make precise distinctions between abuse and dependence.) To make matters more complicated, a recent American adoption study found that alcoholism was heritable, and that the heritability was equal for both sexes (Cadoret et al., 1986).

At this stage all we can say is that the existence of a heritable factor in alcoholism is a strong possibility for males, but the issue remains uncomfortably ambiguous for females because a genetic factor cannot decisively be demonstrated or excluded. There is good evidence to indicate that influences outside the family have a much greater impact on the development of female alcoholism (Cloninger et al., 1978). For example, we know that future female alcoholics begin heavy drinking several years later than future male alcoholics. Since females are more closely supervised, they are unlikely to begin heavy drinking when under their parents' roof. After leaving home, they are much freer to drink in response to stress or social influences.

TREATMENT OF ALCOHOLISM

The search for an effective treatment for alcoholism continues unabated. Many treatments emphasize a physiological route while others emphasize psychological and social factors. No treatment or treatment combination can yet lay claim for superiority, although it is clear that treatment is better than no treatment. There are sporadic publications of well-controlled studies that indicate benefits of a particular treatment over either no treatment or a control treatment (Miller & Hester, 1986). But replications are not always successful, thus preventing any definitive conclusions one way or the other. If there is one principle to be gleaned from these hundreds of treatment studies, it is that initial signs of therapeutic success seem to dissipate with longer follow-ups. That is, the longer the follow-up, the less the advantage of the initially superior treatment. Were alcoholism regarded like a chronic medical disease such as diabetes mellitus, these results would not be surprising. After all, chronic medical conditions do not clear up after time-limited treatment, but often require lifelong therapy.

Clinicians tend to see only the "losers"—those who fail to overcome the addiction without professional help (Schachter, 1982). Some believe that this biased ascertainment may result in an unrealistically pessimistic prognosis for alcoholics in general. Evidence suggests, however, that pessimism is justified. Many undiagnosed alcoholics also abstain for awhile, but eventually relapse. In Valliant and Milofsky's (1982a) longitudinal study of alcohol abusers, which includes a large proportion of previously undiagnosed alcoholics, only 44 percent were abstinent for even a year and only half of the abstinent were "securely abstinent," that is, alcohol-free for at least three years.

Improved treatment methods, however, may lead to somewhat greater abstinence rates at follow-up. For example, aversion therapy can chemically induce nausea or vomiting in association with alcohol. In a recent study of aversion therapy, 45 percent of the alcoholics remained abstinent for at least twelve months (Cannon et al., 1986). A control group was not employed, but a 45 percent rate of abstinence is surely promising.

When addicts enter treatment, they often are depressed or antisocial. Moreover, many are unemployed, divorced, and generally doing poorly. Many of these debilities are the effects rather than causes of the addiction. To illustrate, Table 19.3 gives some findings from a prospective longitudinal study of 456 young teenagers followed until 47 years old (Vaillant & Milofsky, 1982a). Among the subjects were seventy-one who eventually became dependent on alcohol and 260 who were only social drinkers. As adults, the alcoholics had lower social class, more unemployment, and more symptoms of psychopathology. Yet as children, corresponding differences between the two groups were far less apparent, suggesting that at least some of the very large adult differences between alcoholics and nonalcoholics are effects, not causes of alcoholism.

It is interesting to review the histories of people who were once diagnosed as alcoholic but who later became social drinkers or abstainers for at least one year. Figure 19.6 from the Vaillant and Milofsky (1982a) study arranges them according to the severity of their original alcohol abuse. Only the most mildly alcoholic ever returned securely to social drinking; the severely alcoholic all became abstainers if they were not going to remain alcoholics. It would appear that for most severe alcoholics, a return to social drinking is unlikely, and abstinence seems to be a more realistic goal. People with initially milder alcoholism, however, might have some prospect of returning to social drinking.

TABLE 19.3   ADULT VARIABLES THAT ARE MORE A RESULT THAN A CAUSE OF ALCOHOLISM

Variable	Social drinkers, % (N = 260)	Alcohol-dependent, % (N = 71)
Adult		
Lowest adult social class	4	21
Unemployed more than 10 years	4	24
Never completed high school	56	41
High psychopathology score	24	51
Corresponding childhood		
Lowest parent's social class	32	30
Multiproblem families	11	14
IQ of less than 90	28	30
Childhood emotional problems	32	30

Source: From Vaillant, G. E., & Milofsky, E. (1982). The etiology of alcoholism. *American Psychologist, 37,* 494–503. Copyright © 1982 by the American Psychological Association. Reprinted by permission.

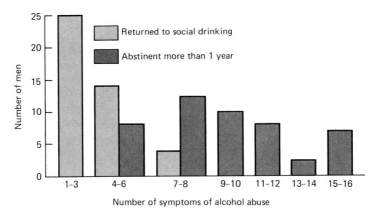

FIGURE 19.6 Number of men who became social drinkers or abstinent classified by the prior severity of their alcohol abuse. From Vaillant, G. E., & Milofsky, E. S. (1982). Natural history of male alcoholism IV: Paths to recovery. *Archives of General Psychiatry, 39,* 127–133. Copyright © 1982, American Medical Association.

Vaillant asked the abstaining alcoholics why they had quit drinking. Most abstainers explained that they had acquired a substitute dependency, including new love relationships, religious involvement, and Alcoholics Anonymous (AA). But this does not prove that alcoholism arose out of unmet dependencies. The demoralization of alcoholism could create dependencies that are relieved by substitutes. It is also interesting that few former alcoholics say that specific treatments were responsible for their recovery (Offord, 1986). Many alcoholics have had to "hit bottom" before they made a sincere and sustained effort to resist the urge to relapse.

Psychological Treatment

Because humans have ideas and feelings arising independently of current external events, internal states that might motivate relapse cannot be controlled simply by rearranging the external environment. If these autonomous internal states are conditioned to the withdrawal symptoms that motivate drinking, a cure is bound to be difficult. One cannot expect great strides in psychological treatment unless the alcoholic breaks the conditioned association of these feelings with withdrawal symptoms. This might be done through cognitive therapies that help the alcoholic reinterpret the meaning of his experience or through therapies that provide better coping skills so that the feelings do not arise. One interesting approach does neither of these. Rather, it tries to train the alcoholic to drink less.

Controlled Drinking The question of whether alcoholics can become controlled drinkers is critical for practical reasons. If alcoholics could be taught to drink moderately—for example, by sipping drinks slowly—the heroic requirement to resist temptation could be finessed. Unfortunately, the evidence indicates that training severe alcoholics to drink in a controlled fashion doesn't usually work (Pendery, Maltzman, & West, 1982; but see Sobell & Sobell, 1984). The "natural" course of events for people receiving more conventional treatments for alcoholism also implies a dim prospect for controlled drinking. In a survey of 387 alcoholics, fewer than 2 percent had become moderate drinkers in the three years following treatment (Helzer et al., 1985). Relaxing the criteria to include mainly abstinence interspersed with episodes of moderate drinking brought it up to only 6 percent.

Alcoholics Anonymous Started in 1935 by a physician and a former alcoholic stockbroker, the tenets of the organization are embodied in Twelve Steps and Twelve Traditions. Essentially, these tenets require unambiguously admitting one's alcoholism, putting faith in God, and making amends to those who have been harmed. If the alcoholic adheres faithfully to the tenets and incorporates the belief system, the former alcoholic is unlikely to resume drinking. Unfortunately, the vast majority of people who have attended AA meetings drop out. Many people have bridled at AA's religious fervor, and others have objected because it substitutes one dependency for another. As we have seen, there appears to be some truth to this latter point. Nevertheless, there are positive aspects that counterbalance these objections. Involvement in AA includes helping others in distress and provides a sense of purpose and worth, qualities that are often sadly lacking in the alcoholic.

Medical Treatment

No dependable medical treatment exists for preventing relapse, although cooperative patients can take a pill containing disulfiram, which can serve as a temporary deterrent to drinking. Disulfiram—or Antabuse, as it is commonly called—inhibits alcohol dehydrogenase, an enzyme important in breaking down alcohol. If the patient then drinks, the consequence is violent nausea and a sudden drop in blood pressure. Unfortunately, a single pill is effective for only three or four days, so that an alcoholic can simply resume drinking after waiting awhile. Indeed, if Antabuse is merely made easily available without ensuring that it is taken, it is an ineffective deterrent to relapse (Shuckit, 1985; Fuller et al., 1986).

Goodwin (1982) nevertheless recommends that alcoholics be told about the pill, especially after being detoxified. The alcoholic may benefit at least temporarily and there need be no permanent heroic commitment to abstinence. Antabuse is not meant to be a total treatment, but rather a temporary assist to give the alcoholic hope. If during this period of sobriety the patient can find substitute pleasures or learn to live without alcohol, perhaps relapse can be delayed or prevented.

OPIATE ADDICTION

Opium, a juice from the poppy, has been praised for centuries for its medicinal properties. It is the only naturally occurring analgesic, a substance capable of relieving intense pain. It also has been celebrated for its capacity to induce a drowsy euphoria when smoked and this is where its powerful addictive potential becomes evident.

In the early 1800s morphine was identified as the primary analgesic in opium (it also contains codeine). Although morphine is addictive, it is not as widely abused as heroin because it is less able to cross the blood-brain barrier quickly, a barrier that prevents large molecules from leaving the blood stream and entering the brain. But a synthetic alteration of the morphine molecule produces heroin, which does cross the blood-brain barrier rapidly, and within ten seconds produces an intense rush that some people have described as an "abdominal orgasm."

Subjective and Behavioral Aspects

After a single injection of heroin, the person may show not only euphoria, but also analgesia, constipation, pupil constriction, a need to urinate, and decreases in temperature, heart rate, respiration, and blood pressure. Nausea, vomiting, and fainting are also common. In the addict these noxious symptoms associated with the euphoria are known as "a good sick" (Wikler, 1980).

A rush lasts for a few minutes, followed by indifference to external events. The heroin addict seems to alternate in reverie between rest and mild arousal, sometimes referred to as being "on the nod." Sexual desire and aggression are usually minimal or absent. But within hours of the last dose, the addict usually becomes irritable and would like more. This is the first sign of withdrawal. By twelve hours the addict is yawning, sneezing, sweating, and tearing, with pupil dilation, trembling, loss of appetite, and the "gooseflesh" nicknamed "cold turkey." After thirty-six hours of abstinence, uncontrollable twitching and muscle cramps develop, accompanied by more restlessness, vomiting, and diarrhea. During withdrawal the addict typically becomes pessimistic and argumentative, with much crying and cursing, and occasional suicidal gestures (Kolb & Brodie, 1982).

It is useful to distinguish dependence from addiction when referring to opiates (Dole, 1980). It is an easy matter to free the opiate addict from symptoms of withdrawal, one of the main criteria for dependence. But most opiate users relapse, suggesting that they still have urges to use the substance and therefore are still addicted.

Heroin addicts tend to come from minority groups and those living in underprivileged urban environments. Availability, peer pressures, and the lack of an achievement orientation are often responsible for initiation into the drug culture. What these factors do not explain, however, is why most people residing in such environments escape addiction. The majority of diagnosed narcotic addicts manifest some form of psychopathology, especially depression and/or antisocial personality disorder. A particularly poignant illustration of antisocial behavior was given by a former addict:

> In the middle of the night my wife begins to have labor pains and I take her to this dinky little hospital. . . . I held my wife's hand and assured her that all was well . . . in the back of my head I'm trying to figure out how I can get at some of the dope (Demerol) the nurse pumped into my wife's arm. . . . Here I am trying to be lovingly concerned with my wife's welfare, help with delivery, and at the same time get hold of the dope. My wife is screaming her head off. . . . I finally snatched the bottle of Demerol and tucked it safely away. . . . Now I feel comfortable, and am ready to help deliver my child (Yablonsky, 1965, p. 10).

It is important also to recognize that drug addiction can make some otherwise normal people antisocial and self-centered. Indeed, some studies have mistaken antisocial tendencies as a cause rather than an effect of opiate addiction (Rounsaville et al., 1982), just as some of the antisocial characteristics of alcoholics have been mistaken as causes.

Medical Treatment

The addict first must be relieved of acute withdrawal symptoms. This can be accomplished by detoxification by tapering the dose or by enforcing abstinence for ten days; that is, going cold turkey. A popular alternative to abstinence is methadone maintenance. This involves an orally administered synthetic opiate which does not produce the euphoria but, more importantly, permits the addict to function with little behavioral impairment.

Some experts believe that methadone maintenance is also the preferred long-term treatment (Dole, 1980). In contrast to morphine or heroin, blood levels of methadone remain fairly constant throughout the day. When the dose is properly adjusted, methadone reduces, but does not eliminate, the desire for heroin.

No doubt methadone maintenance programs have permitted many addicts to function more normally, but the addict is still dependent on a drug. The treatment is not foolproof because patients still pal around with other heroin users and inject heroin occasionally or regularly. Moreover, many are still criminally active despite methadone (Hartnoll et al., 1980).

Social Psychological Treatment

Other treatments emphasize psychological factors in the context of stringent behavioral controls. The therapeutic community has arisen as one form of treatment of this kind. Here addicts live in a well-structured environment, maintaining mutual social control because they know the tricks of their fellows.

A particularly renowned treatment program of this sort is the one followed by Synanon (Yablonsky, 1965). Started in the late 1950s by a charismatic former alcoholic, Charles Dederich, the program had received much acclaim.

Addicts were required to live in an authoritarian environment in which most of their daily activities were controlled. Although they could leave voluntarily, this was strongly discouraged. In the context of a supportive environment and a genuine desire to keep the addict free of drugs, Synanon members relentlessly scrutinized all aspects of the addict's behavior. The most dramatic example involved "haircut" sessions in which the group verbally attacked members who had violated Synanon's rules. Although dropout rates were extremely high, those who submitted to these rules often became productive citizens within Synanon. Leaving the therapeutic community, however, was associated with high relapse rates, not much different from relapse rates for those leaving federal detoxification centers. As a result, members were encouraged to stay within the community, where excesses could be curbed.

Other less authoritarian therapeutic communities have arisen which vary in their similarity to Synanon. As with Alcoholics Anonymous and Synanon, dropout rates are very high. In one study, for example, 50 percent of the subjects who stayed at least one week in such communities had dropped out in less than two months. By four months, only 25 percent were left (Bale et al., 1980).

Endorphins and Opiates

During the 1970s new techniques enabled investigators to identify those areas of the brain to which opiates bind (Snyder, 1978). It turns out that the body manufactures its own opiatelike substances collectively called *endorphins*— which bind to the same receptors and similarly are capable of ameliorating pain. The periaqueductal gray in the brain stem, which was discussed earlier as an area that mediates physical withdrawal symptoms, is the site at which these endorphins are manufactured. The endorphins have sparked an enormous research effort because they may help to elucidate the mechanisms of pain. Opiate administration suppresses endorphin manufacture (Kosterlitz & Hughes, 1975), suggesting that former opiate users may have endorphin deficiencies caused by taking opiates and these deficiencies could be responsible for some of the distress of withdrawal. One interesting finding is that the body secretes endorphins in response to pain, and perhaps even anticipated pain. For example, Figure 19.7 gives endorphin levels both before and during exploratory surgery of the abdomen (Pickar et al., 1982). Endorphin levels increased during surgery. Surprisingly, those with high endorphin levels during surgery spontaneously requested less morphine for pain relief in the following twenty-four hours. Individual differences in the amount of endorphin secreted may account for variations in pain sensitivity.

Apparently, both placebo effects and the positive results of acupuncture relate to endorphin levels. For example, opiate antagonists such as *naloxone*, which block the action of opiates at the receptors, can eliminate both placebo effects in pain studies and the salutary effects of acupuncture (Clement-Jones & Besser, 1983). These studies suggest that placebo effects, in which inert sub-

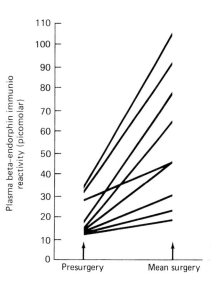

FIGURE 19.7 The effect of surgical stress on levels of plasma beta-endorphin in nine patients with regional malignancy undergoing exploratory abdominal surgery. *Presurgery* represents preanesthesia levels and *surgery* is the mean of all levels during surgical procedures. From Pickar, D. et al. (1982). Clinical studies of the endogenous opiod system. *Biological Psychiatry, 17,* 1243–1276. Copyright © 1984 by Elsevier Science Publishing Co., Inc.

stances relieve pain, may actually operate through changes in endorphin levels induced by anticipation of their pain-relieving effects.

Future research on addiction and its treatment is going to have to contend with a multiplicity of factors that cause addictions and relapse. It is not an area of research that is likely to lead to simple principles of treatment. Preventing or discouraging exposure to addictive substances undoubtedly would be the most effective way to eliminate addictive possibilities, but in a society that prides itself on making accessible almost everything that is pleasurable, prohibition alone is unlikely to work.

SUMMARY

Addictions are drug-related dependencies and preoccupations. Theories of how they arise can be classified into three categories. The first category focuses on the specific effects of addictive substances. All addictive substances are capable of producing rapid changes in affect that probably act on specific pleasure centers in the brain or alter cellular physiology in ways that require more of the drug simply to feel good. Other theories focus on preexisting personality traits, including the symptoms of personality disorder, for which the drug is a kind of self-medication. Still other theories emphasize conditioning and the learning of addictive behavior. Conditioning theories acknowledge the specific properties of addictive drugs, but point out that internal and external cues can come to elicit withdrawal symptoms that drive addictive behavior.

There are surely multiple causes of addiction, and different types of addiction may have different kinds of causes. For all addictions, drug use is obviously a prerequisite. But given that the drug is used, what determines who becomes addicted? For alcoholism, high initial tolerance and few negative symptoms from using alcohol are likely etiological factors. The consequence is that higher doses of alcohol are required to achieve desired effects. It is this overuse with consequent changes in physiology that gets the person into a addictive cycle in which more of the drug is required just to feel normal. These people might drink for the same reasons that less tolerant people drink; that is, there may be nothing special about their motives for drinking. It is simply that they need more alcohol to achieve the desired effect, and this produces pathological changes in physiology.

Alcohol tolerance probably has a hereditary component, one reason for the familiality of alcoholism. However, a substantial fraction of other alcoholics have preexisting personality traits that make them alcoholic prone and that are partly heritable. The personality traits include childhood hyperactivity and antisocial conduct problems. For these people alcohol is especially effective in relieving distress, perhaps because alcohol tends to "normalize" the EEG, producing concomitant feelings of relaxation. Both hyperactivity and conduct problems are associated with EEG aberrations, and it may simply be that these people benefit more than others from the normalizing effects of alcohol.

Opiate addiction is also discussed in this chapter. The etiology of opiate addiction includes living in environments that promote the use of drugs. But an important feature is that opiates themselves are generally extremely pleasurable and their abuse may depend more on the pleasure of using the drug than on preexisting psychopathology. Although the majority of heroin users are not addicted, it seems clear that an addiction can arise from its overuse and it is safer not even to try it. By the time the addict comes to treatment, psychopathology exists. However, evidence indicates that the addiction itself can transform people, so that the psychopathology might best be thought of as an effect rather than a cause of the addiction.

Treatments of addiction generally have not been very successful. Although addicts easily can be relieved of physical dependencies on the drugs, relapse is most often the rule because of psychological and conditioning factors.

Psychosexual Deviations

NATURE OF SEXUALITY

In the panoply of drives none is more insistent than sex. When awakened, it prompts fantasy, courtship, and other sexual activities. When consummated, it produces intense pleasurable experiences. Indeed, this is nature's way of ensuring avidity in pursuing species preservation. But expressions of sexuality and the sexual problems that trouble each of the two sexes are often quite different. Differences in sexual attitudes of the two sexes also can be very large. Eysenck (1976) administered a sexual attitude questionnaire to unmarried British college students; sex differences on some items are given in Table 20.1. The table indicates that females are more likely than males to see sex and love as intimately related, while males are more willing to have sexual relations apart from affectional commitments.

This chapter will describe a variety of psychosexual deviations and how they are differently expressed in men and women. But to understand the often

TABLE 20.1 SEX-RELATED ATTITUDES

Question	Affirmative responses	
	Males, %	Females, %
Sex without love ("impersonal sex") is highly unsatisfactory	49	80
I do not need to respect or love someone in order to enjoy petting and/or intercourse	43	12
It is all right to seduce a person who is old enough to know what he or she is doing	73	35
The thought of a sex orgy is disgusting to me	18	75
Pornographic writing should be freely allowed to be published	59	32
Prostitution should be legal	62	32

Source: Excerpted from H. J. Eysenck, *Sex and Personality,* copyright © 1976 and reprinted by permission of The University of Texas Press.

enormous sex differences in their expression, we need to appreciate the nature of sexual arousal and the biology of sexual development.

Sexual Mechanisms

The sexual mechanisms pertinent to sexual deviations involve the friction and fantasy systems of sexual arousal and desire, as well as the role of certain hormones in sexual development.

Friction and Fantasy   Humans have two sex systems; one responds to friction, the other to fantasy (Kaplan, 1974). The friction system involves reflex arcs between the sex organs and lower regions of the spinal cord. The reflexive nature of the friction system is demonstrable in males when spinal cord damage prevents genital sensations from reaching the brain. If the genitals are stimulated by rubbing, it is possible for erection and orgasmic capacity to be retained for awhile. In contrast, females with comparable spinal damage lose orgasmic responsiveness (Masters, Johnson, & Kolodny, 1982).

The fantasy system is more susceptible to cultural influences and personal experience. In Victorian times the sight of a lady's ankle could excite passion and poetry, though nowadays it seems that something more is usually required. We often have difficulty recognizing the importance of cultural traditions in shaping the fantasy system. For example, many people mistakenly believe that an innate connection exists between kissing and sexual arousal, but erotic arousal from kissing is largely cultural in origin, and the idea of kissing is repugnant to certain preliterate peoples, who prefer the rubbing of cheeks. Most psychosexual disorders are associated with peculiarities of the fantasy system. An exception to this general rule is that psychosexual dysfunctions involving deficiencies in desire, potency, or orgasm often arise from disorders of the *reflex system*. A substantial fraction of impotent males, for example, have an organic condition such as poor blood circulation to the genitals or endocrine deficiencies that could explain an erectile dysfunction.

Endocrine Regulation   The endocrine system produces hormones for sexual development and the maintenance of sexual emotions. Figure 20.1 provides a simplified diagram of the neuroendocrine regulation of sexual physiology. The hypothalamus releases a substance called *gonadotropin-releasing hormone* (GRH) which signals the pituitary to secrete two hormones. *Luteinizing hormone* (LH) in the male stimulates the testes to manufacture testosterone; in the female it triggers ovulation. *Follicle-stimulating hormone* (FSH) prepares the ovaries for ovulation, and, in cooperation with testosterone, stimulates sperm production. Testosterone is responsible for the masculinization of the fetal brain, the embryological differentiation of the penis, and the later maintenance of sexual desire.

The *androgen insensitivity syndrome* vividly illustrates the importance of testosterone for male development. This syndrome arises from a genetic defect

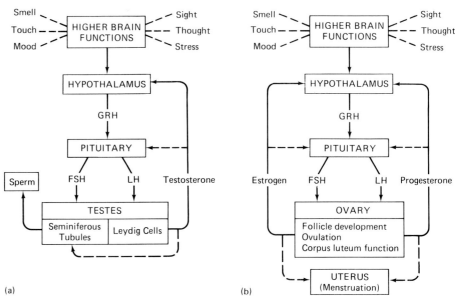

FIGURE 20.1 Endocrine regulation in the male (a) and female (b). From *Human Sexuality* by William H. Masters, Virginia E. Johnson, and Robert C. Kolodny. Copyright © 1982 by William H. Masters, Virginia E. Johnson, and Robert C. Kolodny. Reprinted by permission of Scott, Foresman and Company.

that prevents target tissues from responding to the hormone (Figure 20.2). Males with this rare defect have a female appearance and are reared as girls, though physical examination will reveal undescended testes in the abdomen and a lack of ovaries and a uterus. Psychological identity is also feminine and the child appears to be perfectly healthy. Only upon failure to menstruate in adolescence does the syndrome usually become apparent. As adults, these people are well-adjusted and behave as typical females. The syndrome exemplifies a principle of sexual development; namely, that in the absence of either testosterone or the capacity of tissue to respond to the hormone, sexual differentiation will be female. Not surprisingly, more than normal amounts of testosterone can masculinize a genetically female fetus and produce typically masculine behavior. For example, studies of genetic females who were exposed to excessive testosterone during fetal development have a high incidence of tomboyism during childhood and a homosexual or bisexual orientation later (Reinisch, 1981; Money, Schwartz, & Lewis, 1984; Ehrhardt et al., 1985).

The testosterone surge accompanying puberty in males appears to have profound effects on certain aspects of cognitive performance, especially those involving spatial ability. Although normal males generally outperform females on spatial tests, males with a preadolescent-onset testosterone deficiency often do very poorly (Hier & Crowley, 1982). In such males, the size of the testes

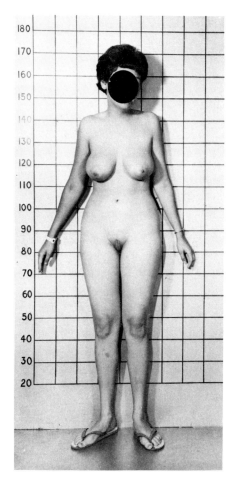

FIGURE 20.2 Androgen-insensitivity syndrome. Note absence of pubic hair, but otherwise normal female external appearance. From H. S. Kupperman, The endocrine status of the transsexual patient. *Transactions of the New York Academy of Sciences,* 1967, *29,* 439.

correlates with spatial ability; the larger the testes the better the performance. Results such as these suggest that sex differences in spatial performance are not due solely to differences in rearing experiences or vocational interests.

The other major sex hormone, estrogen, is manufactured in greater amounts in the ovaries and in lesser amounts in the testes and adrenals. In females, estrogen maintains tonus and lubrication of the vagina and preserves breast elasticity. During puberty, an estrogen surge produces the physically conspicuous signs of being female. The function of estrogen in males is unknown, but hypersecretion can produce breast enlargement and the buildup of excessive fatty tissue around the hips. Males with Klinefelter's syndrome, a disorder in which the male has two X chromosomes in addition to a Y (see Chapter 7, pp. 180–181), often have these two symptoms (Figure 20.3). With this brief overview of the role of hormones in sexual and psychological development, we can now turn to psychosexual disorders.

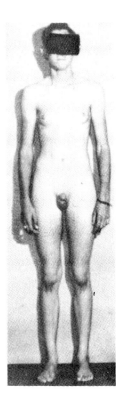

FIGURE 20.3   Klinefelter syndrome (XXY). Note tallness, fat around the hips, small testes, and breast enlargement. From J. J. Nora & F. C. Fraser, *Medical Genetics: Principles and practice* (2d ed.), Philadelphia: Lea & Febiger, 1981, p. 80.

Concept of Psychosexual Disorder

Psychosexual disorders occupy a peculiar place in psychopathological theory. Many involve sexual preferences that are important to the individual, but have no deleterious consequences for the self or for others. However, it has been argued that the presence of sexual peculiarities are themselves signs of mental disorder even in the absence of more traditional signs such as psychosis, anxiety, depression, antisocial personality, or compromised social and occupational functioning. But on what grounds, for example, does homosexuality in the absence of these other signs warrant a diagnosis of disorder? To be sure, homosexuality is a deviation in the sense of being relatively rare. But the concept of abnormality, as we said in Chapter 1, also requires a judgment of maladaption. Without this judgment, a deviation—even one with an established biological basis—is just a difference. In sum, for a disorder to be judged a *mental* disorder, behavioral criteria of maladaption must be applicable.

This question has been hotly debated and few compelling arguments exist on behalf of a *mental disorder* or a *mental disease* concept for some of the conditions to be described. We have chosen the term sexual deviation for the chapter title to reflect our own uncertainty about this question. In a spirit of openness we also have included the topic of homosexuality because many people believe that it is an abnormality, even though it is explicitly excluded in *DSM-III-R* as a mental disorder. Moreover, homosexuality has considerable etiological similarity to transsexuality, which is included in the *DSM-III-R,* and about which the same debate could arise.

GENDER IDENTITY DISORDER: TRANSSEXUALITY

Gender identity disorders are revealed by the incongruence between anatomical sex and *gender identity,* the psychological sense of being male or female. The transsexual feels trapped in the body of the other sex and desires sex reassignment surgery. One such individual is shown in Figures 20.4 and 20.5. Her history follows:

> [A] twenty-three-year-old, single, attractive ''female'' nightclub entertainer who presented herself in such tasteful, feminine attire that no one suspected that ''she'' was an anatomical male. The patient had already had breast implants and had used female hormones regularly. She had dressed, lived and worked exclusively as a female for three years with a begrudging, then supporting approval from her parents. Her femininity was convincing and casual without being exaggerated. She had a fiance and many girlfriends with whom she enjoyed ''girl talk.'' She liked wearing fashionable slacks, had a décolleté and wore some jewelry on her well-manicured hands. Self-assured and intelligent, she had no discomfort whatever. The single purpose of her visit was to gain support for her transsexual surgery. She needed only minimal facial electrolysis, as she had practically no facial hair growth. . . . Sexually, she related exclusively to men. Her sexual gratification resulted not so much from her own orgasm as from ''having fulfilled the role of the female'' and having provided satisfaction to her partner. . . . The results of a full psychological testing were evaluated by two independent psychologists, one of whom was unaware of the patient's problem. Some egocentricity and narcissism were present; one of the psychologists suspected some personality disorder. All other psychiatric and physical examinations were normal, except for [a] mild . . . problem of FSH levels (Koranyi, 1980, pp. 80–81).

FIGURE 20.4 Feminine hand of transsexual male. From E. Koranyi (1980), p. 81. *Transexuality in the male.* Courtesy of Charles C Thomas, Publisher, Springfield, Illinois.

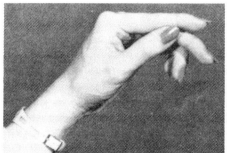 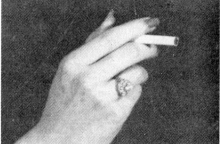

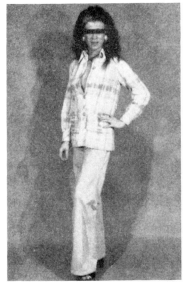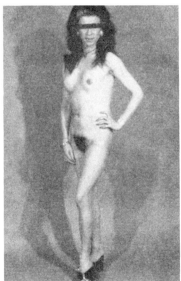

(a)

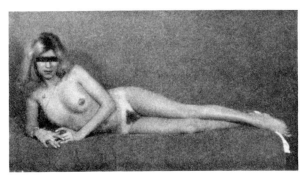

(b)

FIGURE 20.5   Male transsexual before (a) and after (b) transsexual surgery. From E. Koranyi (1980), p. 83). *Transexuality in the male.* Courtesy of Charles C Thomas, Publisher, Springfield, Illinois.

One might think that a peculiar belief like being trapped in the body of the opposite sex is delusional and that other aspects of thinking or perception should also reveal signs of a thought disturbance. The fact is that this patient and many other transsexuals have no peculiar ideas except those concerning their transsexuality, and in some sense they are right in claiming that they feel trapped in a body of the other sex.

It is useful to distinguish between primary and secondary transsexuals. *Primary* transsexuals have a childhood history of a cross-sex gender identity and are essentially conflictfree. As far back as they can remember, they have always thought they were really of the opposite sex. They do not report erotic arousal from cross-dressing. The administration of antitestosterone drugs or even castration does not diminish their transsexual feelings. Psychological problems like depression often occur in primary transsexuals, however, because they are trying to adjust in a society that doesn't understand them.

In contrast, *secondary* transsexuals have a childhood history of a masculine gender identity and erotic arousal from cross-dressing, and perhaps a third or more are diagnosable as psychotic (Lothstein, 1983). These people are usually not accepted knowingly into reputable programs for eventual surgical reassignment.

Etiology

The etiology of primary transsexualism is unknown. Many theories emphasize learning or psychogenic components. One hypothesis is that mothers of future male transsexuals envied the infant's maleness and jealously punished expressions of masculinity. By contrast, future female transsexuals were reinforced for masculine behaviors by their fathers (Stoller, 1980). Other theories emphasize prenatal organic or endocrine factors or some combination of these (see Hoenig & Kenna, 1974).

The endocrine factors can be divided into those that influence prenatal development and those that are influential later. Prenatal testosterone and other androgens have a determinative influence on the development of maleness, both in anatomy and in the growth of certain brain structures. But adult levels of circulating male hormones are not accurate indications of what has occurred prenatally. Moreover, differences in hormone receptor sensitivity must also be considered, along with differences in circulating hormone levels. For example, differences among men in heaviness of beard growth are unrelated to circulating testosterone, but rather depend on the cell receptors of certain target tissues.

Many studies have examined the role of circulating levels of testosterone and other sex hormones in transsexuals and homosexuals (see Gladue, 1987, for a review). The results are decidedly unclear, but the better controlled studies have shown no adult differences in circulating hormone levels among male heterosexuals, male transsexuals, and male homosexuals. A few studies provide evidence of slightly higher levels of circulating testosterone among lesbians than among same-sex controls.

If the critical hormonal events for transsexuality or homosexuality occurred prenatally, however, these studies would not be expected to reveal large differences. A more sensitive way to measure what might have happened prenatally is to study differences in responsiveness to hormonal challenges among men and women differing in their sexual orientation. Unfortunately, the picture here is also somewhat mixed (Gladue, 1987), but there are some positive findings that could point to a prenatal basis, at least among some transsexual and homosexual men (Gladue et al., 1984; Kula, 1986). At this stage it is mainly theory and a small amount of empirical evidence that drives the belief that prenatal influences are contributory, if not determinative, to sexual orientation within each sex (Ellis & Ames, 1987).

Development

Follow-up studies of extremely effeminate boys indicate that about 11 percent will become adult transsexuals and 50 to 78 percent will become homosexuals (Money & Russo, 1979; Leitenberg, 1983; Zuger, 1984; Green, 1987). Corresponding data for the eventual sexual preferences of tomboys is unfortunately sparse. The published literature describes only four very masculine girls who have been followed beyond puberty: one became a transsexual, two became varsity athletes whose gender identities or sexual preferences are unknown, and one was a heterosexual (Green, 1979). The actual rate of transsexualism in the general population is unknown, but an estimate derived from a centralized facility for transsexuals applying for surgical reassignment in the Netherlands indicates rates of one per 18,000 in males and one per 45,000 in females (Eklund, Gooren, & Bezemer, 1988). Given such low base rates, it would appear that extreme cross-gender behavior is a relatively good predictor of later transsexualism.

Cross-gender behavior includes cross-dressing, mannerisms more characteristic of the other sex, preferences for playmates of the other sex, predilections for gender-incongruent toys, and less often, desires to change one's sex. Green (1974) found that all the feminine boys in his study were cross-dressing before age six, most prior to age four. Although the parents once might have regarded this as "cute," they eventually became quite concerned. Moreover, many pediatricians fail to appreciate the significance of cross-gendering, particularly in male children. You can see this in the following history from a mother of a six year-old effeminate boy.

> . . . about the time I separated from my husband . . . [at age three] he started running around with all kinds of hand movements, and dressing up in little girls' clothes. . . . I didn't think much of it, and . . . my pediatrician . . . said, "When he reaches puberty and he starts wearing dresses, then you know you've got a problem." . . . Everything is girls this, girls that, and this psychologist told me that if he wanted to do those things, just send him to another room. . . . He's always in with girls playing, and they've tried to get him away from the clothes, and even made him a sailor suit. . . . And at home he's always putting on a blanket, you know, as a cape. He has put on my bathrobe, my nightgown, and things like that. I've caught him in a slip every once in a while, a half-slip that looks like a skirt. He puts on my shoes. I thought it was a little normal stage. A lot of kids like to dress up (Green, 1974, pp. 151–152).

Keep in mind that gender identity, however arising, does not correlate perfectly with eventual *sexual orientation*; that is, to whom the person is sexually attracted. Nearly half of male-to-female transsexuals still are sexually attracted to females even after sex reassignment surgery (Blanchard, Steiner, &

Clemmensen, 1985). This pattern does not appear to occur among female-to-male transsexuals, all of whom prefer women as sexual partners.

Treatment

Primary transsexuals express no desire to make their gender identity congruent with their anatomical sex. Rather, their therapeutic goal is to alter their anatomical sex to make it congruent with their gender identity. Preparation for surgical sex reassignment requires a period of one or two years living in the future role ("the real-life test") and the administration of feminizing or masculinizing hormones (Leitenberg, 1983). If the transsexual passes the real-life test, surgery can be initiated (see Koranyi, 1980, for a description of surgical techniques).

We have only a few careful follow-up studies of sex reassignment (Green, 1982; Blanchard et al., 1985). The consensus, while not unanimous, is that reassignment frequently has improved their quality of life and that most are satisfied with the operation (Abramowitz, 1986).

HOMOSEXUALITY

Homosexuality is defined as a spontaneous and enduring erotic response to people of the same sex. Like heterosexuality, homosexuality has its causes. In both, the full causal picture is unknown. But one thing seems certain; by late adolescence neither is merely an option in the same way that one chooses pizza over burger. Although causality is ambiguous, it seems clear that the groundwork for developing a homosexual orientation is laid before puberty, often in early childhood.

Behavioral Aspects

Alfred C. Kinsey, a pioneer in American sex research, believed that sexual orientation varies along a continuum (Kinsey et al., 1953). He devised a seven-point scale ranging from 0 (exclusive heterosexual experience) to 6 (exclusive homosexual experience) to characterize that continuum. The midpoint (3) represented bisexuality, or equal proportions of heterosexual and homosexual contacts or fantasies. One's score on this continuum is correlated not only with overt sexual experiences, but also with fanstasy life.

Consider the findings of Bell and Weinberg (1978), who interviewed nearly a thousand San Francisco homosexuals about many aspects of their sexual behavior. Besides being asked about general aspects of homosexual lifestyle, subjects rated their sexual feelings and overt behaviors on the Kinsey scale. Table 20.2 provides some highlights from this study. One can see that the Kinsey scale scores are associated with sometimes substantial differences in fantasy and sexual behavior.

Male and female homosexuals differ dramatically in the number of sexual partners. Whereas 43 percent of the males reported sexual experiences with

TABLE 20.2 SEXUAL BEHAVIOR OF HOMOSEXUALS

	Males, %	Females, %
Behaviors		
Number of different sexual partners		
Fewer than 10	3	58
More than 500	43	0
Proportion of partners who were strangers		
More than one-half	79	6
Percentage who ever had heterosexual coitus by Kinsey Scale Rating		
Kinsey 6	56	77
Kinsey 5	93	93
Feelings		
Had heterosexual sex dreams		
Kinsey 6	20	34
Kinsey 5	40	75
Had heterosexual masturbatory fantasies		
Kinsey 6	37	19
Kinsey 5	68	50

Source: From *Homosexualities: A study of diversity among men and women.* Copyright © 1978 by Alan P. Bell and Martin S. Weinberg. Reprinted by permission of Simon & Schuster, Inc.

more than 500 different partners, none of the lesbians had that many experiences. Not surprisingly, a large proportion of male homosexual partners were strangers, accentuating the typical male-female difference in emotional involvement with partners. This difference in involvement is seen most clearly in observational studies of homosexuals (Masters & Johnson, 1979). Lesbians are much more likely to engage in whole body contact and gay males more likely to move directly to the genitals. Symons (1979) compares heterosexual and homosexual behavior this way:

> I am suggesting that heterosexual men would be as likely as homosexual men to have sex more often with strangers, to participate in anonymous orgies in public baths, and to stop off in public restrooms for five minutes of fellatio on the way home if women were interested in these activities (p. 300).

Except for a higher incidence of suicide attempts, the frequency and distribution of other mental disorders is about the same in homosexuals and heterosexuals. Saghir and Robins (1973), using psychiatric interviews, found that homosexuals had no excess of psychopathology, except for the suicide attempts. Bell and Weinberg (1978) confirmed this observation, finding that homosexual males were six and homosexual females 2 1/2 times more likely to have attempted suicide than matched heterosexual controls. When queried, about 40 percent said that their suicide attempts were specifically related to homosexuality. It is quite possible that these suicide attempts might reflect depression in adjusting a homosexual lifestyle to a heterosexual world. Homosexuals often enter psychotherapy because of negative and intolerant societal attitudes about their sexual orientation. It is demoralizing to be labeled "queer," "fag," "butch," "dyke," and to hear that homosexual feelings are unnatural and should be "cured" (Davison & Neale, 1982).

Etiology

The causes of homosexuality are enigmatic, but homosexuality seems to arise from a developmental matrix similar to that of transsexuality. Like transsexuals, most prehomosexual boys and girls are effeminate and tomboyish, respectively. Moreover, adult male homosexuals often report fantasies about being and dressing as females (Freund et al., 1973).

Psychodynamic Theory Freud believed that homosexuality expresses an inherent bisexuality that is normally resolved during the oedipal phase of psychosexual development when the child begins to identify with the same-sex parent. ("I want a girl just like the girl who married dear old Dad.") Failures to achieve resolution and identify with the same-sex parent were believed to stem from unsatisfactory parent-child relations.

Male homosexual *patients,* as compared with heterosexual patients, are more likely to report a close, binding relationship with their mother but a distant, hostile, or absent father, as Freud suspected (Bieber, 1964). However, *female* homosexuals also report closer relationships with their mothers (Bell et al., 1981), making doubtful any hypothesis about identification with the opposite-sex parent as a causal factor in homosexuality.

Effeminacy Perhaps the most important early sign of future homosexuality in boys is effeminacy. About three-quarters of effeminate boys studied as children become homosexual adults (Green, 1987). Retrospective studies of childhood effeminacy in adult male homosexuals also yield empirical results that agree with those of Green. For example, Whitam (1980) asked homosexuals and heterosexuals six questions about feminine behavior in childhood: Interested in dolls? Liked to dress in women's clothing? Preferred the company of girls to the company of boys? Preferred being around older women than older men? Were regarded as a sissy? Preferred sex play with boys rather than girls? The vast majority (85 percent) of homosexuals endorsed more than one of these childhood items as against only 6 percent of heterosexuals (Table 20.3). Thus, the evidence indicates that extreme femininity in boys is a precursor of homosexual preference. The limited data for extreme tomboyishness in girls also suggest an increased likelihood for a homosexual orientation in adulthood, although these data are much slimmer and the base rate for childhood tomboyism, even in heterosexual females, is so high as to make tomboyism a less powerful predictor of eventual homosexuality.

One speculation is that effeminancy represents an instinctive expression of subordination or fear. Male animals often adopt a feminine posture—normal for females—in the presence of a more dominant male. For example, threat-

TABLE 20.3   SEXUAL ORIENTATION AS RELATED TO NUMBER OF CHILDHOOD INDICATORS

Number of childhood indicators present	Homosexual		Heterosexual	
	N	%	*N*	%
All 6	18	16.8	0	0
5	14	13.1	0	0
4	18	16.8	0	0
3	20	18.7	2	2.9
2	21	19.6	2	2.9
1	13	12.2	10	14.7
0	3	2.8	54	79.4
	107	100.0	68	100.0

Source: From Whitam, "The pre-homosexual child in three societies," *Archives of Sexual Behavior, 9*, 87–99. Copyright © 1980. Reprinted with permission of Plenum Publishing Corporation.

ened male rodents and primates will present their rear ends as if for copulation in order to inhibit aggression. Perhaps by his feminine mannerisms, the prehomosexual boy indicates that he is not a competitive threat to his father. How this expression of subordination translates into a homosexual orientation is unknown, however. Whatever its psychological mechanism, homosexuality is evidently absent in lower animals because they do not prefer sex with other males when given free access to females.

How *might* early effeminacy translate into an eventual homosexual orientation? In contrast to preheterosexual children, effeminate boys prefer opposite-sex playmates, perhaps because they do not like the rough-and-tumble play so common to boys (Green, 1987; Whitam, 1980). Could intimacy with opposite-sex playmates provide a sense of familiarity that later discourages interest in them as erotic objects?

Support for the idea that early intimacy produces disinterest comes from a study of thousands of marriages of children reared in Israeli kibbutzim (Shepher, 1971). Boys and girls of the same age were reared together from birth in intimate groups away from their parents, freely sharing toilet and shower facilities until puberty. Upon reaching adulthood, none of these children married each other, although they often married those in older or younger age groups. When queried, subjects remarked that romantic involvement and sharing a toilet since childhood were mutually contradictory. In short, homosexual and heterosexual erotic arousal might be explained by sex patterning in early friendships. For example, young boys who preferred the company of girls early might lose interest in them when sexual desire is awakened later.

Heredity   The heritability of homosexuality is uncertain, although male homosexuality does run in families (Pillard & Weinrich, 1986; Bell et al., 1981). About 22 percent of the brothers of predominantly homosexual men are bisexual or homosexual in contrast to only about 4 percent of the brothers of heterosexual men. The sisters of these two groups of men do not differ in their rates of homosexuality. Since siblings share both genetic and environmental backgrounds, however, it is not possible from these data to determine why male homosexuality is familial.

Heston and Shields (1968) reported higher concordance rates for homosexuality in identical (MZ) sets than fraternal (DZ) sets in a small study, suggesting a hereditary factor. A report of two pairs of male MZs and four pairs of female MZs *separated* early in life found one of the male sets concordant but all of the female sets discordant for homosexuality (Eckert et al., 1986). A remarkable set of unseparated MZ twins followed up from childhood because of one twin's effeminacy (the other twin was quite masculine as a child) revealed that both were concordant for bisexuality in adulthood (Green, 1987).

While the male data are at least consistent with a hypothesis of a genetic component to homosexuality, the complete discordance among the female MZ sets suggests that unique postnatal environmental factors are more important for female homosexuality. One argument *against* a genetic basis to even male homosexuality, however, is that significantly lower rates of reproduction should have caused its eventual disappearance. A population frequency of 3 or 4 percent for male homosexuality is thus inconsistent with a simple genetic explanation.

Prenatal Factors   Shared intrauterine hormonal abnormalities also could account for greater MZ than DZ concordance for male homosexuality yet not require a genetic hypothesis. MZ twins in comparison to DZ twins could be more similarly affected by hormonally mediated embryological events. Evidence on behalf of a hormonal hypothesis exists. Male rat offspring of mothers stressed during the last week of pregnancy show feminized behavior (Ward, 1984). When confronted with a dominant male, they often assume the feminine receptive posture and, in the presence of an estrous female, are less effective copulators. These behavioral deviations are unaccompanied by any obvious abnormalities in anatomy or physiology. The feminized behavior, however, does not lead to a homosexual orientation. Indeed, it is claimed (on the basis of limited observation [Tyler, 1984]) that an exclusive homosexual orientation in vertebrates lower than humans seems not to exist (Beach, 1978).

Components of feminine behavior can be observed in lower animals, however. Ward discovered a prenatal hormonal correlate of later feminized behavior in the male rats. Prenatal stress delayed the onset of the normal surge of fetal androgen so that it occurred on days 20 and 21 instead of days 18 and 19, as is typical for nonstressed fetuses. Perhaps the androgen surge simply came too late for proper brain masculinization to have taken place. Interestingly, administration of testosterone during the last week of pregnancy and soon after birth will prevent the feminized behavior (Dorner, Gotz, & Docke, 1983). No comparable behavioral or anatomical abnormalities occurred in female fetuses subjected to the same stress. We should keep in mind that even if feminine behavior can be produced in male rats, its connection to human homosexuality remains unclear.

It is noteworthy that one study also suggests that mothers of male homosexuals were exposed to more prenatal stress—for example, an unwanted pregnancy or death of the father—than were the mothers of bisexuals, who in turn were exposed to more prenatal stress than the mothers of heterosexuals. Since stress generally reduces androgen levels, it seems quite plausible that prenatal stress could feminize the human male fetus (Dorner et al., 1983). Unfortunately, the study was based on retrospective reports and it is unclear how much the homosexual subjects knew about the researchers' hypothesis when they reported on prenatal stresses. A more powerful test of the hypothesis would have mothers of homosexual and control subjects report on the pregnancies of their children, especially when they do not know their children's sexual orientation.

Perhaps the clearest support for an endocrine influence in male homosexuality comes from a study by Gladue, Green, and Hellman (1984). They injected an estrogen compound into male homosexuals and male and female heterosexuals. Normally, in females there is a slight fall and then a conspicuous rise in luteinizing hormone (LH) over the next four days; in males, however, there is an initial fall followed by a slow return to baseline. As Figure 20.6 indicates, the response of male homosexuals to the estrogen challenge is intermediate to the two heterosexual groups. It is generally believed that sex differences in the LH response are present at birth. Presumably, the hypothalamic-pituitary axis of the homosexuals was prenatally altered by an unusual hormonal milieu. We

FIGURE 20.6 Changes in luteinizing hormone (LH) following an injection of an estrogenic substance. From B. A. Gladue, R. Green, & R. E. Hellman (1984). Neuroendocrine response to estrogen and sexual orientation. *Science, 225,* p. 1496. Copyright © 1984 by the AAAS.

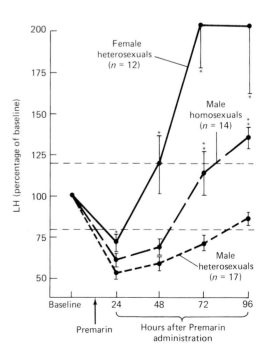

should keep in mind, however, that only nine of the fourteen homosexuals showed this pattern, suggesting multiple pathways to male homosexuality. This study, like others, leaves unsaid how such a possible hypothalamic-pituitary difference translates into a homosexual orientation (Ellis & Ames, 1987).

Treatment

The question of whether extreme childhood effeminacy and/or adult homosexuality should be "treated" has been the subject of much debate. Proponents have argued, for example, that effeminate boys are targets of derision and suffer as a result of their deviant sexual preferences; to prevent these unhappy consequences, it seems only proper to make treatment available. On the other hand, many gay activists object because "treatment" implies the existence of a dysfunction which cannot be demonstrated. Nonetheless, some effeminate boys have received therapy to discourage effeminacy and encourage masculine behavior.

The efficacy of therapy thus far appears to be nil. In Green's (1987) follow-up of effeminate boys, three-quarters of those treated became gay adults, a rate no different from the rate for those who had not been in therapy. Claims of therapeutic success for adult homosexuality are also questionable (for example, Masters & Johnson, 1979) because the successfully treated have usually been bisexuals with a history of heterosexuality prior to treatment. In short, there is little or no evidence for an effective psychological "treatment" for homosexuality.

PARAPHILIAS

Paraphilias can be defined as unusual or bizarre imagery or acts necessary for sexual excitement. Paraphilias tend to be insistently and involuntarily repetitive, generally involving either (1) preference for use of a nonhuman object for sexual arousal, (2) repetitive sexual activity with humans involving real or simulated suffering or humiliation, or (3) repetitive sexual activity with nonconsenting partners (American Psychiatric Association, 1980, p. 226).

Table 20.4 provides brief descriptions of the paraphilias. Collectively, they represent sexual fantasies and behaviors that deviate from the ways people usually achieve sexual arousal. Paraphilias are almost always a male problem, and according to Freud (1927, 1959) the driving force behind them is that "no male human being is spared the terrifying shock of threatened castration at the sight of the female genitals" (p. 201). In Freud's theory, the boy's recognition that the mother lacks a penis indicates that something bad has happened; in an effort to stave off fears that something worse will happen to her, he constructs elaborate fantasies that emphasize perfection and avoids direct con-

TABLE 20.4 PARAPHILIAS

Disorder	Definition
Fetishism	Preference for nonliving objects for achieving sexual excitement.
Transvestism	Recurrent, persistent, or compulsive cross-dressing by a heterosexual male for purposes of sexual excitement. Intense frustration if cross-dressing interfered with.
Zoophilia	Act or fantasy of engaging in sexual activity with animals as a preferred method of achieving sexual excitement.
Pedophilia	The act or fantasy of engaging in sexual activity with prepubertal children as the preferred or exclusive method of achieving sexual excitement.
Exhibitionism	Repetitive acts of exposing genitals to an unsuspecting stranger for the purpose of achieving sexual excitement with no attempt at greater sexual involvement with the stranger.
Voyeurism	Repeatedly observing others naked, while disrobing, or engaging in sexual activity, though no sexual activity is sought. Peeping is the preferred or exclusive method of sexual arousal.
Sexual masochism	Preferred or exclusive mode of sexual excitement is to be humiliated, bound, beaten, or otherwise made to suffer.
Sexual sadism	One of the following: (1) Without consent of the partner, the sadist intentionally inflicts psychological or physical punishment in order to achieve sexual excitement, (2) with a consenting partner, the preferred or exclusive mode of achieving sexual excitement combines humiliation with simulated or mildly injurious bodily suffering, or (3) on a consenting partner, extensive bodily injury is inflicted in order to achieve sexual excitement.
Atypical paraphilia	A residial category including coprophilia (feces), frotteurism (rubbing), klismaphilia (enema), mysophilia (filth), necrophilia (corpse), telephone scatologia (lewdness), and urophilia (urine).

frontation with the fact that females lack a penis (Becker, 1973). Even if one doesn't buy Freud's psychoanalytic hypothesis, the question remains why all paraphilias are strikingly more frequent in males. An alternative explanation may have something to do with the typical male tendency to focus on the most conspicuous target of sexual arousal to the neglect of the larger aspects of the relationship.

Consider a fetishist treated by Boss (1949):

> Whenever he saw or touched [ladies boots] "the world changed miraculously," he said. What had just appeared as "grey and senseless within the dreary, lonely and unsuccessful everyday, then suddenly drifts away from me, and light and glamour radiate from the leather to me." . . . Naked women or a woman's hand without a glove or especially a woman's foot without a shoe . . . seemed to be like lifeless pieces of meat in a butcher shop . . . (in Becker, 1973, pp. 235–236).

According to Becker, by not acknowledging the mother's mortal imperfections, the fetishist can avert anxiety about losing her. Although his explanation of fetishes is interesting, there are no empirical data for the idea.

More often than not, paraphilias are exaggerations of preliminary or accessory components of normal sexual activities. The compulsive desire to achieve sexual arousal through enemas appears bizarre, but there is a rational physiological basis for such a compulsion; namely, that the anus and anal sphincter muscle are innervated by the same neuronal systems as the sex organs. During orgasm they rhythmically contract at the same frequency (0.8 per second) as the sexual muscles.

Fetishes

Fetishes are objects associated with isolated accoutrements of female sexuality such as hair, undergarments, and shoes. Fetishes come to be preferred to actual heterosexual contact or are required accessories to achieve high levels of sexual arousal in heterosexual relations. Although a person may have only one fetish, often he has multiple fetishes as well as other paraphilias. The following fetishist was sexually aroused not only by leather gloves and rubber objects, but also by enemas, withholding his urine, sexual sadism, and sexual masochism.

> At nine years of age he succumbed to a desire for the possession of his mother's brown leather gloves, took them to bed with him, pressed them against his perineum between the anus and the scrotum, and then put them on and masturbated. . . . In the same box with the gloves, he also found some rubber tubes . . . [which] he would . . . wind . . . around his penis. . . . About this time he began to develop an interest in women's gloves and would dance only with the girls who wore kid gloves. He liked gray gloves pretty well, but the woollen ones the dancing teacher wore left him cold. . . . At 12 years . . . the glove . . . took on an increased sexual importance. Whenever he would feel the leather of the glove he would get an erection and would begin to think of girls who could wear them. . . . He would give himself enemas. . . . In addition to gaining pleasure from touching leather or rubber goods, he also liked to smell them . . . . At 16 he would tie rubber bands together and then bind his penis and his scrotum with the elastic. . . . He also had the desire to masturbate with such gloves or to cohabit with the women who wore them. To suit him they must be tight-fitting without a single crease, and absolutely clean. He cannot tolerate any defects in them (Stekel, 1930, pp. 102–103).

This man married and sired children, but his wife's refusal to partake in his leather and rubber preoccupations left little sexual spark. He located a prostitute who would play both sadistic and masochistic roles. Though his fetishes were irresistible and consuming, he was still an active member in clubs, exercised, and performed in plays, always in a woman's role. A significant fraction of fetishists are aroused by rubber and leather. It is tempting to note the similarity of these materials to skin—indeed, leather is skin—and speculate on their symbolic capacity to re-create close physical contact with the mother. But in truth, the reasons for their special attraction are unknown.

Transvestism

This paraphilia involves a childhood or adolescent history of sexual arousal achieved by cross-dressing. However, many adult transvestites no longer report sexual arousal by cross-dressing, saying that it now gives them only tension relief; nevertheless, experimental studies of penile tumescence in these subjects suggests that sexual arousal from cross-dressing still occurs. Perhaps only 20 percent of cross-dressers are homosexually oriented and many are married. Transvestism, like other paraphilias, is almost exclusively a male abnormality. Only three female transvestites have ever been reported; all had been tomboys and became lesbians or bisexuals (Stoller, 1982).

Transvestism can appear very early. Green (1974) interviewed a 5-year-old boy about his cross-dressing:

> *Doctor*: Is it hard to stop dressing up once you've already started it?
> *Boy*: Yeah.
> *Doctor*: How does it make you feel when you dress up?
> *Boy*: Nice, sometimes and boring others.
> *Doctor*: When you dress up, like a girl, does it ever make your penis stand up stiff and straight?
> *Boy*: Yeah.
> *Doctor*: It always does? What other times does your penis get stiff and stand up?
> *Boy*: Right after I've gone to the bathroom sometimes.
> *Doctor*: Any other times?
> *Boy*: No.
> *Doctor*: But always when you put on girls' clothing?
> *Boy*: Yeah.
> *Doctor*: How does it feel when it stands up like that?
> *Boy*: It really hurts.
> *Doctor*: It hurts?
> *Boy*: Yeah.
> *Doctor*: What do you do?
> *Boy*: Take off the clothing.
> *Doctor*: And then what happens?
> *Boy*: And then it goes down again.
> *Doctor*: Then it goes down again?
> *Boy*: Yeah.
> *Doctor*: Does it make your penis feel like you want to play with it when it stands up like that?
> *Boy*: Yeah.
> *Doctor*: Do you play with it?
> *Boy*: Yeah.
> *Doctor*: And how does that feel?
> *Boy*: That's—that feels funny.
> *Doctor*: Is it a—You're smiling. Is it a nice feeling?
> *Boy*: Yeah.
> *Doctor*: When you do play with it, when you put on girls' clothing and it stands up, does that feel good?
> *Boy*: Yeah.

The boy's account clearly indicates a compulsive sexual motive behind cross-dressing, but we do not know if he will become a tranvestite, transsexual, homosexual, or heterosexual as an adult. Even at this early age, the boy cannot provide an explanation for the origin of the cross-dressing, reminding us that adult explanations about childhood origins of their sexual peculiarities also are suspect.

Psychiatric interviews with members of cross-dressing associations have found excesses of definite depression (22 percent) and alcoholism (14 percent), but no elevation in parental psychopathology (Croughan et al., 1981). These other disorders, however, usually precede transvestism and are probably causally insignificant.

Behavior therapies seem modestly successful in eliminating cross-dressing or reducing its frequency (see Langevin, 1983, for a review). But many cross-dressers have not sought therapy or believe transvestism to be a problem. Sometimes the best approach is to reduce conflict and anxiety over the behavior. If a spouse is involved, it often helps to explain to her that transvestism does not imply homosexuality.

Exhibitionism and Voyeurism

These two paraphilias seem to be opposite sides of the same coin. Both involve preferences for visual contact—being seen and seeing—rather than tactile contact. The exhibitionist is erotically aroused by surprising unsuspecting females while exposing his penis. He may masturbate in front of the victim or afterwards. Usually, the surprise component figures in the erotic fantasy.

One theory suggests that exhibitionism might be associated with efforts to cope with feelings of inferiority. Consider the following self-report:

> . . . I usually spend my Saturdays in the bar and this week I had a date that evening with a nice girl. When I was in the bar, I picked up this other girl and went to her place and had sex. Then I went out with my date that evening and had sex with her too. Would you believe I exposed on the way home? Now that's stupid! (Langevin, 1983, p. 330).

Unfortunately, his feelings about the evening's conventional heterosexual encounters are unknown. They probably were unsatisfactory, either because of doubts about sexual adequacy or because a consenting partner does not provide enough thrill. Exposing can be more exciting than actual encounters because the fantasy script need never be blemished by interpersonal problems. Concerns about self-esteem, inferiority, and cleanliness are prominent in exhibitionists (Langevin et al., 1979), but can be completely finessed by avoiding actual physical contact.

The voyeur is aroused by secretly observing females undressing or in the act of sexual intercourse. To be aroused by observing sexuality is normal, indeed, the pornography industry thrives on it. What makes voyeurism a paraphilia is that it is preferred to heterosexual activity.

Exhibitionists and voyeurs are often married and having regular sexual intercourse with their wives. Thus, it is not for lack of a heterosexual outlet that these paraphilias occur. Rather, the fantasy system is insufficiently sparked by the idea of routine marital sex. This alone is not surprising because sexual novelty is generally more exciting than familiarity. But to cope with this, exhibitionists short-circuit the usual courtship process by going immediately to the display of genitals. Some hope that the target will reciprocate:

Patient: What I really like is some nice young thing to expose to me too and then maybe we could go somewhere and have sex.

Doctor: You have been exposing since you were 15 on the average of 4–5 times a week and that means that you have exposed over 1600 times now. Right? Has a woman ever offered you sex or exposed to you?

Patient: (long pause)—-No, but one might (Langevin, 1983, pp. 329–330)!

The kind of "show-and-tell" that seems to motivate exhibitionists and voyeurs has a childlike quality. One wonders how much Western attitudes toward sexuality figure in their origins. Exhibitionism has not been reported in preliterate societies, but we do not know much about voyeurism. Perhaps more permissive attitudes toward childhood sexuality and routine genital exposure provide the sense of familiarity that discourages these sexual deviations.

Pedophilia

Literally, pedophilia refers to love of children, but as a paraphilia, it refers to adult erotic preferences for children. Pedophiles may be heterosexual, homosexual, or "indifferent" in their erotic preferences. The types of sexual activities engaged in with the children may range from surreptitious self-masturbation and fondling to fellatio and vaginal or anal intercourse. Some pedophiles prefer the immature child because they can be dominant. Some claim disgust for adult genitalia and secondary sexual characteristics, preferring physically immature genitals and the absence of pubic hair. Explanations for pedophilia include feelings of low self-esteem, early modeling, fears of adult contact, and impulse disorder (Finkelhor & Araji, 1986), but no specific explanation commands much attention.

Evidence indicates that child molesters and normal people respond to the same erotic stimuli, the important difference between the two groups being largely one of degree. Slides of nude prepubescent girls produce a slight erectile response even in normal male adults, although the response is much more intense in the pedophile (Langevin, 1983). Pedophiles may have dozens of sexual encounters without getting caught. Very often the children are acquaintances, but because of fear of reprisal or appreciation of the benefits provided, they keep the events secret.

Apprehended child molesters report an astonishingly varied array of other paraphilias and sex crimes (Abel et al., 1983). For example, 10 to 20 percent are also rapists and one-fifth are exhibitionists. A large proportion of pedophiles arrested for either homosexual or heterosexual acts with children also are involved with children of the other sex (40 percent or more). This indifference to the sex of the object implies a depersonalization of the child and the domination of sexual desire over all else. Unfortunately, the rate of child sexual abuse appears to be growing (Abel, 1984). Increasing divorce rates expose more young children to men who date the mother and the swelling representation of women in the marketplace leaves more children unsupervised or under the care of strangers.

Sexual Masochism and Sadism

The idea of obtaining sexual pleasure from aggressive acts or humiliation seems foreign to everyday sexual experience. Yet for many animals biting, clawing, and other seemingly violent acts are intimately involved in copulation. Moreover, biting, scratching, and wrestling are not uncommon during human copulation. It thus appears that like child molesters, sadomasochists are sexually more responsive than normals to the same cues.

Aggressive acts and moderately painful experiences have nonspecific arousal components that can potentiate sexual arousal. For example, gently pinching the tail of a male rat can elicit sexual behavior in the presence of a receptive female (Antelman & Caggiula, 1980). As Gebhard (1983) pointed out, aggression "has definite neurophysiological value in establishing, or reinforcing many of the physiological concomitants of sexual arousal such as increased pulse and blood pressure, hyperventilation, and muscular tension" (p. 36). It appears more thrilling to be the masochist than the sadist, though taking turns is often necessary to maintain enduring relationships. It is much more difficult to locate sadists than masochists, and the latter will travel hundreds of miles to meet a female willing to administer "discipline."

Sadomasochistic encounters often involve elaborate theatrical stagings of the sexual events; canes, whips, bonds, leather, boots, and torture apparatus are required props, reminding us that a fantasy is being acted out as in other paraphilias. A delicate balance exists between the partners—the sadist should not inflict too much pain, although copious amounts of humiliation are permitted.

The first sadomasochistic encounter may not occur until adolescence, but earlier childhood fantasies of sadomasochism can often be elicited. For example, one sadomasochist had childhood fantasies of being sexually and otherwise manipulated and controlled by machines; as an adult he enjoyed being bound and whipped (Kamel & Weinberg, 1983).

Although sadism requires a partner, masochism can be practiced alone. Unfortunately, things can get out of hand, resulting in serious injury or death—for example, unintended lethal hangings may occur as the masochist zealously attempts to heighten sexual arousal. These people may use asphyxiation and certain sedative hypnotics such as chloral hydrate to release lower brain centers from normal cortical inhibitory controls. This allows for an otherwise rare intensity of experience perhaps comparable only to the vividness of the erotic dream.

General Comments

That multiple paraphilias often exist in the same individual strains the idea of one-to-one correspondences between a specific childhood experience and a specific paraphilia. It would require too great a variety of specific sexually exciting experiences to be plausible. A more parsimonious hypothesis involves a compulsive sexual preoccupation that has arisen or generalized from one or a few significant experiences.

One gets the impression that the paraphilias are associated with an excess of chromosomal, neurological, or hormonal abnormalities (Berlin, 1983). These abnormal conditions may compromise inhibitory mechanisms that would otherwise prevent acting out of sexual fantasies. Nevertheless, since the causes of the paraphilias are probably varied, we should be reluctant to adhere closely to any single etiological theory. An unanswered question is whether anyone could be made a paraphiliac through conditioning, or whether a special predisposition is required.

Collectively, the paraphilias signify the ascendance of peculiar sexual fantasies which come to dominate erotic life. Most begin early, when the child is impressionable and lacks cognitive capacities to cope with sexually arousing or frightening experiences. Stimulation arising from bathing, enemas, or toilet training, for example, could prompt sexual stirrings that produce a powerful affective charge that does not take its proper place within emotional life, but arrests sexual development before a more balanced orientation can be achieved. Unfortunately, this hypothesis is incomplete because it cannot explain why the paraphilias are almost exclusive to males. Childhood sexual arousal also occurs in girls, yet it does not produce the paraphilias. There might be something different about the brains, anatomy, or hormonal functioning of the two sexes that figures in the paraphilias, but what this is remains a mystery.

RAPE

Rape is a varying mixture of aggression and sex. Intercourse occurs in upward of 80 or 90 percent of rapes (Holmstrom & Burgess, 1980) and intravaginal ejaculation occurs in at least half (Thornhill & Thornhill, 1983), suggesting that rape is not exclusively an act of aggression. Although murder during rape is relatively rare (one per thousand), violence and humiliation are commonly imposed.

Rape is terrifying. Understandably, normal individuals tend to distance themselves psychologically from rapists, but like the paraphilias, there are continuities between rapists and others. For example, a third of a sample of American males say they might rape if there were no chance of getting caught (Malamuth & Check, 1981). Moreover, when the social reins are removed, as in war, rape may become endemic (Brownmiller, 1975). The extent to which a widespread tolerance exists for the idea of rape is evident in the high prevalence of "rape myths," that is, attitudes held by many males and females which increase the "acceptability" of sexual violence toward women.

To see this, consider the items in Table 20.5 excerpted from a lengthier "Rape Myth Acceptance Scale" devised by Burt (1980). Endorsement of these items means that consent is irrelevant to heterosexual intercourse; if she puts herself in a compromising position, she deserves what she gets. In a representative sample of adult Minnesotans of both sexes, Burt found that over half agreed with the idea that "In the majority of rapes, the victim is promiscuous or has a bad reputation." Not only are beliefs like this factually incorrect, they suggest widely held negative attitudes toward women among members of both sexes.

Categorical Distinctions

Rapists are not alike and the differences among them will have to be acknowledged if treatment is ever to be successful. Rape does not exist as a distinct diagnostic entity; it is a form of criminal behavior and not yet a psychiatric term. Rapists can be classified into three broad categories. *Sadistic rapists* have had violent fantasies since childhood and commit multiple rapes if not incarcerated or successfully treated. Another group could be classified as *paraphilic rapists* because, like sexual sadists, they have persistent rape fantasies and commit multiple rapes. Unlike the sexual sadist, however, they are not specifically aroused by the victim's terror. During rape they employ only the force necessary to subdue the victim. Finally, some rapists are *antisocial personalities* with neither persistent rape fantasies nor a high rate of rapes. They rape during the course of another crime, taking callous advantage of an opportunity.

Often the idea of power rather than sex sparks the thrill of rape. Consider the following from a convicted rapist:

TABLE 20.5	ITEMS FROM THE RAPE MYTH ACCEPTANCE SCALE

Any healthy woman can successfully resist a rapist if she really wants to.

When women go around braless or wearing short skirts and tight tops, they are just asking for trouble.

In the majority of rapes, the victim is promiscuous or has a bad reputation.

If a girl engages in necking or petting and she lets things get out of hand, it is her own fault if her partner forces sex on her.

Women who get raped while hitchhiking get what they deserve.

A woman who is stuck-up and thinks she is too good to talk to guys on the street deserves to be taught a lesson.

Many women have an unconscious wish to be raped, and may then unconsciously set up a situation in which they are likely to be attacked.

Source: From M. A. Burt (1980). Cultural myths and support for rape. *Journal of Personality and Social Psychology, 38,* 217–230. Copyright © 1980 by the American Psychological Association. Adapted by permission.

It was one of the most satisfying experiences I've ever had. I got more pleasure out of being aggressive, having power over her, her actions, her life. It gave me pleasure knowing there was nothing she could do. It like built me up. I had been driving around thinking about sex and searching for someone. I was looking for someone I could get my feelings out on. My feelings were a mixture of sex and anger. I wanted pleasure, but I had to prove something, that I could dominate a woman. I felt exhilarated during the rape. It was so intense that it took away from the sex itself. The sex part wasn't very good at all (Groth, 1979, p. 95).

Groth (1979) remarked of his interviews with convicted rapists that none felt that rape was sexually more rewarding than consenting sex. Rather, it had an irresistible quality that promised more than it delivered. This promise never diminished, even in recidivists who had already experienced the disappointments.

Recidivism   About 18 percent of all sex criminals are rearrested for another sex crime within 2½ years of release (Miller et al., 1976). Recidivism rates for rapists of adults are somewhat higher (30 percent), but the new sexual offense is rape only half the time. The remainder are rearrested for sex crimes such as exhibitionism and pedophilia. Since the likelihood of being apprehended for a single crime is low, the actual recidivism rates are probably much higher than the official rates. Indeed, estimates suggest that rapists and child molesters commit an additional two to five times more sex offenses that do not result in arrest (Groth, Longo, & McFadin, 1982). Many rapists have arrest records for nonsex crimes as well, confirming the idea that rapists are often antisocial personalities (Tracy et al., 1983).

Psychophysiological Arousal   What is there about the act of rape that excites rapists? Unfortunately, this question is difficult to answer because most rapists are reluctant to reveal fantasies or additional crimes for which they were not apprehended. However, provided the rapist is moderately cooperative, erectile responses can be used to identify stimuli to which they are aroused. Rapists and nonrapists have been presented with audiotaped narrations of consenting intercourse and violent rape (Abel et al., 1977). Both groups are aroused about equally to consenting sex, but differ dramatically in the sexual response to rape. Whereas nonrapists tend to inhibit erection to scenes of sexual violence, rapists are aroused to about the same degree as with consenting sex (Figure 20.7). Moreover, the degree to which rapists respond to rape scenes is correlated with the violence and number of their past rapes.

Predicting Rape   Youthful sexual aggression may be an especially good marker of the future rapist. Consider a young man charged with two rapes:

[F]or three years prior to his rapes he has been assaulting women in parking lots . . . he would grab their genital areas and then run away. This behavior persisted over a year, eventually occurred in his high school, and led to his expulsion. Ignored, his grabbing of women persisted, and eventually he followed women into of-

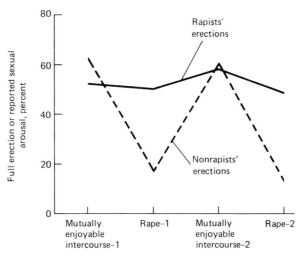

FIGURE 20.7 Comparison of sexual responses in rapists and nonrapists to audiotapes of mutually consenting intercourse and of rape. From G. G. Abel, D. H. Barlow, E. B. Blanchard, & D. Guild (1977). The components of rapists' sexual arousal. *Archives of General Psychiatry, 34,* 895–903, p. 900. Copyright © 1977, American Medical Association.

fice buildings and escalated his sexual behavior to rape . . . his family and school officials did not respond to his early grabbing behavior, even though this behavior duplicated four of the aggressive aspects of rape: hands on victim, aggressive attacks, unconsenting victim, and repetition. His behavior differed in only one aspect: his immediate escape from the victim once she had been touched. . . . Everyone appeared to be waiting for Henry's problem to get serious (Abel, 1983, pp. 244–245).

It doesn't require a prophet to have foreseen that this boy was likely to do great harm. Unfortunately, no effective prevention was instituted. This state of affairs is not unusual; many antisocial children are not provided with treatments that are effective and one seems to wait for the inevitable disaster to happen before being forced to take action.

Treatment

Few rapists or other sex offenders get effective treatment while incarcerated, in part because the judicial system militates against sexual revelations by the inmate. But more importantly, there are no treatments, either physical or psychological, that can guarantee elimination of the urge. Nowadays, surgical and chemical treatments are receiving much attention. They are predicated on the idea that testosterone maintains the sexual appetite of sex offenders and that decreasing testosterone levels will diminish the sex drive.

Two antitestosterone drugs (Androcur and Depo Provera) have been used in an effort to prevent recidivism in sex offenders. These drugs reduce circulating testosterone levels to less than one-fifth of normal. Most patients on the drug report reduced sex drive and erectile difficulties, although adjusting the dosage can take the edge off the sex drive without markedly impairing erectile responsiveness (Langevin, 1983). It appears that some individuals with harmful or dangerous paraphilias can be helped by the drugs, but much more follow-up research is needed (Money & Bennett, 1981).

If the primary urge to rape is nonsexual—if it is triggered by hostility or inferiority feelings—it seems unlikely that such treatments would eliminate recidivism. Castration has been employed as a treatment for sexual offenders in Europe with some success (Heim, 1981). Since the adrenals normally secrete a small amount of testosterone, the hormone is not eliminated entirely by castration, however, and some sexual arousal may remain (Quinsey & Marshall, 1983).

While psychological treatments of all kinds have been tried, including aversion and psychodynamic therapies, none convincingly demonstrates effectiveness in preventing recidivism. Abel (1983), however, says that if rapists and other sex offenders can be encouraged to reveal their fantasies, treatment success rates might increase dramatically, using principles of conditioning.

The Rape Victim

Rape is an extreme violation of personal space. Victims not only are terrorized but, because of a lack of support, may feel humiliated by having succumbed. These feelings can last indefinitely and over half the victims of sexual assaults report new feelings of shame, helplessness, and nightmares (Becker, Skinner, & Abel, 1983). Moreover, the majority of rape victims report sexual problems that had not existed before, especially problems of diminished sexual desire. Unfortunately, the victim's family often does little to ameliorate the dysphoria. Many of these women would benefit from supportive counseling, especially if other family members were included. Some family members mistakenly believe the rape myths and secretly think the victim could have done more to prevent the rape, but education and therapy can be used to correct these erroneous ideas.

PSYCHOSEXUAL DYSFUNCTIONS

Psychosexual dysfunctions comprise a melange of disturbances in the normal sexual response cycle of desire, arousal, orgasm, and resolution (relaxation or fatigue). Dysfunctions usually occur in the absence of diagnosable psychopathology, but can nevertheless be traced to anxiety, hostility, and fixed mistaken ideas about the nature of sexual arousal and copulation. Although the reflex sex system can operate through friction alone—indeed, the genitals of comatose patients can react to friction—it seldom does. Instead, it is abetted or inhibited by higher cognitive functions.

Description

Like sexual arousal, anxiety and hostility involve activation of the autonomic nervous system. These emotions and the accompanying autonomic reactions can potentiate or inhibit sexual responses. If the emotions accelerate the cycle, as in premature ejaculation, then the sexual partners are out of sync, leaving at least one member dissatisfied with the sexual episode. In long-term commitments, these dysfunctions spill over into general unhappiness. Table 20.6 provides an abbreviated listing of the various forms of psychosexual dysfunction.

Treatment

Masters and Johnson (1970), pioneers in the treatment of psychosexual dysfunction, work with *couples*, because both members are inevitably affected

TABLE 20.6 SEXUAL DYSFUNCTIONS

Sexual desire disorders	*Hypoactive sexual desire disorder* refers to a deficiency or absence of sexual fantasies or desire for sexual activity *Sexual aversion disorder* refers to an avoidance of nearly all genital contact with a partner
Sexual arousal disorders	*Female sexual arousal disorder* refers to a complete or partial failure to maintain sexual lubrication during sexual activity or the lack of a subjective sense of excitement and pleasure during sexual activity *Male erectile disorder* refers either to a failure to maintain erection until completion of sexual activity or to a lack of a subjective sense of sexual excitement and pleasure during sexual activity
Orgasm disorders	*Inhibited female orgasm* refers to a recurrent delay or inability to achieve orgasm even when sexually aroused *Inhibited male orgasm* refers to a recurrent delay or inability to achieve orgasm even if sexually aroused *Premature ejaculation* refers to persistent or recurrent ejaculation before or shortly after penetration and before the person wishes it
Sexual pain disorders	*Dyspareunia* refers to genital pain before, during, or after sexual intercourse (can occur in either gender) *Vaginismus* is an involuntary spasm of the musculature of the outer third of the vagina that interferes with intercourse

Source: After *DSM-III-R*, pp. 293–295.

even when only one is dysfunctional. Two general concepts inform their treatment methods: (1) sex is a natural function controlled largely by reflexes; and (2) fears of performance inadequacy and "spectatoring" are often central to sexual dysfunction. By spectatoring they mean becoming overly attentive to one's own sexual performance, thereby infusing it with anxiety instead of spontaneity. In the initial phase of treatment, explicit sexual contact leading to orgasm is banned. This allows couples tactile exploration of each other's body without the necessity of achieving orgasmic goals.

Regardless of the specific psychosexual dysfunction, all couples begin by using the method of *sensate focus*. This technique emphasizes nonverbal exploration of each other's body; communication between partners is via touch or nonverbal expression. It consists of four phases:

1 In two sessions, each partner takes turns exploring the other's body, except that the genitals and breasts are off limits.

2 Touching is expanded to include breasts and genitals, but sexual arousal is not permitted to end in orgasm.

3 There is then mutual and simultaneous exploration, but still no orgasm is permitted.

4 Finally, the female rides atop the male and brings the penis in apposition to the vagina, but does not attempt deep insertion of the penis.

Many dysfunctional couples will be quite aroused by this time. Nevertheless orgasm is explicitly discouraged. This procedure allows partners nonanxiously to rediscover each other's body and become more aware of their own sexual responsiveness. Sometimes, sensate focus exercises along with discussions about the experience are sufficient to clear up some long-standing disturbances, especially if the major problem is boredom. Studies using surrogate partners—for example, prostitutes as therapists—has revealed that many men who are dysfunctional with their regular partners perform normally with the surrogate (Cole, 1985). Results such as these suggest that many dysfunctions of drive and desire are partner-specific, arising from boredom, habituation, anxiety, or hostility.

Treatments for each of the psychosexual dysfunctions can be found in Kaplan (1974; 1979). Included are the squeeze technique for premature ejaculation in which the female applies pressure to the frenulum—the ventral portion behind the tip of the penis—just before ejaculation, and the use of tension-relaxation exercises and vaginal dilators for vaginismus. Some sexual problems may be more complex and require individual psychotherapy.

Although there is more than a little controversy surrounding the definition of cure in sex therapy (Zilbergeld & Evans, 1980; Cole, 1985), the general impression is that treatment success rates are somewhat higher than for other disorders. In one recent study about 60 to 80 percent of those completing treatment were cured or nearly so, 10 percent showed some improvement, and the remainder showed no change (Hawton, 1982). Three-month follow-ups indicated occasional regressions, so that cures or near-cures averaged about 50 to 70 percent.

In this chapter we have reviewed a variety of sexual disturbances that do not fit neatly into one theoretical picture. In part, this is because sexual peculiarities involve hormones, anatomy, childhood experiences, cultural attitudes, and the hostilities and anxieties that arise in normal interpersonal relationships. Moreover, there is debate about whether homosexuality and psychosexual dysfunctions should even qualify as abnormalities or mental disorders. One of the remarkable features of sexuality is that statistically deviant sexual tastes and habits can have little adverse spillover into other aspects of affective or cognitive life. In the absence of additional signs of psychopathology such as psychosis, anxiety, or depression, it is therefore often unclear whether some of these deviations belong in a book on psychopathology. Nevertheless, there is one striking consistency that cries out for a unifying explanation, namely, why are almost all paraphilias virtually exclusive to males?

SUMMARY

Psychosexual deviations are categorized into three broad groups: *gender identity disorders* such as transsexualism, *paraphilias* such as fetishes, and *psychosexual dysfunctions* such as psychogenic impotence. In the gender identity disorder transsexualism, the person feels trapped in the body of the other sex. Male transsexuals—biological males who feel female—have a childhood history of extreme effeminacy, while female transsexuals were more likely to have been tomboys. Although homosexuality is not officially classified as a mental disorder, it is somewhat similar to transsexuality, especially in shared histories of early effeminacy or tomboyism.

The paraphilias, involving unusual and often bizarre imagery or acts required for sexual excitement, include fetishism, cross-dressing, exhibitionism, voyeurism, pedophilia, sexual masochism, and sexual sadism. All the paraphilias appear to have their origins in childhood, but the exact causes are unknown.

Psychosexual dysfunctions refer to disturbances in one or more of the components of the sexual response cycle: desire, arousal, orgasm, resolution. These dysfunctions typically arise because of anxiety about sexuality and are relatively more responsive to treatment than the psychosexual deviations.

Rape involves both the rapist's psychopathology and the victim's problems in coping with the trauma. Some rapists also have paraphilias, suggesting that rape is only the most conspicuous and censurable of his activities. Others have antisocial personalities, where rape is incidental to other antisocial acts. In any case, recidivism rates are high and treatment compromised because rapists are unwilling to reveal the extent and intensity of their rape fantasies. Victims of rape may develop chronic psychosexual problems, often accentuated by unsympathetic societal attitudes.

Except for the psychosexual dysfunctions involving problems of desire, arousal, and orgasm, virtually all the sexual disorders are more frequent in males, sometimes strikingly so. No ready explanation is available to account for this, but presumably hormones and anatomy figure importantly.

CHAPTER 21

Child and Adolescent Psychopathologies

OUTLINE

Childhood behavior problems depend on many things: specific causes, the age of onset, the context in which the problem occurs, the child's prior level of emotional and cognitive development, and the developmental tasks yet to be accomplished. The existence of so many confounding factors has historically separated the study of childhood-onset disorders from the study of adult-onset disorders. It seems rather strange, though a usual practice, to include in one chapter disorders that have in common only the fact that they tend to occur in childhood or adolescence.

This chapter focuses first on some central issues about the causes and nature of various forms of childhood psychopathology and then considers various specific disorders as examples that cover the range of psychopathologies observed in children. We start the discussion of general issues by focusing on the biological aspects of early development, because the seeds of childhood psychopathology can begin before birth, when the fetus is primarily a biological organism.

BIOLOGICAL ASPECTS

Many childhood behavioral problems reflect not only abnormal heredity, but also abnormal embryological events occurring during pregnancy. Often these abnormal events can only be inferred, because it is difficult to assess the health of a fetus. However, biological markers may reveal specifically when in fetal life something went awry. For example, palm print patterns are completely formed by 4 months of fetal life; therefore, distinctively different prints on an infant's two palms indicates the occurrence of an abnormal event prior to that time (Rose, Reed, & Bogle, 1987).

Being a physically healthy child is quite an achievement. Only about three-quarters of successfully implanted embryos live long enough to be born (Polani, 1981), and more than a third of those who spontaneously abort have chromosome anomalies (Warburton, 1987); the remainder succumb to infections and unknown causes. Of those born alive, about 6 per 1000 have chromosome errors, 4 percent have birth defects, and a substantial fraction are in future jeopardy because of prematurity. Very premature infants are especially susceptible to brain hemorrhages because of bleeding due to immature blood vessels (Volpe & Hill, 1983). Moreover, the prematurity itself may indicate that the womb was not providing an optimal environment for the fetus. Premature infants, especially those of very low birth weight, may be at an especially high risk for neurological dysfunctions and learning disabilities (Nichols & Chen, 1981). We should be alert to the possibility that childhood behavior problems may actually have subtle antecedents associated with abnormal events occurring during pregnancy.

Minor Physical Anomalies

Minor physical anomalies (MPAs) provide one example of how events during pregnancy may be associated with later behavioral problems. The long list of MPAs includes oversized incisor teeth, index finger longer than the middle finger, fine electric hair that will not comb down, two or more hair whorls, and a high-steepled palate (Waldrop & Halverson, 1971). These anomalous features originally were presumed to be of no serious medical or cosmetic consequence (Smith, 1970), yet they eventually proved to be anatomic markers of pathology arising from genetic or early prenatal causes such as infection. Fortunately, the onset of the original aberration can be established with a fair degree of confidence because we know the schedule for various embryological events such as when the palate is formed.

Many studies have shown that hyperactive, mentally retarded, and psychotic children have an excess of MPAs (see Krouse & Kauffman, 1982). For example, Firestone and Prabhu (1983) found more MPAs among hyperactive than control children. Moreover, the first-degree relatives of the hyperactives often showed an excess of MPAs themselves. Thus, some of the MPAs seem to derive from genes activated during early prenatal development and are not simply the result of infection, physical, or nutritional problems arising during fetal life. Interestingly, many adult schizophrenics also have high MPA scores (Gualtieri et al., 1982; Guy et al., 1983), suggesting an embryological antecedent even for a disorder that typically is diagnosed only in adulthood.

Prenatal and perinatal factors constitute a vast reservoir of potential and usually obscure causes of behavioral abnormality, but practical limitations in invading the womb and jeopardizing the health of the fetus hamper research progress. Nevertheless, with increasing prenatal diagnostic sophistication, as illustrated by new technologies like sonograms (sound waves) for visualizing the fetus and increasing ability to make diagnoses from amniotic fluid, we can justifiably expect more progress. For example, one study revealed that newborns with relatively high, but still "normal," levels of lead in their umbilical cords had slightly lower scores (about seven IQ points) on a test of cognitive development when tested at age 2. It would not be surprising if their slight intellectual disadvantage continued for life (Bellinger et al., 1987).

At the time the child comes to professional attention, dysfunctions can easily be misattributed to faults in child rearing. After all, no insightful parents can in retrospect deny some child-rearing "mistakes." It is an empirical question whether these mistakes are responsible for the debilities observed, however. We must come to appreciate the possibility of subtle negative influences on development, especially during fetal life. Compared to the adult, the rapidly developing embryo and fetus can be many times more vulnerable to various environmental contaminants such as heavy metals (not only lead) that are endemic in the environment or to diseases such as German measles (rubella) that might produce little or no visible effects in the pregnant woman herself. These hidden prenatal influences may help to explain why it is often so difficult to identify "errors" in child rearing that might explain behavioral abnormalities.

Normal and Abnormal Development

Unfortunately, the limited behavioral repertoire of infants and toddlers also makes difficult the detection of early signs of dysfunction. What are parents to think of an infant who does not cuddle, smile, or otherwise engage in reciprocal social transactions? Do these behavioral peculiarities reflect normal variations in temperament or sociability, or something pathological? Parents and professionals often can only hope for the best.

Empirical norms for the age at which various behavioral accomplishments are supposed to occur can help determine whether a particular behavior is deviant. For example, a normal infant is expected to begin smiling socially between 1 and 2 months of age. Delays beyond 3 months usually indicate that something is wrong. Consider the Babinski reflex, a slow upward extension of the great toe and splaying by the other toes in response to stroking the sole. Presence of the Babinski reflex after age 1 indicates that the cortex is not performing its normal inhibitory functions and therefore may be a sign of brain damage.

Coordination difficulties are especially common in children with certain kinds of psychopathology. For example, 90 percent of 4-year-olds can hop, but those who cannot are about twice as likely to have neurological abnormalities and 45 percent more likely to be called hyperactive-impulsive at age 7 (Nichols & Chen, 1981). At age 6 or 7 children are expected to be able to make fairly rapid alternating hand and foot movements. Children who cannot do this speedily are often poor readers, suggesting a more generalized neurological abnormality not confined to reading (Rudel, 1980; Wolff, Gunnoe, & Cohen,

1985). In sum, children with poor coordination, immature reflexes, and sensori-motor problems show an excess of learning disabilities, hyperactivity, conduct disturbances, and impulsivity (Holden, Tarnowski, & Prinz, 1982).

Ecopathology

Many children grow up in homes that are less than optimal for healthy development. For example, perhaps 80,000 injuries and 800 deaths per year can be attributed to physical abuse of children (Herskowitz & Rosman, 1982). Sexual abuse of children is also quite common. Fourteen percent of college females report some form of childhood sexual abuse and 1 percent even report an incestuous relationship (Finkelhor, 1977). These figures apply to the general population as well. In a San Francisco survey, 12 percent of women reported intrafamilial sexual abuse before the age of 14 (Russell, 1983).

These traumatic events in childhood can alter one's future in disastrous ways. For example, it is not unusual to see physically and sexually abused children turn out to be poor students or delinquents, and to have difficulties in interpersonal relationships. Also, about 30 percent of abused children will be child abusers when they become parents, a rate of child abuse estimated to be about six times that in the general population (Kaufman & Zigler, 1987).

Children reared under adverse social conditions are also less likely than children reared under more desirable circumstances to show behavioral recovery following a head injury. A study of new behavioral disorders arising in children who had suffered a head injury two years earlier revealed that one-third of the children developed new behavioral abnormalities, the most conspicuous being impulsiveness (Brown et al., 1981). The telling point was that the children living in broken homes or with parents having unhappy marriages or psychiatric disorders developed the greatest incidence of new behavioral abnormalities (see Figure 21.1). Unfortunately, there is little known about the specific qualities that promote recovery in the better homes.

FIGURE 21.1 New behavioral disorders in head-injured children as a function of psychosocial adversity. (After B. Brown et al., 1981)

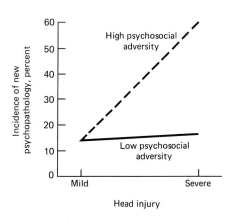

Assessing Childhood Psychopathology

Until recently, disorders of childhood and adolescence were viewed merely as miniature versions of adult disturbances. Consequently, little attention was given to the effects of physical, cognitive, and emotional immaturity on symptom expression. But the relative degree of maturity will affect the kinds of symptoms observed. For example, one does not expect a troubled preschooler to develop paranoid symptoms because such symptoms generally require a near-adult level of cognitive capacity. The implication is that age norms are required to establish whether a particular child is deviant because the specific symptoms expressed will depend greatly on the age at which the problem occurs.

Most children brought to clinics for behavioral problems fall into nine major and reliably differentiable categories (Quay, 1986b). These nine categories and some of their most prominent behavioral correlates are given in Table 21.1. The *DSM-III-R* contains some additional rarely occurring conditions as well as some that are often confused with each other (Werry et al., 1983). The unreliability suggested by the confusion indicates that more work is required to bring the childhood disorders to a level of reliability equal to that obtained for most adult-onset disorders.

Rates for childhood/adolescent disorders are difficult to obtain and vary across samples, diagnostic criteria, and raters. One of the most comprehensive surveys of specific behavior problems such as nightmares, as opposed to disorders, at least provides useful baseline figures. Achenbach and Edelbrock (1981) did home interviews of a representative sample of parents in the Washington, D.C., area and surveyed mental health agencies on the East Coast. Interviewers asked about 118 behavioral problems among children aged 4 to 16 years.

The results from a sample of those items are shown in Figure 21.2. Data are displayed by sex, age, and whether or not they were referred for treatment. Not surprisingly, children referred for treatment had more behavioral problems. Some symptoms showed substantial declines with age—for example, nightmares, speech problems, and bedwetting. But others—compulsions and setting fires, for example—showed negligible changes with age. Those items that show declines with age are probably related to physical and cognitive weaknesses such as defective neural inhibitory control systems that seem to mature with age, but those items that show no changes with age probably reflect enduring neurotic or conduct problems, the cures for which are not dependent on increasing maturity, at least during the years covered by these statistics.

We turn now to specific disorders of childhood and adolescence. There are too many to cover adequately in the space available, so we consider only a few of them in depth here. The disorders we describe cover the range from severe behavioral debility such as mental retardation to those that usually produce relatively short-lived debilities such as school phobia.

TABLE 21.1 DIMENSIONS OF CHILDHOOD PROBLEMS AND THEIR FREQUENTLY ASSOCIATED CHARACTERISTICS

Conduct Disorder	Stomachaches
Fighting, hitting	Muscle aches and pains
Disobedient, defiant	Elimination problems
Temper tantrums	Socialized Aggression
Destructiveness	Has "bad" companions
Impertinent, impudent	Truant from home
Uncooperative, resistant	Truant from school
Attention Problems	Steals in company with others
Poor concentration, short attention span	Loyal to delinquent friends
Daydreams	Belongs to a gang
Clumsy, poor coordination	Anxious-Depressed Withdrawal
Preoccupied, stares into space	Anxious, fearful, tense
Fails to finish, lacks perseverance	Shy, timid, bashful
Impulsive	Withdrawn, seclusive
Motor Overactivity	Depressed, sad, disturbed
Restless, overactive	Hypersensitive, easily hurt
Excitable, impulsive	Feels inferior, worthless
Squirmy, jittery	Schizoid Unresponsive
Overtalkative	Won't talk
Hams and makes other odd noises	Withdrawn
Social Ineptness	Sad
Poor peer relations	Stares blankly
Likes to be alone	Confused
Is teased, picked on	Psychotic Disorder
Prefers younger children	Visual hallucinations
Shy, timid, lacks self-confidence	Auditory hallucinations
Stays with adults, ignored by peers	Bizarre, odd, peculiar
Somatic Complaints	Strange ideas and behavior
Headache	Incoherent speech
Vomiting, nausea	Repetitive speech

Source: From Quay (1986b).

AUTISTIC DISORDER

Seldom has a rare disorder sparked as much interest as autistic disorder. Kanner (1943) described eleven children "whose condition differs so markedly and uniquely from anything reported so far, that each case merits . . . a detailed consideration of its fascinating peculiarities." Kanner's (1943/1973) first case displayed the following patterns of behavior.

> He wandered about smiling, making stereotyped movements with his fingers, crossing them about in the air. He shook his head from side to side, whispering or humming the same three-note tune. He spun with great pleasure anything he could seize upon to spin. . . Most of his actions were repetitions carried out exactly the same way in which they had been performed originally. If he spun a block, he must always start with the same face uppermost . . . repeating something that had obviously been said to him often, he said to his mother, "Eat it or I won't give you tomatoes." . . . He paid no attention to persons around him. When taken into a room,

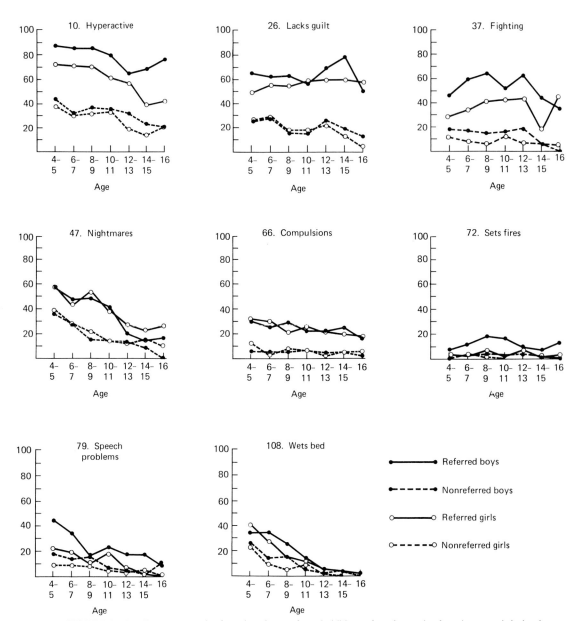

FIGURE 21.2 Percentage of referred and nonreferred children of each gender for whom each behavior problem was reported. (From T. M. Achenbach & C. S. Edelbrock, *Monographs of the Society for Research in Child Development,* 1981, *46,* No. 188)

he completely disregarded the people and instantly went for objects, preferably those that could be spun (1943/1973, pp. 4–5).

This child could accurately sing tunes at age 1. A year or so later he was reciting short poems; he had learned the Twenty-third Psalm and could repeat the twenty-five questions and answers of the Presbyterian catechism.

Most autistic children have peculiar mannerisms including toe walking, hand flapping, whirling, and repetitive rocking. They may be overresponsive or underresponsive to sounds, and are often thought to be deaf. Among the more socially disruptive excesses of autistic children are tantrums and self-injurious behavior. About 70 percent of autistic children are mentally retarded. Studies of these children require the use of mentally retarded controls so that one can be sure that the presumed signs of autism are truly distinct and not simply a consequence of mental retardation. This has not always been done and there is currently some debate about whether the diagnostic signs of autism are really as rare as previously believed in mentally retarded children.

Description

Autistic Triad   Autistic children, all of whom display signs of pathology in infancy, have the autistic triad of symptoms: (1) autistic aloneness, (2) speech and language disturbances, and (3) an obsessive desire for sameness. *Autistic aloneness* is manifested in a lack of social attachment or bonding. Autistic toddlers neither follow their parents about the house nor acknowledge their entrances and exits (Rutter, 1982). They neither make postural adjustments in anticipation of being picked up nor seek bodily contact for pleasure or reassurance. *Autistic speech* is often devoid of conventional meaning or the rhythm and inflection of normal speech. Autistics often parrot back what they have heard, a phenomenon called echolalia. Their memory for detail may be prodigious, but they seem to lack a capacity for abstraction, instead focusing almost totally on the physical qualities of objects. For example, the word "chair" may refer to a specific chair only. Pronoun reversals, in which they refer to themselves as "you" rather than "I," are quite common. Finally, the *obsessive desire for sameness* is the insistent demand that situations be repeated exactly as they had previously occurred. Even a slight rearrangement of furniture or toys, for example, can occasion inconsolable tantrums alleviated only by precisely reproducing the original arrangement.

Autistic disorder has attracted widespread attention for two reasons: (1) the first cases all came from highly intelligent parents, providing a rare but socially provocative example of deficiencies associated with the upper classes, and (2) many of the children had "islands of excellence"; that is, extraordinary abilities in the context of these severe disabilities.

Course   About two-thirds of autistic children are unable to function independently in adulthood. The majority reside in institutions unless the family can care for them. Only about 10 percent eventually achieve a rudimentary social life and occupation. The two most powerful predictors of adult adjustment are IQ and language skills. IQs below 60 or impaired language after age 5 is almost always associated with a dire prognosis (Rutter & Garmezy, 1983).

Diagnostic Criteria   Modern criteria generally conform to Kanner's original description, but without requiring that the children have islands of excellence. The *DSM-III-R* emphasizes three major classes of criteria: (1) qualitative impairment in reciprocal social interaction (for example, marked lack of awareness of the existence or feelings of others); (2) impaired verbal and nonverbal communication (for example, no history of babbling, peculiar facial expressions and gestures); and (3) a markedly restricted repertoire of activities and interests (for example, stereotyped movements or persistent preoccupations with parts of objects and virtually no interest in people).

Pathology and Etiology

For many years it was erroneously believed that faulty maternal child-rearing styles were responsible for infantile autism. Mothers of such children were called "emotional refrigerators" and blamed for their child's defects. In 1964 Bernard Rimland published an award-winning book that persuasively challenged the evidence for any shred of psychosocial causation in autistic disorder. Rimland (1964) argued that infantile autism arose from neuropathology which adversely affected cognitive functioning.

Cognitive Factors   About 70 percent of autistics score in the mentally retarded range (IQ less than 70), though their pattern of intellectual performance is usually quite uneven. They are more likely to score low on verbal than on nonverbal visual-spatial measures, but this is not universally observed. As a general rule autistic children are much better at spatial than verbal tasks (O'Connor & Hermelin, 1978). Their capacity for near-normal performance on spatial tasks is illustrated in a study that presented autistic, mentally retarded, and chronologically younger normal children an embedded figure task in which a target was to be located in a complex figure (Figure 21.3). The autistic, retarded, and normal children achieved 82, 55, and 63 percent correct, respectively. Clearly the autistic children were superior to both groups of controls (Shah and Frith, 1983).

FIGURE 21.3   Examples of complex figure in which the child is to find the target design.

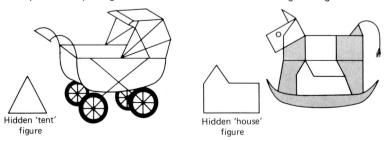

Hidden 'tent' figure

Hidden 'house' figure

A remarkable example of a visual-spatial island of excellence, shown in Figure 21.4, comes from a 5-year-old autistic child named Nadia (Selfe, 1977). Nadia could not speak in sentences, was echolalic, and was poorly coordinated. Yet Nadia's drawings, numbering in the thousands, were far beyond the talents of normal children her age and exceeded the capabilities of most adults.

FIGURE 21.4 This drawing was made by Nadia when she was about 5 years and 6 months old. (From L. C. Selfe (1977). *A case of extraordinary drawing ability in an autistic child.* Academic Press.)

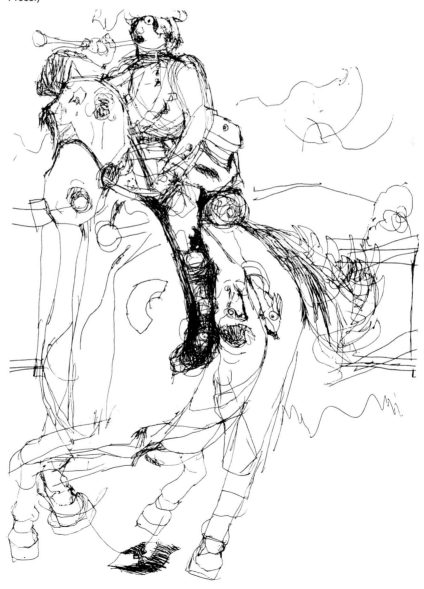

Only about 10 percent of autistic children display such islands of excellence (Rimland, 1978). Unfortunately, we do not know much about these 10 percent, except that they often have highly intelligent or talented parents. Perhaps these autistic children inherited innately superior neural tissue, some of which remains undamaged and free from interference. All we know for certain is that superior talent can co-exist with serious debilitation in some of these children.

Biological Factors In comparison to controls, autistic children are more than twice as likely to have been exposed to pregnancy and birth complications (Gillberg & Gillberg, 1983). Higher maternal age, bleeding during pregnancy, and prematurity are especially frequent. Moreover, congenital rubella (German measles) during fetal life is associated with a hundredfold increase in risk for autism. An elevated rate of minor physical anomalies in autistic children also suggests that something has gone awry prenatally (Coleman, 1978).

Neurological abnormalities are found in many autistic children (see Gillberg & Svedsen, 1983). For example, a substantial minority of autistic children develop epilepsy during adolescence—as many as 35 percent (Gillberg & Wahlstrom, 1985). An abnormality of the left hemisphere has been inferred from the autistic language peculiarities, but brain abnormalities, if detected, are not always left-sided. Many autistic children display no signs of cerebral damage (Williams et al., 1980), but recent reports suggest damage to specific parts of the cerebellum (Bauman & Kemper, 1985; Courchesne, Yeung-Courchesne, Press, Hesselink, & Jernigan, 1988). The Courchesne et al. report, using magnetic resonance imaging, found that between ten and fourteen (depending on stringency of the criterion) of eighteen autistic people had abnormally small lobules VI and VII of the posterior cerebellum, while the other six lobules of the cerebellum were of normal size. Lobules VI and VII are the latest to develop in embryogenesis (Altman, 1987), so that the results point to a developmental anomaly occurring late in pregnancy. By virtue of their extensive interconnections with other brain areas, these lobule abnormalities may interfere with many aspects of sensory information processing, learning, memory, and emotional regulation that take place primarily in other areas of the brain.

Etiological theories about the biological origins of autism have generally suggested a cortical or brain stem defect (although we have just seen that the primary defect could arise in another area that connects to the cortex or brain stem). Although older autistic children display conspicuous cognitive and language abnormalities, suggesting a cortical abnormality, younger autistic children often have reflex abnormalities suggesting damage to lower brain centers (Ornitz, 1985). For example, after being spun in a centifugelike device, autistics do not show the normal amount of postrotational nystagmus, an involuntary jerking of the eyeballs. This reflex deficit is believed to reflect an abnormality in the brain stem. Not all autistics show this abnormality, however, implying multiple etiologies for autism.

Others theories of autism have focused on neurotransmitter abnormalities. Nearly a dozen neurochemical studies of autistic children have revealed elevations and greater variability in blood serotonin levels than in controls (Anderson & Hoshino, 1987). Serotonin is an important neurotransmitter involved in sleep, mood, temperature regulation, appetite, and hormone release, but it is difficult to see how dysfunctions in any of these areas would lead to autistic behavior. The fact that serotonin studies of autistic children reveal much more variability from one autistic child to the next suggests that only some autistic children have excessive amounts of serotonin. Perhaps a neurochemical defect is central to the disorder in some autistic children, while in others the basic defect is neuroanatomical.

Autism occurs at a rate of 2 to 4 per 10,000 births, with males being affected about three times more often than females. About 25 percent of autistic children have a sex chromosome defect called the fragile X, associated with mental retardation (Gillberg & Wahlstrom, 1985) and described later in the chapter. About 2 percent of the siblings of autistics are also affected (Rutter & Garmezy, 1983). This rate, at least fifty times that of the general population, implies a genetic factor. Folstein and Rutter (1977) suggested a genetic factor in a study of twenty-one sets of twins, each with an autistic member. Using broad criteria for concordance, ten of the eleven identical, but only one of the ten fraternal, co-twins either were autistic or had other cognitive defects.

These results seem to be confirmed by Ritvo et al. (1985) in a larger study of forty twin pairs containing at least one autistic member. They found a 96 percent concordance rate for autism among the MZ pairs and a 23 percent rate among the DZ pairs. Although their twin results are consistent with a genetic hypothesis for autism, fewer than 2 percent of the singleton siblings of the twins in this study were also autistic. Although a 1.7 percent rate for the singleton siblings is still very high, it differs significantly from the 23 percent rate for the DZ twins, despite equal degrees of genetic overlap. This result clearly implicates shared prenatal factors in addition to possible genetic causes.

In sum, the evidence suggests multiple origins for infantile autism, including chromosome defects, neuroanatomical deviations probably associated with birth complications, MPAs, and nonspecific neurological signs. The implication is that the autistic syndrome reflects the final common path for a variety of insults.

Treatment

Many believe that no treatment can make an autistic child normal. However, behaviorally oriented therapy can partly ameliorate excesses such as tantrums, self-injury, and deficits such as deviant speech and lack of cooperation. Punishment has been found especially effective for self-injurious behavior such as head banging. Although this treatment may seem inhumane, less efficient treatments may ultimately result in more damage to the child.

A study by Lovaas (1987) challenges the extreme pessimism about the prospects for normal recovery. After a monumental treatment program for nineteen autistic preschoolers between the ages of 2 and 4, nine were regarded as normal by their second-grade public school teachers and indistinguishable from other children in the classroom, while only two were still regarded as autistic and retarded. The remaining eight were in special education classes. These results can be compared with those obtained for two control groups, in which only one of forty autistic children was regarded as fully recovered and twenty-one were still diagnosed as autistic and retarded.

The behavioral treatment program was of an intensity seldom achieved before, requiring an army of dedicated student therapists, using behavioral methods for a minimum of forty hours per week for two years. The comparison groups received either ten hours per week of this treatment or no systematic behavioral treatment, with no differences between the two comparison groups. While the time and money invested in this project make it inaccessible to most families with autistic children, Lovaas points out that a full-time special education teacher would cost $40,000 for a two-year period as against $2 million for lifelong maintenance in an institution.

There no doubt will be many criticisms of this study—for example, the reliance on schoolteachers' judgments of normality when more sensitive diagnostic techniques are available. These results will be scrutinized carefully because they run counter to the prevailing pessimism about cure. Lovaas has attempted to anticipate the critics by careful diagnosis of the autistic cases and by documenting the gains that the children have made, but confirmatory follow-ups with unbiased and more sophisticated diagnostic techniques will be necessary before most authorities are convinced.

ATTENTION-DEFICIT HYPERACTIVITY DISORDER

The most frequent symptom patterns of childhood maladjustment generally fall into one of two broad classes: overcontrolled or undercontrolled (Achenbach, 1982). Overcontrolled children are shy, inhibited, fearful, or anxious. They often have disturbances in which anxiety is the most prominent feature. Undercontrolled children tend to be hyperactive or have conduct disorder, the childhood version of antisocial personality disorder. We focus here on attention-deficit hyperactivity disorder (ADHD) as an example of undercontrolled behavior because conduct disorder is discussed in Chapter 18. Later in the chapter school phobia will be discussed as an example of overcontrolled behavior. Among the nonpsychotic disorders of childhood, ADHD is one of the most enduring and disruptive, affecting not only the individual, but family and society as well.

Description

Attention-deficit hyperactivity disorder has been called many things: hyperactive child syndrome, hyperkinesis, minimal brain damage, minimal cerebral dysfunction, and minimal brain dysfunction. Research published before 1980 usually refers to hyperactivity instead of ADHD. The *DSM-III* distinguished between attention deficit disorder with and without hyperactivity. That distinction has been abolished in the *DSM-III-R*, which calls it Attention-Deficit Hyperactivity Disorder (ADHD) because almost all of these children are hyperactive.

Hyperactive Features Children with ADHD always have their motor running. They get into trouble because of boundless energy, impulsivity, and an inability to stick to a task. Although they are not easy to distinguish from other active children on the playground, when quiet recreation, rest, or sustained attention is required, their hyperactivity stands out. Relations with playmates are compromised because of fighting and inability to cooperate. The house also needs to be "child-proofed" to protect valuables and reduce the risk of harm. Accidents are quite common—for example, poisoning from ingesting dangerous liquids. The slightest lapse in parental vigilance can result in untoward consequences. Not surprisingly, parents are often exhausted and on a short fuse trying to keep the child occupied and safe.

Parents often recall difficulties even in infancy because of colic, irritability, and irregular sleep habits. Activity monitors attached to sleeping hyperactive children reveal that they are more restless than normal children even when asleep (Porrino et al., 1983). This is an important observation because hyperactivity during sleep implies that the conspicuous attentional difficulties are secondary to a more basic physiological disturbance involving inhibitory dysfunction.

ADHD children also show metabolic hypoactivity in frontal lobe white matter when measured by regional cerebral blood flow techniques (Lou, Henriksen, & Bruhn, 1984), suggesting an anatomical locus for the inhibitory dysfunction. We noted in Chapter 18 that ADHD children often become juvenile delinquents or antisocial adults, and observed that many adult antisocials show signs of frontal-lobe dysfunction. It would be interesting to divide adults with antisocial personality disorder into those with or without a history of ADHD to see whether they differ on tests of frontal lobe function. Perhaps disputes about the presence or absence of frontal abnormalities in antisocials arise because of differing proportions of subjects with a history of ADHD in each study.

During the school years hyperactive behavior patterns become more ominous because of increased social demands for conformity. These children cannot sit still, quarrel with teachers and peers, and often progress slowly in school. They get bored easily and teachers must sustain a fast pace in order to maintain the child's interest.

Diagnosis Diagnostic criteria emphasize attentional deficits, restlessness, fidgeting, overtalkativeness, and impulsivity as essential features of ADHD. Hyperactivity generally declines with age, as does overactivity in normal children, but signs of attentional and inhibitory difficulties often continue into adolescence and beyond. The ADHD diagnosis is at least six times more frequent in boys than in girls and is believed to affect about 3 percent of American children.

Perhaps three-quarters of the children diagnosed with ADHD are also diagnosed with conduct disorder (Quay, 1986b). Follow-ups of hyperactive youngsters even without an initial diagnosis of conduct disorder indicate that nearly half of them will be diagnosed as having a conduct disorder as teenagers (Gittelman et al., 1985). Although the two disorders are difficult to distinguish from each other, "pure" cases of each can be found.

Deficits   The diagnosis of ADHD assumes a basic impairment in attentional processes, but it is difficult to be more specific (Douglas, 1983). If stimuli are intrinsically interesting, varied, and novel, many ADHDs can attend about as well as normal controls, at least for awhile. But they quickly become fatigued, bored, or distracted. Unfortunately, schoolwork is often less than exciting and ADHD children seem particularly inept when they must generate the proper interest.

Biological Aspects and Etiology

Many ADHD children are clumsy (Nichols & Chen, 1981), suggesting nonspecific neurological involvement, and many have an excess of MPAs (Deutsch, 1983; Firestone & Prabhu, 1983; Gualtieri et al., 1982). Table 21.2 shows excess anomalies in autistic and hyperactive children in comparison to normal children. While both autism and hyperactivity are associated with MPA aberrations occurring during fetal life, no MPAs are specific to one or the other disorder. It is possible to reproduce some of the behavioral features of ADHD in rats by preventing the proper embryological development of small neurons in the hippocampus and the cerebellum, leading to the suggestion that this disorder may arise from prenatal abnormalities (Altman, 1987).

A genetic etiology is also suggested because hyperactivity runs in families (Willerman, 1973; Deutsch, 1983). Deutsch, for example, compared the incidence of hyperactivity in biologically and adoptively related siblings of hyperactive children. In contrast to only 0 to 4 percent of the adoptively related siblings, 26 percent of the biologically related siblings were also hyperactive.

TABLE 21.2   MINOR PHYSICAL ANOMALIES IN HYPERACTIVE, AUTISTIC, AND NORMAL CHILDREN

Diagnostic group	Mean score	Five or more anomalies, %
Normal children (N = 76)	2.0	3
Hyperactive children (N = 50)	2.8	18
Autistic children (N = 39)	3.7	23

Source: From Gualtieri et al. (1982). *American Journal of Psychiatry, 139,* 427–441. Copyright © 1982, The American Psychiatric Association. Reprinted by permission.

There are surely multiple etiologies for hyperactivity and there is little reason to expect that a single form of treatment will always be satisfactory. For example, Deutsch (1983) found that hyperactive children who improved when given stimulant medication were less likely to have MPAs than those who showed no improvement with stimulants. The implication is that stimulant responders and nonresponders differ in the etiology of their hyperactivity. Perhaps nonresponders have a structural neurological problem that cannot be improved by drugs that alter only neurotransmission.

Treatment

Parents and teachers find hyperactive children to be extremely disruptive. The children are noncompliant and are the target of much criticism from virtually everyone around them. Many of the children are chronically unhappy and want to improve their behavior, but seem unable to control themselves. Thus, affected children and their parents have eagerly sought an effective treatment.

Pharmacological Treatment Up to 75 percent of hyperactive children benefit from stimulants such as dextroamphetamine or methylphenidate (Ritalin). These drugs increase the availability of dopamine and norepinephrine by blocking their reuptake into the presynaptic neuron (Solanto, 1984) and improve concentration as well as reduce purposeless activity and impulsivity (Weiss, 1983). Moreover, stimulants enhance performance on measures of vigilance as indexed by faster reaction times and fewer errors of "commission" (Rapoport, 1983). Commission errors are responses that should have been inhibited, and are regarded as a measure of impulsivity.

Stimulants have positive behavioral effects on many laboratory cognitive and behavioral tests, but they do not facilitate performance on IQ and achievement tests (Gittelman, 1983) or make for a more positive adult prognosis (Weiss, 1983). For example, follow-ups of treated children indicate that while overt hyperactivity generally declines with age, one still observes restlessness, nervousness, unstable job histories, and an excessive number of automobile accidents (Borland & Heckman, 1976; Weiss, 1983). About 46 percent of hyperactive children given only stimulants for treatment are arrested for two or more felonies by the time they are 18 years old (Satterfield, Satterfield, & Schell, 1987) It has been argued that continued administration of stimulants would have prevented some of the undesirable outcomes in adulthood (Wender et al., 1981), but these stimulants may lose their effectiveness when the children reach maturity (Taylor, 1986).

Since 25 percent or more of hyperactive children do not benefit from stimulants, a dopamine- or norepinephrine-related abnormality seems an unlikely explanation for all hyperactivity. It seems probable that some hyperactive children have anatomical brain defects that are unresponsive to stimulant medication or have anxiety problems that produce inattention and hyperactivity for reasons that have little to do with brain malfunction. It is for these latter children that a behavioral approach to treatment would seem especially appropriate.

Behavioral Treatment   Behavioral treatments, alone or in conjunction with stimulants, are warranted because even favorable stimulant responders often fail to benefit scholastically or interpersonally. Behavioral approaches have used a variety of techniques, including self-control procedures which teach the child to think before acting; for example, many hyperactive children are taught to say to themselves, "I must stop and look." These procedures work quite well in the laboratory, but do not seem to generalize beyond the specific testing situation (Devany & Nelson, 1986). However, a treatment combining stimulants and behavioral interventions tailored to each child's specific problems—for example, aggression or scholastic inadequacies—has shown long-term positive effects (Satterfield, Satterfield, & Schell, 1987).

Some experts believe that stimulants can improve schoolwork even in the absence of specific scholastic remediation provided the dosage is properly adjusted. Unfortunately, the stimulant dose that makes the child quieter and more compliant exceeds the dose for improving scholastic performance. It has been suggested that lowering the typical dose would produce greater scholastic gains but at the cost of making the child less tractable in the classroom (Pelham et al., 1985).

SCHOOL PHOBIA

Many forms of psychopathology involve irrational anxiety that dominates thinking to the point of severe inhibition or even outright panic. The central features of all the childhood anxiety disorders are feelings of insecurity, especially fears of separation from the mother. Whenever required to venture out, the children show extreme shyness, worry, tantrums, or panic. In *avoidant disorder,* the most conspicuous feature is a fear of strangers. In *overanxious disorder,* the child has pervasive anxiety, including unrealistic worries about future events, doubts of self-competence, and excessive needs for reassurance. In *separation anxiety disorder,* conspicuously intense fears appear when the mother is absent. If the separation anxiety involves refusal to attend school, it is called school phobia, but children can be diagnosed with a separation anxiety disorder even in the absence of any specific fears about attending school.

Descriptive Aspects

Strictly speaking, school phobia is not a phobia at all. The child is not afraid of school, but of maternal abandonment. It is associated with a history of overdependence and lack of individuation from a generally close-knit family. Parents have overprotected the child, perhaps because of their own insecurities or perception of the child's fragility as indicated by a history of extreme timidity, psychosomatic complaints, and unwillingness to go to sleep alone.

Generally, two types of school phobia are observed (see Table 21.3). The early-onset cases tend to occur abruptly in younger children and to begin on Mondays. The later-onset cases tend to occur in older children, have a more chronic course, and are associated with more familial and personal psychopathology. Many late-onset cases have neurotic and phobic symptoms when followed into young adulthood (Berg, 1984). Before making a school refusal diagnosis, however, it is first necessary to ensure that the child is not actually reluctant to tell you about a strict teacher or a threatening classmate.

Treatment

Many early-onset school phobias are readily treated. Kennedy (1965) outlines the following steps for rapid treatment:

1 Instruct parents to be optimistic and unswerving in their adherence to the regime.
2 Ignore somatic complaints (for example, nausea).
3 Force the child to attend school no matter how vehement the protestations.
4 Present the parents with the formula for effective treatment.

The formula is as follows: Do not discuss school attendance over the weekend. Give the child only a light breakfast to diminish problems of nausea and hand

---

TABLE 21.3 TWO TYPES OF SCHOOL PHOBIA

Early onset	**Late onset**
1. Present illness is the first episode	1. Second, third, or fourth episode
2. Monday onset, following illness the previous Thursday or Friday	2. Monday onset not especially common
3. Acute onset	3. Incipient onset
4. Lower grades most prevalent	4. Upper grades most prevalent
5. Expressed concern about death	5. Death theme not present
6. Mother's physical health in question: actually ill or child thinks so	6. Health of mother not an issue
7. Good communication between parents	7. Poor parental communication
8. Mother and father well adjusted	8. Mother shows neurotic behavior; father, a character disorder
9. Father competitive with mother in household management	9. Father shows little interest in household or children
10. Parents achieve understanding of dynamics easily	10. Parents difficult to work with

Source: From W. A. Kennedy, (1965). School phobia: Rapid treatment of fifty cases. *Journal of Abnormal Psychology, 70,* 285–289. Copyright © 1965 by the American Psychological Association. Reprinted by permission.

the child over to the school authorities. Compliment the child on whatever successes were achieved that day and follow the same routine on successive days. Kennedy's data suggest that uncomplicated school refusal will stop in a few days. However, this conclusion is probably too optimistic, since the children in his study had been referred for treatment soon after phobia onset. Less positive results are to be expected in a group containing more chronic cases and those whose onset is at an older age.

ENURESIS

Delayed control of bladder and bowel function can be a source of frustration, inconvenience, and shame to both the affected child and the parents. Enuretic children often refuse to go to school, and bitter relations can arise as the family tries to cope with the problem. Enuresis is included here because it illustrates how a disorder with a substantial genetic-physiological component can be ameliorated through behavioral therapy.

Enuresis is usually defined as urinary incontinence twice monthly in 5- to 6-year-olds and at least once monthly in older children. Boys are more frequently affected than girls, as are more children from lower than higher social class (Gross & Dornbusch, 1983).

There are striking physiological, intellectual, and behavioral correlates of enuresis. Enuretics have younger than normal bone ages, suggesting delayed maturation; and during the early teenage years they are slower to enter puberty. Moreover, a significant fraction have smaller bladder capacities. Enuretics also have slightly lower IQ and achievement test scores than nonenuretic controls. They are described by their parents as being high-strung and intemperate.

Etiology

Much about the etiology of enuresis is unknown, but it clearly has a genetic component. More identical than fraternal twins are concordant for enuresis, and in comparison to control parents, a formerly enuretic parent has three times the risk of having an enuretic child. If both parents were enuretic, the risk increases fivefold over control values (Bakwin, 1971).

While many have blamed faulty parental child-rearing practices, it appears that enuresis runs in families even when parents play a smaller than usual role in child rearing. Among 4-year-old children reared in Israeli communal settings (kibbutzim), where children are cared for by professional caretakers and sleep in houses away from their parents, 67 percent of the enuretics had an older sibling who was also enuretic. In contrast, only 22 percent of the dry children had an enuretic older sibling (Kaffman & Elizur, 1977).

These authors also found that hyperactivity and aggression were very frequent in the enuretics. These excesses may help to explain an oft-reported observation that children who set fires have a history of enuresis (Yarnell, 1940). The association between enuresis and setting fires has prompted psychoanalytic speculation that sexual feelings are involved in causing a fire and then drowning it out. Recent studies of those who set fires show that they are likely to have disorders of undercontrol, especially ADHD and conduct disorder. It seems more plausible that the connection between setting fires and enuresis arises via these disorders of undercontrol than as a consequence of perverted sexual desires (Kolko, Kazdin, & Meyer, 1985; Kuhnley, Hendren, & Quinlan, 1982).

Treatment

There are two major approaches to treating enuresis. The behavioral approach employs an alarm device that, triggered by urine, immediately awakens the sleeping child. A buzzer powered by a hearing aid battery is attached to the shoulder of the pajama top and is connected to a sensor in a small plastic card sewn into ordinary underpants. A version of such a device is shown in Figure 21.5. From 60 percent to 90 percent of children benefit from the alarm, although relapses requiring a repeat treatment are often necessary (Dische et al., 1983; Gross & Dornbusch, 1983).

The only drugs of proven effectiveness against enuresis are tricyclic antidepressants such as imipramine. Other types of antidepressants, amphetamines, tranquilizers, and anticonvulsant drugs are not useful (Gross & Dornbusch, 1983). Because the side effects of tricyclics include dry mouth, drowsiness, weight gain, dizziness, sleep disturbances, and nightmares, it seems more judicious to try a behavioral method first.

EATING DISORDERS

When food is in scarce supply, plumpness confers social status. When food is in abundance, slimness is prized. Females bear the brunt of these changing

FIGURE 21.5 Wet-stop enuresis alarm.

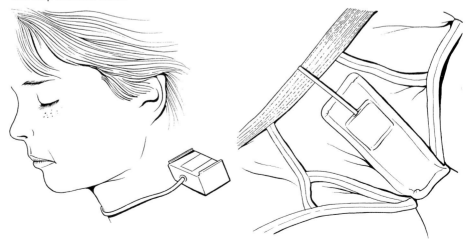

norms. Nowadays, to achieve "ideal" weight and increase their attractiveness, women are much more likely than men to diet, to belong to weight-reducing clubs, and to use amphetamines as appetite suppressants.

Anorexia Nervosa

Trendsetters in Western society place a premium on being thin. At the same time, there is an abundance of good-tasting but fattening food. Many people have great difficulty resisting these caloric temptations and as a consequence use "unnatural" means of controlling weight gain. For example, nearly 7 percent of females attending a family planning clinic in England reported self-induced vomiting in order to control their weight (Cooper & Fairburn, 1983).

In modern society, one disorder stands out because of apparent voluntary starvation in the midst of plenty. Called *anorexia nervosa*—literally, a loss of appetite caused by nervousness—it is characterized by a preoccupying pursuit of slimness accompanying a bizarre and often delusional conviction of being overweight. The consequence is marked weight loss endangering survival, usually with a failure to acknowledge even severe undernourishment (see Figure 21.6). Frequency of the disorder is around 0.5 to 1 percent among young white females ranging in age from 12 to 25. About 95 percent of those affected are female and most are of middle-class background.

Description Typically a perfectionistic middle-class girl voluntarily decides to diet. Becoming extremely pleased by her rapid successes and the admiration received, she presses forward. Relatives become alarmed, pleading with her to desist, but the dieting passion is too intense. She may discover that self-induced vomiting, laxatives, and frenetic exercise permit her to eat yet continue to lose weight. As starvation continues, urine output increases, menses disappear, heart rate and basal metabolism decrease, the latter causing her to feel chilly, and a fine hair (lanugo) begins to cover the body as a physiological adaptation to being cold. Medical complications are often quite serious. The self-induced vomiting erodes tooth enamel, and the catastrophic metabolic aberrations brought on by the starvation causes death in up to 18 percent of cases in long-term follow-ups. Suicide attempts are also elevated for anorectic patients. Here is a description of an anorexic girl.

> . . . awe-inspiring to the onlooker, is the iron determination with which anorexics pursue their goal of ultimate thinness, not only through food restriction but also through exhausting exercise. . . . In spite of the weakness associated with such a severe weight loss, they will drive themselves to unbelievable feats to demonstrate that they live by the ideal of "mind over body." Cora took up swimming, increasing the number of laps from day to day finally spending five to six hours at it. In addition she would play tennis for several hours, run instead of walking whenever possible, and became an expert at fencing. She also worked many hours on her school assignments to achieve the highest grades. She kept busy twenty-one hours, reducing her sleeping time to three hours (Bruch, 1978, p. 5).

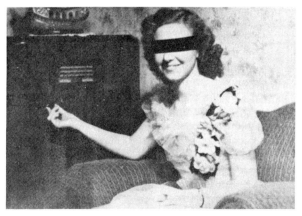

(a)

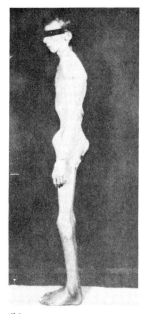

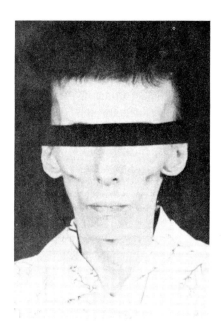

(b)

FIGURE 21.6 At 18 years of age this woman weighed 120 pounds, but became anorexic following her marriage that year. At age 37 she weighed only 47 pounds. In the University of Virginia Hospital she was placed in a controlled setting in which she was allowed mail, television, shampoos, and social contacts only if she ate. After about three months she had gained 17 pounds and was released, only to relapse (Bachrach, Erwin, & Mohr, 1965).

Preanorectics are described as introverted, conscientious, and well-behaved. Curiously, many preanorectics apparently cease menstruating before dieting, suggesting a type of hypothalamic-pituitary dysregulation that is often associated with depression (Bemis, 1978). Following the starvation, certain additional hypothalamic-pituitary defects occur. For example, a normal response to sex hormones is lost, reappearing only after a return to normal weight (Palmer, 1980), but regular menstruation often requires another two years (Richardson & Tolis, 1984).

The diagnosis of anorexia nervosa according to the *DSM-III-R* requires:

1 An intense fear of obesity, even if underweight
2 Flagrant distortion of body image such that the slightest signs of fat are exaggerated out of all proportion
3 Marked weight loss of at least 15 percent of normal body weight or a refusal to make expected weight gain during growth, leading to a weight 15 percent below that expected
4 In females, absence of at least three consecutive menstrual cycles

Nearly half of those with anorexia nervosa also binge by consuming enormous quantities of highly caloric junk food (Garfinkel, Moldofsky, & Garner, 1980). The bingeing, usually followed by remorse, vomiting, and laxative abuse, may increase weight by as much as nine pounds in a single episode. Bingeing can exist alone as well, in which case the diagnosis is *bulimia nervosa,* a disorder to be considered momentarily.

Etiology Two facts stand out as distinctive in anorexia: (1) the elevated frequency in middle-class females and (2) the excess of affective disorder, not only in the patients themselves, but also in their first-degree relatives (Cantwell et al., 1977; Hudson et al., 1983). Indeed, the frequency of affective disorder in the relatives of anorectics differs little from the frequency in relatives of patients with bipolar affective disorder. Both of these groups have significantly more affective disorder in their family background than do schizophrenics or borderline personalities (Hudson et al., 1983; Rivinus et al., 1984). Moreover, a genetic component in anorexia is implicated by a 55 percent MZ and a 7 percent DZ concordance rate (Holland et al., 1984).

Preoccupation with slimness is quite frequent among higher social class females; thus they would be more likely to diet and to be emotionally invested in the outcome. Yet, inexplicably, only a small fraction of those who diet become anorectic. It appears that females with eating disorders, even more than other females, have accepted the cultural stereotype of thinness as an ideal (Striegel-Moore, Silberstein, & Rodin, 1986), but it is not known whether the enthusiastic acceptance of the ideal precedes or follows the onset of the disorder.

Clinical reports imply a pathological transformation after the initiation of dieting, suggesting that dieting alone can unintentionally precipitate the disorder (Bruch, 1978). In other words, a seemingly unexceptional attempt to diet undergoes a pathological metamorphosis into a compulsive dedication to thinness and delusional distortions of body image; incredibly, a patient may actually perceive her emaciated mirror image as fat. This morbid transformation is difficult to explain. Perhaps by insisting that she is too fat, the anorexic is defensively rationalizing an irresistible urge to diet whose origins she actually does not know.

Treatment At the point that weight loss endangers life, there is little alternative to hospitalization. Under strict regimes where the patient is closely watched to prevent vomiting or purging, weight gain may occur without forcefeeding. More problematic is getting the patient to eat after leaving the hospital. Behavioral and psychodynamic treatment approaches are of questionable value (Bruch, 1978), but family therapy has achieved some modest success with younger, though not older, anorectic patients (Russell et al., 1987).

Antidepressant drugs for anorexia are at best only moderately successful (Pope & Hudson, 1984). Their relative ineffectiveness contrasts to the efficacy of antidepressants for bulimia. This finding puts into jeopardy the view that anorexia nervosa and bulimia nervosa are alternative expressions of the same underlying condition.

Bulimia Nervosa

The distinctive feature of bulimia is binge eating of enormous quantities of high caloric food. Bingeing typically produces stupor or sleep, but may be followed by vomiting or purging as well as remorse and guilt. Because they vomit or purge, many binge eaters never become overweight. Here is the story of one severely bulimic college female.

> I would go out, almost driven like a machine, to the supermarket . . . and buy a gallon, or maybe even two gallons of maple-walnut ice cream and a couple of packages of fudge brownie mix—enough to make seventy two brownies. . . . I would always be convinced that I was just getting the mix to make brownies for my roommates, and I always swore to myself that I would eat only one or two brownies myself. . . . I'd hurry up the apartment stairs with the urge for more bingeing growing stronger by the minute. Still, I'd keep myself under the illusion that I was making brownies for my roommates. I'd hastily mix up the brownie mix and get the brownies in the oven, usually managing to eat a fair amount of the mix myself as I was going along. Then, while they were cooking, I'd hit the ice cream. Only by constantly eating ice cream could I bear the delay until the brownies came out of the oven. Sometimes I'd finish the whole gallon even before the brownies were done, and I'd take the brownies out of the oven while they were still baking. At any rate I'd start eating brownies, even though by this time I was feeling sick, intending to stop after two or three. Then it would be five or six. Pretty soon, I'd have put away fifteen or twenty of the brownies, and then I'd be overcome with embarrassment. . . . Seventy-two brownies later, the depression would begin to hit. I'd go to the bathroom, stick my finger down my throat, and make myself throw up. I was so good at it that it was almost automatic— no effort necessary, just instant vomiting, over and over until there was nothing coming out of my stomach except clear pale-green fluid. . . . I'd be sitting alone in the

apartment. . . . No one to talk to, no one to turn to. I'd sit there and think. You idiot, you disgusting idiot, why did you do that? And I'd swear I'd not do it again. But I knew in my heart that the cycle would repeat itself the next day, and the next, and the next (Pope & Hudson, 1984, pp. 12–13).

DSM-III-R criteria for bulimia nervosa include recurrent binges, a feeling of lack of control over eating during binges, the regular use of self-induced vomiting, laxatives, strict dieting, or vigorous exercise in order to prevent weight gain, a minimum of two binges a week for at least three months, and a persistent concern with body shape and weight. The frequency of bulimia is about 4.5 percent in American female college freshman and 0.5 percent in freshmen males using criteria similar to these.

Bulimics, like anorectics, seem to show a familial excess of affective disorder (Lee, Rush, & Mitchell, 1985). Unlike anorectics, however, many bulimics respond favorably to antidepressant medication (Pope & Hudson, 1984). No one knows why anorectics and bulimics respond differently to antidepressants. Perhaps the hormonal upheavals in anorexia prevent the antidepressants from working.

Many investigators have focused on psychological characteristics commonly observed in bulimics. These include impulsivity, low self-esteem, and depression. Unfortunately, the data come almost exclusively from bulimic patients, so it is not clear that these factors play a causal role in the disorder rather than reflect mental transformations arising as a result of the bulimia.

Chemical dysregulation of appetite is implicated in bulimia. Curiously, junk foods, appetite-suppressing drugs, and antidepressants all increase serotonin within brain synapses. Wurtman (1983) reports that patients often feel anxious, tense, or depressed before eating carbohydrates, feeling peaceful and relaxed afterward. But other neurotransmitters also affect appetite. For example, norepinephrine injections in the hypothalamus increase carbohydrate intake even in sated rats (Leibowitz, 1984). Cravings for carbohydrate-rich foods probably arise in bulimics because of serotonin deficiencies or norepinephrine excesses, although it seems implausible that these neurotransmitter abnormalities arise without psychological provocation. We pointed out in Chapter 8 that the hypothalamus acts as a mediator between psychological experiences and endocrine function. Perhaps psychological stress can produce hypothalamically mediated endocrine and neurotransmitter dysfunctions that take on a life of their own, bulimia being a conspicuous behavioral consequence.

MENTAL RETARDATION

Mental retardation, as defined by the American Association of Mental Deficiency, "refers to significantly subaverage intellectual functioning existing concurrently with deficits in adaptive behavior and manifested during the developmental period" (Grossman, 1973, p. 11). This definition is also followed in the *DSM-III-R,* which places mental retardation on Axis II along with personality disorders and autistic disorder since they are all presumed to have their origins in early childhood.

The most important point about this definition of mental retardation is that the diagnosis requires deficits in intellectual *and* adaptive behaviors. Adaptive behaviors refer to performances of various duties and social roles appropriate to age and sex. Among preschoolers, for example, self-help skills like getting dressed or going to the bathroom would be important; for the adult, adaptive behavior might be measured by the capacity to work independently on a job. Intellective behaviors are generally assessed by intelligence tests. People scoring more than two standard deviations below the mean—that is, obtaining an IQ score of less than 70—are regarded as intellectually retarded.

The requirement that adaptive deficits be included in the formal diagnosis of mental retardation is controversial. Zigler (1984) argues that only IQ should enter into the definition because judgments of adaptation are usually ill-defined and depend on circumstances—for example, whether the retarded person has a job. Zigler believes that adaptive behaviors are best viewed as correlates of IQ rather than as a criterion for the diagnosis.

Epidemiology

The IQ distribution in the general population is given in Figure 21.7. It appears to be composed of two hypothetical underlying distributions, the larger one with a mean of 100 and the other with a mean of 35. In the larger "normal" distribution, extreme scores represent genetic and environmental variations of the same sort that enter into IQs of 100. Presumably, favorable or unfavorable combinations of genetic and environmental factors are responsible for scores higher or lower than 100. The smaller distribution reflects more purely biological factors: genetic and chromosomal abnormalities or brain damaging traumatic events such as birth complications and prenatal infectious diseases.

FIGURE 21.7 Hypothetical distribution of IQs in the population, showing two types of mental retardation.

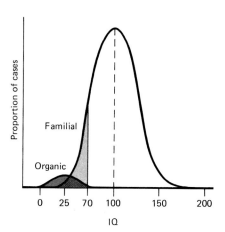

Two sources of evidence support the hypothesis of two broad and discontinuous classes of mental retardation. First, social class is correlated with IQ for individuals above 50 IQ, but not for those below 50 (Abramowicz & Richardson, 1975); that is, children with IQs below 50 are no more likely to come from a lower than from a higher social class. Second, Roberts (1952) has shown that the moderately retarded (IQs ranging from 50 to 70) have siblings with IQs averaging around 80 IQ, while siblings of the severely retarded average about 100 IQ (see Figure 21.8). The implication is that severe retardation arises from rare and relatively unpredictable causes, whereas moderate retardation reflects the lower end of the normal distribution arising from a combination of normally distributed biological and social factors, some of which may have a genetic basis. We now consider three examples of the more than 300 major chromosome or genetic defects causing discontinuous forms of mental retardation (McKusick, 1978).

Down's Syndrome

Down's syndrome (DS), formerly called mongolism, accounts for 10 percent of all cases of mental retardation. The sequence of intellectual and social development is similar for normal and DS children, although the rate of intellectual development and the ultimate level achieved by the DS children is lower. Children with DS often have endearing personalities. When reared in a nurturant environment, they are affectionate and generally happier than other retarded children.

The characteristic visible signs of DS are well known, especially the epicanthic skin fold over the nasal portion of the eye and the flattened facial features that remind one of mongoloid traits (see Figure 21.9). But they also have a peculiar crease on the palms, short and stubby hands, muscle flaccidity, and short stature. Congenital heart defects occur in about half the cases (Nora & Fraser, 1981). The mental retardation in Down's syndrome is believed

FIGURE 21.8   Frequency distributions of the IQs of 562 siblings of 149 moderately retarded and 122 severely retarded individuals. (From Roberts, 1952)

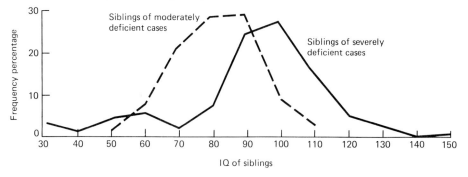

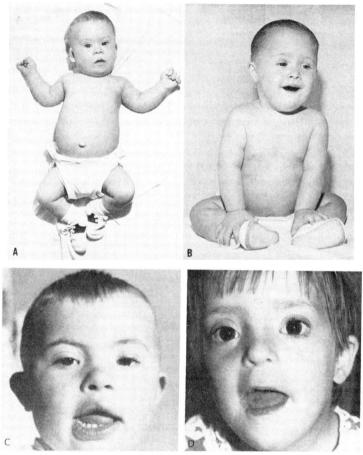

FIGURE 21.9 Unrelated 1-year-olds and unrelated older children with Down's syndrome. (From J. Nora & F. Clarke Fraser (1981). *Medical genetics: Principles and practice (3rd ed.). Copyright © 1989 and reprinted by permission of Lea and Febiger.)*

to arise from elevated levels of certain chemicals called purines (Patterson, 1987).

Most children with DS have IQs below 50. In all instances the disorder is due to an extra copy of a gene called *Gart* on the long arm of chromosome 21. In 93 percent of DS cases the extra *Gart* gene occurs because there are three rather than two copies of chromosome 21 (Nora & Fraser, 1981). In the remaining cases the critical *Gart* fragment of chromosome 21 is attached to another chromosome. The extra copy of genetic material arises because of *nondisjunction* when two chromosomes 21 from one parent—usually the mother—combine with one chromosome 21 from the other parent during fertilization.

The incidence of nondisjunction DS is strongly related to maternal age (see Figure 21.10). Only 1 per 1000 females under age 30 gives birth to a child with DS; the corresponding rate is about ten times greater for 40-year-old women. The other two causes of DS (mosaicism and translocation) will not be considered here, except to note that these forms are unrelated to maternal age. Currently, there is no biological treatment for DS, but now that the gene has been identified, a prenatal test for its presence may become available, as well as a therapy to regulate the *Gart* gene controlling purine metabolism (Patterson, 1987).

Phenylketonuria

Many disorders leading to mental retardation are associated with *autosomal recessive* genes. Phenylketonuria (PKU) is one of the few autosomal recessive

FIGURE 21.10 Frequency of Down's syndrome as a function of maternal age. (From Trimble & Baird, 1978)

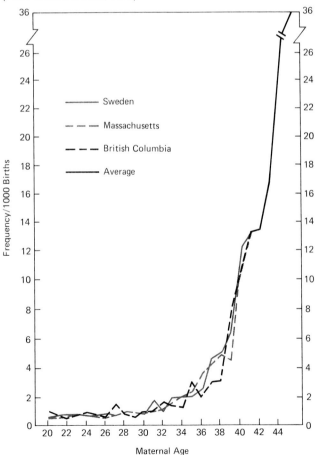

disorders for which there is a treatment. The enzymatic defect is in the conversion of phenylanine to tyrosine, which causes deficiencies of tyrosine and dopamine and an excess of phenylpyruvic acid.

The disorder can be identified by a urine test just before the newborn leaves the hospital. The test is not perfectly reliable, so that a positive result warrants a more definitive blood test before a definite diagnosis of PKU is made. About 1 in 10,000 whites is affected, but the incidence in blacks is much lower.

The untreated newborn looks normal but begins to show development delays within the first few months. Seizures often begin after six months, with a precipitous drop in intellectual functioning. If untreated, 90 percent will eventually have IQs below 50 (Tourian & Sidbury, 1978). Untreated children are hyperactive and irritable, with increased muscle tone, awkwardness, and purposeless repetitive movements. The skin is rough and dry; complexion, hair, and eye color are lighter than expected. A deficiency in tyrosine is responsible for the lighter color because this amino acid is also the precursor of melanin pigment.

A special diet low in phenylalanine but properly balanced in other respects can prevent most of the sequelae of PKU, although the treated children will still average about five IQ points below their unaffected siblings (Koch et al., 1984). The diet must be initiated very early and followed scrupulously because the longer treatment is delayed, the more severe the retardation (Knox, 1966). Unfortunately, the diet is not palatable and the PKU child is tempted by what other children eat. Usually the special diet is stopped around the time of adolescence.

The offspring of even successfully treated PKU adult females, however, are at great risk for various physical and mental defects, including microcephaly, heart abnormalities, and mental retardation. This is because the developing fetus is exposed to high circulating levels of phenylalanine unless the PKU mother resumes the special diet during the pregnancy.

Fragile X Syndrome

The fragile X syndrome probably equals Down's syndrome in the frequency with which it causes mental retardation, and it is largely responsible for a 25 percent excess of males in institutions for the retarded. The syndrome gets its name from the observation that when the X chromosome is stained for visualization, either of two things happens: an unstained area remains near the tip of the long arm or that portion of the long arm is broken off. In either case, the tip of the long arm appears to be, or actually is, fragmented (see Figure 21.11).

In males the fragile X syndrome is usually associated with moderate retardation (average IQs around 50), although intellectual deficiencies can range from mild to severe. Females with fragile X are usually less severely affected because the adverse consequence of the defect is mitigated by the female's other, usually normal, X chromosome (Paul et al., 1984). About one-quarter of boys with infantile autism have the fragile X chromosome (Gillberg &

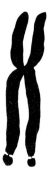

FIGURE 21.11 Fragile X chromosome appears to fragment near the tip of the long arm. (From J. Nora & F. Clarke Fraser (1982). *Medical genetics: Principles and practice (3rd ed.). Copyright © 1989 and reprinted by permission of Lea and Febiger.)*

Wahlstrom, 1985), so that this aberration is not simply associated with mental retardation, but may also play a role in autism.

Most affected adults appear to be physically normal, but they often have a large forehead, prominent chin, and large ears (Figure 21.12). When a child reaches puberty the scrotum often becomes enlarged because of edema. Unfortunately, there is no established therapy for the fragile X syndrome.

We have omitted a discussion of familial mental retardation largely because the specific causes have not been identified. Yet these cases constitute the bulk of the mentally retarded, exacting a substantial cost in personal, familial, and societal disability. Presumably, many cases of familial mental retardation represent the unfortunate side of the normal distribution of genetic and environmental factors contributing to intelligence. It may not be possible to identify a simple cause of these deficiencies and therefore specific remediation of one kind or another may be difficult to achieve.

SUMMARY

The character and consequence of childhood disorders are affected by the cognitive and maturational level of the child, so that the same cause can have different consequences at different ages. Because of dependency and cognitive immaturity, ecopathological factors such as physical and sexual abuse can have enduring and widespread consequences. Many of the disorders first evident in childhood seem to be associated with hereditary factors, neurological impairments, and minor physical anomalies (MPAs) indicative of aberrations arising during fetal life. As more insight is being acquired about infectious and other prenatal agents that can affect the fetus, we can expect substantial increases in understanding about their origins.

Several disorders discussed in this chapter—autistic disorder, attention deficit hyperactivity disorder, and enuresis or bedwetting—appear to have genetic and prenatal antecedents. Identical twin concordance rates for these disorders are elevated and, at least for the first two of them, many affected children have MPAs. Children with autistic disorder all have language disturbances and dis-

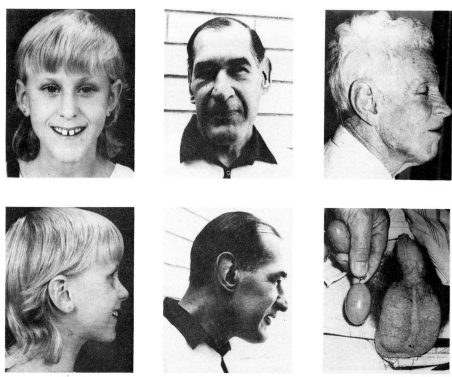

FIGURE 21.12 Facial appearance of retarded individuals with the fragile X syndrome. Note the enlarged size of testes in relation to a "normal" comparison model. (Courtesy of G. R. Sutherland).

play an obsessive desire for sameness. Most are mentally retarded but about 10 percent of these retarded have "islands of excellence," or specific areas of cognitive superiority. As many as 35 percent have epilepsy and 25 percent have the fragile X chromosome anomaly usually associated with mental retardation.

Children with attention deficit hyperactivity disorder always seem to have their motors running; they get bored easily, cannot sit still, and exhaust parents and teachers. Stimulant medication is successful in up to three-quarters of the cases, but the remainder do not seem to benefit. The implication is that hyperactivity has multiple etiologies and that other forms of treatment will need to be devised.

School refusal—so-called school phobia—is one example of a common childhood disorder that is readily treatable. It often arises in a closely knit family from which the child fears separation. The most effective treatment involves taking the child to school, supporting the school authorities in keeping the child there, and being firm if the child refuses to return.

Two adolescent-onset eating disturbances, anorexia nervosa and bulimia nervosa, are considered in this chapter: Anorexia is characterized by an obsessive pursuit of slimness, usually in girls from middle-class backgrounds, and bulimia is distinguished by excessive binge eating involving high-caloric foods. Anorexics and bulimics often have a family history of depression, suggesting a biopsychological link to affective disorder. Unfortunately, the etiological picture remains unclear because antidepressants, which appear moderately effective for bulimia, are much less effective for anorexia nervosa.

Perhaps the most widespread and debilitating disorders are those that produce mental retardation. Many different genetic and chromosomal abnormalities can be identified. Down's syndrome, phenylketonuria (PKU), and the fragile X syndrome are given as examples here. While Down's and the fragile X syndrome are currently untreatable, the mental retardation caused by PKU can be avoided by the early introduction of a diet low in phenylalanine. This disorder is an example of a specific and well-understood genetic biochemical abnormality whose deleterious effects can now be ameliorated by a rationally designed nutritional therapy.

Treatment Evaluation

OUTLINE

After exhausting all easy options, psychologically troubled people seek out experts to relieve their distress. In preliterate societies the experts are called shamans or witch doctors; in modern societies they are religious figures or clinical professionals trained to use specific treatments (Frank, 1973). This chapter will describe and evaluate several major psychological and somatic types of therapy. Moreover, we attempt to gauge the extent of improvement to be expected from the therapies with respect to achieving normal levels of functioning. Most established therapies are at least moderately effective in producing improvement, but they do not necessarily "cure" people of their ailments.

In practice, psychological therapies are time-limited. Patients are seldom seen for more than fifty sessions, and most are seen for fewer than ten. The implication is that with "successful" therapy, people will acquire the resources to cope effectively with the problems that might befall them. For some types of mental disorders, however, this view may not be applicable. If some mental disorders are more akin to chronic illnesses like diabetes mellitus or rheumatoid arthritis, time-limited therapy is currently unrealistic. Chronic conditions like schizophrenia, bipolar illness, alcoholism, and certain personality disorders may require lifelong treatment, and even a year of intensive therapy will not cure the sufferer. Consequently, relapses during follow-up can be expected. These relapses do not necessarily imply that therapy is without value, but rather that the disorder requires continued treatment.

A recent count revealed more than 250 psychotherapies (Corsini, 1984), not to mention numerous drug and other somatic therapies, making it impossible to discuss all of them. We will therefore concentrate on the major classes of psychological therapy (behavioral, cognitive, and psychodynamic), drug therapies, and electroconvulsive therapy. We will start our discussion with psychological forms of therapy.

METHODS OF PSYCHOLOGICAL THERAPY

Psychotherapy, broadly construed, involves a therapist interacting with a troubled person to bring about beneficial changes in feelings, cognitions, and behaviors. As Strupp (1978) puts it:

> . . . psychotherapy is a *collaborative* endeavor or a partnership, in which the patient, almost from the beginning, is expected to play an active part. . . . In a sense, psychotherapy is a learning process and the role of the therapist is analogous to that of a teacher or mentor . . . psychotherapy is seen by some as a "psychosocial treatment," by others as a special form of education, and by still others as a means of promoting personality growth and self-actualization (pp. 4–5).

In a similar vein, Frank (1982) says that:

> Psychotherapy is a planned, emotionally charged, confiding interaction between a trained, socially sanctioned healer and a sufferer. During this interaction the healer seeks to relieve the sufferer's distress and disability through symbolic communication, primarily words, but also sometimes bodily activities (p. 10).

These descriptions are somewhat more applicable to the psychodynamic therapies in which the interpersonal relationship between the patient and therapist is paramount for uncovering conflict and unconscious mechanisms than for the behavioral therapies. Behaviorally oriented therapies spend more time on external environmental stimuli that elicit abnormal behavior while using observational learning, conditioning, and extinction to reshape behavior in more adaptive ways. We begin by describing the most widely used behavioral and psychodynamic therapies before launching into an evaluation of their efficacy.

Behavioral Therapies

We will quickly tour the major forms of behavior therapy and highlight some of the differences between them. All the behavioral therapies share the following features according to Wilson (1984):

1 An assumption that abnormal behavior is acquired and maintained through learning and reinforcement in the same manner as normal behavior
2 Emphasis on current rather than on past determinants
3 Detailed behavioral analysis of the problem, with treatment procedures targeted at specific components
4 An assumption that understanding etiology is not essential for producing behavioral change; conversely, changing behavior does not imply an understanding of etiology

Behavior therapies differ in their emphasis, depending on the problem to be treated and the outcome desired. Some behavioral therapies emphasize the extinction of maladaptive behavior through repeated nonreinforcement of feared stimuli while others focus on altering inappropriate appetitive motivations such as being sexually attracted to children.

Systematic Desensitization   Systematic desensitization can best be understood by considering a "natural" therapy used routinely by parents to alleviate unwarranted childhood fears. If a child is afraid of a dog, the parent first keeps the dog leashed at a distance while reassuring the child that it is safe, making the child more relaxed in the presence of the dog. As anxiety diminishes, the dog is brought closer, always with the reassuring (anxiety-reducing) presence of the parent. Eventually, with enough exposure, modeling, and reassurance, the child may feel comfortable enough to touch, and eventually even be alone with, the dog.

Systematic desensitization is very similar to this treatment (Wolpe, 1982). First, the client is trained in relaxation techniques by a therapist. Then a hierarchy of frightening imaginary scenes graded in severity is constructed by the client in collaboration with the therapist. The scene that produces the least anxiety is first imagined while the client relaxes. When the client gets to the point that no anxiety is experienced by imagining that scene, the next more frightening scene is imagined, and so on. Eventually, the client is able to imagine even the most frightening scenes without anxiety, and the therapist then gets the client actually to experience the feared stimuli in the real world.

The original explanation for the effectiveness of systematic desensitization was that the relaxation response is physiologically incompatible with the high arousal of anxiety—what has been called counterconditioning. If the client can remain relaxed in the presence of the aversive conditioned stimulus, or CS, the latter will eventually lose its anxiety-arousing properties. This seems to make a lot of sense, but more recent evidence indicates that relaxation is actually not necessary for systematic desensitization to be effective. Instead, the critical ingredient for anxiety reduction is *exposure* to the anxiety-arousing situation (Marks, 1987). Moreover, it may not be necessary to imagine a hierarchy of feared stimuli or even to start with the least anxiety-provoking stimulus. Instead, the therapist can encourage real-world or in vivo exposure early in therapy. Indeed, most experts argue that in vivo exposure hastens treatment dramatically (Emmelkamp, 1982).

Flooding   Unlike systematic desensitization, flooding has the client imagine or actually experience the most frightening stimuli head-on, with full force, right from the beginning. A compulsive hand washer, for example, is persuaded to soil his hands while prevented from washing. After a series of these high-impact, traumatic confrontations with the feared stimulus, anxiety gradually diminishes. Flooding therapy is not always for the faint of heart. Just imagine trying to master a fear of cockroaches by putting your hand in a box of roaches and letting them crawl about for many minutes.

You can see that exposure to feared stimuli is an essential ingredient of both systematic desensitization and flooding. Exposure is even more effective if the person is also prevented from performing anxiety-reducing avoidance or escape responses, such as hand washing. The basic idea is that avoidance and escape responses serve to attenuate anxiety; but when the escape responses are prevented, the person experiences the anxiety-arousing situation with full force and comes to learn that these responses are unnecessary. An example of this form of treatment follows:

> Exposure treatment included two hours per day of deliberate contact with the discomfort-evoking stimuli during therapy sessions and four additional hours of exposure as a homework assignment. For example, a patient who feared contamination by cancer-associated objects was gradually confronted with increasingly disturbing objects. In the sixth session, the patient was taken to a cancer ward. Individuals in this group were allowed to wash or clean as they wished, but after each washing during the six hours of exposure, they were recontaminated immediately. Response prevention treatment consisted of strict and continuous blocking of ritualistic cleaning and washing; no contact with water was allowed throughout treatment excepting one supervised ten-minute shower every fifth day. Avoidance of contaminants was permitted. Treatment sessions included discussion of daily avoidance patterns, incidental contamination, and urges to wash; no deliberate exposure was implemented. All patients were supervised continuously by a relative or, if hospitalized, by a hospital staff member. Four days after this phase, both groups received a combination of exposure and response prevention for an additional ten sessions (Steketee, Foa, & Grayson, 1982, p. 1366).

Aversion Therapy In aversion therapy, the therapist helps the patient establish a connection between a stimulus to which the person is inappropriately "attracted"—cigarettes, alcohol, fetishes, for example—and a noxious unconditioned stimulus such as electric shock or a chemical that induces nausea. The goal of this classical conditioning approach is to reduce attraction to the subjectively positive but otherwise inappropriate stimulus. Aversion therapy can be thought of as a reverse of systematic desensitization or exposure therapy. In aversion therapy the goal is to turn a positive stimulus into a negative or an anxiety-provoking stimulus. In systematic desensitization or exposure, the goal is to make an anxiety-provoking or negative stimulus into a neutral stimulus.

Cognitive Therapy Cognitive therapies are based on two ideas: cognitions are prime movers of behavior, so changing the way a person thinks is the key to meaningful and lasting improvement. Although other therapies also endeavor to change how a person thinks, cognitive approaches focus specifically on thinking habits, many of which are out of awareness. Generally, cognitive therapy is devoted to discovering maladaptive thinking habits by a detailed analysis of the current thoughts motivating certain behaviors. In contrast, psychodynamic therapy focuses on the defensive and metaphorical aspects of the patient's thoughts, especially as they relate to specific childhood experiences. The cognitive approach also differs from the behavioral approach, which focuses mainly on changing behavior through the modification of the external environment by altering reinforcement contingencies or using mechanisms of habituation. However, many therapists now attempt to combine what they see as the best parts of cognitive and behavioral therapy.

The first formal cognitive-behavioral therapy was devised by Albert Ellis in 1955. The fundamental premise of his rational-emotive approach is that much misery derives from hidden irrational and often childish assumptions, such as that you must always be loved or you must always be obedient. For example, normally one feels slightly dysphoric if an acquaintance does not reciprocate your "Hello." According to Ellis, the hidden connection between this disappointment and dysphoria involves an irrational and catastrophic self-statement about being bad and therefore "worthless." He believes that certain people, especially those with neurotic disorders, typically misconstrue, exaggerate, and negatively misinterpret their behaviors and the behaviors of others, making emotional mountains out of innocuous molehills. These biased catastrophic cognitions, resulting in anxiety, depression, and a poor self-concept, are what the therapist tries to change.

People with anxiety problems (neurotics) tend to catastrophize because of a preoccupation with security. As Angyal (1965) puts it:

> For the neurotic, almost his entire life is devoted to the pursuit of safety.... When ... making decisions his considerations are overwhelmingly on the dangers to be avoided rather than on the objective to be achieved.... It is not "I would like to do this or that," but "I must do it *or else.*" ... For a healthy person, consummation is the important aspect of experience.... The neurotic does things not for the sake of enjoyment but in order to prove or disprove something (1965, pp. 81–82).

Therapy requires detecting and disputing these hidden irrational beliefs, trying to make persons realize the negative and often hidden assumptions behind their irrational actions. Ellis believes that most clients tend to exaggerate the consequences of a frustration or disappointment because they mistake preferences for needs. Presumably, by exposing to critical scrutiny these irrationalities, the client will acquire more rational self-statements (Ellis, 1984).

A popular form of cognitive-behavioral therapy was devised by Beck. The difference between the cognitive aspects of the Ellis and Beck therapies is largely that the former emphasizes disputation and verbal argument while the latter uses a more Socratic approach, with the idea of helping people discover their irrationalities and false beliefs themselves. Also, Beck's approach explicitly requires homework assignments where the person must realistically confront that which is feared, whereas Ellis does not necessarily require homework assignments.

Both Ellis and Beck were originally trained in psychodynamic approaches but became doubtful about the necessity of discovering the childhood origins of current maladaptive behaviors. And it is undeniably true that the original motives for a behavior may have little to do with the current motives for maintaining that behavior. For example, a child might have found that faking illness was advantageous for avoiding school. Within the cognitive approach, it is unnecessary to recall that childhood event in order to deter that person as an adult from habitually playing sick. Psychodynamic therapists would argue that unless sick-role episodes in childhood are brought into consciousness, the adult will tend to "get sick" when the going gets rough even if made aware through cognitive therapy that it is a defense against anxiety. Empirical evidence, however, does not support the necessity for uncovering the childhood origins of adult maladaptive behavior to sustain therapeutic improvement.

Psychodynamic Therapy

Psychodynamic therapies are predicated on the central role of unconscious conflict and fantasies as causes of psychological problems, and the need to achieve conscious insight about them in order to overcome abnormal behavior. The methods by which one acquires insight include the analysis of free associations, dreams, and defenses, often with the symbolic interpretation of experiences. In keeping with psychoanalytic ideas about the prepotent role of repressed childhood experiences shaping adult behavior, the therapy focuses on the analysis of the "transference"; that is, infantile feelings, thoughts, and behaviors now expressed toward the therapist. Psychodynamic therapists believe that the analysis of the transference is the key to discovering childhood reactions to the parents and thus the source of the adult problem. In sum, the therapeutic goal of the psychodynamic method is to achieve insight about inappropriate motives, with the idea that behavior will change because the cognitive maturity of the adult can now replace the infantile thoughts.

Example   We give here a synopsis of a fairly brief and relatively successful psychodynamically oriented treatment for illustration. Keep in mind that few cases show such rapid improvement after revelations of a repressed experience.

A college-educated woman in her late 20s complained of extreme passivity, interpersonal alienation, and obsessive thoughts of wanting to harm her young children. Therapy made slow progress and the cause of these feelings remained mysterious until her mother happened to give away a childhood violin. She then became very angry, revealing that the violin had been a gift from the father just before he died. Following this, she now remembered with photographic precision and intense emotion her father's lingering illness and death, facts she had previously insisted could not be recalled.

Between that therapy session and the next, she vented considerable anger at her husband and reported the absence of hostile feelings toward her children. She then came to see her therapist in a more realistic light, now citing numerous therapeutic errors he had made. This was important because she seemed to have idolized her therapist earlier, an indication of her transference misperceptions.

Discussing her father's death revealed deep feelings of loss and resentment about his illness and its disruption of her life. When he died, she felt that her hostile fantasies were responsible, with the consequence that all her expressions of anger brought on feelings of guilt and a sense of imminent danger. By examining the original feelings from a more mature perspective, she was able to become appropriately assertive in current interpersonal relationships without apprehension.

This woman had completed the MMPI after the second therapy session and again at termination, about thirty sessions later. Her before- and after-therapy scores are shown in Figure 22.1. Scores of greater than 70 or less than 30 on each scale are seen only rarely in the normal population.

The before-therapy profile shows distinct elevations on the Depression (D) and Psychopathic deviate (Pd) scales, suggesting dysphoric mood, alienation,

FIGURE 22.1 MMPI profile before and after therapy.

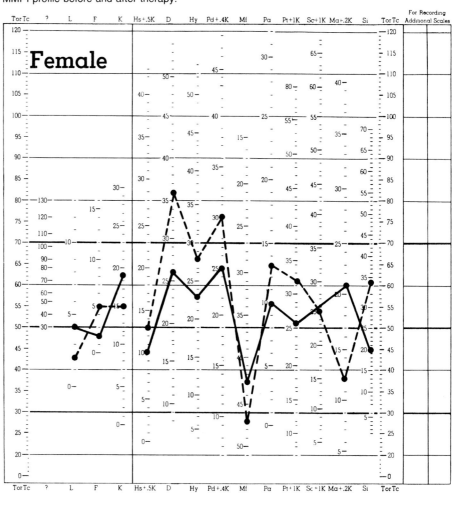

- - - - After 2nd session
of therapy

——— At termination
of therapy

and conflict with those around her. The trough on the Masculinity-femininity (Mf) scale signifies strong identification with stereotypic "feminine" roles and attitudes, including excessive passivity and submissiveness.

The after-therapy profile exhibits some normalization, with extreme deviations less evident. The score on the Hypomania (Ma) scale is higher and the score on the Social Introversion (Si) scale is lower. This combination suggests expansiveness, energy, and social participation, qualities quite different from the symptoms of alienation at the time of beginning therapy. The overall personality configuration nevertheless remains easily recognizable because many of the MMPI items ask about past events and thus would not be expected to change, even with the improvements observed.

Comment   Freud was at once both ambitious and pessimistic about his approach to treatment. In a discussion written on the subject just two years before his death, he noted that chance factors could re-create a neurosis in a seemingly cured patient and that congenital frailties of the personality often limit the extent to which recovery could be expected. One case of hysteria Freud (1937) describes had

> . . . been cut off from life by an inability to walk, owing to acute pain in her legs. Her condition was obviously hysterical in character and it had resisted various kinds of treatment. After an analysis lasting nine months the trouble disappeared. . . . In the years following her recovery she was consistently unfortunate: there were disasters in her family, they lost their money and, as she grew older, she saw every hope of happiness in love and marriage vanish. But this woman . . . stood her ground valiantly and was a support to her people. [Unfortunately, more than a decade later, a tumor was discovered which necessitated a hysterectomy and prompted a relapse into neurosis.] She proved inaccessible to a further attempt at analysis, and to the end of her life she remained abnormal (p. 323).

Perhaps the original treatment was incomplete because it did not inoculate the patient against all eventualities. On the other hand, it may be unrealistic to expect that a therapy can completely eradicate old ways of behaving when the going gets rough. After all, no therapy is designed to produce amnesia for past maladaptive ways of behaving.

EVALUATION OF PSYCHOTHERAPEUTIC OUTCOME

Assessment of treatment effectiveness is one of the most controversial topics in psychology. Because each of the many schools of psychotherapy often claims to be the most effective, the consumer can be at a loss in selecting either the right therapy or the right therapist. In fact, the relative success of various therapies often depends on who is doing the evaluation, the factors being rated, the weights given to each outcome factor, the diagnosis of the patient being treated, and the type of control group employed.

Complexities and Controversies

Different Perspectives Different therapeutic schools emphasize different procedures in evaluating the success of therapy. Indeed, some therapists are antagonistic to any evaluation of their work, thus making it especially difficult to assess efficacy.

Therapists differ in the kinds of problems they treat. Therefore, estimates of therapeutic efficacy will be confounded with the nature and seriousness of the problem. People with circumscribed problems such as simple phobias are more likely to seek behavioral or cognitive therapy. People who are not getting much joy from life but have only vague ideas about their specific problems are more likely to enter dynamic therapy. Even behavior therapists choose dynamic therapies for such vaguely formulated problems. A survey of twenty behavior therapists in personal treatment revealed that not one was in behavior therapy, and half were in psychoanalytic therapy (Lazarus, 1971)!

In contrast to behaviorally oriented therapists, psychoanalytically oriented therapists generally downplay the importance of specific symptoms. You can see this clearly in the first major study of psychoanalytic therapy done at the Berlin Psychoanalytic Institute (Fenichel, 1930).

> We were most particular in what was understood as "cure." Included were only such cases where success meant *not merely the disappearance of symptoms, but also the manifestation of analytically acceptable personality changes* (italics ours, quoted in Bergin & Lambert, 1978, p. 141).

Contemporary psychoanalysts feel similarly about symptomatic improvement.

> The patient . . . may have been cured of more conditions than he had complained about when he first started; previously unforeseen possibilities of self-fulfillment may have been realized . . . psychoanalysis tries to help the patient effect the best possible solution of his difficulties that circumstances will allow. It seeks to achieve the most stable equilibrium possible between the various forces of conflict. . . . How well that equilibrium is sustained will also depend on how favorably life treats the patient during and after treatment (Arlow, 1984, p. 37).

In contrast to dynamic therapists, behavior therapists believe that the focus should be on specific maladaptive behaviors rather than on the presumptive inner conflict. The behavioral emphasis is exemplified in a classic behavioral approach to treating a schizophrenic woman who stole food, hoarded towels, and wore twenty-five pounds of clothing (Ayllon, 1963). By the use of behavioral techniques, this woman reduced her weight from 250 to 150 pounds, went from hoarding 600 towels to hoarding only a few, and began to wear the proper amount of clothing. These quite dramatic improvements helped considerably in day-to-day management and demonstrated powerful effects of behavioral treatment. A ten-year follow-up indicated that she was dressing appropriately and only occasionally hoarding, but that she weighed 270 pounds and was still hospitalized with psychotic delusions about fires and Jesus in her body (Sherwood & Gray, 1974).

Apparently the treatment had a substantial effect on significant target symptoms while having no impact on the basic disorder. In this case the symptoms were emblematic of the more basic schizophrenic dysfunction. Of course, even staunch advocates of behavioral approaches would agree that in the case of schizophrenia, there is something more underneath the peculiar maladaptive behaviors that makes management troublesome.

How to Evaluate Improvement An important and controversial question is how much improvement is required to achieve normalization. You can get a simplified answer by examining Table 22.1. This Health-Sickness Rating Scale reduces the multifaceted nature of health and sickness to a single 100-point dimension of overall functioning (Luborsky, 1962). In constructing the scale the author attempted to balance such factors as self-sufficiency, subjective discomfort, and quality of interpersonal relationships. People with various psychotic and borderline disturbances achieve a score no higher than 35 on this scale. Consequently, even a "successful" therapy that improves scores ten or fifteen points may not get patients close to the score of 76 representing minimally satisfactory adjustment. For people with higher initial scores, a ten- or fifteen-point improvement may be all that is necessary.

Most studies of therapeutic effectiveness use as controls untreated patients with similar diagnoses rather than people with normal levels of functioning. Because of this, it is difficult to tell whether a "successful" therapy has resulted in complete normalization rather than just improvement. An analogy might help here. A therapy for severe mental retardation might raise IQs from 20 to 50, surely a substantial improvement. Yet none of the treated retarded patients would approach intellectual normality (100 IQ).

We should also keep in mind that ratings along a single dimension of mental health/sickness does injustice to the complex multifaceted nature of psychological problems. It is quite possible that some aspects of behavior and experience may be improved by therapy while other aspects remain unchanged or even deteriorate. Consider the following examples:

1 A patient enters therapy because of an inability to achieve orgasm. After therapy, the patient is still inorgasmic, but is no longer distressed about it.

2 Following drug treatment, a schizophrenic no longer has persecutory delusions, but develops tardive dyskinesia, a debilitating and disfiguring neurological condition caused directly by the antipsychotic drugs.

3 A patient is no longer depressed after therapy, but the spouse complains that the husband is now extremely argumentative and unloving toward the children.

Each of these cases shows clear benefits of therapy, but the consequences either to self or others can yield a mixed picture of gains and losses.

Now is a time of great turmoil in therapy evaluation, spurred both by new quantitative methods for analyzing therapeutic outcome (Smith, Glass, &

TABLE 22.1   HEALTH-SICKNESS RATING SCALE

Definition of scale points

At 100: An ideal state of complete functioning integration, resiliency in the face of stress, happiness, and social effectiveness

(99 to 76: Degrees of "everyday" adjustment. Few of these people seek treatment.)

At 75, inhibitions, symptoms, character problems become severe enough to cause more than "everyday" discomfort. May occasionally seek treatment.

At 65, generally functioning pretty well but have *focalized* problem or more generalized lack of effectiveness without specific symptoms.

At 50, definitely needs treatment to continue work satisfactorily and has increasing difficulty in maintaining himself automatically (even without expressed or recognized need for formal treatment). Patient may either be in a stable unsatisfactory adjustment (where most energy is bound in the conflicts) or an unstable adjustment from which he will very likely regress.

At 25, person obviously unable to function autonomously. Needs hospital protection (or would need it if it were not for the support of the therapist). (The fact that the patient is in the hospital does not mean he *must* be rated at this point—he may have changed since admission or be in for a variety of reasons.)

(24 to 1: Increased loss of contact with reality; need for protection of patient or others from the patient; high degree of regression.)

At 10, extremely difficult to make any contact with patient. Needs closed ward care. Not much chance of continued existence without care.

At 0, any condition which, if unattended, would quickly result in the patient's death, but not necessarily by his own hand.

Examples of scale points

100	(Some patients who complete treatment and some patients who come for and need only "situational" counseling will fall within this range.)
75	Very mild neuroses or mild addictions and behavior disorders *begin here* and go on down, depending on severity.
65	Clearly neurotic conditions (most phobias, anxiety neuroses, neurotic characters).
50	Severe neuroses such as severe obsessive-compulsiveness may be rated at 50 or lower, rarely below 35. Some *compensated* psychoses. Many character disorders, neurotic depressions.
35	*Most* borderline schizophrenics; severe character problems. Psychotic depressions may be this high, or go all the way to 0.
25	Most clear-cut, overt psychoses, psychotic characters, severe addictions (which require hospital care).
10	Closed ward patients such as chronic schizophrenics, excited manics, profound suicidal depressives.
0	Completely regressed schizophrenics, incontinent, out of contact, who require complete nursing care, tube feeding.

Miller, 1980), and by insurance companies who want evidence that therapy is beneficial. Patients and others have a right to know about the effectiveness of therapy and about the relative merits and demerits of different forms of treatment. Unfortunately, there are neither firm conclusions nor final answers, though researchers seem to be making progress.

The complexities of therapy evaluation can be exemplified with one famous controversy. When Eysenck (1952) reevaluated the Berlin study of psychoanalytic therapy described earlier, he concluded that only 39 percent of the patients were "improved," a figure that does not inspire confidence in psychoanalytic therapy. On the other hand, Bergin's (1971) reanalysis of the same data concluded that 91 percent of the same patients in the Berlin study improved! This striking difference arose mainly because of a correspondingly radical difference in how the data were tabulated. Eysenck included "premature dropouts" as treatment failures and placed those patients originally classified as "improved" in a category ultimately considered as failures. Bergin, on the other hand, eliminated dropouts and considered "improved" cases as "successes."

One cannot easily decide whose reanalysis is closer to the truth. Patients drop out from therapy for various reasons, including the perception that the therapy was useless or that they have already benefited sufficiently (Frank, 1982). Nevertheless, a high percentage of dropouts is no credit to any therapy. Moreover, we must ask whether improvement, no matter how slim, warrants the label of success. Patients enter therapy demoralized and distressed. When placed on a waiting list, for example, patients may still improve because of hope instilled by the prospect of eventually receiving therapy.

The search for *absolute* categories of improvement is fruitless because any specific cutoff points for cure or even moderate improvement are arguable. The best strategy is to evaluate outcomes using continuous scales which permit statistics such as means and standard deviations. The advantage of continuous scales is that absolute or discrete categories of improvement need not be imposed and debatable judgments can be avoided.

Meta-Analysis: Concept and Measurement

Until the mid-1970s, treatment evaluation was dominated by two approaches: the narrative and the box score. The narrative approach provided detailed reviews of studies pertinent to whatever therapy was being evaluated, while the box score provided tallies of positive and negative results to yield some overall statistical summary. Neither approach was entirely satisfactory because each suffered from two major flaws: potential biases in study selection and primitive statistical analyses that failed to consider not only whether one therapy was better than another, but also how much better it was.

Effect Size

Perhaps the major problem in interpreting the effects of therapy was the noncomparability of different studies. Studies differed not only in the types of patients seen and the type of therapy, but also in the types of measures used to assess outcome. Gene V. Glass (1976) developed a quantitative method for systematically rendering diverse studies statistically comparable. Any group of scores—what psychologists often call a distribution—can be described statistically by its *mean*, or central tendency, and its *standard deviation* (SD), the variability of the individual scores around the mean. Glass first takes the difference between the means of the treatment group and the control group. Then he divides this mean difference by the SD of the control group.

To illustrate, suppose subjects in a therapy study were randomly assigned either to a treatment or control condition and later given a test to evaluate treatment outcome. If the treatment group obtained a mean of 6 while the control group obtained a mean of 5, we could do much more than summarize the difference by saying that the treated group was, on the average, one point higher. In fact, this one-point difference doesn't really mean anything without some standard against which we can evaluate it. This is where the SD of the control group comes in. If the control SD equaled 2, our one-point difference could be translated into an *effect size* (ES) of .5, or the one-point mean difference divided by the two-point standard deviation.

An effect size can be evaluated concretely by using a statistical table that converts effect sizes to percentiles that indicate how well one group is doing *relative* to another group. For example, an ES of .85, the average improvement of treated over untreated patients in Glass's review, is equal to the eightieth percentile; this means that the *average person* in the treated group exceeded the scores of 80 percent of the subjects in the control group. Had the treated group averaged one SD better than the control group, the average treated person would have had a score at the eighty-fourth percentile; that is, a score exceeded eighty-four of one hundred control subjects. Note that if therapy has neither positive nor negative effects (ES = 0), the average person in therapy would exceed 50 percent of those not receiving therapy, that is, points on the treated and control group curves would overlap 100 percent.

By looking at Figure 22.2 you can see just what a .85 SD difference means graphically. Each point on the control group distribution represents a percen-

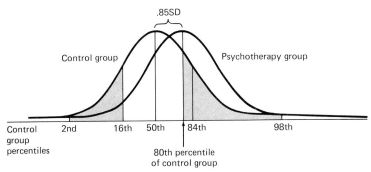

FIGURE 22.2 Illustration of an effect size of .85 assuming the outcome measure is normally distributed. The average patient in therapy achieves a score equivalent to the eightieth percentile of the control group. If there were 100 people in the control group, the average treated patient would exceed eighty of them.

tile ranking. The .85 effect size is equivalent to a treatment that raised mean IQs by thirteen points or increased the average height of adult males by 2.5 inches.

After computing effect sizes for individual studies it is possible to get an average effect size for all studies. Moreover, it becomes possible to group the effect sizes according to different types of therapy or patients. Thus, one can tell if psychodynamic therapy produced a bigger effect size than other forms of therapy. The averaging of effect sizes over many different studies is called *meta-analysis*.

Research Findings

In 1980, Smith, Glass, and Miller published an important meta-analysis of 475 therapy outcome studies. The studies were classified along many dimensions, but we shall single out only a few here: type of therapy, type of disorder, and reactivity and specificity of the outcome measures.

Type of Treatment Table 22.2 gives an abbreviated summary of effect sizes for a variety of psychological therapies in comparison to control groups that received no treatment (Smith, Glass, & Miller, 1980). The overall effect size for all forms of psychological therapy was .85, indicating that the average person at the end of treatment is better off than 80 percent of the controls. The largest effect sizes (ES > 1) seem to come from behavioral and cognitive therapies.

In fifty-six of the studies evaluated by Smith et al., a verbal therapy was compared directly to both a behavioral therapy and a no-treatment control. Since the same outcome measures were used within each study, we can assess

TABLE 22.2   AVERAGE EFFECT SIZES FOR EACH THERAPY TYPE

Type of therapy	Average effect size	No. of effects
Other cognitive therapies	2.38	57
Hypnotherapy	1.82	19
Cognitive-behavioral therapy	1.13	127
Systematic desensitization	1.05	373
Dynamic-eclectic therapy	.89	103
Eclectic-behavioral therapy	.89	37
Behavior modification	.73	201
Psychodynamic therapy	.69	108
Rational-emotive therapy	.68	50
Implosion	.68	60
Gestalt therapy	.64	68
Client-centered therapy	.62	150
Placebo treatment	.56	200
Total	.85	1761

their relative effectiveness. Comparison of the two types of therapy gave an edge to the behavioral (ES = .96) over the verbal therapies (ES = .77). This difference translates into about six percentile points. The average individual in behavioral treatment exceeded 83 percent of the untreated controls, while the average individual in a verbal treatment exceeded 77 percent of the untreated controls. Keep in mind that if chance alone were operating the average treated patient would exceed 50 percent of the untreated controls. In commenting on these results, Glass and Kliegl (1983) reflected that:

> This difference . . . between verbal and behavioral therapies struck us as quite small, and our saying so appears to have offended those who seem to believe that the psychotherapy Olympics were long since over and the laurels were theirs [the behavioral therapists], even as it pleased those (Freudians and Rogerians) who once believed that the race had been lost (p. 32).

Studies rarely compare specific types of therapy with each another (Shapiro & Shapiro, 1982; Stiles, Shapiro, & Elliott, 1986). However, when a variety of cognitive therapies were compared specifically to systematic desensitization (Miller & Berman, 1983), no significant difference in effectiveness was found. This is interesting because desensitization has a theoretical perspective *opposite* to those of cognitive behavioral therapies; that is, it concentrates on changing affective responses first, with the expectation that cognitions will follow. Given these results, one wonders about the relationship of the specific theory to the actual reasons that patients improve.

Type of Disorder Studies in the Smith et al. (1980) meta-analysis included disorders of varying severity. Nevertheless, whether some diagnostic groups benefited from treatment more than others could not be resolved by analyzing effect sizes (see also Andrews & Harvey, 1981). Even psychotic patients benefited significantly. A recent meta-analysis did find phobic symptoms more amenable to therapy than either anxiety or depression (Shapiro & Shapiro, 1982). But anxiety and depression are found in virtually every disorder; and it therefore would be important to know whether the anxiety or depression was a primary or secondary diagnosis. It does appear, however, that borderline or psychotic patients require more psychotherapy than neurotics before achieving significant improvement (Howard et al., 1986).

Reactivity and Specificity *Reactivity* is the extent to which an outcome measure is susceptible to distortion by personal bias or the desire to appear in a favorable light. Included among highly reactive measures would be a patient's self-report of improvement. Among the least reactive would be changes in physiological responsiveness. Outcomes will differ, depending on the reactivity of the measures used to assess outcome, with the more reactive measures showing larger effect sizes for treatment.

Specificity is the degree to which the outcome measure is directly related to the target symptoms of treatment. The least specific measures would include a broad-band instrument like the Rorschach test, which is not used to make specific diagnoses and covers many areas of the patient's functioning, including those not directly related to the patient's problems. At the most specific level are measures targeted precisely for a particular patient's symptoms. As a general rule, the more specific the outcome to the focus of treatment, the greater the change.

It is impossible to determine *the* effect of psychotherapy because effect size varies with the reactivity and specificity of outcome measures, and there is no general answer to which outcomes should be given preeminence. Outcomes tailored to directly treated symptoms seem to show larger effect sizes (Casey & Berman, 1985). In the context of behavior therapy, this is as it should be. Any additional benefit beyond remission of target symptoms—improved interpersonal relationships, for example—is regarded as a bonus.

Glass's quantitative approach has not escaped criticism from behaviorally oriented psychologists (Rachman & Wilson, 1980; Searles, 1985), perhaps because the effect sizes for behavioral approaches were not that much larger than for psychodynamic approaches. The critics believe that without detailed evaluation of each study, results of a meta-analysis will obey the principle of "garbage in, garbage out." For example, the results of any study using unskilled therapists and/or unreliable measures will blur actual differences among treatments. If both good and bad studies are lumped, the true effect size will be underestimated.

Types of Treatment Failure

Treatment failures can arise because of refusal to participate, dropping out, ineffective treatment, or relapse (Foa et al., 1983). Refusal usually stems from the perception that a treatment will be too stressful or ineffective. While there are constraints on what can be done to increase motivation, a confident, competent, and sensitive therapist will probably have fewer refusals.

Treatment is ineffective not only when the treatment is technically inappropriate, but also when patients cannot commit themselves to the procedure. Indeed, defensive maneuvers can foil even quite appropriate treatments. Foa et al. (1983), for example, describe flooding therapy with a patient burdened by a morbid phobia of urine. Drops of urine were placed on her arms but, after a momentary panic, she rapidly calmed down. She indicated an ability to "freeze" the contaminated spot mentally, and thus prevent it from spreading. The rapid reduction of discomfort arose not from the intended habituation to the fear-inducing stimulus, but from dissociation, in which she imagined the urine to be isolated from the rest of her body and therefore no longer frightening. Failure of emotional processing, which prevents her from bearing the full brunt of the fear-inducing stimulus, is a major reason for unsuccessful treatment (Rachman, 1983).

Follow-up

Patients and therapists often find that initial therapeutic gains deteriorate by the time of follow-up. This would seem to be almost the rule for severe addictions, but not for disorders in which mild depression and anxiety dominate (Nicholson & Berman, 1983). This is good news for two reasons: (1) gains seem to persist and (2) costly follow-ups for such disorders may be unnecessary. This is not to say that the treated patients fully recover. Some may, but treatment effectiveness is determined by comparison with nonnormal controls. The issue of full recovery is a separate matter and may be extremely rare or impossible for some disorders.

For example, prospects for full recovery are much dimmer for the psychological treatment of chronic schizophrenia because of the gross disintegration of personality. The most ambitious demonstration of the benefits of treatment for severe schizophrenia will illustrate how limited the outlook for recovery is. Paul and Lentz (1977) took "the most severely debilitated chronically institutionalized adults ever subject to systematic study" and exposed them to one of three treatments: *social learning, milieu therapy,* or a *hospital comparison.* The social learning treatment encouraged self-help skills, regular chores, and responsible behavior. The staff scrupulously reinforced these behaviors with the idea of gradually increasing the patients' independence. The milieu treatment promoted positive expectancies and encouraged desirable thoughts, feelings, and behaviors through suitable feedback and group cohesiveness. The hospital comparison control was quite similar to routine state hospital treatment using chemotherapy with little additional psychological treatment.

Results indicated greater behavioral improvements in the social learning and milieu therapy groups than in the hospital comparison group, both in and out of the hospital. For example, after discharge, 97 percent of the residents in the social learning program stayed out of the hospital for at least ninety days, whereas only 45 percent of the hospital comparison group did this well. The milieu therapy group fell in between: 71 percent stayed out of the hospital for at least that long.

Considering that the average patient in this study had been hospitalized for a total of seventeen years, this is a significant accomplishment. Yet, if we ask how well they functioned on the outside, only about 10 percent of those in the social learning or milieu therapy conditions ever achieved a measure of self-support and independent functioning in contrast to zero percent in the hospital comparison condition. Most of the patients had been discharged to boarding homes that placed few demands on them. Thus, from the perspective of a return to normal function, even the most successful treatment was limited.

Placebo Effects and Positive Expectations

Given the acrimony between adherents of the psychodynamic and behavioral schools, it is surprising that large differences in therapeutic efficacy often cannot be found. Frank (1973) anticipated this when pointing out that patients' expectancies of therapeutic benefit figure prominently in improvement. He concluded that all brands of psychotherapy engender positive expectations by four common ingredients:

1 The therapist has certain healing skills.
2 Patients are treated in socially sanctioned settings dedicated to healing.
3 All psychotherapies have "rationales" to explain maladjustment.
4 All psychotherapies have procedures that, if followed, are designed to benefit the patient.

The role of positive expectancies is shown in the placebo response, in which an inert substance relieves distress (Frank, 1973). Placebo therapy shows an effect size of .56, indicating that the average placebo client improves to the seventy-first percentile relative to no-treatment controls (see Table 22.2). Explanation of the placebo response in psychotherapy centers around its anti-demoralization effects. Many who seek psychotherapy are already dispirited by an inability to cope or a fear of going crazy. The therapist's "treatment" induces positive expectations and significantly ameliorates anxiety.

The power of positive expectation is illustrated in a study by Berman and Wenzlaff (1983) who devised a bogus "test" that allegedly could identify rapid responders to psychotherapy. The test—actually a symptom checklist—was administered to clients coming to a university counseling center before their first therapy session. Their therapist was then led to believe that a particular client would be a rapid responder (positive expectation) or that the test could not make a prediction (neutral expectation). Each client was followed for six therapy sessions with periodic therapists' ratings of improvement and clients' independent completion of the symptom checklist.

Figure 22.3 shows selected results from this study. Therapists given the positive expectation reported significantly more improvement through the six sessions. More importantly, the clients in the positive condition actually reported less anxiety and depression than those in the neutral condition, although none of the clients had been given the "test" results. Positive expectations had no impact, however, on obsessive-compulsive, interpersonal, or somatic problems.

The positive expectancy effect thus was limited to those reactive aspects of demoralization which can be alleviated by hope. As yet it is not clear how the therapists' positive expectations were communicated to the client. They could have exuded more confidence or been more sensitive to the client's condition. However caused, a therapist's own beliefs about the efficacy of therapy play a role in the client's relief.

DRUG TREATMENT

From time immemorial, drugs have been used to treat an assortment of mental ailments. A large fraction of these medicaments were useless, harmful, or effective only because of positive expectancies. Just 160 years ago, the bag of

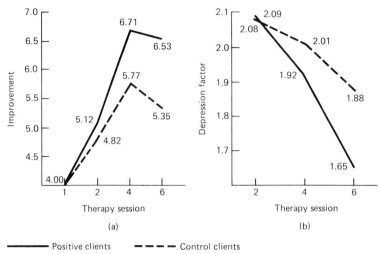

FIGURE 22.3   (a) Therapists' reports of client improvement as a function of whether the therapist was told in advance that the client would respond favorably to psychotherapy. (b) Clients' ratings of their depression as a function of whether or not their therapists were told that they would respond favorably to psychotherapy. (From J. S. Berman, & R. M. Wenzlaff, The impact of therapist expectancies on the outcome of psychotherapy. Paper presented at the August 1983 meeting of the American Psychological Association.)

psychiatric treatments was quite limited (see Table 22.3). Many of the recommendations in Table 22.3 are without merit or cruel by contemporary standards. It is clear that Pinel's earlier ideas about the humane treatment of the insane (see Chapter 2, pp. 47–48) had not yet been generally accepted. One can only concur with Oliver Wendell Holmes, a physician and Supreme Court Justice who said in 1860 that if most drugs used by doctors "could be sent to the bottom of the sea, it would be all the better for mankind and all the worse for the fishes."

Effects of Drug Treatment

Emil Kraepelin is regarded as the father of modern psychopharmacology (Spiegel & Aebi, 1983). His 1892 textbook of psychiatry reports many behavioral experiments on the effects of alcohol, sedative-hypnotics, and stimulants. Some date the modern era of psychopharmacological treatment to 1951, with the discovery of the antipsychotic effects of chlorpromazine. But Bradley's 1937 discovery of the use of benzedrine for hyperactivity and Cade's 1949 discovery of lithium salts for mania could also be the starting date. Prior to the advent of these drugs, medication consisted largely of opiates, hypnotics, and stimulants which might sedate or energize, but did little specific for the condition being treated.

TABLE 22.3   MATERIA MEDICA (PSYCHIATRIC TREATMENTS OF THE EARLY 19TH CENTURY)

Antagonists (For use in cases of excessive nervous sensitivity or insufficient physical sensitivity)
A. Remedies promoting nausea and vomiting:
Internal: Various emetics
External: Revolving machine, revolving chair, swing, red-hot iron, whips with nettles, cupping glasses, suppurating head wounds, gentle rubbing of the skin
Enemas, mustard plasters, blistering plasters, ants, scabies
Cold baths, snow baths, sudden immersion, ice bags, tepid baths
B. Cathartics (laxatives): Psychic disturbances are often located in the abdomen
Medicaments, some of which are still in use today

Antiphlogistics (Temperature-reducing measures)
Medical
Surgical (e.g., bleeding, cupping)

Narcotic Agents (Calming agents)
A. Narcotics:
Saffron, thorn apple, henbane, tobacco, alraun, prussic acid, opium
B. Strong narcotics:
Belladonna, hemlock, foxglove, verbena
C. External agents:
Sack, cupboard, hollow wheel, straightjacket, straight cradle

Excitants, Analeptics (Nerve-invigorating agents)
A. Internal remedies:
Camphor, sage, rosemary, lavender, balm mint, filix, valerian, green tea, arnica, cinnamon oil, juniper oil, cumin, fennel, aniseed, peppermint, and turpentine oil
Musk, castoreum, Spanish fly
Many spices
Naphthalene, old wines
B. External remedies:
Hot compresses on the head
Sneezing powder, intake of irritants
Electricity, galvanism, magnetism

Source: From P. J. Schneider (1824). In R. Spiegel & H.J. Aebi, *Psychopharmacology: An introduction.* Copyright © 1983 by John Wiley and Sons, Inc.

Side Effects   In normal people, the antipsychotic and the antidepressant drugs usually produce unpleasant subjective experiences, including dullness, lethargy, and confused thought; they also impair performance on tests of perceptual, motor, and mental speed (Spiegel & Aebi, 1983) and, in low doses, they can sometimes induce sedation.

Because of debilitating side effects (see Table 22.4), potential benefits to patients must be balanced against the probable costs of taking these drugs. However, some critics focus on the debilitating effects to the exclusion of the benefits obtained.

The widespread use of the most potent psychiatric drugs—the major tranquilizers— has created a public health menace of great proportions. These drugs are known to produce a permanent, disfiguring neurological disease, *tardive dyskinesia,* in a large

TABLE 22.4   COMMON SIDE EFFECTS OF NEUROLEPTICS AND ANTIDEPRESSANTS

Side effects of neuroleptics

1. Vegetative symptoms (particularly with sedative neuroleptics)
   Orthostatic (i.e., occurring on getting up) drop in blood pressure
   Rise in pulse rate, changes in ECG
   Sweating, dryness of the mouth, constipation
   Disturbed potency, other disturbances in sexual function
2. Extrapyramidal motor symptoms (particularly after having a pronounced antipsychotic action)
   Early dyskinesia (uncontrolled movements which may arise at the commencement of therapy)
   Spasms of the tongue, visual spasms, pharyngospasms
   Grimacing, stiff neck, trismus
   Gyratory and rotatory movements of the upper extremities
   Neuroleptic parkinsonoid (after several weeks' treatment)
   Restriction of motor movement (akinesia)
   Loss of facial expression (hypomimia), festinating gait
   Increased muscle tension (rigor); trembling (tremor)
   Akathisia (after prolonged treatment)
   Restlessness, inability to remain seated
   Urge to move continuously
   Tardive dyskinesia (after prolonged treatment and particularly in older patients)
   Involuntary chewing, smacking of lips, swallowing, and rolling movements of the tongue
   Gyratory and flailing movements of the extremities

Side effects of antidepressants

1. Psychic symptoms
   Tiredness, pronounced daytime sedation; sleep disturbances
   Delirium (following overdosage, particularly in elderly patients)
2. Somatic symptoms
   Dryness of the mouth, constipation, urinary retention, disturbance of potency
   Difficulty in focusing the eyes
   Orthostatic hypotension, collapse (in elderly patients)
   Dizziness, headache, palpitations
   Increased sweating
   Depending on the initial vegetative situation, opposing symptoms may also arise:
   hypersalivation, diarrhea, rise in blood pressure, etc.
3. Complications
   Transition from depression to mania (in bipolar depression)
   attempted suicide (particularly with drive-enhancing antidepressants)

Source: From R. Spiegel & H. J. Aebi, *Psychopharmacology: An introduction.* Copyright © 1983 by John Wiley and Sons, Inc.

percentage of cases. Still more ominous, the same drugs permanently damage the higher centers of the brain, producing irreversible psychoses, apathy, generalized brain dysfunction, dementia, and other effects similar to those resulting from lobotomy (Breggin, 1983, p. 2).

Drugs versus Placebo in Schizophrenia Neuroleptics are effective for psychotic ideation at dose levels far short of sedation. Davis (1975) reviewed twenty-four controlled comparisons of neuroleptics and placebos. In every instance the drug was more effective in preventing relapse, but sometimes the advantage of neuroleptics over placebos was not great (Crow et al., 1986).

A significant fraction (about 15 percent) of schizophrenics do not relapse even on placebos. They tend to be the good-premorbid, acute-onset cases with initially florid symptoms. While neuroleptic drugs are effective against their psychotic symptoms, they are really unnecessary after these symptoms disappear. Aside from lower relapse risk in acute patients, attempts to predict which patients would not relapse have been unsuccessful. We hope that the people who would not require it may one day be spared unnecessary maintenance medication.

One cannot predict from a patient's symptoms which neuroleptic will be most effective. Except for the observation that all neuroleptics block dopamine transmission, the specific mechanism by which they work remains speculative (see Chapter 12, pp. 325–327). Moreover, one of the biggest puzzles about drug efficacy is the apparent absence of a dose-response curve for a range of doses of the antipsychotic drugs; in other words, a predictable relationship between the amount of the dose and its effectiveness in bringing about symptom remission does not exist (Donaldson, Gelenberg, & Baldessarini, 1983). Of course, very high doses do have a great impact, but this is deceptive because high doses produce overall sedation rather than reduce specific psychotic symptoms.

Lithium and Antidepressants The effectiveness of lithium for severe unipolar or bipolar disorder is not disputed. In nine studies the rate of relapse was much lower with lithium (Davis, 1976). However, lithium's effectiveness was not related to a unipolar versus bipolar diagnosis, nor did lithium prevent the recurrence of mania more often than the recurrence of depression. It appears that lithium has "normalizing" effects on mood, but it is not specific to mania as originally believed. Lithium, in combination with tricyclic antidepressants, is especially effective in patients otherwise resistant to tricyclics alone (de Montigny et al., 1983; Heninger, Charney, & Steinberg, 1983).

Antidepressants for depression are superior to placebo in controlled comparisons of tricyclics and placebo (Davis, 1976). However, their side effects, shown in Table 22.4, make them not entirely benign. Additionally, they may induce mania in depressed bipolar individuals, a rebound effect which is poorly understood.

Drugs and Psychotherapy Combined

Since psychological therapy and drug therapy have each proven effective for the relief of many disorders, it seems reasonable that combining both forms of treatment would result in even greater benefits. Surprisingly, this prediction has not been clearly supported.

Depression   Most experts believe that bipolar depression has a endo-genously determined physiological etiology and thus is relatively unaffected by ecopathology. Consequently, virtually no controlled psychotherapy research is done with bipolar patients. Since unipolar depressions more often appear to have a significant environmental component, they have been the main target of psychotherapy studies of depression. Evidence indicates that psychotherapy, whether behavioral or dynamic, is at least as effective as if not more effective than, tricyclic antidepressants in relieving unipolar depressions (Smith et al., 1980; Steinbrueck, Maxwell, & Howard, 1983).

How can the mixed bag of depressed mood and negative attitudes be ame-nable to such radically different modes of treatment? Adding to the uncertainty is the observation that the time course for improvement is similar, whether de-pressed patients are treated by tricyclics, cognitive behavior therapy, or a combination of the two. Consider findings from two studies of tricyclics and cognitive behavior therapy for moderately to severely depressed unipolar pa-tients (Murphy et al., 1984; Simons, Garfield, & Murphy, 1984). Both studies found that patients treated with either tricyclics or psychological therapy im-proved about equally, and Murphy et al. found that a combination of the two was neither more nor less effective than either alone. Figure 22.4 gives the re-sults from the Murphy et al. study, in which psychological therapy alone and in combination with tricyclics or placebo was compared with tricyclics alone. The two outcome measures used are standard self-report scales for depres-sion, the Beck Depression Inventory and the Hamilton Rating Scale, in which high scores reflect more depressive symptoms.

Regardless of the therapeutic method employed, all patients improved about the same degree and at the same rate. In discussing similar findings from another study, Simons et al. (1984) argue that either psychological therapy or medication provides a point of entry into the loosely related cognitive and veg-etative functions. We admit that this argument is hardly more than a restate-ment of the data; nevertheless, this important problem deserves more atten-tion than it has received thus far.

We hesitate to suggest that expectancies such as placebo effects are solely responsible for the resemblance between pharmacological and psychological therapy because this requires expectancy effects to be precisely the same re-gardless of therapeutic method used. Follow-up of these patients has indicated that psychological therapy was associated with fewer relapses than drug ther-apy, however (Simons et al., 1986). The study suggests that new exacerbations of depressive symptoms cause patients who had been in psychological therapy to reinstitute the coping strategies that they had learned earlier. Drug patients had not learned these strategies, and therefore they returned for more medi-cation.

Schizophrenia   Although the efficacy of neuroleptics for the positive symp-toms of schizophrenia is only rarely disputed, there is less clarity about the combination of drugs and psychological therapy. Since low-stress environ-

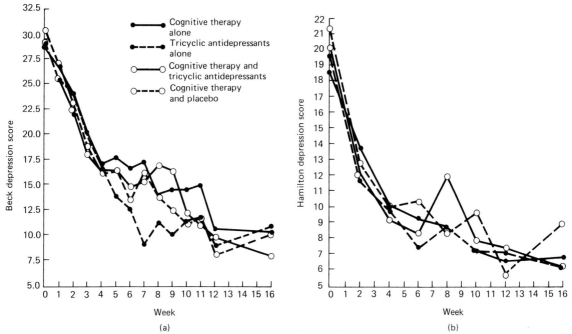

FIGURE 22.4 (a) Mean Beck Depression Inventory scores for four treatment groups over sixteen weeks. (From G. E. Murphy, A. D. Simons, R. D., Wetzel, & P. J. Lustman. Cognitive therapy and pharmacotherapy. *Archives of General Psychiatry, 41,* 33–41. Copyright © 1984, American Medical Association. (b) Mean Hamilton Rating Scale Depression scores for four treatment groups over sixteen weeks. (From G. E. Murphy, A. D. Simons, R. D., Wetzel, & P. J. Lustman. Cognitive therapy and pharmacotherapy. *Archives of General Psychiatry, 41,* 33–41. Copyright © 1984, American Medical Association.

ments seem to be associated with lower relapse rates (see Falloon & Liberman, 1983), psychotherapeutic inoculation against stress should result in even more benefit. Nowadays, schizophrenics must live under artificially restrictive conditions in order to deter relapse. Scattered findings suggest that combined therapies may be more effective for treating schizophrenia than either psychothrapy or drug therapy alone (Falloon & Liberman, 1983).

Panic and Agoraphobia Panic and agoraphobia appear to respond to different kinds of therapeutic approaches. Antidepressants and benzodiazepines seem to reduce the frequency of panic attacks, and their discontinuation often leads to relapse. On the other hand, these drugs do not substantially reduce the frequency of agoraphobic avoidance. Exposure therapy, while of less utility for panic, does seem to be effective for agoraphobic avoidance (Marks, 1987).

Apparently, behavioral therapy also enables patients to cope with problems arising after treatment has been completed. One might expect that combining the two forms of treatment—drugs for panic and exposure for avoidance—might produce the best overall outcomes (Telch, 1988).

ELECTROCONVULSIVE THERAPY

People never come to mental health professionals because of a dysfunctional physiological system (for example, an overactive hypothalamus, a defective frontal lobe, a deficiency of a neurotransmitter). Rather they come because of distress and deficient or disorganized behavior. If physiological impairments are discovered and successfully corrected, we are inclined to believe that the physical condition was the root of the mental problem. This is a perfectly reasonable inference, but without clear correspondences between physiological and mental impairments, the inference is empirical only and not based on a sound theory. Electroconvulsive therapy (ECT) is a good example of an empirically successful treatment lacking a rational theory for its effectiveness.

History

Convulsive therapies had their origins in the observation that mental patients would incidentally lose their symptoms following a spontaneous seizure. In 1934 von Meduna deliberately induced convulsions in mental patients by injecting camphor in oil. Later he switched to a synthetic camphor (Metrazol) because the timing of the convulsion could be better controlled. These and other chemical inductions of seizures have now been replaced by ECT because of fewer medical complications, though it is doubtful that the chemically induced seizures were less effective.

ECT was first introduced in Italy in 1938 by Cerletti and Bini, with widespread use in the United States almost from the beginning. Much controversy has surrounded its application, in part because it was originally called electroshock therapy, but also because the violent seizures produced were quite frightening. The early history of ECT is lamentably laden with excess and misuse. Patients were given too many treatments, electrical currents were often poorly controlled, oxygenation and sedation were not employed, and the convulsion itself was frightening. Even in the modern era, ECT is frequently misadministered (see Weiner, 1984).

Nowadays the oxygenated patient is sedated and a paralysis-inducing muscle relaxant is injected. Electrodes placed bilaterally or unilaterally at various locations around the skull permit an electric current to be passed for about a half second. In the absence of muscle relaxants, this immediately produces a grand mal convulsion consisting of a tonic phase in which the patient stiffens for about ten seconds followed by a clonic phase composed of alternating stiffenings and relaxations lasting for another forty seconds.

Since the introduction of muscle relaxants to prevent bone fractures, the convulsive manifestations of the seizure are hardly apparent, though there is a slight flexion of the feet. After the seizure has stopped a short period of anoxia occurs because spontaneous breathing is temporarily lost—hence the oxygen respirator. Early versions of ECT did not administer oxygen, and it is quite possible that unnecessary brain damage sometimes resulted.

The patient regains consciousness in a few minutes but is in a clouded state for about a half hour, perhaps with nausea and headaches. If treatment is on an outpatient basis, patients can be taken home after an hour. Patients typically undergo a series of thrice-weekly treatments lasting two to four weeks.

Evaluation

Currently, more than 80 percent of patients receiving ECT have been diagnosed with depression (Weiner, 1984), the vast majority being drug-nonresponders, adverse responders, or in immediate danger because of suicidal or homicidal impulses. The remainder have been diagnosed as manic, schizophrenic, or schizoaffective.

Effectiveness   The short-term efficacy of ECT for depression is not in much dispute. More than 80 percent of depressed drug-nonresponders show rapid mood improvements with ECT (DeCarolis et al., 1964). Equally clear, however, is that while ECT often produces a speedy remission, it is not a cure. Comparisons of depressives on ECT, drugs, and/or placebos reveal a substantial initial advantage for ECT, but six or eight months later the groups are not discernibly different (Clinical Research Centre, 1984). The difference vanishes because the non-ECT patients receive other forms of therapy in the interim or spontaneously improve, or the ECT patients relapse. ECT is nevertheless useful for obtaining relatively quick improvements in a patient's mood and is widely used when a suicide attempt seems imminent.

ECT increases hypothalamic activation for selected hormones, and limbic arousal may be important in producing mood changes. However, the fact that the treatment excites so many brain areas makes it difficult to tell how the treatment works.

Adverse Effects   Assertions that ECT causes brain damage and memory impairments are probably the main reason that ECT is typically a treatment of last resort. Roger Breggin, a vociferous opponent of all biological therapies, asks:

> What is the improvement seen following ECT [electroconvulsive treatment]? It is the direct effect of the acute organic brain syndrome, which not only blunts patients' memory and awareness of their problems, but produces a corresponding artificial apathy or euphoria. . . . The nurses . . . notes on the ward, however, will show that the patient is no longer able to focus attention, remember everyday details, or carry out complex tasks. Why doesn't the cure last? Because the gross effects gradually subside, and as the patients' brain function approximates normal again, their problem again becomes apparent (Breggin, 1984, p. 25).

Acute EEG slowing and psychological impairments suggest that ECT produces an organic delirium for several days with perhaps minor signs of memory loss for as long as three months. Initially, patients show confusion, disorientation, and amnesia for the events around the time of the ECT. While the confusion and disorientation rapidly dissipate, some amnesia may remain. It is not the durable loss of memory for the ECT itself that sustains the controversy, but the question of more generalized memory loss.

Most of the evidence for the permanent brain damage argument stems from evocative case histories and uncontrolled studies. Controlled studies reveal no evidence of sustained or serious memory impairment aside from the events surrounding the ECT itself (Fink, 1984; Weiner, 1984). Defenders of ECT suggest that the depressed are prone to exaggerate real or imagined deficiencies. These defenders are in an awkward position, however, because it is impossible to prove that something does not cause brain damage; after all, a more sensitive test might reveal a previously undetected impairment.

PERFECTABILITY THROUGH THERAPY?

This chapter has focused on the evaluation of therapy for a large variety of disorders, but what about therapeutic interventions for everyday depressive thoughts and dissatisfying feelings that life promises more than it delivers? For a variety of historical and economic reasons, Americans are perhaps overly optimistic about achieving improvement. We have many times our share of therapists and self-help books purveying expectations for a more joyous and fulfilling life. This is not just money-making flim-flam by the mental health community, for therapists themselves are among the biggest consumers.

Some therapists are grandiose about the prospects for psychotherapy. Even a former president of the American Psychiatric Association has said that "...no less than the entire world is a proper catchment area for present-day psychiatry, and psychiatry need not be appalled by the magnitude of the task" (in Zilbergeld, 1983, p. 91). Zilbergeld points out that "what attracts most people are promises of personal change—radiant health, peace of mind, better communication and relationships, more satisfying sex, development of potentials, and an end to addiction and bad feeling, and, in a word, happiness" (p. 6).

We have no quarrel with utopian aspirations; indeed, many even benefit from therapies with no scientific basis. To learn that others have similar problems, or at least that they understand, may provide welcome relief. But consumers should know that even proven psychotherapies rarely warrant extravagant claims made by charismatic therapists or enthusiastic clients. This is illustrated by those who go from one therapy to another as a way of life, proclaiming the latest to be just what was needed. That one therapy after another has been sought out suggests quite the opposite conclusion, namely, that none has done the job. Claims of modest efficacy usually are more realistic.

SUMMARY

This chapter concentrates on the evaluation of treatment, discussing only a few of the available therapies for mental disorders. The exclusively psychological therapies, psychodynamic, behavioral, and cognitive, each has advocates who often claim more than their therapies can deliver. Distressed individuals coming to a therapist are usually demoralized, having exhausted their own internal coping resources. The therapist provides solace by offering the possibility that treatment may be effective. This often has the immediate positive effect of reducing the demoralization that had accentuated the seriousness of other debilities.

Most behavioral therapists pragmatically focus on symptoms rather than hypothetical psychopathology; according to them, little is gained by going beneath the surface. Cognitive therapists are somewhat closer to their dynamic brethren, believing that the individual's understanding of the situation figures importantly in both etiology and treatment. Dynamic therapists treat symptoms as expressions of underlying conflict, emphasizing the need to free the individual from conflict, especially of infantile origin, before substantial personal change can occur.

Despite the often vast theoretical chasms among therapies, large differences in therapeutic efficacy are difficult to demonstrate. Overall, behaviorally oriented therapies (including cognitive therapy) are slightly more effective. The average individual after therapy exceeds about 80 percent of untreated controls, indicating a modest degree of therapeutic efficacy.

One must also consider, however, the efficacy of therapy with respect to achieving normal function. Here the results are not quite so positive. It seems clear that seriously disturbed patients—for example, psychopaths or schizophrenics—still have a long way to go before achieving normalcy. This is true whether therapy is psychological or pharmacological. If therapies cannot cure, they at least often result in improved functioning and decreased rates of relapse, themselves worthy accomplishments.

BIBLIOGRAPHY

Aalpoel, P. J., & Lewis, D. J. (1984). Dissociative disorders. In H. E. Adams & P. B. Sutker (Eds.), *Comprehensive handbook of psychopathology* (pp. 223–249). New York: Plenum.

Abel, G. (1984, October). Precautions against child molesters. *Physician & Patient, 12–17.*

Abel, G., Mittelman, M. S., Becker, J. V., Cunningham-Rathner, J., & Lucas, L. (1983, December). The characteristics of men who molest young children. Paper presented at the World Congress of Behavior Therapy, Washington, D. C.

Abel, G. G., Barlow, D. H., Blanchard, E. B. & Guild, D. (1977). The components of rapists' sexual arousal. *Archives of General Psychiatry, 34,* 895–903.

Abeles, M., & Schilder, P. (1935). Psychogenic loss of personal identity. *Archives of Neurology and Psychiatry, 34,* 587–604.

Abramovicz, H. K., & Richardson, S. A. (1975). Epidemiology of severe mental retardation in children. *American Journal of Mental Deficiency, 80,* 18–39.

Abramowitz, S. I. (1986). Psychosocial outcomes of sex reassignment surgery. *Journal of Consulting and Clinical Psychology, 54,* 183–189.

Abrams, R., Taylor, M. A., & Gaztanaga, P. (1974). Manic-depressive illness and paranoid schizophrenia. A phenomenologic, family history, and treatment-response study. *Archives of General Psychiatry, 31,* 640–642.

Abramson, L. Y., Seligman, M. E. P., & Teasdale, J. D. (1978). Learned helplessness in humans: Critique and reformulation. *Journal of Abnormal Psychology, 87,* 49–74.

Abse, W. (1982). Multiple personality. In A. Roy (Ed.), *Hysteria* (pp. 165–184). Chichester, England: Wiley.

Achenbach, T. M. (1982). *Developmental psychopathology* (2nd ed.). New York: Wiley.

Achenbach, T. M., & Edelbrock, C. S. (1981). Behavioral problems and competencies reported by parents of normal and disturbed children aged four through sixteen.

Monographs of the Society for Research in Child Development, Vol. *8,* Serial No. 188.

Adler, A. (1927). *Practice and theory of individual psychology.* New York: Harcourt.

Adler, L. E., Waldo, M. C., & Freedman, R. (1985). Neurophysiologic studies of sensory gating in schizophrenia: Comparison of auditory and visual responses. *Biological Psychiatry, 20,* 1284–1296.

Akiskal, H. (1979). A biobehavioral approach to depression. In R. A. Depue (Ed.), *The psychobiology of the depressive disorders: Implications for the effects of stress* (pp. 409–437). New York: Academic Press.

Akiskal, H. S. (1985). Anxiety: Definition, relationship to depression, and proposal for an integrative model. In A. H. Tuma & J. D. Maser (Eds.), *Anxiety and the anxiety disorders* (pp. 787–797). Hillsdale, N. J.: Laurence Erlbaum.

Akiskal, H. S., Bitar, A. H., Puzantian, V. R., Rosenthal, T. L., & Walker, P. W. (1978). The nosological status of neurotic depression: A prospective three- to four-year follow-up examination in light of the primary-secondary and unipolar-bipolar dichotomies. *Archives of General Psychiatry, 35,* 756–766.

Akiskal, H. S., Djenderdejian, A. H., Rosenthal, R. H., & Khani, M. K. (1977). Cyclothymic disorder: Validating criteria for inclusion in the bipolar affective group. *American Journal of Psychiatry, 134,* 1227–1233.

Akiskal, H. S., Yerevanian, B. I., Davis. G. C., King, D., & Lemmi, H. (1985). The nosological status of borderline personality: A clinical and polysomnographic study. *American Journal of Psychiatry, 142,* 192–198.

Al-lssa, I. (1982). *Culture and psychopathology.* Baltimore: University Park Press.

Albert, M. S., Butters, N., & Levin, J. (1979). Temporal gradients in the retrograde amnesia of patients with alcoholic Korsakoff's disease. *Archives of Neurology, 36,* 211–216.

Aldenhoff, J. B., & Lux, H. D. (1981). Effects of lithium on calcium-dependent processes in nerve cells. In C. Perris, G. Struwe, & B. Jansson (Eds.), *Biological psychiatry 1981* (pp. 649–652). Amsterdam: Elsevier/North-Holland.

Alldridge, P. (1979). Hospitals, madhouses, and asylums: Cycles in the care of the insane. *British Journal of Psychiatry, 134,* 321–334.

Allen, M. G. (1976). Twin studies of affective illness. *Archives of General Psychiatry, 33,* 1476–1478.

Allport, G. W. (1937). *Personality: A psychological interpretation.* New York: Henry Holt.

Alpert, M., & Friedhoff, A. J. (1980). An un-dopamine hypothesis of schizophrenia. *Schizophrenia Bulletin, 6,* 387–392.

Altman, J. (1987). Morphological and behavioral markers of environmentally induced retardation of brain development: An animal model. *Environmental Health Perspectives, 74,* 153–168.

Altman, J. H., & Wittenborn, J. R. (1980). Depression-prone personality in women. *Journal of Abnormal Psychology, 89,* 303–308.

Ambelas, A. (1987). Life events and mania: A special relationship? *British Journal of Psychiatry, 150,* 235–240.

American Psychiatric Association (APA) (1980). *Diagnostic and statistical manual of mental disorders* (3rd ed.) (*DSM-III*). Washington, D. C.: American Psychiatric Association.

American Psychiatric Association (APA) (1987). *Diagnostic and statistical manual of mental disorders* (3rd ed., Revised) (*DSM-III-R*). Washington, D. C.: American Psychiatric Association.

APA Task Force on Laboratory Tests in Psychiatry (1987). The dexamethasone suppression test. An overview of its current status in psychiatry. *American Journal of Psychiatry, 144,* 1253–1262.

Anderson, G. M., & Hoshino, Y. (1987). Neurochemical studies of autism. In D. J. Cohen & A. M. Donnellan (Eds.), *Handbook of autism and pervasive developmental disorders* (pp. 166–191). New York: Wiley.

Anderson, K. E. Lytton, H., Romney, D. M. (1986). Mothers' interactions with normal and conduct-disordered boys. Who affects whom? *Developmental Psychology, 22,* 604–609.

Andreasen, N. C. (1979). Thought, language, and communication disorders: II. Diagnostic significance. *Archives of General Psychiatry, 36,* 1325–1330.

Andreasen, N. C. (1980). Posttraumatic stress disorder. In H. I. Kaplan, A. M. Freedman, & B. J. Sadock (Eds.), *Comprehensive textbook of psychiatry/III* (3rd Edition) (Vol. 2., pp. 1517–1525). Baltimore: Williams & Wilkins.

Andreasen, N. C. (1982). Negative symptoms in schizophrenia: Definition and reliability. *Archives of General Psychiatry, 39,* 784–788.

Andreasen, N. C. (1986). Scale for the assessment of thought, language, and communication (TLC). *Schizophrenia Bulletin, 12,* 473–481.

Andreasen, N. C., & Grove, W. (1979). The relationship between schizophrenic language, manic language, and aphasia. In J. Gruzelier & P. Flor-Henry (Eds.), *Hemisphere asymmetries of function in psychopathology* (pp. 373–390). Amsterdam: Elsevier/North-Holland Biomedical Press.

Andreasen, N. C., & Olsen, S. (1982). Negative and positive schizophrenia: Definition and validation. *Archives of General Psychiatry, 39,* 789–794.

Andrews, G., & Harvey, R. (1981). Does psychotherapy benefit neurotic patients? A reanalysis of the Smith, Glass, & Miller data. *Archives of General Psychiatry, 38,* 1202–1208.

Angst, J., Felder, W., & Frey, R. (1979). The course of unipolar and bipolar affective disorders. In M. Schon & E. Stromgren (Eds.), *Origin, prevention and treatment of affective disorders* (pp. 215–226). London: Academic Press.

Angst, J., Felder, W., & Lohmeyer, B. (1979). Schizoaffective disorders: Results of genetic investigations, I. *Journal of Affective Disorders, 1,* 139–153.

Angst, J., Grigo, H., & Lanz, M. (1981). A genetic validation of diagnostic concepts for schizo-affective psychoses. In C. Perris, G. Struwe, & B. Jansson (Eds.), *Biological psychiatry, 1981* (pp. 486–495). Amsterdam: Elsevier/North-Holland.

Angyal, A. (1965). *Neurosis and treatment: A holistic theory.* New York: Viking.

Antelman, S. M., & Caggiula, A. R. (1980). Stress-induced behavior: Chemotherapy without drugs. In J. M. Davidson & R. J. Davidson (Eds.), *The psychobiology of consciousness* (pp. 65–104). New York: Plenum.

Arana, G. W., Baldessarini, R. J., & Ornsteen, M. (1985). The dexamethasone suppression test for diagnosis and prognosis in psychiatry: Commentary and review. *Archives of General Psychiatry, 42,* 1193–1204.

Arlow, J. A. (1984). Psychoanalysis. In R. J. Corsini (Ed.), *Current psychotherapies* (pp. 14–55). Itasca, IL: F. E. Peacock Publishers, Inc.

Arnhoff, F. N. (1975). Social consequences of policy toward mental illness. *Science, 188,* 1277–1281.

Asarnow, R. F., & MacCrimmon, D. J. (1978). Residual performance deficit in chronically remitted schizophrenics: A marker of schizophrenia? *Journal of Abnormal Psychology, 87,* 597–608.

Asarnow, R. F., Steffy, R. A., MacCrimmon, D. J., & Cleghorn, J. M. (1978). An attentional assessment of foster children at risk for schizophrenia. In L. C. Wynne, R. L. Cromwell, & S. Matthysse (Eds.), *The nature of schizophrenia: New Approaches to research and treatment* (pp. 339–358). New York: Wiley.

Astrachan, B. M., Brauer, L., Harrow, M., & Schwartz, C. (1974). Symptomatic outcomes in schizophrenia. *Archives of General Psychiatry, 31,* 155–160.

Ayllon, T. (1963). Intensive treatment of psychotic behavior by stimulus satiation and food reinforcement. *Behavior Research and Therapy, 1,* 53–61.

Baker, S. L. (1980). Traumatic war disorders. In H. I. Kaplan, A. M. Freedman, & B. J. Sadock (Eds.), *Comprehensive textbook of psychiatry/III* (3rd Edition) (Vol. 2, pp. 1829–1842). Baltimore: Williams & Wilkins.

Baker, T. B. Morse, E., & Sherman, J. E. (1987). The motivation to use drugs: A psychobiological analysis of urges. In P. C. Rivers (Ed.), *Nebraska symposium on motivation, 1986: Alcohol and addictive behavior* (pp. 257–322). Lincoln, Nebraska: The University of Nebraska Press.

Bakwin, H. (1971). Enuresis in twins. *American Journal of Diseases of Children, 121,* 222–225.

Baldessarini, R. J. (1975). The basis for amine hypotheses in affective disorders. *Archives of General Psychiatry, 32,* 1087–1093.

Bale, R. N., Van Stone, W. W., Kuldau, J. M., Engelsing, T. M. J., Elashoff, R. M., & Zarcone, V. P., Jr. (1980). Therapeutic communities vs. methadone maintenance. *Archives of General Psychiatry, 37,* 179–193.

Bandura, A. (1968). A social learning interpretation of psychological functions. In P. London & D. Rosenhan (Eds.), *Foundations of abnormal psychology* (pp. 293–344). New York: Holt, Rinehart & Winston.

Bandura, A. (1986). *Social foundations of thought and action: A social cognitive theory.* Englewood Cliffs, N. J.: Prentice-Hall.

Bandura, A., & Walters, R. H. (1959). *Adolescent aggression.* New York: Ronald Press.

Barber, T. X. (1969). *Hypnosis: A scientific approach.* New York: Van Nostrand Reinhold.

Barbizet, J. (1970). *Human memory and its pathology.* San Francisco: W. H. Freeman.

Barlow, D. H. (1985). The dimensions of anxiety disorders. In A. H. Tuma & J. D. Maser (Eds.), *Anxiety and the anxiety disorders* (pp. 479–500). Hillsdale, N. J.: Lawrence Erlbaum.

Barlow, D. H. (1988) *Anxiety and its disorders: The nature and treatment of anxiety and panic.* New York: Guilford.

Barnett, P. A., & Gotlib, I. H. (1988). Psychosocial functioning and depression: Distinguishing among antecedents, concomitants, and consequences. *Psychological Bulletin, 104,* 97–126.

Baron, M., Risch, N., Hamburger, R., Mandel, B., Kushner, S. et al. (1987). Genetic linkage between X-chromosome markers and bipolar affective illness. *Nature, 326,* 289–292.

Barsky, A. J., Wyshak, G., & Klerman, G. L. (1986). Hypochondriasis: An evaluation of the DSM-III criteria in medical outpatients. *Archives of General Psychiatry, 43,* 493–500.

Bassett, A. S., McGillivray, B. C., Jones, B. D., & Pantzar, J. T. (1988, April 9). Partial trisomy chromosome 5 cosegregating with schizophrenia. *Lancet,* 799–801.

Bassuk, E. L. (1984, July). The homeless problem. *Scientific American, 251,* 40–45.

Bauman, M., & Kemper, T. L. (1985). Histoanatomic observations of the brain in early infantile autism. *Neurology, 35,* 866–874.

Beach, F. A. (1978). Cross-species comparisons and the human heritage. In F. A. Beach (Ed.), *Human sexuality in four perspectives* (pp. 296–316). Baltimore: Johns Hopkins University Press.

Bear, D. M., & Fedio, P (1977). Quantitative analysis of interictal behavior in temporal lobe epilepsy. *Archives of Neurology, 34,* 454–467.

Bebbington, P. E., Brugha, T., MacCarthy, B., Potter, J., Sturt, E., Wykes, T., & McGuffin, P. (1988). The Camberwell Collaborative Depression Study: I. Depressed probands: Adversity and the form of depression. *British Journal of Psychiatry, 152,* 754–765.

Beck, A. T. (1967). *Depression: Clinical, experimental, and theoretical aspects.* New York: Harper & Row (Hoeber Medical Division).

Beck, A. T., & Emery, G. (1985). *Anxiety disorders and phobias: A cognitive perspective.* New York: Basic Books.

Beck, A. T., & Greenberg, R. L. (1977). Depression: Clinical aspects. In A. Frazer & A. Winokur (Eds.), *Biological bases of psychiatric disorders* (pp. 199–205). New York: Spectrum.

Beck, A. T., Steer, R. A., Kovacs, M., & Garrison, B. (1985). Hopelessness and eventual suicide: A 10-year study of patients hospitalized with suicidal ideation. *American Journal of Psychiatry, 142,* 559–563.

Becker, E. (1973). *The denial of death.* New York: The Free Press.

Becker, J. V., Skinner, L. J., & Abel, G. G. (1983). Sequelae of sexual assault: The survivor's perspective. In J. G. Greer & I. R. Stuart (Eds.), *The sexual aggressor: Current perspectives on treatment* (pp. 240–266). New York: Van Nostrand Reinhold Co.

Beers, C. W. (1981). *A mind that found itself: An autobiography* (1907). Pittsburgh: University of Pittsburgh.

Beidel, D., & Turner, S. M. (1986). A critique of the theoretical bases of cognitive-behavioral theories and therapy. *Clinical Psychology Review, 6,* 177–197.

Bell, A. P., & Weinberg, M. S. (1978). *Homosexualities: A study of diversity among men and women.* New York: Simon & Schuster.

Bell, A. P., Weinberg, M. S., & Hammersmith, S. K. (1981). *Sexual preference: Its development in men and women.* Bloomington: Indiana University Press.

Bell, R. Q. (1968). A reinterpretation of the direction of effects in studies of socialization. *Psychological Review, 75,* 81–95.

Bellak, L. (1954). *The Thematic Apperception Test and the Children's Apperception Test in clinical use.* New York: Grune & Stratton.

Bellinger, D., Leviton, A., Waternaux, C., Needleman, H., & Rabinowitz, M. (1987). Longitudinal analyses of prenatal and postnatal lead exposure and early cognitive development. *New England Journal of Medicine, 316,* 1037–1043.

Belsher, G., & Costello, C. G. (1988). Relapse after recovery from unipolar depression. A critical review. *Psychological Bulletin. 104,* 84–96.

Bemis, K. M. (1978). Current approaches to the etiology and treatment of anorexia nervosa. *Psychological Bulletin, 85,* 593–617.

Benes, F. M., Majocha, R., Bird, E. D., & Marotta, C. A. (1987). Increased vertical axon numbers in cingulate cortex of schizophrenics. *Archives of General Psychiatry, 44,* 1017–1021.

Benson, D. F., Miller, B. L. & Signer, S. F. (1986). Dual personality associated with epilepsy. *Archives of Neurology, 43,* 471–474.

Berg, I. (1984). School refusal. *British Journal of Hospital Medicine, 31,* 59–62.

Berger, M., Reimann, D., Höchli, D., & Spiegel, R. (1989) The cholinergic rapid eye movement sleep induction test with RS-86: State or trait marker of depression? *Archives of General Psychiatry, 46,* 421–428.

Berger, P. A., & Tinklenberg, J. R. (1977). Treatment of abusers of alcohol and other addictive drugs. In J. D. Barchas, P. A. Berger, R. D. Ciaranello, & G. R. Elliot (Eds.), *Psychopharmacology: From theory to practice* (pp. 355–385). New York: Oxford University Press.

Bergin, E. C. (1971). The evaluation of therapeutic outcomes. In A. E. Bergin & S. L. Garfield (Eds.), *The handbook of psychotherapy and behavior change.* New York: Wiley.

Bergin, A. E., & Lambert, M. J. (1978). The evaluation of therapeutic outcomes. In S. L. Garfield & A. E. Bergin (Eds.), *Handbook of psychotherapy and behavior change* (pp. 139–189). New York: Wiley.

Berlin, F. S. (1983). Sexual offenders: A biomedical perspective and a status report on biomedical treatment. In J. G. Greer & I. R. Stuart (Eds.), *The sexual aggressor: Current perspectives on treatment* (pp. 83–123). New York: Van Nostrand Reinhold Co.

Berman, J. S., & Wenzlaff, R. M. (1983). The impact of therapist expectancies on the outcome of psychotherapy. Paper presented at the Annual Meeting of the American Psychological Association.

Bernheim, K. F., & Lewine, R. J. (1979). *Schizophrenia: Symptoms, causes, treatment.* New York: Norton.

Berntson, G. G., Tuber, D. S., Ronca, A. E., & Bachman, D. S. (1983). The decerebrate human: Associative learning. *Experimental Neurology, 81,* 77–88.

Bertelsen, A. (1979). A Danish twin study of manic-depressive disorders. In M. Schou & E. Stromgren (Eds.), *Origin, prevention and treatment of affective disorders* (pp. 227–239). London: Academic Press.

Bertelsen, A., Harvald, B., & Hauge, M. (1977). A Danish twin study of manic-depressive disorders. *British Journal of Psychiatry, 130,* 330–351.

Bieber, I. *Homosexuality* (1964). New York: Basic Books.

Birch, H. G. (1964). The problem of brain damage. In H. G. Birch (Ed.) *Brain damage in children* (pp. 3–12). Baltimore: Williams & Wilkins.

Birnbaum, K. (1914). *Die psychopathischen verbrecker.* Leipzig: Thieme.

Blakemore, C. (1977). *Mechanics of the mind.* Cambridge: Cambridge University Press.

Blanchard, R., Steiner, B. W., & Clemmensen, L. H. (1985). Gender dysphoria, gender reorientation, and the clinical management of transsexualism. *Journal of Consulting and Clinical Psychology, 53,* 295–304.

Bland, R. C., Newman, S. C., & Orne, H. (1986). Recurrent and nonrecurrent depression: A family study. *Archives of General Psychiatry, 43,* 1085–1089.

Blane, H. T. (1979). Middle-aged alcoholics and young drinkers. In H. T. Blane & M. E. Chafetz (Eds.), *Youth, alcohol and social policy* (pp. 5–38). New York: Plenum Press.

Blashfield, R. K. (1984). *The classification of psychopathology: Neo-Kraepelinian and quantitative approaches.* New York: Plenum.

Blashfield, R. K. (1986). Structural approaches to classification. In T. Millon & G. L. Klerman (Eds.), *Contemporary directions in psychopathology: Toward the DMS-IV* (pp. 363–380). New York: The Guilford Press.

Blehar, M. C., & Rosenthal, N. E. (1989). Seasonal affective disorders and phototherapy: Report of a National Institute of Mental Health-sponsored workshop. *Archives of General Psychiatry, 46,* 496–474.

Bleuler, E. (1950). *Dementia praecox or the group of schizophrenias* (1911). New York: International Universities Press.

Bleuler, M. E. (1978). The long-term course of schizophrenic psychoses. In L. C. Wynne, R. L. Cromwell, & S. Matthysse (Eds.), *The nature of schizophrenia: New approaches to research and treatment* (pp. 631–636). New York: Wiley.

Bliss, E. L. (1980). Multiple personalities: A report of 14 cases with implications for schizophrenia and hysteria. *Archives of General Psychiatry, 37,* 1388–1397.

Bliss, E. L. (1984a). A symptom profile of patients with multiple personalities, including MMPI results. *Journal of Nervous and Mental Disease, 172,* 197–202.

Bliss, E. L. (1984b). Hysteria and hypnosis. *Journal of Nervous and Mental Disease, 172,* 203–206.

Bliss, E. L. (1984c). Spontaneous self-hypnosis in multiple personality disorder. In B. G. Braun (Ed.), Symposium on multiple personality. *Psychiatric Clinics of North America, 7,* 135–148.

Blodgett, H. C. (1929). The effect of the introduction of reward upon the maze performance of rats. *University of California Publications in Psychology, 4,* 113–135.

Bloom, F. E., Lazerson, A., & Hofstadter, L. (1985). *Brain, mind, and behavior,* New York: W. H. Freeman.

Blumer, D. (1975). Temporal lobe epilepsy and its psychiatric significance. In D. F. Benson & D. Blumer (Ed.), *Psychiatric aspects of neurological disease.* (pp. 171–197). New York: Grune & Stratton.

Blumer, D., & Benson, D. F. (1975). Personality changes with frontal and temporal lobe lesions. In D. F. Benson & D. Blumer (Eds.), *Psychiatric aspects of neurological disease* (pp.. 151–170). New York: Grune & Stratton.

Bockoven, J.S. (1963). *Moral treatment in American psychiatry.* New York: Springer.

Bohman, M., Cloninger, C. R., Sigvardsson, S., & von Knorring, A-L. (1982). Predisposition to petty criminality in Swedish adoptees. I. Genetic and environmental heterogeneity. *Archives of General Psychiatry, 39,* 1233–1241.

Bohman, M., Cloninger, C. R., von Knorring, A-L., & Sigvardsson, S. (1984). An adoption study of somatoform disorders: III. Cross-fostering analysis and genetic relationship to alcoholism and criminality. *Archives of General Psychiatry, 41,* 872–878.

Bolles, R. C. (1979). The nonextinction of fear: Operation bootstrap. (Open peer commentary on a paper by Eysenck). *The Behavioral and Brain Sciences, 2,* 167–168.

Bond, T. C. (1980). Recognition of acute delerious mania. *Archives of General Psychiatry, 37,* 553–554.

Bonn, J. A., Readhead, C. P., & Timmons, B. H. (1984). Enhanced adaptive behavioural response in agoraphobic patients pretreated with breathing retraining. *The Lancet, 8404,* 665–669.

Boor, M. (1982). The multiple personality epidemic: Additional cases and inferences regarding diagnosis, etiology, dynamics, and treatment. *Journal of Nervous and Mental Disease, 170,* 302–304.

Boorstein, D. J. (1983). *The discoverers.* New York: Random House.

Boring, E. G. (1950). *A history of experimental psychology.* New York: Appleton-Century-Croft.

Borland, B. L., & Heckman, H. K. (1976). Hyperactive boys and their brothers. *Archives of General Psychiatry, 33,* 669–675.

Bortner, M., & Birch, H. G. (1970). Cognitive capacity and cognitive competence. *American Journal of Mental Deficiency, 74,* 735–744.

Boss, M. (1949). *Meaning and content of sexual perversions.* New York: Grune & Stratton.

Bouchard, T. J. Jr., & McGue, M. (1981). Familial studies of intelligence: A review. *Science, 212,* 1055–1059.

Bower, G. H. (1981). Mood and memory. *American Psychologist, 36,* 129–148.

Bowers, K. S. (1984). On being unconsciously influenced and informed. In K. S. Bowers & D. Meichenbaum (Eds.), *The unconscious reconsidered* (pp. 227–272). New York: Wiley.

Bowers, M. K., Brecher-Marer, S., Newton, B. W. Piotrowski, Z., Spyer, T. C., Taylor, W. S., & Watkins, J. G. (1971). Therapy of multiple personality. *International Journal of Clinical and Experimental Hypnosis, 19,* 57–65.

Bowlby, J. (1969). *Attachment and loss, Vol. 1: Attachment.* New York: Basic Books.

Bowlby, J. (1980). *Attachment and loss, Vol. 3: Loss, sadness, and depression.* New York: Basic Books.

Boyd, J. H., Burke, J. D. Jr., Gruenberg, E., Holzer, C. E., III, Rae, D. S. et al. (1984). Exclusion criteria of DSM-III. *Archives of General Psychiatry, 41,* 983–989.

Boyd, J. H., & Weissman, M. M. (1982). *Epidemiology.* In E. S. Paykel (Ed.), *Handbook of affective disorders* (pp. 109–125). New York: Guilford Press.

Bradley, C. (1937). The behavior of children receiving benzedrine. *American Journal of Psychiatry, 94,* 577–585.

Braff, D. L., & Saccuzzo, D. P. (1985). The time course of information-processing deficits in schizophrenia. *American Journal of Psychiatry, 142,* 170–174.

Breed, W., & Huffine, C. L. (1979). Sex differences in suicide among older white Americans: A role and developmental approach. In O. J. Kaplan (Ed.), *Psychopathology of aging* (pp. 289–309). New York: Academic Press.

Breggin, P. R. (1983). *Psychiatric drugs: Hazards to the brain.* New York: Springer Publishing Co.

Breggin, P. R. (1984). *Electroshock therapy and brain damage: The acute organic brain syndrome as treatment. The Behavioral and Brain Sciences, 7,* 24–25.

Breier, A., Charney, D. S., & Heninger, G. R. (1984). Major depression in patients with agoraphobia and panic disorder. *Archives of General Psychiatry, 41,* 1129–1135.

Breier, A., Charney, D. S., & Heninger, G. R. (1986). Agoraphobia with panic attacks: Development, diagnostic stability, and course of illness. *Archives of General Psychiatry, 43,* 1029–1036.

Brenner, C. (1955). *An elementary textbook of psychoanalysis.* New York: Doubleday/ Anchor, 1957 (Originally published by International Universities Press).

Brewin, C. R. (1985). Depression and causal attributions: What is their relation? *Psychological Bulletin, 98,* 297–309.

Brickman, A. S., McManus, M., Grapentine, W. L., & Alessi, N. (1984). Neuropsychological assessment of seriously delinquent adolescents. *Journal of American Academy of Child Psychiatry, 23,* 453–457.

Brill, A. A. (1938). *The basic writings of Sigmund Freud.* New York: Modern Library.

Bromet, E., Harrow, M., & Kasl, S. (1974). Premorbid functioning and outcome in schizophrenics and nonschizophrenics. *Archives of General Psychiatry, 30,* 203–207.

Brown, G., Chadwick, O., Shaffer, D., Rutter, M. & Traub, M. (1981). A prospective study of children with head injuries: III. Psychiatric sequelae. *Psychological Medicine, 11,* 63–78.

Brown, G. W. (1979). The social etiology of depression-London Studies. In R. Depue (Ed.), *The psychobiology of the depressive disorders: Implications for the effects of stress* (pp. 263–289). New York: Academic Press.

Brown, G. W., & Birley, J. L. T. (1968). Crises and life changes and the onset of schizophrenia. *Journal of Health and Social Behavior, 9,* 203–214.

Brown, G. W., Bone, M., Dalison, B., & Wing, J. K. (1966). *Schizophrenia and social care.* Maudsley Monograph No. 17. London: Oxford University Press.

Brown, G. W., Harris, T. O., & Copeland, J. R. (1977). Depression and loss. *British Journal of Psychiatry, 130,* 1–18.

Brown, R., & Herrnstein, R. J. (1975). *Psychology.* Boston: Little, Brown.

Browne, A., & Finkelhor, D. (1986). Impact of child sexual abuse: A review of the research. *Psychological Bulletin, 99,* 66–77.

Brownmiller, S. (1975). *Against our will: Men, women and rape.* New York: Simon & Schuster.

Bruch, H. (1978). *The golden cage: The enigma of anorexia nervosa.* Cambridge, MA: Harvard University Press.

Bryer, J. B., Nelson, B. A., Miller, J. B., & Krol, P. A. (1987). Childhood sexual and physical abuse as factors in adult psychiatric illness. *American Journal of Psychiatry, 144,* 1426–1430.

Buchsbaum, M. S., & Rieder, R. O. (1979). Biologic heterogeneity and psychiatric research. *Archives of General Psychiatry, 36,* 1163–1169.

Buglass, D., Clarke, J., Henderson, A. S., Kreitman, N., & Presley, A. S. (1977). A study of agoraphobic housewives. *Psychological Medicine, 7,* 73–86.

Burt, M. R. (1980). Cultural myths and supports for rape. *Journal of Personality and Social Psychology, 38,* 217–230.

Buss, A. (1966). *Psychopathology.* New York: Wiley.

Butcher, J. N., & Bemis, K. M. (1984). Abnormal behavior in cultural context. In H. E. Adams & P. B. Sutker (Eds.), *Comprehensive handbook of psychopathology* (pp. 111–139). New York: Plenum.

Butcher, J. N., & Finn, S. (1983). Objective personality assessment in clinical settings. In M. Hersen, A. E. Kazdin, & A. S. Bellack (Eds.), *The clinical psychology handbook* (pp. 329–344). New York: Pergamon.

Cadoret, R. J., Troughton, E., O'Gorman, T. W., & Heywood, E. (1986). An adoption study of genetic and environmental factors in drug abuse. *Archives of General Psychiatry, 43,* 1131–1136.

Caine, E. D. (1981). Pseudodementia. *Archives of General Psychiatry, 38,* 1359–1364.

Cameron, N. (1963). *Personality development and psychopathology.* Boston: Houghton Mifflin.

Cameron, N. S. (1938). Reasoning, regression and communication in schizophrenics. *Psychological Monographs, 50,* No. 1 (Whole No. 221).

Campbell, M., Small, A. M., Green, W. H., Jennings, S. J., Perry, R., Bennett, W. G., & Anderson, L. (1984). Behavioral efficacy of haloperidol and lithium carbonate: A comparison of hospitalized aggressive children with conduct disorder. *Archives of General Psychiatry, 41,* 650–656.

Campbell, S. B., & Werry, J. S. (1986). Attention deficit disorder (hyperactivity). In H. C. Quay & J. S. Werry (Eds.), *Psychopathological disorders of childhood* (3rd ed.) (pp. 111–155). New York: John Wiley & Sons.

Cannon, D. S., Baker, T. B., Gino, A., & Nathan, P. E. (1986). Alcohol-aversion therapy: relation between strength of aversion and abstinence. *Journal of Consulting and Clinical Psychology, 54,* 825–830.

Cannon, W. B. (1939). *The wisdom of the body.* New York: W. W. Norton & Co., Inc.

Cantwell, D. P., Sturzenberger, S., Burroughs, J., Salkin, B., & Green, J. K. (1977). Anorexia nervosa: An affective disorder? *Archives of General Psychiatry, 34,* 1087–1093.

Caporael, L. (1976). Ergotism: The satan loosed in Salem? *Science, 192,* 21–26.

Carey, G., & Gottesman, I. I. (1981). Twin and family studies of anxiety, phobic and obsessive disorders. In D. F. Klein & J. Rabkin (Eds.), *Anxiety: New research and changing concepts* (pp. 112–136). New York: Raven.

Carlson, N. R. (1980). *Physiology of behavior.* Boston: Allyn and Bacon.

Carpenter, W. T., Jr., Strauss, J. S., & Bartko, J. J. (1973). A flexible system for the identification of schizophrenia: A report from the W.H.O. International Pilot Study of Schizophrenia. *Science, 182,* 1275–1278.

Carpenter, W. T., Jr., Strauss, J. S., & Mulch, S. (1973). Are there pathognomonic symptoms in schizophrenia? An empiric investigation on Schneider's first rank symptoms. *Archives of General Psychiatry, 28,* 847–852.

Carpenter, W. T., Jr., & Stephens, J. H. (1979). An attempted integration of information relevant to schizophrenic subtypes. *Schizophrenia Bulletin, 5,* 490–506.

Carr, A. T. (1974). Compulsive neurosis: A review of the literature. *Psychological Bulletin, 81,* 311–318.

Carter, C. O. (1977). Multifactorial genetic disease. In V. A. McKusick & R. Claiborne (Eds.), *Medical genetics* (pp. 199–208). New York: Hospital Practice Publishing Co.

Casey, R., & Berman, J. S. (1985). The outcome of psychotherapy with children. *Psychological Bulletin, 98,* 388–400.

Chafetz, M. E. (1975). Alcoholism and alcoholic psychoses. In A. M. Freedman, H. I. Kaplan, & B. J. Sadock (Eds.). *Comprehensive textbook of psychiatry/II* (pp. 1331–1348). Baltimore: Williams and Wilkins Co.

Chambless, D. L. (1982). Characteristics of agoraphobics. In D. L. Chambless & A. J. Goldstein (Eds.), *Agoraphobia: Multiple perspectives on theory and treatment* (pp. 19–42). New York: Wiley-Interscience.

Chapman, J. (1966). The early symptoms of schizophrenia. *British Journal of Psychiatry, 112,* 225–251.

Chapman, L. J. (1958). Intrusion of associative responses into schizophrenic conceptual performance. *Journal of Abnormal and Social Psychology, 56,* 374–379.

Chapman, L. J., & Chapman, J. P. (1973). *Disordered thought in schizophrenia.* New York: Appleton-Century-Croft.

Chapman, L. J., Edell, W. S., & Chapman, J. P. (1980). Physical anhedonia, perceptual aberration, and psychosis proneness. *Schizophrenia Bulletin, 6,* 639–653.

Charney, D. S. (1982). Depression and agoraphobia: Chicken or egg? In R. L. DuPont (Ed.), *Phobia: A comprehensive summary of modern treatments* (pp. 126–132). New York: Bruner/Mazel.

Chodoff, P. (1974). The depressive personality: A critical review. In R. J. Friedman & M. M. Katz (Eds.), *The psychology of depression: Contemporary theory and research* (pp. 55–70). Washington, D. C.: V. H. Winston & Sons.

Chodoff, P., & Lyons, H. (1958). Hysteria, the hysterical personality and hysterical conversion. *American Journal of Psychiatry, 114,* 734–740.

Ciompi, L. (1980). Catamnestic long-term study on the course of life and aging of schizophrenics. *Schizophrenia Bulletin, 6,* 606–618.

Clarfield, A. M. (1988). The reversible dementias: Do they reverse? *Annals of Internal Medicine, 109,* 476–486.

Clarke, A. M., & Clarke, A. D. B. (1976). *Early experience: Myth and evidence.* New York: The Free Press.

Clayton, P. J. (1982). Bereavement. In E. S. Paykel (Ed.), *Handbook of affective disorders* (pp. 403–415). New York: Guilford Press.

Cleckley, H. (1950). *The mask of sanity.* St. Louis: Mosby.

Clement-Jones, V. & Besser, G. M. (1983). Clinical perspectives on opioid peptides. *British Medical Bulletin, 39,* 95–100.

Clinical Research Centre (1984). The Northwick Park ECT trial: Predictors of response to real and simulated ECT. *British Journal of Psychiatry, 144,* 227–237.

Cloninger, C. R. (1978). The link between hysteria and sociopathy: An integrative model of pathogenesis based on clinical, genetic, and neurophysiological observations. In H. Akiskal (Ed.), *Psychiatric diagnosis: Explorations of biological predictors* (pp. 189–218). New York: Spectrum Publications.

Cloninger, C. R. (1983). Antisocial behavior. In H. Hippius & G. Winokur (Eds.), *Clinical psychopharmacology* (pp. 33–370). Princeton, NJ: Excerpta Medica Publisher.

Cloninger, C. R. (1987). Neurogenetic adaptive mechanisms in alcoholism. *Science, 236,* 410–415.

Cloninger, C. R., Bohman, M., & Sigvardsson, S. (1981). Inheritance of alcohol abuse: Cross-fostering analysis of adopted men. *Archives of General Psychiatry, 38,* 861–868.

Cloninger, C. R., Christiansen, K. O., Reich, T., & Gottesman, I. I. (1978). Implications of sex differences in the prevalences of antisocial personality, alcoholism, and criminality. *Archives of General Psychiatry, 35,* 941–953.

Cloninger, C. R., & Gottesman, I. I. (1987). Genetic and environmental factors in antisocial behavior disorders. In S. A. Mednick & T. Moffitt (Eds.), *Biosocial bases of antisocial behavior* (pp. 92–109). New York: Cambridge University Press.

Cloninger, C. R., & Guze, S. B. (1970). Psychosomatic illness and female criminality: The role of sociopathy and hysteria in the antisocial woman. *American Journal of Psychiatry, 127,* 303–311.

Cloninger, C. R., Sigvardsson, S., von Knorring, A-L., & Bohman, M. (1984). An adoption study of somatoform disorders: II. Identification of two discrete somatoform disorders. *Archives of General Psychiatry, 41,* 863–871.

Cohen, A. Y. (1972). The journey beyond trips: Alternatives to drugs. In D. E. Smith & G. R. Gay (Eds.), *It's so good, don't even try it once: Heroin in perspective* (p. 186). Englewood Cliffs, NJ: Prentice-Hall.

Cohen, D. B. (1979). *Sleep and dreaming: Origins, nature and functions.* Oxford, England, Pergamon.

Cohen, J. A. (1960). A coefficient of agreement for nominal scales. *Educational and Psychological Measurement, 20,* 37–46.

Cohen, M. E., Robins, E., Purtell, J. J., Altman, M. W., & Reid, D. E. (1953). Excessive surgery in hysteria. *Journal of the American Medical Association, 151,* 977–986.

Cole, L. E. (1970). *Understanding abnormal behavior.* Scranton, Pennsylvania: Chandler.

Cole, M. (1985). Sex therapy—A critical appraisal. *British Journal of Psychiatry, 147,* 337–351.

Coleman, M. (1978). Biochemical and organic abnormalities associated with the cognitive defects of autism. In G. Serban (Ed.), *Cognitive defects in the development of mental illness* (pp. 3–23). New York: Brunner/Mazel.

Colligan, M. J., Pennebaker, J. W., & Murphy, L. R. (Eds.) (1982). *Mass psychogenic illnesses: A social psychological analysis.* Hillside, NJ: Laurence Erlbaum.

Colter, N., Battal, S., Crow, T. J., Johnstone, E. C., Brown, R., & Burton, C. (1987). White matter reduction in the parahippocampal gyrus of patients with schizophrenia. *Archives of General Psychiatry, 44,* 1023.

Combs, G. Jr., & Ludwig, A. M. (1982). Dissociative disorders. In J. H. Greist, J. W. Jefferson, & R. L. Spitzer (Eds.), *Treatment of mental disorders* (pp. 309–319). New York: Oxford University Press.

Comings, D. E., & Comings, B. G. (1985). Tourette syndrome: Clinical and psychological aspects of 250 cases. *American Journal of Human Genetics, 37,* 435–450.

Conel, J. L. (1939–1963). *The postnatal development of the human cerebral cortex.* Volumes I through VI. Cambridge, MA: Harvard University Press.

Connolly, J., Hallam, R. S., & Marks, I. M. (1976). Selective association of fainting with blood/injury phobias. *Behavior Therapy, 7,* 8–13.

Conrad, A. J., & Scheibel, A. B. (1987). Schizophrenia and the hippocampus: The embryological hypothesis extended. *Schizophrenia Bulletin, 13,* 577–587.

Cook, M., Mineka, S., Wolkenstein, B., & Laitsch, K. (1985). Observational conditioning of snake fear in unrelated rhesus monkeys. *Journal of Abnormal Psychology, 94,* 591–610.

Coons, P. M. (1988). Psychophysiological aspects of multiple personality disorder. *Dissociation, 1,* 47–53.

Coons, P. M., Milstein, V., & Marley, C. (1982). EEG studies of two multiple personalities and a control. *Archives of General Psychiatry, 39,* 825.

Cooper, B. (1978). Epidemiology. In J. K. Wing (Ed.), *Schizophrenia: Towards a new synthesis* (pp. 31–51). New York: Grune & Stratton.

Cooper, J. E., Kendell, R. E., Gurland, B. J., Sharp, L., Copeland, J. R. M., & Simon, R. (1972). *Psychiatric diagnosis in New York and London.* London: Oxford University Press.

Cooper, P. J., & Fairburn, C. G. (1983). Binge-eating and self-induced vomiting in the community: A preliminary study. *British Journal of Psychiatry, 142,* 139–144.

Coppen, A., Metcalfe, M., & Wood, K. (1982). Lithium. In E. S. Paykel (Ed.), *Handbook of affective disorder* (pp. 276–285). New York: Guilford Press.

Corsini, R. J. (Ed.) (1984). *Current psychotherapies* (3rd ed.). Itasca, IL: F. E. Peacock Publishers Inc.

Coryell, W. (1980). A blind family history study of Briquet's syndrome. *Archives of General Psychiatry, 37,* 1266–1269.

Coryell, W., Endicott, J., Andreasen, N. C., Keller, M. B., Clayton, P. J., Hirschfeld, M. A., Scheftner, W. A., & Winokur, G. (1988). Depression and panic attacks: The significance of overlap as reflected in follow-up and family study data. *American Journal of Psychiatry, 145,* 293–300.

Costello, C. G. (1970). Dissimilarities between conditioned avoidance responses and phobias. *Psychological Review, 7,* 250–254.

Costello, C. G. (1978). A critical review of Seligman's laboratory experiments on learned helplessness and depression in humans. *Journal of Abnormal Psychology, 87,* 21–31.

Cotton, N. S. (1979). The familial incidence of alcoholism: A review. *Journal Studies of Alcohol, 40,* 89–116.

Courchesne, E., Yeung-Courchesne, R., Press, G. A., Hesselink, J. R., & Jernigan, T. L. (1988). Hypoplasia of cerebellar vermal lobules VI and VII in autism. *New England Journal of Medicine, 318,* 1349–1354.

Cousins, N. (1984). Taking charge of your health. *Science 84* (Special Supplement), July/August, pp. 79–85.

Cox, A. (1976). The association between emotional disorders in childhood and neuroses in adult life. In H. M. van Praag (Ed.), *Research in neurosis* (pp. 40–58). Utrecht, The Netherlands: Bohn, Scheltema & Holkema.

Coyle, J. T., Price, D. L., & DeLong, M. R. (1983). Alzheimer's disease: A disease of cortical cholinergic innervation. *Science, 219*, 1184–1190.

Coyne, J. C., Aldwin, C., & Lazarus, R.S. (1981). Depression and coping in stressful episodes. *Journal of Abnormal Psychology, 90*, 439–447.

Coyne, J. C., & Gotlib, I. H. (1983). The role of cognition in depression: A critical appraisal. *Psychological Bulletin, 94*, 472–505.

Coyne, J. C., & Gotlib, I. (1986). Studying the role of cognition in depression: Well-trodden paths and cul-de-sacs. *Cognitive Therapy, 10*, 695–705.

Creer, C., & Wing, J. (1981). Living with a schizophrenic patient. In S. Crown, (Ed.), *Practical psychiatry, Vol. 1.* (pp. 122–126). London: Northwood Books.

Critchley, M. (1979). *The divine banquet of the brain.* New York: Raven Press.

Cromwell, R. L., & Pithers, W. D. (1981). Schizophrenic/paranoid psychosis: Determining diagnostic divisions. *Schizophrenia Bulletin, 7*, 674–688.

Cronbach, L. J. (1970). *Essentials of psychological testing* (3rd ed.). New York: Harper & Row.

Crook, T., & Eliot, J. (1980). Parental death during childhood and adult depression: A critical review of the literature. *Psychological Bulletin, 87*, 252–259.

Croughan, J. L., Saghir, M., Cohen R., & Robins, E. (1981). A comparison of treated and untreated male cross-dressers. *Archives of Sexual Behavior, 10*, 515–528.

Crow, T. J. (1980). Positive and negative schizophrenic symptoms and the role of dopamine. *British Journal of Psychiatry, 137*, 383–386.

Crow, T. J. (1985). The two-syndrome concept: Origins and current status. *Schizophrenia Bulletin, 11*, 471–485.

Crow, T. J., Macmillan, J. F., Johnson, A. L., & Johnstone, E. C. (1986). II. A randomized controlled trial of prophylactic neuroleptic treatment. *British Journal of Psychiatry, 148*, 120–127.

Crowe, R. (1974). An adoption study of antisocial personality. *Archives of General Psychiatry, 31*, 785–791.

Crowe, R. R., Noyes, R., Pauls, D. L., & Slymen, D. (1983). A family study of panic disorder. *Archives of General Psychiatry, 40*, 1065–1069.

Culliton, B. J. (1976). Psychosurgery: National commission issues surprisingly favorable report. *Science, 194*, 299–301.

Dakof, G. A., & Mendelsohn, G. A. (1986). Parkinson's disease: The psychological aspects of a chronic illness. *Psychological Bulletin, 99*, 375–387.

Dalby, J. T., Morgan, D., & Lee, M. L. (1986). Schizophrenia and mania in identical twin brothers. *Journal of Nervous and Mental Disease, 174*, 304–308.

Dan, A. J. (1980). Free-associative versus self report measures of emotional change over the menstrual cycle. In A. J. Dan, E. A. Graham, & C. P. Beecher (Eds.), *The menstrual cycle. Vol. 1. A synthesis of interdisciplinary research* (pp. 115–120). New York: Springer.

Darnton, R. (1968). *Mesmerism and the end of the Enlightenment in France.* Cambridge, Massachusetts: Harvard University Press.

Darwin, C. (1859). *The origin of species by means of natural selection or the preservation of favoured races in the struggle for life.* London: John Murray. (New York: New American Library, 1958).

Darwin, C. (1871). *The descent of man and selection in relation to sex.* London: John Murray.

Davidson, R. J., Schwartz, G. E. Saron, C., Bennet, J., & Goleman, D. J. (1979). Frontal versus parietal EEG asymmetry driving positive and negative affect. *Psychophysiology, 16,* 202–203.

Davidson, J., Swartz, M., Storck, M., Krishnan, R., & Hammett, E. (1985). A diagnostic and family study of posttraumatic stress disorder. *American Journal of Psychiatry, 142,* 90–93.

Davis, J. M. (1975). Overview: Maintenance therapy in psychiatry: I. Schizophrenia. *American Journal of Psychiatry, 132,* 1237–1245.

Davis, J. M. (1976). Overview: Maintenance therapy in psychiatry: II. Affective disorders. *American Journal of Psychiatry, 133,* 1–13.

Davis, K. L., Berger, P. A., Hollister, L. E., & Defraites, E. (1978). Physostigmine in mania. *Archives of General Psychiatry, 35,* 119–122.

Davison, G. C., & Neale, J. M. (1982). *Abnormal psychology: An experimental clinical approach.* New York: Wiley & Sons.

DeCarolis, V., Gibertz, F., Roccatagliata, G., Rossi, R., & Venutti, G. (1964). Imipramine and electroshock in the treatment of depression. *Sistema Nervosa, 16,* 29–42.

DeLisi, L. E., Mirsky, A. F., Buchsbaum, M. S., van Kammen, D. P., Berman, K. F., Phelps, B. H., Karoum, F., Ko, G. N., Korpi, E. R., Linnoila, M., Sheinan, M. (1984). The Genain Quadruplets 25 Years later: A diagnostic and biochemical followup. *Psychiatry Research, 13,* 59–76.

deMontigny, C., Cournoyer, G., Morissette, R., Langlois, R., & Caille, G. (1983). Lithium carbonate addition to tricyclic antidepressant-resistant unipolar depression. *Archives of General Psychiatry, 40,* 1327–1334.

Depue, R. A., Slater, J. F., Wolfstetter-Kansch, H., Klein, D., Goplerud, E., & Farr, D. (1981). A behavioral paradigm for identifying persons at risk for bipolar depressive disorder: A conceptual framework and five validation studies. *Journal of Abnormal Psychology, 90,* 381–437.

Derry, P. A., & Kuiper, N. A. (1981). Schematic processing and self-reference in clinical depression. *Journal of Abnormal Psychology, 90,* 286–297.

Devany, J. M., & Nelson, R. O. (1986). Behavioral approaches to treatment. In H. C. Quay & J. S. Werry (Eds.), *Psychopathological disorders of childhood* (3rd ed). (pp. 523–557). New York: John Wiley & Sons.

DiChiara, G., & Imperato, A. (1988). Drugs abused by humans preferentially increase synaptic dopamine concentrations in the mesolimbic system of freely moving rats. *Proceedings National Academy of Sciences, U.S.A., 85,* 5274–5278.

Dimond, S. J. (1980). *Neuropsychology: A textbook of systems and psychological functions in the brain.* London: Butterworths.

Dixon, N. F. (1981). *Preconscious processing.* Chichester, England: Wiley.

Dole, V. P. (1980, December). Addictive behavior. *Scientific American, 245,* 136–143.

Donaldson, S. R., Gelenberg, A. J., & Baldessarini, R. J. (1983). The pharmacologic treatment of schizophrenia: A progress report. *Schizophrenia Bulletin, 9,* 504–527.

Dorner, G., Gotz, F., & Docke, W. D. (1983). Prevention of demasculinization and feminization of the brain in prenatally stressed male rats by perinatal androgen treatment. *Experimental and Clinical Endocrinology, 81,* 88–90.

Dorner, G., Schenk, B., Schmiedel, B., & Ahrens, L. (1983). Stressful events in prenatal life and bi- and homosexual men. *Experimental and Clinical Endocrinology, 81,* 83–87.

Douglas, V. I. (1983). Attentional and cognitive problems. In M. Rutter (Ed.), *Developmental neuropsychiatry* (pp. 280–329). New York: Guilford Press.

Draguns, J. G. (1982). Methodology in cross-cultural psychopathology. In I. Al-Issa (Ed.), *Culture and psychopathology* (pp. 33–70). Baltimore: University Park Press.

Drake, R. E., & Vaillant, G. E. (1985). A validity study of Axis II of DSM-III. *American Journal of Psychiatry, 142,* 553–558.

Dunham, H. W., Phillips, P., & Srinivasan, B. (1966). A research note on diagnosed mental illness and social class. *American Sociological Review, 31,* 223–227.

Durkheim, E. (1897). *Suicide: A study in sociology.* In Contemporary Civilization Staff, Columbia College (Eds.), *Man in contemporary society, Vol. 1* (pp. 384–402). New York: Columbia University Press, 1955.

Dworkin, R. H., & Lenzenweger, M. F. (1984). Symptoms and the genetics of schizophrenia: Implications for diagnosis. *American Journal of Psychiatry, 141,* 1541–1546.

Eagly, A. H., & Carli, L. L. (1981). Sex of researchers and sex-typed communications as determinants of sex differences in influenceability: A meta-analysis of social influence studies. *Psychological Bulletin, 90,* 1–20.

Easser, R. & Lesser, S. (1965). Hysterical personality: A reevaluation. *Psychoanalytic Quarterly, 34,* 390–402.

Eaves, E., & Rush, A. J. (1984). Cognitive patterns in symptomatic and remitted unipolar depression. *Journal of Abnormal Psychology, 93,* 31–40.

Eckert, E. D., Bouchard, T. J., Jr., Gottesman, I. I., Segal, N., Wilcox, K. et al. (1986). Homosexuality in monozygotic twins reared apart. *British Journal of Psychiatry, 148,* 421–425.

Eckert, E. D., Heston, L. L., & Bouchard, T. J., Jr. (1981). MZ twins reared apart: Preliminary findings of psychiatric disturbances and traits. In L. Gedda, P. Parisi, & W. E. Nance (Eds.), *Twin research 3: Part B. Intelligence, personality, and development* (pp. 179–188). New York: Alan R. Liss, Inc.

Efron, R. (1957). Conditional inhibition of uncinate fits. *Brain, 80,* 561–566.

Egeland, J. A., & Sussex, J. N. (1985). Suicide and family loading for affective disorders. *Journal of the American Medical Association, 254,* 915–918.

Egeland, J. A., Gerhard, D. S., Pauls, D. L., Sussex, J. N., Kidd, K. K. et al. (1987). Bipolar affective disorders linked to DNA markers on chromosome 11. *Nature, 325,* 783–787.

Ehrhardt, A. A., Meyer-Bahlburg, H. F. L., Rosen, L. R., Feldman, J. F., Veridiano, N. P., Zimmerman, I., & McEwen, B. S. (1985). Sexual orientation after prenatal exposure to exogenous estrogen. *Archives of Sexual Behavior, 14,* 75–77.

Eisdorfer, C., Cohen, D., & Keckich, W. (1981). Depression and anxiety in the cognitively impaired aged. In D. F. Klein & J. Rabkin (Eds.), *Anxiety: New research and changing concepts* (pp. 425–430). New York: Raven.

Eitinger, L., & Strom, A. (1973). *Mortality and morbidity after excessive stress.* New York: Humanities Press.

Eklund, P. L. E., Gooren, L. J. G., & Bezemer, P. D. (1988). Prevalence of transsexualism in the Netherlands. *British Journal of Psychiatry, 152,* 638–640.

Ellenberger, H. F. (1970). *The discovery of the unconscious: The history and evolution of dynamic psychiatry.* New York: Basic Books.

Elliot. F. A. (1978). Neurological aspects of antisocial behavior. In W. H. Reid (Ed.), *The psychopath* (pp. 146–189). New York, Brunner/Mazel Publishers.

Ellis, A. (1962). *Reason and emotion in psychotherapy.* New York: Lyle Stuart.

Ellis, A. (1984). Rational-emotive therapy. In R. J. Corsini (Ed.), *Current psychotherapies* (pp. 196–238). Itasca, IL: F. E. Peacock.

Ellis, A. (1987). The impossibility of achieving consistently good mental health. *American Psychologist, 42,* 364–375.

Ellis, L., & Ames, M. A. (1987). Neurohormonal functioning and sexual orientation: A theory of homosexuality-heterosexuality. *Psychological Bulletin, 101,* 233–258.

Emmelkamp, P. M. G. (1982). *Phobic and obsessive-compulsive disorders.* New York: Plenum Press.

Enna, S. J. (1982). The role of neurotransmitters in the pharmacologic actions of benzodiazepines. In R. J. Mathew (Ed.), *The biology of anxiety* (pp. 107–122). New York: Brumer/Mazel.

Enoch, M. D., & Trethowan, W. H. (1979). *Uncommon psychiatric syndromes* (2nd ed.). Bristol, England: John Wright & Sons.

Erdelyi, M. H. (1974). A new look at the new look: Perceptual defense and vigilance. *Psychological Review, 81,* 1–25.

Erdelyi, M. H. (1985). *Psychoanalysis: Freud's cognitive psychology.* New York: Freeman.

Erikson, E. H. (1963). *Childhood and society.* New York: Norton.

Erlenmeyer-Kimling, L. Marcuse, Y., Cornblatt, B., Friedman, D., Rainer, J. D., & H. G. Rutschmann. "The New York High-Risk Project." (1984). In N. F. Watt, E. J. Anthony, L. C. Wynne, & J. E. Rolf (Eds.), *Children at risk for schizophrenia* (pp. 169–189). Cambridge, England: Cambridge University Press.

Evarts, E. V. (1979). Brain mechanisms of movement. *Scientific American, 241,* 164–179.

Evarts, E. V., Kimura, M., Wurtz, R. H., & Hikosaka, O. (1984). Behavioral correlates of activity in basal ganglia neurons. *Trends in Neuroscience, 7,* 447–453.

Exner, J. E., Jr. (1986). *The Rorschach: A comprehensive system. Vol. 2: Basic foundations* (2nd ed.). New York: Wiley-Interscience.

Ey, H. (1982). History and analysis of the concept. In A. Roy (Ed.) *Hysteria* (pp. 3–19). Chichester, England: Wiley.

Eysenck, H. J. (1952). The effects of psychotherapy: An evaluation. *Journal of Consulting Psychology, 16,* 319–324.

Eysenck, H. J. (1976). *Sex and personality.* Austin, TX: University of Texas Press.

Eysenck, H. J. (1982). A psychological theory of hysteria. In A. Roy (Ed.), *Hysteria* (pp. 57–80). Chichester, England: Wiley.

Eysenck, H. J. (1986). A critique of contemporary classification and diagnosis. In T. Millon & G. L. Klerman (Eds.), *Contemporary directions in psychopathology: Toward the DSM-IV* (pp. 73–98). New York: The Guilford Press.

Eysenck, H. J., & Rachman, S. (1965). *The causes and cures of neurosis.* San Diego: Knapp.

Fagan, J. & McMahon, J. J. (1984). Incipient multiple personality in children. *Journal of Nervous and Mental Disease, 172,* 25–36.

Falk, J. L., Dews, P. B., & Schuster, C. R. (1983). Commonalities in the environmental control of behavior. In P. K. Levinson, D. R. Gerstein, & D. R. Maloff (Eds.), *Commonalities in substance abuse and habitual behavior* (pp. 47–110). Lexington, MA: D. C. Heath.

Falloon, I. R. H., Boyd, J. L., McGill, C. W., Williamson, M., Razani, J., Moss, H. G., Gilderman, A. M., & Simpson, G. M. (1985). Family management in the prevention of morbidity of schizophrenia. Clinical outcome of a two-year longitudinal study. *Archives of General Psychiatry, 42*, 887–896.

Falloon, I. R. H., & Liberman, R. P. (1983). Interactions between drugs and psychosocial therapy in schizophrenia. *Schizophrenia Bulletin, 9*, 543–554.

Farde, L., Wiesel, F. A., Hall, H., Halldin, C., Stone-Ellander, S., & Sedval, G. (1987). No D_2 receptor increase in PET study of schizophrenia. *Archives of General Psychiatry, 44*, 671–672.

Faris, R. E. L., & Dunham, H. W. (1939). *Mental disorders in urban areas: An ecological study of schizophrenia and other psychoses.* Chicago: University of Chicago Press.

Farmer, A. E., McGuffin, P., & Gottesman, I. I. (1987). Twin concordance for DSM III schizophrenia: Scrutinizing the validity of the definition. *Archives of General Psychiatry, 44*, 634–641.

Farrington, D. P., & West, D. J. (1981). The Cambridge study of delinquent development. In S. A. Mednick & A. E. Baert (Eds.), *Prospective longitudinal research: An empirical basis of primary prevention of psychosocial disorders* (pp. 137–145). Oxford: Oxford Univ. Press, 1981.

Fedio, P. (1986). Behavioral characteristics of patients with temporal lobe epilepsy. In R. M. Restak (Ed.), *The psychiatric clinics of North America, 9*, 267–281.

Fehr, F. S., & Stern, J. A. (1970). Peripheral physiological variables and emotion: The James-Lange theory revisited. *Psychological Review, 74*, 411–424.

Feighner, J. P., Robins, E., Guze, S. B., Woodruff, R. A., Winokur, G., & Munoz, R. (1972). Diagnostic criteria for use in psychiatric research. *Archives of General Psychiatry, 26*, 57–63.

Fenichel, O. (1930). *Ten years of the Berlin Psychoanalytic Institute, 1920–1930,* Vienna: International Psychoanalytic Press.

Fenichel, O. (1945). *The psychoanalytic theory of neurosis.* New York: Norton.

Fenton, G. W. (1982). Hysterical alterations of consciousness. In A. Roy (Ed.), *Hysteria* (pp. 229–246). Chichester, England: Wiley.

Fenton, G. W. (1986). Epilepsy and hysteria. *British Journal of Psychiatry, 149*, 28–37.

Fenz, W., & Epstein, S. (1967). Gradients of psychological arousal in parachutists. *Psychosomatic Medicine, 29*, 33–51.

Ferguson-Smith, M. A. (1988). Genes on the X and Y chromosomes controlling sex: Genetic sex is a matter of quantity. *British Medical Journal, 297*, 635–636.

Finger, S., & Stein, D. G. (1982). *Brain damage and recovery: Research and clinical perspectives.* New York: Academic Press.

Fink, M. (1981). Dexamethasone suppression test and outcome with ECT. In C. Perris, G. Struwe, & B. Jansson (Eds.), *Biological psychiatry 1981* (pp. 1075–1077). Amsterdam: Elsevier/North-Holland Biomedical Press.

Fink, M. (1984). ECT-verdict: Not guilty. *The Behavioral and Brain Sciences, 7*, 26–27.

Finkelhor, D. (1979). *Sexually victimized children.* New York: Free Press.

Finkelhor, D., & Araji, S. (1986). Explanations of pedophilia: A four factor model. *The Journal of Sex Research, 22*, 145–161.

Finn, S. E. (1982). Base rates, utilities, and DSM-III: Shortcomings of fixed-rule systems of psychodiagnosis. *Journal of Abnormal Psychology, 91*, 294–302.

Firestone, P., & Prabhu, A. N. (1981). Minor physical anomalies and obstetrical complications: Their relationship to hyperactive, psychoneurotic, and normal children and their families. *Journal of Abnormal Child Psychology, 11*, 207–216.

Fischer, M. (1973). Genetic and environmental factors in schizophrenia: A study of schizophrenic twins and their families. *Acta Psychiatrica Scandinavica*, Supplement 238.

Fischer, M., Gottesman, I. I., & Bertelsen, A. (1985). Investigation of children whose parents have both been hospitalized for psychiatric disorders. *Ugeske Laeger, 147,* 327–330.

Fish, B. (1977). Neurobiologic antecedents of schizophrenia in children: Evidence for an inherited, congenital neurointegrative defect. *Archives of General Psychiatry, 34,* 1297–1313.

Fish, B. (1984). Characteristics and sequelae of the neurointegrative disorder in infants at risk for schizophrenia: 1952-1982. In N. F. Watt, E. J. Anthony, L. C. Wynne, & J. E. Rolf (Eds.), *Children at risk for schizophrenia: A longitudinal perspective* (pp. 423–439). Cambridge: Cambridge University Press.

Fisher, S., & Greenberg, R. P. (1977). *The scientific credibility of Freud's theories and therapy*. New York: Basic Books.

Flament, M. F., Rapoport, J. L., Berg, C. J., Sceery, W., Kilts, C., Mellstrom, B., & Linnoila, M. (1985). Clomipramine treatment of childhood obsessive-compulsive disorder: A double-blind controlled study. *Archives of General Psychiatry, 42,* 977–983.

Flor-Henry, P. (1976). Lateralized temporal-limbic dysfunction and psychopathology. *Annals of the New York Academy of Sciences, 280,* 777–797.

Flor-Henry, P. (1983). Hemisyndromes of temporal lobe epilepsy: Review of evidence relating psychopathological manifestations in epilepsy to right- and left-sided epilepsy. In M. S. Myslobodsky (Ed.), *Hemisyndromes: Psychobiology, neurology, psychiatry* (pp. 149–174). New York: Academic Press.

Foa, E. B., Steketee, G., Grayson, J. B., & Doppelt, H. G. (1983). Treatment of obsessive-compulsives: When do we fail? In E. B. Foa & P. M. G. Emmelkamp (Eds.), *Failures in behavior therapy* (pp. 10–34). New York: Wiley.

Foa, E. B., Steketee, G., & Young, M. C. (1984). Agoraphobia: Phenomenological aspects, associated characteristics, and theoretical considerations. *Clinical Psychology Review, 4,* 431–457.

Folstein, S. E., & Rutter, M. (1977). Infantile autism: A genetic study of 21 twin pairs. *Journal of Child Psychology and Psychiatry, 18,* 297–321.

Ford, C. V. (1983). *The somatizing disorders: Illness is a way of life*. New York: Elsevier Biomedical.

Ford, C. V., King, B. H., & Hollender, M. H. (1988). Lies and liars: Psychiatric aspects of prevarication. *American Journal of Psychiatry, 145,* 554–562.

Forrest, M. S., & Hokanson, J. E. (1975). Depression and autonomic arousal reduction accompanying self-punitive behavior. *Journal of Abnormal Behavior, 84,* 346–357.

Foulds, G. A. (1965). *Personality and personal illness*. London: Tavistock Publications.

Fowler, R. C. (1978). Remitting schizophrenia as a variant of affective disorder. *Schizophrenia Bulletin, 4,* 68–77.

Frances, A. (1982). Categorical and dimensional systems of personality diagnosis: A comparison. *Comprehensive Psychiatry, 23,* 516–527.

Frank, G. H. (1965). The role of the family in the development of psychopathology. *Psychological Bulletin, 64,* 191–205.

Frank, J. D. (1982). *Persuasion and healing*. Baltimore: Johns Hopkins University Press.

Frank, J. D. (1982). Therapeutic components shared by all psychotherapies. In J. H.

Harvey, & M. M. Parks (Eds.), *Psychotherapy research and behavior change* (pp. 5–37). Washington, DC: American Psychological Association.

Frankel, M., Cummings, J. L., Robertson, M. M., Trimble, M. R., Hill, M. A., & Benson, D. F. (1986). Obsessions and compulsions in Gilles de la Tourette syndrome. *Neurology, 36,* 378–382.

Franzen, G., & Ingvar, D. H. (1975). Abnormal distribution of cerebral activity in chronic schizophrenia. *Journal of Psychiatric Research, 12,* 199–214.

Frazier, S. H. (1980). Headache. In H. I. Kaplan, A. M., Freedman, & B. J. Sadock (Eds.), *Comprehensive textbook of psychiatry/III* (3rd ed.), *Vol. 2* (pp. 1957–1960). Baltimore: Williams & Wilkins.

Freeman, T. (1969). *Psychopathology of the psychoses.* New York: International Universities Press.

Freud, S. (1893a). Charcot. In S. Freud, *Collected papers, Vol. 1* (pp. 9–23). New York: Basic Books, 1959.

Freud, S. (1893b). On the physical mechanisms of hysterical phenomena. In S. Freud, *Collected Papers, Vol. 1* (pp. 42–58). New York: Basic Books, 1959.

Freud, S. (1895). Obsessions and phobias: Their psychical mechanisms and their etiology. In S. Freud, *Collected papers, Vol. 1* (pp. 128–137). New York: Basic Books, 1959.

Freud, S. (1896). The aetiology of hysteria. In S. Freud, *Collected papers, Vol. 1* (pp. 183–219). New York: Basic Books, 1959.

Freud, S. (1900). *The interpretation of dreams.* New York: Basic Books, 1953. Reprint of Hogarth Press *Standard Edition* version.

Freud, S. (1901). *The psychopathology of everyday life.* New York: Norton, 1960.

Freud, S. (1905). Three contributions to a theory of sex. In A. A. Brill (Ed.), *The basic writings of Sigmund Freud,* New York: Modern Library, 1938.

Freud, S. (1908). Character and anal eroticism. In S. Freud, *Collected papers. Volume 2* (pp. 45–58). New York: Basic Books, 1959.

Freud, S. (1917). Mourning and melancholia. In S. Freud, *Collected papers, Vol. 4* (pp. 152–170). New York: Basic Books, 1959.

Freud, S. (1923). *The ego and the id.* New York: Norton, 1960.

Freud, S. (1926). *Inhibition, symptoms and anxiety. Standard Edition, 20* (pp. 87–172). London: Hogarth Press, 1959.

Freud, S. Analysis terminable and interminable. In J. Strachey (Ed.), *Collected papers, Vol. 5,* New York: Basic Books, 1959.

Freund, K., Nagler, E., Langevin, R., Zajac, A., & Steiner, B. (1974). Measuring feminine gender identity in homosexual males. *Archives of Sexual Behavior, 3,* 249–260.

Friedman, D., Erlenmeyer-Kimling, L., & Vaughn, H. G. Jr. (1984). Event-related potential (ERP) methodology in high-risk research. In N. F. Watt, E. J. Anthony, L. C. Wynne, & J. E. Rolf (Eds.), *Children at risk for schizophrenia: A longitudinal perspective* (pp. 190–197). Cambridge: Cambridge University Press.

Friedrich, W. N., & Boriskin, J. A. (1976). The role of the child in abuse: A review of the literature. *American Journal of Orthopsychiatry, 46,* 580–590.

Fuller, J. L., Church, A. C., & Dann, L. (1976). Ethanol consumption by mice selected for high and low ethanol sleep times. *Behavior Genetics, 7,* 59 (Abstract).

Fuller, J. L., & Thompson, W. R. (1978). *Foundations of behavior genetics.* St. Louis: C. V. Mosby.

Fuller. R. C. (1982). *Mesmerism and the American cure of souls.* Philadelphia: University of Pennsylvania Press.

Funkenstein, D. H. (1966). The physiology of fear and anger. In S. Coopersmith (Ed.), *Frontiers of psychological research: Readings from Scientific American* (pp. 71–75). San Francisco: Freeman.

Gabrielli, W. F., Jr., Mednick. S. A., Volavla, J., Pollock, V. E., Schulsinger, F. & Itil, T. (1982). Electroencephalograms in children of alcoholic fathers. *Psychophysiology, 19,* 404–407.

Galaburda, A. M., & Kemper, T. L. (1979). Cytoarchitectonic abnormalities in developmental dyslexia: A case study. *Annals of Neurology, 6,* 94–100.

Galaburda, A. M., Sherman, G. F., Rosen, G. D., Aboitiz, F., & Geschwind, N. (1985). Developmental dyslexia: Four consecutive patients with cortical anomalies. *Annals of Neurology, 18,* 222–233.

Gallup, G. G., Jr., & Maser, J. D. (1977). Tonic immobility: Evolutionary underpinnings of human catelepsy and catatonia. In J. D. Maser & M. E. P. Seligman (Eds.), *Psychopathology: Experimental models* (pp. 334–357). San Francisco: W. H. Freeman.

Gardner, H. (1974). *The shattered mind.* New York: Vintage Books, 1974.

Garfinkel, P. E., Moldofsky, H., & Garner, D. M. (1980). Heterogeneity of anorexia nervosa: Bulimia as a distinct subgroup. *Archives of General Psychiatry, 37,* 1036–1040.

Garmezy, N. (1966). Process and reactive schizophrenia: Some conceptions and issues. In M. M. Katz, J. O. Cole, & W. E. Barton (Eds.), *The role of methodology of classification in psychiatry and psychopathology* (pp. 419–466). (Public Health Service Publication No. 1584). Washington, DC: U.S. Department of Health, Education and Welfare/National Institute of Mental Health.

Garmezy, N. (1983). Stressors of childhood. In N. Garmezy & M. Rutter (Eds.), *Stress, coping, and development in children* (pp. 43–84). New York: McGraw-Hill.

Gawin, F. A., Ellinwood, E. H. (1988). Cocaine and other stimulants. *New England Journal of Medicine, 318,* 1173–1182.

Gebhard, P. H. (1983). Sadomasochism. In T. Weinberg & G. W. Levi Kamel (Eds.), *S and M: Studies in sadomasochism* (pp. 36–39). Buffalo, NY: Prometheus Books.

Gelinas, D. J. (1983). The persisting negative effects of incest. *Psychiatry, 46,* 312–332.

Gersh, F. S., & Fowles, D. C. (1979). Neurotic depression: The concept of anxious depression. In R. A. Depue (Ed.), *The psychobiology of depressive disorders: Implications for the effects of stress* (pp. 81–104). New York: Academic Press.

Gershon, E. S., Hamovit, J., Guroff, J. J., Dibble, E., Leckman, J. F. et al. (1982). A family study of schizoaffective, bipolar I, bipolar II, unipolar, and normal control probands. *Archives of General Psychiatry, 39,* 1157–1167.

Gershon, E. S., DeLisi, L. E., Hamovit, J., Nurnberger, Jr., J. I., Maxwell, M. E., Schreiber, J., Dauphinais, D., & Dingman, C. W. II (1988). A controlled family study of chronic psychoses: Schizophrenia and schizoaffective disorder. *Archives of General Psychiatry, 45,* 328–336.

Geschwind, N. (1979). Specializations of the human brain. *Scientific American, 241,* 180–199.

Geschwind, N. (1981). The pervasiveness of the right hemisphere. *The Behavioral and Brain Sciences, 4,* 106–107.

Giles, D. E., Biggs, M. M., Etzel, B. A., Rush, J. A., Kupfer, D. J., & Roffwarg, H. A. (1988). Secular trend in unipolar depression. *Sleep Research, 17,* 122.

Gillberg, C., & Gillberg, I. C. (1983). Infantile autism: A total population study of reduced optimality in the pre-, peri-, and neonatal period. *Journal of Autism and Developmental Disorders, 13,* 153–166.

Gillberg, C., & Svedson, P. (1983). Childhood psychosis and computed tomographic brain scan findings. *Journal of Autism and Developmental Disabilities, 13*, 19–32.

Gillberg, C., & Wahlstrom, J. (1985). Chromosome abnormalities in infantile autism and other childhood psychoses: A population study of 66 cases. *Developmental Medicine and Child Neurology, 27*, 293–304.

Gillin, J. C., & Borbely, A. (1985, December). Sleep: A neurobiological window on affective disorders. *Trends in Neuroscience*, 537–542.

Gittelman, R., & Kanner, A. (1986). Psychopharmocotherapy. In H. C. Quay & J. S. Werry (Eds.), *Psychopathological disorders of childhood* (3rd ed.) (pp. 455–494). New York: John Wiley & Sons.

Gittelman, R., & Klein, D. F. (1985). Childhood separation anxiety and adult agoraphobia. In A. H. Tuma & J. Maser (Eds.), *Anxiety and the anxiety disorders* (pp. 389–402). Hillsdale, New Jersey: Laurence Erlbaum.

Gittelman, R., Mannuzza, S., Shenker, R., & Bonagura, N. (1985). Hyperactive boys almost grown up. I. Psychiatric status. *Archives of General Psychiatry, 42*, 937–947.

Gladue, B. A. (1987). Psychobiological contributions. In L. Diamant (Ed.), *Male and female homosexuality* (pp. 129–153). Washington, DC: Hemisphere Publishing Corp.

Gladue, B. A., Green, R., & Hellman, R. E. (1984). Neuroendocrine response to estrogen and sexual orientation. *Science, 225*, 1496–1499.

Glaser, G. H. (1975). Epilepsy: Neuropsychological aspects. In M. F. Reiser (Ed.), *American handbook of psychiatry, Vol. 4* (pp. 314–355). New York: Basic Books.

Glass, G. V. (1976). Primary, secondary, and meta-analysis of research. *Educational Research, 5*, 3–8.

Glass, G. V., & Kliegl, R. H. (1983). An apology for research integration in the study of psychotherapy. *Journal of Consulting and Clinical Psychology, 51*, 28–41.

Glueck, S., & Glueck, E. (1956). *Physique and delinquency.* New York: Harper & Brothers.

Gold, P. W., Goodwin, F. K., & Chrousos, G. P. (1988). Clinical and biochemical manifestations of depression: Relation to the neurobiology of stress. (First of two parts) *New England Journal of Medicine, 319*, 348–352.

Gold, P. W., Goodwin, F. K., & Chrousos, G. P. (1988a). Clinical and biochemical manifestations of depression: Relation to the neurobiology of stress. (Second of two parts) *New England Journal of Medicine, 319*, 413–420.

Goldberg, S. C. (1985). Negative and deficit symptoms in schizophrenia do respond to neuroleptics. *Schizophrenia Bulletin, 11*, 453–456.

Goldstein, K. (1975). Functional disturbances in brain damage. In M. F. Reiser (Ed.) *American handbook of psychiatry: Organic disorders and psychosomatic medicine* (pp. 183–207). New York: Basic Books.

Goleman, D. (1988a, November 29). Behind abnormal fears, normal aches and pains: New insight on sensitivity helps fight hypochondria. *New York Times*, pp. 23, 26.

Goleman, D. (1988b, June 28). Probing the enigma of multiple personality. *New York Times*, pp. 21–27.

Golub, S. (1980). Premenstrual changes in mood, personality, and cognitive emotion. In A. J. Dan, E. A. Graham, & C. P. Beecher (Eds.), *The menstrual cycle: Vol. 1. A synthesis of interdisciplinary research* (pp. 237–246). New York: Springer.

Goodwin, D. W. (1982). Substance induced and substance use disorders: Alcohol. In J. H. Griest, J. W. Jefferson, & R. Spitzer (Eds.), *Treatment of mental disorders* (pp. 44–61). New York: Oxford University Press.

Goodwin, D. W., & Guze, S. B. (1979). *Psychiatric diagnosis* (2nd ed.). New York: Oxford University Press.

Goodwin, D. W., Schulsinger, F., Hermansen, L., Guze, S. B., Winokur, G. (1973). Alcohol problems in adoptees raised apart from alcoholic biological parents. *Archives of General Psychiatry, 28,* 238–243.

Goodwin, D. W., Schulsinger, F., Knop, J., Mednick, S., & Guze, S. B. (1977). Alcoholism and depression in adopted-out daughters of alcoholics. *Archives of General Psychiatry, 34,* 751–755.

Goodwin, F. K. (1979). On the biology of depression. In R. J. Friedman & M. M. Katz (Eds.), *The psychology of depression: Contemporary theory and research* (pp. 240–251). New York: V. H. Winston & Sons.

Goodwin, J. (1988). Munchausen's syndrome as a dissociative disorder. *Dissociation, 1,* 54–60.

Gorenstein, E. E. (1982). Frontal lobe functions in psychopaths. *Journal of Abnormal Psychology, 91,* 368–379.

Gorenstein, E. E., & Newman, J. P. (1980). Disinhibitory psychopathology: A new perspective and a model for research. *Psychological Review, 87,* 301–315.

Gotlib, I. H., & Cane, D. B. (1987). Construct accessibility and clinical depression: A longitudinal investigation. *Journal of Abnormal Psychology, 96,* 199–204.

Gottesman, I. I., Bouchard, T. J., Jr., & Carey, G. (1984, May). *The Minnesota Study of Twins Reared Apart.* Meeting of the Behavior Genetics Association, Bloomington, Indiana.

Gottesman, I. I., & Carey, G. (1983). Extracting meaning and direction from twin data. *Psychiatric Developments, 1,* 35–50.

Gottesman, I. I., & Shields, J. (1982). *Schizophrenia: The epigenetic puzzle.* Cambridge: Cambridge University Press.

Gough, H. (1960). Theory and measurement of socialization. *Journal of Consulting Psychology, 24,* 23–30.

Gould, R., Miller, B. L., Goldberg, M. A., & Benson, D. F. (1986). The validity of hysterical signs and symptoms. *Journal of Nervous and Mental Disease, 174,* 593–597.

Grant, I., Yager, J., Sweetwood, H. L., & Olshen, R. (1982). Life events and symptoms: Fourier analysis of time series from a three-year prospective inquiry. *Archives of General Psychiatry, 39,* 598–605.

Gray, J. A. (1981). A critique of Eysenck's theory of personality. In H. J. Eysenck (Ed.), *A model for personality* (pp. 246–276). New York: Springer.

Gray, J. A. (1985). Issues in the neuropsychology of anxiety. In A. H. Tuma & J. Maser (Eds.), *Anxiety and the anxiety disorders* (pp. 5–25). Hillsdale, New Jersey: Laurence Erlbaum.

Greaves, G. B. (1980). Multiple personality: 165 years after Mary Reynolds. *Journal of Nervous and Mental Disease, 168,* 577–596.

Green, M. F., Satz, P., Gaier, D. J., Ganzell, S., & Kharabi, F. (1989). Minor physical anomalies in schizophrenia. *Schizophrenia Bulletin, 15,* 91–99.

Green, M. F., Satz, P., Soper, H. V., & Kharabi, F. (1987). Relationship between physical anomalies and age at onset of schizophrenia. *American Journal of Psychiatry, 144,* 666–667.

Green, R. (1974). *Sexual identity conflict in children and adults.* New York: Basic Books.

Green, R. (1979). Childhood cross-gender behavior and subsequent sexual preference. *American Journal of Psychiatry, 136,* 106–108.

Green, R. (1982). Gender identity disorders and transvestism. In J. H. Griest, J. W. Jefferson, & R. L. Spitzer (Eds.), *Treatment of mental disorders* (pp. 320–337). New York: Oxford University Press.

Green, R. (1985). Gender identity in childhood and later sexual orientation: Follow-up of 78 males. *American Journal of Psychiatry, 142*, 339–341.

Green, R. (1987). *The "sissy boy syndrome" and the development of homosexuality.* New Haven: Yale University Press.

Gross, R. T., & Dornbusch, S. M. (1983). Disordered processes of elimination: Enuresis. In M. D. Levine, W. B. Carey, A. C. Crocker, & R. T. Gross (Eds.), *Developmental-behavioral pediatrics* (pp. 573–586). Philadelphia: W. B. Saunders Co.

Grossman, H. (Ed.) (1973). *Manual on terminology and classification in mental retardation, 1973 revision.* Washington, DC: American Association on Mental Deficiency.

Grotevant, H. D., Scarr, S., & Weinberg, R. A. (1977). Patterns of interest similarity in adoptive and biological parents. *Journal of Personality and Social Psychology, 35*, 667–676.

Groth, A. N. (1979). *Men who rape.* New York: Plenum Press.

Groth, A. N., Longo, R. E., & McFadin, J. B. (1982). Undetected recidivism among rapists and child molesters. *Crime & Delinquency, 28*, 450–458.

Grove, W. M. (1987). The reliability of psychiatric diagnosis. In C. G. Last, & M. Hersen (Eds.), *Issues in diagnostic research* (pp. 99–119). New York: Plenum.

Grunbaum, A. (1984). *The foundations of psychoanalysis: A philosophical critique.* Berkeley: University of California Press.

Gruzelier, J. H. (1978). Bimodal states of arousal and lateralized dysfunction in schizophrenia: Effects of chlorpromazine. In L. C. Wynne, R. L. Cromwell, & S. Matthysse (Eds.), *The nature of schizophrenia: New approaches to research and treatment* (pp. 167–187). New York: Wiley.

Gualtieri, C. T., Adams, A., Shen, C. D., & Loiselle, D. (1982). Minor physical anomalies in alcoholic and schizophrenic adults and hyperactive and autistic children. *American Journal of Psychiatry, 139*, 640–643.

Gunderson, J. G., & Elliot, G. R. (1985). The interface between borderline personality and affective disorder. *American Journal of Psychiatry, 142*, 277–288.

Gurling, H. M. D., Grant, S., & Dangl, J. (1985). The genetic and cultural transmission of alcohol use, alcoholism, cigarette smoking and coffee drinking: A review and an example using a log linear cultural transmission model. *British Journal of Addiction, 80*, 269–279.

Gusella, J. F., Wexler, N. S., Conneally, R. M., Naylor, S. L. et al. (1983). A polymorphic DNA marker genetically linked to Huntington's disease. *Nature, 306*, 234–238.

Gutheil, T. G. (1985). Medicolegal pitfalls in treatment of borderline patients. *American Journal of Psychiatry, 142*, 9–14.

Guttmacher, L. B., & Nelles, C. (1984). In vivo desensitization of lactate-induced panic: A case study. *Behavioral Therapy, 15*, 369–372.

Guy, J. D., Majorski, L. V., Wallace, C. J., & Guy, M. P. (1983). The incidence of minor physical anomalies in adult male schizophrenics. *Schizophrenia Bulletin, 9*, 571–582.

Guze, S. B., Cloninger, C. R., Martin, R. L., & Clayton, P. J. (1986). A follow-up and family study of Briquet's syndrome. *British Journal of Psychiatry, 149*, 17–23.

Haggerty, R. J. (1980). Life stress, illness and social supports. *Developmental Medicine and Child Neurology, 22*, 391–400.

Halberstadt, L. J., Mukherji, B. R., Metalsky, G. I., & Abramson, L. Y (in press). Cognitive styles among college students: Toward an integration of the cognitive theories of depression with cognitive psychology and descriptive psychiatry. *Journal of Abnormal Psychology*.

Halbreich, V., Endicott, J., & Nee, J. (1983). Premenstrual depressive changes: Value of differentiation. *Archives of General Psychiatry, 40*, 535–542.

Hall, B. K. (1984). Developmental mechanisms underlying the formation of atavisms. *Biological Reviews, 99*, 89–124.

Hall, R. C. (Ed.) (1980a). *Psychiatric presentations of medical illnesses: Somatopsychic disorders*. New York: SP Medical Scientific Books.

Hall, R. C. (1980b). Depression. In R. C. Hall (Ed.), *Psychiatric presentations of medical illness: Somatopsychic disorders* (pp. 37–63). New York: SP Medical & Scientific Books.

Hall, R. C., LeCann, A. F., & Schoolar, J. C. (1978). Amobarbital treatment of multiple personality. Use of structural video tape interviews as a basis for intensive psychotherapy. *Journal of Nervous and Mental Disease, 166*, 666–670.

Hall, R. C. W., Popkin, M. K., DeVanl, R. Faillace, L. A., & Stickney, S. K. (1978). Physical illness presenting as psychiatric illness. *Archives of General Psychiatry, 35*, 1315–1320.

Hamilton, M. (Ed.) (1967). *Abnormal psychology*. Baltimore: Penguin.

Hanna, J. M. (1976). Ethnic groups, human variation, and alcohol use. In W. E. Everett, J. O. Waddell, & D. B. Heath (Eds.), *Cross-cultural approaches to the study of alcohol: An interdisciplinary perspective* (pp. 235–242). The Hague: Mouton Publishers.

Hanson, D. R., Gottesman, I. I., & Heston, L. L. (1976). Some possible childhood indicators of adult schizophrenia inferred from children of schizophrenics. *British Journal of Psychiatry, 129*, 142–154.

Hanson, D. R., Gottesman, I. I., & Meehl, P. E. (1977). Genetic theories and the validation of psychiatric diagnoses: Implications for the study of children of schizophrenia. *Journal of Abnormal Psychology, 86*, 575–588.

Harada, S., Agarwal, D. P., Goedde, H. W., Tagaki, S., & Ishikawa, B. (1982). Possible protective role against alcoholism for aldehyde dehydrogenase isozyme deficiency in Japan. *Lancet II*, 827.

Harding, C. M., Brooks, G. W., Ashikaga, T., Strauss, J. S., & Breier, A. (1987). The Vermont Longitudinal Study of persons with severe mental illness, II. Long-term outcomes of subjects who retrospectively met DSM-III criteria for schizophrenia. *American Journal of Psychiatry, 144*, 727–735.

Hare, R. D. (1965). Temporal gradient of fear arousal in psychopaths. *Journal of Abnormal Psychology, 70*, 442–445.

Hare, R. D. (1978). Electrodermal and cardiovascular correlates of psychopathy. In R. D. Hare & D. Schalling (Eds.), *Psychopathic behaviour: Approaches to research* (pp. 107–143). Chichester, England: Wiley and Sons.

Hare, R. D. (1983). Diagnosis of antisocial personality disorder in two prison populations. *American Journal of Psychiatry, 140*, 888–890.

Hare, R. D. (1984). Performance of psychopaths on cognitive tasks related to frontal lobe function. *Journal of Abnormal Psychology, 93* 133–140.

Hare, R. D. (1985). Comparison of procedures for the assessment of psychopathy. *Journal of Consulting and Clinical Psychology, 53*, 7–16.

Hare, R. D., McPherson, L. M., & Forth, A. E. (1988). Male psychopaths and their criminal careers. *Journal of Consulting and Clinical Psychology, 56,* 710–714.

Harford, T. C., Haack, M. R., & Spiegler, D. L. (1987/88). Positive family history for alcoholism. *Alcohol Health & Research World, 12,* 138–143.

Harrow, M., Carone, B. J., & Westermeyer, J. F. (1985). The course of psychosis in early phases of schizophrenia. *American Journal of Psychiatry, 142,* 702–707.

Harrow, M., Grossman, L. S., Silverstein, J. L., & Meltzer, H. Y. (1982). Thought pathology in manic and schizophrenic patients: Its occurrence at hospital admission and seven weeks later. *Archives of General Psychiatry, 39* 665–671.

Hartmann, E., Russ, D., VanDer Kolk, B., Falke, R., & Oldfield, M. (1981). A preliminary study of the personality of the nightmare sufferer: Relationship to schizophrenia and creativity? *American Journal of Psychiatry, 138,* 794–797.

Hartnoll, R. L., Mitcheson, M. C., Battersby, A., Brown, G., Ellis, M., Fleming, P., & Hedley N. (1980). Evaluation of heroin maintenance in controlled trial. *Archives of General Psychiatry, 37,* 877–884.

Hathaway, S. R., & McKinley, J. C. (1943). *The Minnesota Multiphasic Personality Inventory.* New York: Psychological Corporation.

Hathaway, S. R., & Monachesi, E. D. (1963). *Adolescent personality and behavior.* Minneapolis: University of Minnesota Press.

Hauri, P., & Orr, W. C. (1982). *The sleep disorders.* Kalamazoo, MI: The Upjohn Company.

Hawton, K. (1982). The behavioural treatment of sexual dysfunction. *British Journal of Psychiatry, 140,* 94–101.

Heilman, K. M., Scholes, R., & Watson, R. T. (1975). Auditory affective agnosia: Disturbed comprehension of affective speech. *Journal of Neurology, Neurosurgery & Psychiatry, 38,* 69–72.

Heim, N. (1981). Sexual behavior of castrated sexual offenders. *Archives of Sexual Behavior, 10,* 11–19.

Heinrichs, D. W., & Buchanan, R. W. (1988). Significance and meaning of neurological signs in schizophrenia. *American Journal of Psychiatry, 145,* 11–18.

Helzer, J. E., Robins, L. N., & McEvoy, L. (1987). Post-traumatic stress disorder in the general population: Findings of the Epidemiological Catchment Area Survey. *New England Journal of Medicine, 317,* 1630–1634.

Helzer, J. E., Robins, L. N., Taylor, J. R., Carey, K., Miller, R. H., Combs-Orme, T., & Farmer, A. (1985). The extent of long-term moderate drinking among alcoholics discharged from medical and psychiatric treatment facilities. *New England Journal of Medicine, 312,* 1678–1682.

Hendin, H. (1982). *Suicide in America.* New York: Norton.

Henn, F. A., Bardwell, R., & Jenkins, R. L. (1980). Juvenile delinquents revisited. *Archives of General Psychiatry, 37,* 1160–1163.

Henning, J. J., & Levy, R. H. (1967). Verbal-performance IQ differences of white and Negro delinquents on the WISC and WAIS. *Journal of Clinical Psychology, 23,* 164–168.

Henry, J. P., & Stephens, P. M. (1977). *Stress, health, and the social environment: A sociobiologic approach to medicine.* New York: Springer-Verlag.

Herbert, W. (1982). The three brains of Eve: EEG data. *Science News, 121,* 356.

Hermann, B. P., & Whitman, S. (1984). Behavioral and personality correlates of epilepsy: A review, methodological critique, and conceptual model. *Psychological Bulletin, 95,* 451–497.

Herskowitz, J., & Rosman, N. P. (1982). *Pediatrics, neurology, and psychiatry—Common ground*. New York: Macmillan.

Heston, L. L. (1966). Psychiatric disorders in foster home reared children of schizophrenic mothers. *British Journal of Psychiatry, 112,* 819–825.

Heston, L. L., & Denny, D. (1968). Interactions between early life experience and biological factors in schizophrenia. In D. Rosenthal & S. S. Kety (Eds.), *The transmission of schizophrenia* (pp. 363-376). Oxford: Pergamon.

Heston, L. L., Mastri, A. R., Anderson, V. E., & White, J. (1981). Dementia of the Alzheimer type. *Archives of General Psychiatry, 38,* 1085–1093.

Heston, L. L., & Shields, J. (1968). Homosexuality in twins: A family study and a registry study. *Archives of General Psychiatry, 18,* 149–160.

Hier, D. B., & Crowley, W. F., Jr. (1982). Spatial ability in androgen-deficient men. *New England Journal of Medicine, 306,* 1202–1205.

Hinkle, L. E. (1974). The effect of exposure to culture change, social change, and changes in interpersonal relationships on health. In B. S. Dohrenwend & B. P. Dohrenwend (Eds.), *Stressful life events: Their nature and effects.* New York: Wiley.

Hiroto, D. S. (1974). Locus of control and learned helplessness. *Journal of Experimental Psychology, 102,* 187–193.

Hirschi, T., & Hindelang, M. J. (1977). Intelligence and delinquency: A revisionist review. *American Sociological Review, 42,* 571–587.

Hodgkinson, S., Sherrington, R., Gurling, H., Marchbanks, R., Reeders, S. et al. (1987). Molecular genetic evidence for heterogeneity in manic depression. *Nature, 325,* 805–806.

Hoehn-Saric, R. (1981). Characteristics of chronic anxiety patients. In D. F. Klein & J. Rabkin (Eds.), *Anxiety: New research and changing concepts* (pp. 399–409). New York: Raven Press.

Hoenig, J., & Kenna, J. C. (1974). The nosological position of transsexualism. *Archives of Sexual Behavior, 3,* 273–287.

Hoffman, R. E., Stopek, S., & Andreasen, N. C. (1986). A comparative study of manic vs schizophrenic speech disorganization. *Archives of General Psychiatry, 43,* 831–838.

Hogarty, G. E., McEvoy, J. P., Munetz, M., DiBarry, A. L., Bartone, P., Cather, R., Cooley, S. J., Ulrich, R. F., Carter, M. M. J., Madonia, M. J. et al. (1988). Dose of fluphenazine, familial expressed emotion, and outcome in schizophrenia: Results of a two-year controlled study. *Archives of General Psychiatry, 45,* 797–805.

Hohmann, G. W. (1966). Some effects of spinal cord lesions on experienced emotional feelings. *Psychophysiology, 3,* 143–156.

Holden, C. (1987). A top priority at NIMH. *Science, 235,* 431.

Holden, E. W., Tarnowski, K. J., & Prinz, R. J. (1982). Reliability of neurological soft signs in children: Reevaluation of the PANESS. *Journal of Abnormal Child Psychology, 10,* 163–172.

Holland, A. J., Hal, A., Murray, R., Russell, G. F. M., & Crisp, A. H. (1984). Anorexia nervosa: A study of 34 twin pairs and one set of triplets. *British Journal of Psychiatry, 145,* 414–419.

Hollon, S., & Beck, A. T. (1986). Research on cognitive therapies. In S. L. Garfield & A. E. Bergin (Eds.), *Handbook of psychotherapy and behavior change* (3rd ed.) (pp. 443–482). New York: Wiley.

Holmes, T. H. (1979). Development and application of a quantitative measure of life change magnitude. In J. E. Barrett, R. M. Rose, & G. L. Klerman (Eds.), *Stress and mental disorder* (pp. 37–53). New York: Raven.

Holmes, T. H., & Rahe, R. H. (1967). The social readjustment rating scale. *Journal of Psychosomatic Research, 11,* 213–218.

Holmstrom, L. L., & Burgess, A. W. (1980). Sexual behavior of assailants during reported rapes. *Archives of Sexual Behavior, 9,* 427–439.

Holt, R. R. (1960). Editor's foreward. In D. Rapaport, M. M. Gill, & R. Schafer, *Diagnostic psychological testing* (pp. 1–44). New York: International Universities Press, 1960.

Holzman, P. S., Kringlen, E., Levy, D. L., Proctor, L. R., Haberman, S. J., & Yasillo, N. J. (1977). Abnormal-pursuit eye movements in schizophrenia. *Archives of General Psychiatry, 34,* 802–805.

Holzman, P. S., Kringlen, E., Matthysse, S., Flanagan, S. D., Lipton, R. B., Cramer, G., Levin, S., Lange, K., & Levy, D. (1988). A single dominant gene can account for eye tracking dysfunctions and schizophrenia in offspring of identical twins. *Archives of General Psychiatry, 45,* 641–647.

Holzman, P. S., & Levy, D. L. (1977). Smooth pursuit eye movements and functional psychoses: A review. *Schizophrenia Bulletin, 3,* 15–27.

Holzman, P. S., Levy, D. L., & Proctor, L. R. (1976). Smooth pursuit eye movements, attention, and schizophrenia. *Archives of General Psychiatry, 33,* 1415–1420.

Holzman, P. S., Shenton, M. E., & Solovay, M. R. (1986). Quality of thought disorder in different diagnosis. *Schizophrenia Bulletin, 12,* 360–371.

Homer, A. C., Honavar, M. Lantos, P. L., Hastie, I. R., Kellett et al., (1988). Diagnosing dementia: Do we get it right? *British Medical Journal, 297,* 894–896.

Hoover, C. F., & Insel, T. R. (1984). Families of origin in obsessive-compulsive disorder. *Journal of Nervous and Mental Disease, 172,* 207–215.

Howard, K. I., Kopta, S. M., Krause, M. S., & Orlinsky, D. E. (1986). The dose-effect relationship in psychotherapy. *American Psychologist, 41,* 159–164.

Hudson, J. I., Pope, H. G., Jr., Jones, J. M., & Yurgelun-Todd, D. (1983). Family history study of anorexia nervosa and bulimia. *British Journal of Psychiatry, 142,* 133–138.

Hull, J. G. (1981). A self-awareness model of the causes and effects of alcohol consumption. *Journal of Abnormal Psychology, 90,* 586–600.

Hull, J. G., Levenson, R. W., Young, R. D., & Sher, K. J. (1983). Self-awareness–reducing effects of alcohol consumption. *Journal of Personality and Social Psychology, 44,* 461–473.

Hunt, J. McV. (1961). The effects of feeding-frustration upon adult hoarding in the albino rat. *Journal of Abnormal and Social Psychology, 36,* 338–360.

Hunt, J. McV. (1961). *Intelligence and experience.* New York: Ronald Press.

Hunt, M. (1974). *Sexual behavior in the 1970's.* New York: Dell.

Hutchings, B., & Mednick, S. A. (1974). Registered criminality in the adoptive and biological parents of registered male adoptees. In S. A. Mednick, F. Schulsinger, J. Higgins, & B. Bell (Eds.) *Genetics, environment and psychopathology* (pp. 215–227). New York: Elsevier Publishing Co.

Hymen, B. T., Van Hoesen, G. W., Damasio, A. R., & Barnes, C. L. (1984). Alzheimer's disease: Cell-specific pathology isolates the hippocampal formation. *Science, 225,* 1168–1170.

Insel, T. R., Ninan, P. T., Aloi, J., Jimerson, D. C., Skolnick, P., & Paul, S. M. (1984). A benzodiazepine receptor-mediated model of anxiety. *Archives of General Psychiatry, 41,* 741–750.

Insel, T. R., Zahn, T., & Murphy, D. L. (1985). Obsessive-compulsive disorder: An anxiety disorder? In A. H. Tuma & J. D. Maser (Eds.), *Anxiety and the anxiety disorders* (pp. 577–589). Hillsdale, NJ: Lawrence Erlbaum.

Iversen, L. L. (1979). The chemistry of the brain. *Scientific American, 241*, 134–149.

Jaffe, J. H. (1965). Drug addiction and drug abuse. In L. Goodman & A. Gilman (Eds.), *The pharmacological basis of therapeutics* (3rd ed.) (pp. 285–311). New York: Macmillan.

Jaffe, J. H. (1980). Drug addiction and drug abuse. In A. G. Gilman, L. S. Goodman, & A. Gilman (Eds.), *The pharmacological basis of therapeutics* (6th ed.) (pp. 535–584). New York: Macmillan Publishing Co.

Janet, P. (1920). *The major symptoms of hysteria* (2nd ed.). New York: Macmillan.

Janowsky, D. S., & Judd, L. (1981). The effects of lithium on cholinergic mechanisms. In C. Perris, G. Struwe, & B. Jansson (Eds.), *Biological psychiatry 1981,* (pp. 653–656). Amsterdam: Elsevier/North-Holland.

Jasinski, D. R., Johnson, R. E., & Henningfield, J. E. (1984). Abuse liability assessment in human subjects. *Trends in Pharmacological Sciences, 5,* 196–200.

Jaynes, J. (1976). *The origin of consciousness in the breakdown of the bicameral mind.* Boston: Houghton Mifflin.

Jefferson, J. W., & Marshall, J. R. (1981). *Neuropsychiatric features of medical disorders.* New York: Plenum.

Jeste, D. V., & Wyatt, R. J. (Eds.) (1984). *Neuropsychiatric movement disorders.* Washington, DC: American Psychiatric Press.

John, E. R., Prichep, L. S., & Easton, J. F. (1988). Neurometrics: Computer-assisted differential diagnosis of brain dysfunctions. *Science, 239* 162–169.

Johnstone, E. C., Crow, T. J., Frith, C. D., Stevens, M., Kreel, L., & Husband, J. (1978). The dementia of dementia praecox. *Acta Psychiatrica Scandinavica, 57,* 305–324.

Jones, E. (1964). *The life and work of Sigmund Freud.* Middlesex, England: Penguin.

Jones, M. C. (1968). Personality correlates and antecedents of drinking patterns in adult males. *Journal of Consulting and Clinical Psychology, 32,* 2–12.

Juel-Nelson, N. (1979). Suicide risk in manic-depressive disorders. In M. Schou & E. Stromgren (Eds.), *Origin, prevention and treatment of affective disorders* (pp. 269–276). New York: Academic Press.

Kaffman, M., & Elizur, E. (1977). Infants who become enuretics: A longitudinal study of 161 Kibbutz children. *Monographs of the Society for Research in Child Development, 42,* No. 2.

Kaij, L. (1960). *Alcoholism in twins: Studies on the etiology and sequels of abuse of alcohol.* Stockholm: Almqvist & Wiksell.

Kamel, G. W. L., & Weinberg, T. S. (1983). Diversity in sadomasochism: Four S & M careers. In G. W. L. Kamel & T. S. Weinberg (Eds.), *S & M: Studies in sadomasochism* (pp. 113–118). Buffalo, NY: Prometheus Books.

Kanfer, F. H., & Phillips, J. S. (1970). *Learning foundations of behavior therapy.* New York: Wiley.

Kanner, L. (1943). Autistic disturbances of affective contact. *Nervous Child, 2,* 217–250.

Kaplan, H. I. (1985). Typical signs and symptoms of psychiatric illness. In H. I. Kaplan, A. M. Freedman, & B. J. Sadock, (Eds.), *Comprehensive textbook of psychiatry/IV* (Vol. 1) (pp. 499–501). Baltimore: Williams & Wilkins.

Kaplan, H. S. (1974). *The new sex therapy.* New York: Brunner/Mazel.

Kaplan, H. S. (1979). *Disorders of sexual desire*. New York: Simon & Schuster.

Kaplan, S. J., Pelcovitz, D., Salzinger, S., & Ganeles, D. (1983). Psychopathology of parents of abused and neglected children and adolescents. *Journal of Academy of Child Psychiatry, 22,* 238–244.

Karpmann, B. (1955). Criminal psychodynamics: A platform. *Archives of Criminal Psychodynamics, 1,* 3–100.

Kass, F., Skodol, A. E., Charles, E., Spitzer, R. L., & Williams, J. B. W. (1985). Scaled ratings of DSM-III personality disorders. *American Journal of Psychiatry, 142,* 627–630.

Katon, W. (1982). Depression: Somatic symptoms and medical disorders in primary care. *Comprehensive Psychiatry, 23,* 274–287.

Kaufman, D. M. (1981). *Clinical neurology for psychiatrists*. New York: Grune & Stratton.

Kaufman, J., & Zigler, E. (1987). Do abused children become abusive parents? *American Journal of Orthopsychiatry, 37,* 186–192.

Kazdin, A. E., Esveldt-Dawson, K., French, N. H., & Unis, A. S. (1987). Problem-solving skills training and relationship therapy in the treatment of antisocial child behavior. *Journal of Consulting and Clinical Psychology, 55,* 76–85.

Kemper, T. L. (1984). Asymmetrical lesions in dyslexia. In N. Geschwind & A. M. Galaburda (Eds.), *Cerebral dominance: The biological foundations* (pp. 75–89). Cambridge, Mass.: Harvard University Press.

Kendell, R. E. (1975). *The role of diagnosis in psychiatry*. Oxford, England: Blackwell Scientific.

Kendler, K. S., & Davis, K. L. (1981). The genetics and biochemistry of paranoid schizophrenia and other paranoid psychoses. *Schizophrenia Bulletin, 7,* 689–709.

Kendler, K. S., & Eaves, L. J. (1986). Models for the joint effect of genotype and environment on liability to psychiatric illness. *The American Journal of Psychiatry, 143,* 279–289.

Kendler, K. S., & Gruenberg, A. M. (1984). An independent analysis of the Danish adoption study of schizophrenia: IV. The relationship between psychiatric disorders as defined by DSM-III in the relatives and adoptees. *Archives of General Psychiatry, 41,* 555–564.

Kendler, K. S., Gruenberg, A. M., & Strauss, J. S. (1981). An independent analysis of the Copenhagen sample of the Danish adoption study of schizophrenia: III. The relationship between paranoid psychosis (delusional disorder) and the schizophrenia spectrum disorders. *Archives of General Psychiatry, 38,* 985–987.

Kendler, K. S., Gruenberg, A. M., & Tsuang, M. T. (1985). Psychiatric illness in first-degree relatives of schizophrenics and surgical control patients: A family study using DSM-III criteria. *Archives of General Psychiatry, 42,* 770–779.

Kendler, K. S., Gruenberg, A. M., & Tsuang, M. T. (1988). A family study of the subtypes of schizophrenia. *American Journal of Psychiatry, 145,* 57–62.

Kendler, K. S., & Hays, P. (1981). Paranoid psychosis (delusional disorder) and schizophrenia. *Archives of General Psychiatry, 38,* 547–551.

Kendler, K. S., & Robinette, C. D. (1983). Schizophrenia in the National Academy of Sciences' National Research Council twin registry: A 16-year update. *American Journal of Psychiatry, 140,* 1551–1563.

Kennedy, J. L., Giuffra, L. A., Moises, H. W., Cavalli-Sforza, L. L., Pakstis, A. J. et al. (1988). Evidence against linkage of schizophrenia to markers on chromosome 5 in a northern Swedish pedigree. *Nature, 336,* 167–170.

Kennedy, W. A. (1965). School phobia: Rapid treatment of fifty cases. *Journal of Abnormal Psychology, 70,* 285–289.

Kerckhoff, A. C. (1982). Analyzing a case of mass psychogenic illness. In M. J. Colligan, J. W. Pennebaker, & L. R. Murphy (Eds.), *Mass psychogenic illness: A social psychological analysis* (pp. 5–19). Hillside, New Jersey: Laurence Erlbaum.

Kertesz, A. (1979). *Aphasia and associated disorders.* New York: Grune & Stratton.

Kety, S. S. (1987). The significance of genetic factors in the etiology of schizophrenia: Results from the national study of adoptees in Denmark. *Journal of Psychiatric Research, 21,* 423–429.

Kety, S. S., Rosenthal, D., Wender, P. H., & Schulsinger, F. (1968). The types and prevalence of mental illness in the biological and adoptive families of adopted schizophrenics. In D. Rosenthal & S. S. Kety (Eds.), *The transmission of schizophrenia* (pp. 345–362). Oxford: Pergamon Press.

Kety, S. S., Rosenthal, D., Wender, P. H., & Schulsinger, F. (1978). The biological and adoptive families of adopted individuals who become schizophrenic: Prevalence of mental illness and other characteristics. In L. C. Wynne, R. L. Cromwell, & S. Matthysse (Eds.), *The nature of schizophrenia: New approaches to research and treatment* (pp. 25–37). New York: Wiley.

Keyes, D. (1981). *The minds of Billy Milligan.* New York: Random House.

Kidd, K. K. (1983). Recent progress on the genetics of stuttering. In C. L. Ludlow & J. A. Cooper (Eds.), *Genetic aspects of speech and language disorders* (pp. 197–213). New York: Academic Press.

Kihlstrom, J. F. (1987). The cognitive unconscious. *Science, 237,* 1445–1452.

Kiloh, L. G. (1982). Electroconvulsive therapy. In E. S. Paykel (Eds.), *Handbook of affective disorders* (pp. 264–275). New York: Guilford Press.

Kimble, R., Williams, J. G., & Agras, S. (1975). A comparison of two methods of diagnosing hysteria. *American Journal of Psychiatry, 132,* 1197–1199.

King, M. C., & Wilson, A. C. (1975). Evolution at two levels: Molecular similarities and biological differences between humans and chimpanzees. *Science, 188,* 107–116.

Kinney, D. K., & Jacobson, B. (1978). Environmental factors in schizophrenia: New adoption study evidence. In L. C. Wynne, R. L. Cromwell, & S. Matthysse (Eds.), *The nature of schizophrenia* (pp. 38–51). New York: Wiley & Sons.

Kinsbourne, M. (1971). The minor cerebral hemisphere as a source of aphasic speech. *Archives of Neurology, 29,* 302–306.

Kinsey, A. C., Pomeroy, W. B., Martin, C. E., & Gebhard, P. H. (1953). *Sexual behavior in the human female.* Philadelphia: W. B. Saunders.

Klein, D. (1972). *Psychiatric case studies: Treatment, drugs and outcome.* Baltimore: Williams & Wilkins.

Klein, D. F. (1981). Anxiety reconceptualized. In D. F. Klein & J. Rabkin (Eds.), *Anxiety: New research and changing concepts* (pp. 235–262). New York: Raven Press.

Klein, D. F., Ross, D. C., & Cohen, P. (1987). Panic and avoidance in agoraphobia: Application of path analysis to treatment studies. *Archives of General Psychiatry, 44,* 377–385.

Klein, D. N., Clark, D. C., Dansky, L., & Margolis, E. T. (1988). Dysthymia in the offspring of parents with primary unipolar depression. *Journal of Abnormal Psychology, 97,* 265–274.

Klein, D. N., Depue, R. A., & Slater, J. F. (1985). Cyclothymia in the adolescent offspring of parents with bipolar disorder. *Journal of Abnormal Psychology, 94,* 115–127.

Klein, D. N., Taylor, E. B., Harding, K., & Dickstein, S. (1988). Double depression and episodic major depression: Demographic, clinical, familial, personality, and socioenvironmental characteristics and short-term outcomes. *American Journal of Psychiatry, 145,* 1226–1231.

Klein, G. S. (1976). *Psychoanalytic theory: An exploration of essentials.* New York: International Universities Press.

Kleinman, J. E., Casanova, M. F., & Jaskiw, G. E. (1988). The neuropathology of schizophrenia. *Schizophrenia Bulletin, 14,* 209–216.

Klerman, G. L. (1978). The evolution of a scientific nosology. In J. C. Shershow (Ed.), *Schizophrenia: Science and practice* (pp. 99–121). Cambridge, MA: Harvard University Press.

Kline, P. (1972). *Fact and fantasy in Freudian theory.* London: Methuen.

Kluft, R. P. (1984). Multiple personality in childhood. In B. G. Braun (Ed.), Symposium on multiple personality. *Psychiatric Clinics of North America, 7,* 121–134.

Kluft, R. P. (1987). An update on multiple personality disorder. *Hospital and Community Psychiatry, 38,* 363–373.

Kluft, R. P. (1987b). First-rank symptoms as a diagnostic clue to multiple personality disorder. *American Journal of Psychiatry, 144,* 293–298.

Kluft, R. P., Steinberg, M., & Spitzer, R. L. (1988). DSM-III-R revisions in the dissociative disorders: An exploration of their derivation and rationale. *Dissociation, 1,* 39–46.

Knox, W. E. (1966). Phenylketonuria. In J. B. Stanbury, J. B. Wyngaarden, & D. S. Fredrickson (Eds.), *The metabolic basis of inherited disease* (pp. 258–294). New York: McGraw Hill.

Kobasa, S. C. O., & Puccetti, M. C. (1983). Personality and social resources in stress resistance. *Journal of Personality and Social Psychology, 45,* 839–850.

Koch, R., Azen, C., Friedman, E. G., & Williamson, M. L. (1984). Paired comparisons between early treated PKU children and their matched sibling controls on intelligence and school achievement test results at eight years of age. *Journal of Inherited Metabolic Diseases, 7,* 86–90.

Kocsis, J. H., & Frances, A. J. (1987). A critical discussion of DSM-III dysthymic disorder. *American Journal of Psychiatry, 144,* 1534–1542.

Kohut, H. (1977). *The restoration of the self.* New York: International Universities Press.

Kolb, B., & Whishaw, I. Q. (1985). *Fundamentals of human neuropsychology.* San Francisco: W. H. Freeman.

Kolb, L. C. (1987). A neuropsychological hypothesis explaining posttraumatic stress disorders. *American Journal of Psychiatry, 144,* 989–995.

Kolb, L. C., & Brodie, H. K. H. (1982). *Modern clinical psychiatry* (10th ed.). Philadelphia: W. B. Saunders Co.

Kolko, D. J., Kazdin, A. E., & Meyer, E. C. (1985). Aggression and psychopathology in childhood firesetters: Parent and child reports. *Journal of Clinical and Consulting Psychology, 53,* 377–385.

Koluchova, J. (1976a). Severe deprivation in twins: A case study. In A. M. Clarke & A. D. B. Clarke (Eds.), *Early experience: Myth and evidence* (pp. 45–55). New York: The Free Press.

Koluchova, J. (1976b). A report on the further development of twins after severe and prolonged deprivation. In A. M. Clarke & A. D. B. Clarke (Eds.), *Early experience: Myth and evidence* (pp. 56–66). New York: The Free Press.

Koranyi, E. (1979). Morbidity and rate of undiagnosed physical illness in a psychiatric clinical population. *Archives of General Psychiatry, 36,* 414–419.

Koranyi, E. K. (1980). *Transsexuality in the male.* Springfield, IL: Charles C Thomas.

Kosslyn, S. M. (1988). Aspects of cognitive neuroscience of mental imagery. *Science, 240,* 1621–1626.

Kosterlitz, H., & Hughes, J. (1975). Some thoughts on the significance of enkephalin, the endogenous ligand, *Life Sciences, 17,* 91–96.

Kraepelin, E. (1907). *Clinical psychiatry.* Delmar, New York: Scholars' Facsimiles & Reprints.

Kraines, S. H. (1948). *The therapy of neuroses and psychoses* (3rd ed.). Philadelphia: Lea & Febiger.

Kravis, N. M. (1988). James Braid's psychophysiology: A turning point in the history of dynamic psychiatry. *American Journal of Psychiatry, 145,* 1191–1206.

Krell, R. (1988). Survivors of childhood experiences in Japanese concentration camps. *American Journal of Psychiatry, 145,* 383–384.

Kroll, J. (1973). A reappraisal of psychiatry in the Middle Ages. *Archives of General Psychiatry, 29,* 276–283.

Krouse, J. P., & Kauffman, J. M. (1982). Minor physical anomalies in exceptional children: A review and critique of research. *Journal of Abnormal Child Psychology, 10,* 147–264.

Kuhnley, E. J., Hendren, R. L., & Quinlan, D. M. (1982). Fire-setting by children. *Journal of the American Academy of Child Psychiatry, 21,* 560–563.

Kula, K. (1986). Changes in gonadotropin regulation in both behavioral and phenotypic disturbances of sexual differentiation in men. *Psychoneuroendocrinology, 11,* 61–67.

Kunst-Wilson, W. R., & Zajonc, R. B. (1980). Affective discrimination of stimuli that cannot be recognized. *Science, 207,* 557–558.

Kupfer, D. J. (1976). REM latency: A psychobiologic marker for primary depressive disease. *Biological Psychiatry, 11,* 159–174.

Kupperman, H. S. (1967). The endocrine status of the transsexual patient. *Transactions of the N.Y. Academy of Sciences, 29,* 434–439.

Lacey, B., & Lacey, J. (1974). Studies of heart rate and other bodily processes in sensorimotor behavior. In P. Obrist, A. Black, J. Brener, & L. Dicara (Eds.), *Cardiovascular psychophysiology* (pp. 538–564). Chicago: Aldine.

Lacey, B. C., & Lacey, J. I. (1978). Two-way communication between the heart and the brain: Significance of time within the cardiac cycle. *American Psychologist, 33,* 99–113.

Lacey, J. S., Bateman, D. E., & VanLean, R. (1953). Autonomic response specificity: An experimental study. *Psychosomatic Medicine, 15,* 8–21.

Lachman, S. J. (1972). *Psychosomatic disorders: A behavioristic interpretation.* New York: Wiley.

Lader, M. (1978). Physiological research in anxiety. In H. M. VanPraag (Ed.), *Research in neurosis* (pp. 108–120). Utrecht, The Netherlands: Bohn, Scheltema, & Holkema.

Lane, H. (1976). *The wild boy of Aveyron.* Cambridge, MA: Harvard University Press.

Lang, P. (1968). Fear reduction and fear behavior: Problems in treating a construct. In J. M. Schlien (Ed.), *Research in psychotherapy, 3* (pp. 90–103). Washington, DC: American Psychological Association.

Lang, P. J. (1978). Anxiety: Toward a psychophysiological definition. In H. S. Akiskal & W. L. Webb (Eds.), *Psychiatric diagnosis: Explorations of biological mediators* (pp. 365–389). New York: SP Medical & Scientific Books.

Langevin, R. (1983). *Sexual strands: Understanding and treating sexual anomalies.* Hillsdale, NJ: Lawrence Erlbaum.

Langevin, R., Paitich, D., Ramsay, G., Anderson, C., Kamrad, J., Pope, S., Geller, G., & Newman, S. (1979). Experimental studies in the etiology of genital exhibitionism. *Archives of Sexual Behavior, 8,* 307–331.

Langinvainio, H., Kaprio, J., Koskenvuo, M., & Lonnquist, J. (1984). Finnish twins reared apart III: Personality factors. *Acta Geneticae Medicae Gemellologiae, 33,* 259–264.

Lassen, N. A., Ingvar, D. H., & Skinhoj, E. (1978, October). Brain function and blood flow. *Scientific American,* 63.

Latham, C., Holzman, P. S., Manschreck. T. C., & Tole, J. (1981). Optokinetic nystagmus and pursuit eye movements in schizophrenia. *Archives of Psychiatry, 38,* 997–1003.

Lazarus, A. A. (1971). Where do behavior therapists take their troubles? *Psychological Reports, 28,* 349–350.

Lazarus, R. S. (1981). The stress and coping paradigm. In C. Eisdorfer, D. Cohen, A. Kleinman, & P. Maxim (Eds.), *Models for clinical psychopathology* (pp. 177–214). New York: Spectrum.

Le, A. D., & Kiianma, K. (1988). Characteristic of ethanol tolerance in alcohol drinking (AA) and alcohol avoiding (ANA) rats. *Psychopharmacology, 94,* 479–483.

Lee, N. F., Rush, A. J., & Mitchell, J. E. (1985). Bulimia and depression. *Journal of Affective Disorders, 9,* 231–238.

Leff, J. P., & Vaughn, C. E. (1981). The role of maintenance therapy and relatives' expressed emotion in relapse of schizophrenia: A two-year follow-up. *British Journal of Psychiatry, 139,* 102–104.

Lehrmitte, F., Pillon, B. & Serdaru, M., (1986). Human autonomy and the frontal lobes. Part I: Imitation and utilization behavior: A neuropsychological study of 75 patients. *Annals of Neurology, 19,* 326–344.

Leibowitz, S. F. (1984). Noradrenergic function in the medial hypothalamus: Potential relation to anorexia nervosa and bulimia. In K. M. Pirke & D. Ploog (Eds.), *The psychobiology of anorexia nervosa* (pp. 35–45). New York: Springer-Verlag.

Leitenberg, H. (1983). Transsexuality: The epitome of sexism and homosexual denial. In G. W. Albee, S. Gordon, & H. Leitenberg (Eds.), *Promoting sexual responsibility and preventing sexual problems* (pp. 183–219). Hanover, Vermont: University Press of New England.

Levander, S., Mattsson, A., Schalling, D., & Dalteg, A. (1987). Psychoendocrine patterns within a group of male juvenile delinquents as related to early psychosocial stress, diagnostic classification, and follow-up data. In D. Magnusson & A. Ohman (Eds.), *Psychopathology: An interactional perspective* (pp. 235–252). New York: Academic Press.

Levitt, J. J., & Tsuang, M. T. (1988). The heterogeneity of schizoaffective disorder: Implications for treatment. *American Journal of Psychiatry, 145,* 926–936.

Levy, D. L., Yasillo, N. J., Dorus, E., Shaughnessy, R., Gibbons, R. D., Peterson, J., Janicak, P. G., Gaviria, M., & Davis, J. M. (1983). Relatives of unipolar and bipolar patients have normal pursuit. *Psychiatry Research, 10,* 285–293.

Levy, R. S., & Jankovic, J. (1983). Placebo-induced conversion reaction: A neurobehavioral and EEG study of hysterical aphasia, seizure, and coma. *Journal of Abnormal Psychology, 92,* 243–249.

Lewine, R. R. J. (1984). Stalking the schizophrenia marker: Evidence for a general vulnerability model of psychopathology. In N. F. Watt, E. J. Anthony, L. C. Wynne, &

J. E. Rolf (Eds.), *Children at risk for schizophrenia: A longitudinal perspective* (pp. 545–550). Cambridge: Cambridge University Press.

Lewinsohn, P. M., Mischel, W., Chaplin, W., & Barton, R. (1980). Social competence and depression: The role of illusory self-perception. *Journal of Abnormal Psychology, 89,* 203–212.

Lewinsohn, P. M., Steinmetz, J. L., Larson, D. W., & Franklin, J. (1981). Depression-related cognitions: Antecedent or consequence? *Journal of Abnormal Psychology, 90,* 213–219.

Lewis, S. W., & Murray, R. M. (1987). Obstetric complications, neurodevelopmental deviance, and risk of schizophrenia. *Journal of Psychiatric Research, 21,* 413–421.

Liebowitz, M. R., Fyer, A. J., Gorman, J. M., Dillon, D., Davies, S., Stein, J. M., Cohen, B. S., & Klein, D. F. (1985). Specificity of lactate infusions in social phobia versus panic disorders. *American Journal of Psychiatry, 142,* 947–950.

Liebowitz, M. R., & Klein, D. F. (1979). Hysteroid dysphoria. *Psychiatric Clinics of North America, 2,* 555–575.

Liem, J. H. (1974). Effects of verbal communication of parents and children: A comparison of normal and schizophrenic families. *Journal of Consulting and Clinical Psychology, 42,* 438–450.

Lincoln, N. B., McGuirk, E., Mulley, G. P., Lendrum, W., Jones, A. C., & Mitchell, J. R. A. (1984). Effectiveness of speech therapy for aphasic stroke patients. *Lancet, I,* 1197–1200.

Lindstrom, L., Klockhoff, I., Svedberg, A., & Bergstrom, K. (1987). Abnormal auditory brain stem responses in hallucinating schizophrenic patients. *British Journal of Psychiatry, 151,* 9–14.

Linehan, M. M., Goodstein, J. L., Nielsen, S. L., & Chils, J. (1983). Reasons for staying alive when you are thinking of killing yourself: The Reasons For Living Inventory. *Journal of Consulting and Clinical Psychology, 51,* 276–286.

Link, B., & Dohrenwend, B. F. (1982a). Formulation of hypotheses about the ratio of untreated to treated cases in the true prevalence studies of functional psychiatric disorders in adults in the United States. In B. P. Dohrenwend et al. (Eds.), *Mental Illness in the United States* (pp. 133–149). New York: Praeger Publishers.

Link, B., & Dohrenwend, B. P. (1982b). Formulation of hypotheses about the true prevalence of demoralization in the United States. In B. P. Dohrenwend et al. (Eds.), *Mental illness in the United States* (pp. 114–132). New York: Praeger Publishers.

Linton, R. (1956). *Culture and mental disorders.* Springfield, IL: Charles C Thomas.

Lipowski, Z. J. (1980). Organic mental disorders: Introduction and review of syndromes. In H. I. Kaplan, A. M. Freedman, & B. J. Sadock (Eds.), *Comprehensive textbook of psychiatry/III* (3rd ed.) (pp. 1359–1392). Baltimore: Williams & Wilkins.

Lipowski, Z. J. (1988). Somatization: The concept and its clinical application. *American Journal of Psychiatry, 145,* 1358–1368.

Lipscomb, T. R., Nathan, P. E., Wilson, T., & Abrams, D. B. (1980). Effects of tolerance on the anxiety-reducing function of alcohol. *Archives of General Psychiatry, 37,* 577–582.

Lipsey, J. R., Robinson, R. G., Pearlson, G. D., Rao, K., & Price, T. R. (1983). Mood change following bilateral hemisphere brain injury. *British Journal of Psychiatry, 143,* 266–273.

Lipton, A. A. (1984). Was the "nervous illness" of Schreber a case of affective disorder? *American Journal of Psychiatry, 141,* 1236–1239.

Lipton, R. B., Levy, D. L., Holzman, P. S., & Levin, S. (1983). Eye movement dysfunctions in psychiatric patients: A review. *Schizophrenic Bulletin, 9,* 13–32.

Lishman, W. A. (1978). *Organic psychiatry.* Oxford: Blackwell Scientific Publications.

Liskow, B. L., Clayton, P., Woodruff, R., Guze, S. B., & Cloninger, R. (1977). Briquet's syndrome, hysterical personality, and the MMPI. *American Journal of Psychiatry, 134,* 1137–1139.

Livingstone, M., & Hubel, D. (1988). Segregation of form, color, movement, and depth: Anatomy, physiology, and perception. *Science, 240,* 740–749.

Ljungberg, L. (1957). Hysteria: A clinical, prognostic and genetic study. *Acta Psychiatrica et Neurological Scandinavica, 32,* Supplement 112.

Loeber, R. (1982). The stability of antisocial and delinquent child behavior: A review. *Child Development, 53,* 1431–1446.

Loeber, R., & Dishion, T. (1983). Early predictors of male delinquency: A review. *Psychological Bulletin, 94,* 68–99.

Loehlin, J. C., Horn, J. M., & Willerman, L. (1989). Modeling IQ change: Evidence from the Texas Adoption Project. *Child Development, 60,* 993–1004.

Loehlin, J. C., Horn, J. M., & Willerman, L. (in press). Heredity, environment, and personality change: Evidence from the Texas Adoption Project. *Journal of Personality.*

Loehlin, J. C., Willerman, L., & Horn, J. M. (1982). Personality resemblances between unwed mothers and their adopted-away offspring. *Journal of Social and Personality Psychology, 42,* 1089–1099.

Loranger, A. W. (1981). Genetic independence of manic-depression and schizophrenia. *Acta Psychiat. Scand., 63,* 444–452.

Loranger, A., Susman, V., Oldham, J., & Russakoff, L. M. (1987). Personality disorder examination: A preliminary report. *Journal of Personality Disorders.*

Lorenz, K. (1963). *On aggression.* New York: Harcourt, Brace & World/Bantam, 1966.

Losonczy, M. F., Song, I. S., Mohs, R. C., Mathe, A. A., Davidson, M., Davis, B. M., & Davis, K. L. (1986). Correlates of lateral ventricular size in chronic schizophrenia: II. Biological measures. *American Journal of Psychiatry, 143,* 1113–1118.

Lou, H. C., Henriksen, L., & Bruhn, P. (1984). Focal cerebral hypoperfusion in children with dysphasia and/or attention deficit disorder. *Archives of Neurology, 41,* 825–829.

Lovass, O. (1987). Behavioral treatment and normal educational and intellectual functioning in young autistic children. *Journal of Consulting and Clinical Psychology, 55,* 3–9.

Lovaas, O. I., & Simmons, J. Q. (1969). Manipulation of self-destruction in three retarded children. *Journal of Applied Behavior Analysis, 2,* 143–157.

Lowing, P. A., Mirsky, A. F., & Pereira, R. (1983). The inheritance of schizophrenia spectrum disorders: A reanalysis of the Danish adoptee study data. *American Journal of Psychiatry, 140,* 1167–1171.

Luborsky, L. (1962). Clinicians' judgments of mental health. *Archives of General Psychiatry, 7,* 407–417.

Ludwig, A. M., Brandsma, J. M., Wilbur, C. B., Bendfeldt, F., & Jameson, D. H. (1972). The objective study of a multiple personality: Or, are four heads better than one? *Archives of General Psychiatry, 26,* 298–310.

Ludwig, A. M., Wikler, A., & Stark, L. H. (1974). The first drink: Psychobiological aspects of craving. *Archives of General Psychiatry, 30,* 539–547.

Lum, L. C. (1981). Hyperventilation and anxiety states. *Journal of the Royal Society of Medicine, 74,* 1–4.

Luria, A. R. (1973). The frontal lobes and the regulation of behavior. In K. H. Pribram & A. R. Luria (Eds.), *Psychophysiology of the frontal lobes* (pp. 3–26). N.Y.: Academic Press.

Luria, A. R. (1980). *Higher cortical functions in man* (2nd ed.). New York: Basic Books.

Luria, A. R., & Hutton, T. (1977). A modern assessment of the basic forms of aphasia. *Brain and Language, 4,* 129–151.

Luxenberg, J. S., Swedo, S. E., Flament, M. F., Friedland, R. P., Rapoport, J., & Rapoport, S. I. (1988). Neuroanatomical abnormalities in obsessive-compulsive disorder detected with quantitative X-ray computed tomography. *American Journal of Psychiatry, 145,* 1089–1093.

Lykken, D. (1957). A study of anxiety in the sociopathic personality. *Journal of Abnormal Psychology, 55,* 6–10.

Lykken, D. T. (1982). Research with twins: The concept of emergenesis. *Psychophysiology, 19,* 361–373.

Lykken, D. T., Tellegen, A., & Iacono, W. G. (1982). EEG spectra in twins: Evidence for a neglected mechanism of genetic determination. *Physiological Psychology, 10,* 60–65.

MacDonald, N. (1960). Living with schizophrenia. *Canadian Medical Journal, 82,* 218–221.

Macias-Flores, M. A., Garcia-Cruz, D., Escobar-Lujan, M., et al. (1984). A new form of hypertrichosis inherited as an X-linked dominant trait. *Human Genetics, 66,* 66–70.

MacKinnon, R. A. (1980). Diagnosis and psychiatry: Examination of the psychiatric patient. In H. I. Kaplan, A. M. Freedman, & B. J. Sadock (Eds.), *Comprehensive textbook of psychiatry/III* (3rd ed.), *Vol. 1* (pp. 895–905). Baltimore: Williams & Wilkins.

MacLean, P. D. (1962). New findings relevant to the evolution of psychosexual functions of the brain. *Journal of Nervous and Mental Disease, 135,* 289.

MacLean, P. D. (1964). Man and his animal brains. *Modern Medicine, 3,* 95–106.

MacLean, P. D. (1973). A triune concept of brain and behavior. In Boag, T. & Campbell, D. (Eds.), *The Hincks memorial lectures.* Toronto: University of Toronto Press.

MacLeod, C., Mathews, A., & Tata, P. (1986). Attentional bias in emotional disorders. *Journal of Abnormal Psychology, 95,* 15–20.

MacMillan, J. F., Gold, A., Crow, T. J., Johnson, A. L., & Johnstone, E. C., IV (1986). Expressed emotion and relapse. *British Journal of Psychiatry, 148,* 133–143.

Magnusson, D. (1987). Adult delinquency in the light of conduct and physiology at an early age: A longitudinal study. In D. Magnusson & A. Ohman (Eds.), *Psychopathology: An interactional perspective* (pp. 221–234). New York: Academic Press.

Maher, B. A., & Maher, W. B. (1979). Psychopathology. In E. Hearst (Ed.), *The first century of experimental psychology* (pp. 561–621). Hillsdale, NJ: Lawrence Erlbaum.

Maher, W. B., & Maher, B. A. (1985). Psychopathology: I. From ancient times to the eighteenth century. In G. A. Kimble & K. Schlesinger (Eds.), *Topics in the history of psychology, Vol. 2* (pp. 251–294). Hillsdale, NJ: Lawrence Erlbaum.

Mai, F. M., & Merskey, H. (1980). Briquet's *Treatise on Hysteria:* A synopsis and commentary. *Archives of General Psychiatry, 37,* 1401–1405.

Maier, N. R. F. (1949). *Frustration.* Ann Arbor: University of Michigan Press.

Maier, W., Philipp, M., & Buller, R. (1988). The value of structured clinical interviews. *Archives of General Psychiatry, 45,* 963–964.

Malamuth, N. M., & Check. J. V. P. (1981). Penile tumescence and perceptual responses to rape as a function of victim's perceived reactions. *Journal of Applied Social Psychology, 10,* 528–547.

Malan, D. H., Heath, E. J., Bacal, H. A., & Balfour, H. G. (1975). Psychodynamic changes in untreated patients. II. Apparently genuine improvements. *Archives of General Psychiatry, 32,* 110–126.

Maloney, M. P., & Ward, M. P. (1976). *Psychological assessment: A conceptual approach.* New York: Oxford University Press.

Manosevitz, M., & Stedman, J. M. (1981). Some thoughts on training the novice family therapist in the art of family assessment. *Family Therapy, 13,* 67–76.

Marcus, J., Auerbach, J., Wilkinson, L., & Burack, C. M. (1984). Infants at risk for schizophrenia. The Jerusalem infant development study. In N. F. Watt, E. J. Anthony, L. C. Wynne, & J. E. Rolf (Eds.), *Children at risk for schizophrenia: A longitudinal perspective* (pp. 440–464). Cambridge: Cambridge University Press.

Margraf, J., Ehlers, A., & Roth, W. T. (1986). Biological models of panic disorder—a review. *Behavior Research and Therapy, 24,* 553–567.

Mark, V. H., & Ervin, F. R. (1970). *Violence and the brain.* New York: Harper & Row Publishers.

Marks, I. (1969). *Fears and phobias.* New York: Academic Press.

Marks, I. (1981). *Cure and care of neuroses: Theory and practice of behavioral psychotherapy.* New York: Wiley.

Marks, I. (1987). *Fears, phobias and rituals: Panic, anxiety, and their disorders.* New York: Oxford University Press.

Marks, I. (1988). Blood-injury phobia: A review. *American Journal of Psychiatry, 145,* 1207–1213.

Marshall, J. C., & Newcombe, F. (1980). The conceptional status of deep dyslexia: An historical perspective. In M. Coltheart, K. Patterson, & J. C. Marshall (Eds.), *Deep dyslexia* (pp. 1–21). London: Routledge and Kegan Paul.

Marshall, J. F., Levitan, D., & Stricker, E. M. (1976). Activation-induced restoration of sensorimotor functions in rats with dopamine-depleting brain lesions. *Journal of Comparative and Physiological Psychology, 90,* 536–546.

Martin, B., & Sroufe, L. A., (1970). Anxiety. In C. G. Costello (Ed.), *Symptoms of psychopathology: A handbook* (pp. 216–259). New York: Wiley.

Martin, J. H. (1981). Properties of cortical neurons, the EEG, and the mechanisms of epilepsy. In E. R. Kandel & J. H. Schwartz (Eds.), *Principles of neural science* (pp. 461–471). New York: Elsevier/North-Holland.

Martin, J. H., & Brust, J. C. M. (1981). Imaging the living brain. In E. R. Kandel & J. H. Schwartz (Eds.), *Principles of neural science* (pp. 259–283). New York: Elsevier.

Masling, J. (1960). The influence of situational and interpersonal variables in projective testing. *Psychological Bulletin, 57,* 65–85.

Mason, J. W. (1975). Clinical psychophysiology: Psychoendocrine mechanisms. In S. Arieti (Ed.), *American handbook of psychiatry* (2nd ed.), (Vol. 4) (pp. 553–582). New York: Basic Books.

Masserman, J. (1950/1966). Experimental neurosis. In S. Coopersmith (Ed.), *Frontiers of psychological research* (Readings from Scientific American). San Francisco: Freeman.

Masters, W. H., & Johnson, V. E. (1970). *Human sexual inadequacy.* Boston: Little, Brown.

Masters, W. H., & Johnson, V. E. (1979). *Homosexuality in perspective.* Boston: Little, Brown.

Masters, W. H., Johnson, V. E., & Kolodny, R. C. (1982). *Human Sexuality.* Boston: Little, Brown.

Mathews, A. M., Gelder, M. G., & Johnston, D. W. (1981). *Agoraphobia: Nature and treatment.* New York: Guilford Press.

Mathews, A. M., Johnston, D. W., Lancashire, M., Munby, M., Shaw, P. M., & Gelder, M. G. (1976). Imaginal flooding and exposure to real phobic situations: Treatment outcome with agoraphobic patients. *British Journal of Psychiatry, 129,* 362–371.

Mathews, A. M., & MacLeod, C. (1986). Discrimination of threat cues without awareness in anxiety states. *Journal of Abnormal Psychology, 95,* 131–138.

Matussek, P., Soldner, M. L., & Nagel, D. (1982). Neurotic depression. *Journal of Nervous and Mental Disease, 170,* 588–597.

Mayr, E. (1978). Evolution. *Scientific American, 239,* 47–55.

McCabe, M. S., & Stromgren, E. (1975). Reactive psychoses: A family study. *Archives of General Psychiatry, 32,* 447–454.

McCarley, R. W. (1982). REM sleep and depression: Common neurobiological control mechanisms. *American Journal of Psychiatry, 139,* 565–570.

McCauley, E., Kay, T., Ito, J., & Treder, R. (1987). The Turner syndrome: Cognitive deficits, affective discrimination, and behavior problems. *Child Development, 58,* 464–473.

McClearn, G. E., & DeFries, J. C. (1973). *Introduction to behavioral genetics.* San Francisco: W. H. Freeman.

McClure, J. N., Reich, T., Wetzel, R. D. (1971). Premenstrual symptoms as indicators of bipolar affective disorder. *British Journal of Psychiatry, 119,* 527–528.

McFie, J., & Zangwill, O. L. (1960). Visual-constructive disabilities associated with lesions of the left cerebral hemisphere. *Brain, 83,* 243–260.

McGue, M., Gottesman, I. I., & Rao, D. C. (1983). The transmission of schizophrenia under the multifactorial threshold model. *American Journal of Human Genetics, 35,* 1161–1178.

McGuffin, P., Farmer, A. E., & Gottesman, I. I. (1987). Is there really a split in schizophrenia? The genetic evidence. *British Journal of Psychiatry, 150,* 581–592.

McGuffin, P., Farmer, A. E., Gottesman, I. I., Murray, R. M., & Reveley, A. M. (1984). Twin concordance for operationally defined schizophrenia: Confirmation of familiality and heritability. *Archives of General Psychiatry, 41,* 541–545.

McGuffin, P., Reveley, A., & Holland, A. (1982). Identical triplets: Nonidentical psychosis? *British Journal of Psychiatry, 140,* 1–6.

McGuinness, D., & Pribram, K. (1980). The neuropsychology of attention: Emotional and motivational controls. In M. C. Wittrock (Ed.), *The brain and psychology* (pp. 95–139). New York: Academic Press.

McKenna, P. J. (1984). Disorders with overvalued ideas. *British Journal of Psychiatry, 145,* 579–585.

McKinney, W. T., & Bunney, W. E. (1969). Animal model of depression: I. Review of evidence: Implications for research. *Archives of General Psychiatry, 21,* 240–248.

McKinney, W. T., & Moran, E. C. (1982). Animal models. In E. S. Paykel (Ed.), *Handbook of affective disorders* (pp. 202–211). New York: Guilford Press.

McKinney, W. T., Suomi, S. J., & Harlow, H. F. (1971). Depression in primates. *American Journal of Psychiatry, 127,* 1313–1320.

McKusick, V. (1978). *Mendelian inheritance in man.* Baltimore: Johns Hopkins Press.

McNeil, T. F., & Kaij, L. (1978). Obstetric factors in the development of schizophrenia: Complications in the births of preschizophrenics and in reproduction by schizophrenic parents. In L. C. Wynne, R. L. Cromwell, & S. Matthysse (Eds.), *The nature of schizophrenia: New approaches to research and treatment* (pp. 401–429). New York: Wiley.

Mechanic, D. (1974). Discussion of research programs on relations between stressful life events and episodes of physical illness. In B. S. Dohrenwend & B. P. Dohrenwend (Eds.), *Stressful life events: Their nature and effects* (pp. 87–97). New York: Wiley.

Mednick, S. A., Gabrielli, W. F., Jr., & Hutchings, B. (1984). Genetic influences in criminal convictions: Evidence from an adoption cohort. *Science, 224,* 891–894.

Mednick, S. A., Pollock, V., Volavka, J., & Gabrielli, W. F., Jr. (1982). Biology and violence. In M. E. Wolfgang & N. A. Weiner (Eds.), *Criminal violence* (pp. 21–80). Beverly Hills, CA: Sage Publications.

Mednick, S. A., & Schulsinger, F. (1968). Some premorbid characteristics related to breakdown of children with schizophrenic mothers. In D. Rosenthal & S. S. Kety (Eds.), *The transmission of schizophrenia* (pp. 267–291). New York: Pergamon.

Meehl, P. E. (1962). Schizotaxia, schizotypy, schizophrenia. *American Psychologist, 17,* 827–838.

Meehl, P. E. (1978). Theoretical risks and tabular asterisks: Sir Karl, Sir Ronald, and the slow progress of soft psychology. *Journal of Consulting and Clinical Psychology, 46,* 806–834.

Meehl, P. (1986). Diagnostic taxa as open concepts: Metatheoretical and statistical questions about reliability and construct validity in the ground strategy of nosological revision. In T. Millon & G. L. Klerman (Eds.), *Contemporary directions in psychopathology: Toward the DSM-IV* (pp. 215–231). New York: The Guilford Press.

Megargee, E. I. (Ed.) (1966). *Research in clinical assessment.* New York: Harper & Row.

Megaro, P. A. (1981). The paranoid and the schizophrenic: The case for distinct cognitive style. *Schizophrenia Bulletin, 7,* 632–661.

Meichenbaum, D. (1977). *Cognitive-behavior modification: An integrative approach.* New York: Plenum Press.

Meichenbaum, D., & Genest, M. (1980). Cognitive behavior modification: An integration of cognitive and behavioral methods. In F. H. Kanfer & A. P. Goldstein (Eds.), *Helping people change* (2nd ed.). New York: Pergamon Press.

Meller, W., Kathol, R. G., Jaeckle, R. S., Grambsch, P., & Lopez, J. F. (1988). HPA axis abnormalities in depressed patients with normal response to the DST. *American Journal of Psychiatry, 145,* 318–324.

Mello, N. K., & Mendelson, J. H. (1978). Alcohol and human behavior. In L. L. Iversen, S. D. Iversen, & S. H. Snyder (Eds.), *Handbook of psychopharmacology. Vol. 12: Drug abuse* (pp. 235–317). New York: Plenum Press.

Meltzer, H. Y. (1979). Biochemical studies in schizophrenia. In L. Bellak (Ed.), *Disorders of the schizophrenic syndrome* (pp. 135–345). New York: Basic Books.

Mendelson, J. H., & Mello, N. K. (1979). The treatment of alcoholism: A reevaluation of the rationale for therapy. In J. Mendewicz & H. M. van Praag (Eds.), *Alcoholism: A multidisciplinary approach* (pp. 11–19). Basel, Switzerland: S. Karger.

Mendelson, W. B., Gillin, J. C., & Wyatt, R. J. (1978). *Human sleep and its disorders.* New York: Plenum.

Mendlewicz, J. (1981). Adoption study in affective illness. In C. Perris, G. Struwe, & B. Jansson (Eds.), *Biological psychiatry 1981* (pp. 101–107). Amsterdam: Elsevier/North-Holland.

Mendlewicz, J., & Rainer, J. D. (1977). Adoption study supporting genetic transmission in manic-depressive illness. *Nature, 268,* 327–329.

Merikangas, K. R. (1982). Assortative mating for psychiatric disorders and psychological traits. *Archives of General Psychiatry, 39,* 1173–1180.

Merrill, D. J. (1962), *Evolution and genetics.* New York: Holt, Rinehart & Winston.

Merskey, H. (1986). The importance of hysteria. *British Journal of Psychiatry, 149,* 23–28.

Mesulam, M. M. (1981). Dissociative states with abnormal temporal lobe EEG. *Archives of Neurology, 38,* 176–181.

Metalsky, G. I., Abramson, L. Y., Seligman, M. E. P., Semmel, A., & Peterson, C. (1982). Attributional styles and life events in the classroom: Vulnerability and invulnerability to depressive mood reactions. *Journal of Personality and Social Psychology, 43,* 612–617.

Metalsky, G. I., Halberstadt, L., & Abramson, L. Y. (1987). Vulnerability to depressive mood reactions: Toward a more powerful test of the diathesis-stress and causal mediation components of the reformulated theory of depression. *Journal of Personality and Social Psychology, 52,* 389–393.

Metrakos, J. D., & Metrakos, K. (1960). Genetics of convulsive disorders. I. Introduction, problems, methods, baselines. *Neurology, 10,* 228–240.

Metrakos, J. D., & Metrakos, K. (1961). Genetics of convulsive disorders. II. Genetic and electroencephalic studies in centrencephalic epilepsy. *Neurology, 11,* 474–483.

Meyer, R. J., & Haggerty, R. J. (1962). Streptococcal infection in families: Factors affecting individual susceptibility. *Pediatrics, 29,* 539–549.

Meyer-Bahlburg, H. F. L. (1977). Sex hormones and male homosexuality in comparative perspective. *Archives of Sexual Behavior, 6,* 297–325.

Miles, C. P. (1977). Conditions predisposing to suicide: A review. *Journal of Nervous and Mental Disease, 164,* 231–246.

Miller, F. W., Dawson, R. O., Dix, G. E., & Parnas, R. I. (1976). *The mental health process.* Mineola, NY: The Foundation Press, Inc.

Miller, R. C., & Berman, J. S. (1983). The efficacy of cognitive behavior therapies: A quantitative review of the research evidence. *Psychological Bulletin, 94,* 39–53.

Miller, W. E. (1981). The benzodiazepine receptor: An update. *Pharmacology, 22,* 153–161.

Miller, W. R., & Heather, N. (1986). The effectiveness of alcoholism treatment: What research reveals. In W. R. Miller & Reid K. Hester (Eds.), *Treating addictive behaviors: Processes of change* (pp. 121–174). New York: Plenum Press.

Miller, W. R., Rosellini, R. A., & Seligman, M. E. P. (1977). Learned helplessness and depression. In J. D. Maser & M. E. P. Seligman (Eds.), *Psychopathology: Experimental models* (pp. 104–130). San Francisco: Freeman.

Millon, T. (1969). *Modern psychopathology: A biosocial approach to maladaptive learning and functioning.* Philadelphia: Saunders.

Millon, T. (1975). Reflections on Rosenhan's "On being sane in insane places." *Journal of Abnormal Psychology, 84,* 456–461.

Millon, T. (1981). *Disorders of personality: DSM-III: Axis II.* New York: Wiley.

Millon, T. (1986). On the past and future of the DSM-III: Personal reflections and projections. In T. Millon & G. L. Klerman (Eds.), *Contemporary directions in psychopathology: Toward the DSM-IV* (pp. 29–70). New York: The Guilford Press.

Millon, T., & Klerman, G. L. (1986). *Contemporary directions in psychopathology: Toward the DSM-IV.* New York: The Guilford Press.

Milner, B. (1974). Sparing of language functions after early brain damage. *Neurosciences Research Program Bulletin, 12,* 213–217.

Mineka, S. (1985). Animal models of anxiety-based disorders: Their usefulness and limitations. In J. Maser & A. H. Tuma (Eds.), *Anxiety and the anxiety disorders* (pp. 199–244). Hillsdale, NJ: Lawrence Erlbaum.

Mineka, S., & Cook, M. (1986). Immunization against the observational conditioning of snake fear in Rhesus monkeys. *Journal of Abnormal Psychology, 95,* 307–318.

Mineka, S., Davisdon, M., Cook, M., & Keir, R. (1984). Observational conditioning of snake fear in Rhesus monkeys. *Journal of Abnormal Psychology, 93,* 355–372.

Mineka, S., & Kihlstrom, J. F. (1978). Unpredictable and uncontrollable events: A new perspective on experimental neurosis. *Journal of Abnormal Psychology, 87,* 256–271.

Mineka, S., & Suomi, S. J. (1978). Social separation in monkeys. *Psychological Bulletin, 85,* 1376–1400.

Mirsky, A. F., DeLisi, L. E., Buchsbaum, M. S., Quinn, O. W., Schwerdt, P., Siever, L. J., Mann, L. Weingartner, H., Zec, R., Sostek, A., Alkerman, I., Revere, V., Dawson, S. D., & Zahn, J. P. (1984). The Genain Quadruplets: Psychological studies. *Psychiatry Research, 13,* 77–93.

Mischel, W. (1973). Toward a cognitive social learning reconceptualization of personality. *Psychological Review, 80,* 252–283.

Mischler, E. G., & Waxler, N. E. (1968). *Interaction in families: An experimental study of family processes and schizophrenia.* New York: Wiley.

Mishkin, M., & Appenzeller, T. (1987, May). The anatomy of memory. *Scientific American, 256,* 80–89.

Moffitt, T. (in press). The neuropsychology of juvenile delinquency: A critical review of research and theory. In N. Morris & M. Tonry (Eds.), *Crime and justice: An annual review of research.* Chicago: Chicago University Press.

Moffitt, T., & Silva, P. A. (1988). IQ and delinquency: A direct test of the differential detection hypothesis. *Journal of Abnormal Psychology, 97,* 330–333.

Mohs, R. C., Breitner, J. C. S., Silverman, J. M., & Davis, K. L. (1987). Alzheimer's disease: Morbid risk among first-degree relatives. *Archives of General Psychiatry, 44,* 405–408.

Money, J., & Bennett, R. G. (1981). Postadolescent paraphilic sex offenders: Antiandrogenic and counseling therapy follow-up. *International Journal of Mental Health, 10,* 122–133.

Money, J., & Ehrhardt, A. A. (1972). *Man & woman/boy & girl.* Johns Hopkins University Press.

Money, J., & Russo, A. (1979). Homosexual outcome of discordant gender identity/role in childhood: Longitudinal follow-up. *Journal of Pediatric Psychology, 4,* 29–41.

Money, J., Schwartz, M., & Lewis, V. G. (1984). Adult heterosexual status and fetal hormonal masculinization and demasculinization: 46,XX congenital virilizing adrenal hyperplasia and 46,XY androgen-insensitivity syndrome compared. *Psychoneuroendocrinology, 9,* 405–414.

Monroe, R. R. (1978). The medical model in psychopathy and dyscontrol syndromes. In W. H. Reid (Ed.), *The psychopath* (pp. 190–208). New York: Brunner/Mazel Publishers.

Morneau, R. H., Jr., & Rockwell, R. R. (1980). *Sex, motivation, and the criminal offender.* Springfield, IL: Charles C Thomas.

Morrison, J. R. (1978). Management of Briquet syndrome (hysteria). *Western Journal of Medicine, 128,* 482–487.

Mosher, L. R. (1978). Can diagnosis be nonpejorative? In L. C. Wynne, R. L. Cromwell, & S. Matthysse (Eds.), *The nature of schizophrenia: New approaches to research and theory* (pp. 690–695). New York: Wiley.

Motley, M. T. (1980). Verification of ''Freudian Slips'' and semantic prearticulatory editing via laboratory-induced spoonerisms. In V. A. Fromkin (Ed.), *Errors in linguistic performance: Slips of the tongue, ear, pen, and hand* (pp. 133–147). New York: Academic Press.

Motley, M. T. (1985). Slips of the tongue. *Scientific American, 253,* 116–127.

Mowrer, O. H. (1947). On the dual nature of learning. *Harvard Educational Review, 17,* 102–148.

Mueser, K. T., & Butler, R. W. (1987). Auditory hallucinations in combat-related chronic posttraumatic stress disorder. *American Journal of Psychiatry, 144,* 299–302.

Munford, P. R., & Liberman, R. P. (1982). Behavior therapy of hysterical disorders. In A. Roy (Ed.), *Hysteria* (pp. 287–303). Chichester, England: Wiley.

Munjack, D., & Moss, H. B. (1981). Affective disorder and alcoholism in families of agoraphobics. *Archives of General Psychiatry, 38,* 869–871.

Munro, A. (1982). Paranoia revisited. *British Journal of Psychiatry, 141,* 344–349.

Murphey, R. M. (1983). Phenylketonuria (PKU) and the single gene: An old story retold. *Behavior Genetics, 13,* 141–157.

Murphy, G. E. (1984). The prediction of suicide: Why is it so different? *American Journal of Psychotherapy, 38,* 341–349.

Murphy, G. E., Simons, A. D., Wetzel, R. D., & Lustman, P. J. (1984). Cognitive therapy and pharmacotherapy. *Archives of General Psychiatry, 41,* 33–41.

Murray, H. A. (1940). What should psychologists do about psychoanalysis? *Journal of Abnormal and Social Psychology, 35,* 150–175.

Murray, H. A. (1943). *Manual of Thematic Apperception Test.* Cambridge, MA: Harvard University.

Muse, K. N., Cetel, N. S., Futterman, L. A., & Yen, S. S. (1984). The premenstrual syndrome: Effects of ''medical ovariectomy.'' *The New England Journal of Medicine, 311,* 1345–1349.

Naeser, M. A. (1982). Language behavior in stroke patients. *Trends in Neuroscience, 5,* 53–59.

Naficy, A., & Willerman, L. (1980). Excessive yielding to normal biases is not a distinctive sign of schizophrenia. *Journal of Abnormal Psychology, 89,* 697–703.

Neale, J. M., Oltmanns, T. F., & Davison, G. C. (1982) *Case studies in abnormal psychology.* New York: Wiley.

Neel, J. V., Fajans, S. S., Conn, J. W., & Davidson, R. T. (1965). Diabetes mellitus. In J. V. Neel, M. W. Shaw, & W. J. Schull (Eds.), *Genetics and epidemiology of chronic diseases.* Public Health Service Publication No. 1163, Washington, DC: Government Printing Office.

Nemiah, J. C. (1980a). Dissociative disorders (Hysterical neurosis, dissociative type),

In H. I. Kaplan, A. M. Freedman, & B. J. Sadock (Eds.), *Comprehensive textbook of psychiatry/III* (3rd ed.), Vol. 2 (pp. 1544–1561). Baltimore: Williams & Wilkins.

Nemiah, J. C. (1980b). Phobic disorder (phobic neurosis). In H. I. Kaplan, A. M. Freeman, & B. J. Sadock (Eds.), *Comprehensive textbook of psychiatry/III* (3rd ed.) Vol. 2 (pp. 1493–1504). Baltimore: Williams & Wilkins.

Nemiah, J. C. (1980c). Somatoform disorders. In H. I. Kaplan, A. M. Freedman, & B. J. Sadock (Eds.), *Comprehensive textbook of psychiatry/III* (3rd ed.), Vol. 2 (pp. 1525–1544). Baltimore: Williams & Wilkins.

Neuchterlein, K. H. (1984). Sustained attention among children vulnerable to adult schizophrenia and among hyperactive children. In N. F. Watt, E. J. Anthony, L. C. Wynne, & J. E. Rolf (Eds.), *Children at risk for schizophrenia: A longitudinal perspective* (pp. 304–311). Cambridge: Cambridge University Press.

Neugebauer, R. (1978). Treatment of the mentally ill in medieval and early modern England: A reappraisal. *Journal of the History of the Behavioral Sciences, 14,* 158–169.

Newlin, D. B. (1985). The antagonistic placebo response to alcohol cues. *Alcoholism: Clinical and Experimental Research, 9,* 411–416.

Newman, J. P., & Kosson, D. S. (1986). Passive avoidance learning in psychopathic and nonpsychopathic offenders. *Journal of Abnormal Psychology, 95,* 252–256.

Nichols, P. L., & Chen, T. (1981). *Minimal brain dysfunction.* Hillsdale, NJ: Lawrence Erlbaum.

Nicholson, R. A., & Berman, J. S. (1983). Is follow-up necessary in evaluating psychotherapy? *Psychological Bulletin, 93,* 261–278.

Nielsen, J. M., & Sedgwick, R. P. (1949). Instincts and emotions in an anencephalic monster. *Journal of Nervous and Mental Disease, 110,* 387–394.

Ninan, P. T., Insel, T. M., Cohen, R. M., Cook, J. M., Skolnick, P., & Paul, S. M. (1982). Benzodiazepine receptor-mediated experimental "anxiety" in primates. *Science, 218,* 1332–1334.

Nolen-Hoeksema, S. (1987). Sex differences in unipolar depression: Evidence and theory. *Psychological Bulletin, 101,* 259–282.

Nora, J. J., & Fraser, F. C. (1981). *Medical genetics: Principles and practice.* Philadelphia: Lea & Febiger.

Noyes, Jr., R., Anderson, D. J., Clancy, J., Crowe, R. R., Slymen, D. J., Ghoneim, M. M., & Hinrichs, J. V. (1984). Diazepam and propranolol in panic disorder and agoraphobia. *Archives of General Psychiatry, 41,* 287–292.

Noyes, R., Jr., Clarkson, C., Crowe, R. R., Yates, W. R., & McChesney, C. M. (1987). A family study of generalized anxiety disorder. *American Journal of Psychiatry, 144,* 1019–1024.

Noyes, R., Jr., Crowe, R. R., Harris, E. L., Hamra, B. J., McChesney, C. M., & Chaudhry, D. R. (1986). Relationship between panic disorder and agoraphobia: A family study. *Archives of General Psychiatry, 43,* 227–232.

Ochitill, H. (1982). Somatization disorder. In J. H. Greist, J. W. Jefferson, & R. L. Spitzer (Eds.), *Treatment of mental disorders* (pp. 266–271). New York: Oxford University Press.

O'Connor, N., & Hermelin, B. (1978). *Seeing and hearing and space and time.* New York: Academic Press.

Offord, D. R., & Reitsma-Street, M. (1983). Problems of studying antisocial behavior. *Psychiatric Developments, 2,* 207–224.

Ohman, A. (1979). Fear relevance, autonomic conditioning, and phobias: A laboratory model. In P. O. Sjoden & S. Bates (Eds.), *Trends in behavior therapy* (pp. 107–133). New York: Academic Press.

Ohman, A., Fredrickson, M., Hugdahl, K., & Rimino, P.-A. (1976). The premise of equipotentiality in human classical conditioning: Conditioned electrodermal responses to potentially phobic stimuli. *Journal of Experimental Psychology: General, 105,* 313–337.

Olds, J., & Milner, R. (1954). Positive reinforcement produced by electrical stimulation of septal area and other regions of rat brain. *Journal of Comparative and Physiological Psychology, 47,* 419–427.

Ornitz, E. M. (1985). Neurophysiology of infantile autism. *Journal of American Academy of Child Psychiatry, 24,* 251–262.

Osterweis, M., Solomon, F., & Green, M. (1984). *Bereavement: Reactions, consequences and care.* Washington, DC: National Academy Press.

Pakalnis, A., Drake, M. E., Kuruvilla, J. & Kellum, J. B. (1987). Forced normalization: Acute psychosis after seizure control in seven patients. *Archives of Neurology, 44,* 289–292.

Palmer, R. L. (1980). *Anorexia nervosa: A guide for sufferers and their families.* New York: Penguin Books.

Pals, D. L., Towbin, K. E,. Leckman, J. F., Zahner, E. P., & Cohen, D. J. (1986). Evidence supporting an etiological relationship between Gilles de la Tourette's Syndrome and obsessive compulsive disorder. *Archives of General Psychiatry, 43,* 1180–1182.

Parker, G., Johnston, P., & Hayward, L. (1988). Parental 'expressed emotion' as a predictor of schizophrenic relapse. *Archives of General Psychiatry, 45,* 806–813.

Patterson, D. (1987, August). The causes of Down's syndrome. *Scientific American, 257,* 52–59.

Patterson, G. R. (1986). Performance models for antisocial boys. *American Psychologist, 41,* 432–444.

Paul, G. L., & Lentz, R. J. (1977). *Psychological treatment of chronic mental patients.* Cambridge, MA: Harvard University Press.

Paul, J., Froster-Iskenius, U., Moje, W., Schwinger, E. (1984). Heterozygous female carriers of the marker-X-chromosome: IQ estimation and replication status of fra(X)(q). *Human Genetics, 66,* 344–346.

Paul, S. M., & Skolnick, P. (1981). Benzodiazepine receptors and psychopathological states: Towards a neurobiology of anxiety. In D. F. Klein & J. Rabkin (Eds.), *Anxiety: New research and changing concept* (pp. 215–230). New York: Raven.

Pauls, D. L., & Leckman, J. F. (1986). The inheritance of Gilles de la Tourette's syndrome and associated behaviors. *The New England Journal of Medicine, 315,* 993–997.

Pavlov, I. P. (1927). *Conditioned reflexes: An investigation of the physiological activity of the cerebral cortex.* New York: Dover, 1960.

Paykel, E. S. (1974). Life stress and psychiatric disorder: Applications of the clinical approach. In B. S. Dohrenwend & B. S. Dohrenwend (Eds.), *Stressful life events: Their nature and effects* (pp. 135–149). New York: Wiley.

Paykel, E. S. (1979). Recent life events in the development of the depressive disorders. In R. A. Depue (Ed.), *The psychobiology of the depressive disorders: Implications for the effects of stress* (pp. 245–262). New York: Academic Press.

Pelham, W. E., Bender, M. E., Caddell, J., Booth, S., & Moorer, S. H. (1985). Methylphenidate and children with attention deficit disorder. *Archives of General Psychiatry, 42,* 948–952.

Pendery, M. L., Maltzman, I. M., & West, L. J. (1982). Controlled drinking by alcoholics? New findings and a reevaluation of a major affirmative study. *Science, 217,* 169–175.

Pennington, B. F., Bender, B., Puck, M., Salbenblatt, J., & Robinson, A. (1982). Learning disabilities in children with sex chromosome anomalies. *Child Development, 53,* 1182–1192.

Perley, M. J., & Guze, S. B. (1962). Hysteria—the stability and usefulness of clinical criteria. *New England Journal of Medicine, 266,* 421–426.

Perris, C. (1966). A study of bipolar and unipolar recurrent depressive psychoses. *Acta Psychiatrica Scandinavica, 42,* Supplement 194.

Perse, T. L., Greist, J. H., Jefferson, J. W., Rosenfeld, R., & Dar, R. (1987). Fluvoxamine treatment of obsessive-compulsive disorder. *American Journal of Psychiatry, 144,* 1543–1548.

Petersen, K. G. I., Matousek, M., Mednick, S. A., Volavka, J., & Pollock, V. (1982). EEG antecedents of thievery. *Acta Psychiatrica Scandinavica, 65,* 331–338.

Peterson, D. (Ed.), (1982). *A mad people's history of madness.* Pittsburgh: University of Pittsburgh.

Phillips, L. (1953). Case history data and prognosis in schizophrenia. *Journal of Nervous and Mental Disease, 6,* 515–525.

Phoon, W. H. (1982). Outbreaks of mass hysteria at workplaces in Singapore: Some patterns and modes of presentation. In M. J. Colligan, J. W. Pennebaker, & L. R. Murphy (Eds.), *Mass psychogenic illness: A social psychological analysis* (pp. 21–31). Hillside, NJ: Laurence Erlbaum.

Pickar, D. (1988). Perspectives on a time-dependent model of neuroleptic action. *Schizophrenia Bulletin, 14,* 255–268.

Pickar, D., Cohen, M. R., Naber, D. & Cohen, R. M. (1982). Clinical studies of the endogenous opioid system. *Biological Psychiatry, 17,* 1243–1276.

Pilkonis, P. A., & Frank, E. (1988). Personality pathology in recurrent depression: Nature, prevalence, and relationship to treatment. *American Journal of Psychiatry, 145,* 435–441.

Pillard, R. C., & Weinrich, J. D. (1986). Evidence of familial nature of male homosexuality. *Archives of General Psychiatry, 43,* 808–812.

Pincus, J. H., & Tucker, G. J. (1985). *Behavioral neurology.* New York: Oxford University Press.

Piotrowski, Z. A. (1982). Unsuspected and pertinent microfacts in personology. *American Psychologist, 37,* 190–196.

Piran, N., Bigler, E. D., & Cohen, D. B. (1982). Motoric laterality and eye dominance suggest unique pattern of cerebral organization in schizophrenia. *Archives of General Psychiatry, 39,* 1006–1010.

Pitblado, C., & Cohen, J. (1984). State-related changes in amplitude, latency, and cerebral asymmetry of averaged evoked potentials in a case of multiple personality. *International Journal of Clinical Neuropsychology, 6,* 70.

Polani, P. E. (1981). Chromosomes and chromosomal mechanisms in the genesis of maldevelopment. In K. J. Connolly & H. F. R. Prechtl (Eds.), *Maturation and development* (pp. 50–72). Philadelphia: Lippincott.

Pontius, A. A. (1974). Basis for a neurological test of frontal lobe system functioning up to adolescence—a form analysis of actions expressed in narratives. *Adolescence, 34,* 221–232.

Pope, H. G., Jr., & Hudson, J. I. (1984). *New hope for binge eaters.* New York: Harper & Row.

Pope, H. G., Jr., & Lipinski, J. F. (1978). Diagnosis in schizophrenia and manic-depressive illness: A reassessment of the specificity of 'schizophrenic' symptoms in the light of current research. *Archives of General Psychiatry, 35,* 811–828.

Pope, H. G., Jr., Lipinski, J. F., Cohen, B. M., & Axelrod, D. T. (1980). "Schizoaffective disorder": An invalid diagnosis? A comparison of schizoaffective disorder, schizophrenia, and affective disorder. *American Journal of Psychiatry, 137,* 921–927.

Porrino, L. J., Rapoport, J. L., Behar, D., Sceery, W., Ismond, D. R., Bunny, W. E., Jr. (1983). A naturalistic assessment of the motor activity of hyperactive boys. *Archives of General Psychiatry, 40,* 681–687.

Posner, M. I., Early, T. S., Reiman, E., Pardo, P. J., & Dhawan, M. (1988). Asymmetries in hemisphere control of attention in schizophrenia. *Archives of General Psychiatry, 45,* 814–821.

Posner, M. I., Petersen, S. E., Fox, P. T., & Raichle, M. E. (1988). Localization of cognitive operations in the human brain. *Science, 240,* 1627–1631.

Post, R. M., Rubinow, D. R., Uhde, T. W., Roy-Byrne, P. P. Linnoila, M. et al. (1989). Dysphoric mania: Clinical and biological correlates. *Archives of General Psychiatry, 46,* 353–358.

Pribram, K. H., & McGuiness, D. (1975). Arousal, activation, and effort in the control of attention. *Psychological Bulletin, 82,* 116–149.

Price, R. A., Kidd, K. K., Cohen, D. J., Pauls, D. L., & Leckman, J. F. (1985). A twin study of Tourette syndrome. *Archives of General Psychiatry, 42,* 815–820.

Prince, M. (1906). *The dissociation of a personality: A biographical study in abnormal psychology.* New York: Greenwood Press, 1969.

Procci, W. R. (1976). Schizo-affective psychosis: Fact or fiction: A survey of the literature. *Archives of General Psychiatry, 33,* 1167–1178.

Propping, P. (1978). Alcohol and alcoholism. *Human Genetics, Supplement,* 91–99.

Purtell, J. J., Robins, E., & Cohen, M. E. (1951). Observations on clinical aspects of hysteria. *Journal of the American Medical Association, 146,* 902–909.

Putnam, F. W. (1986). The scientific investigation of multiple personality disorder. In J. M. Queen (Ed.), *Split minds split brains: Historical and current perspectives* (pp. 109–125). New York: New York University Press.

Putnam, F. W., Guroff, J. J., Silberman, E. K., Barban, L., & Post, R. M. (1986). The clinical phenomenology of multiple personality disorder: Review of 100 recent cases. *Journal of Clinical Psychiatry, 47,* 285–293.

Quay, H. C. (1986a). Conduct disorders. In H. C. Quay & J. S. Werry (Eds.), *Psychopathological disorders of childhood* (3rd ed.) (pp. 35–72). New York: John Wiley & Sons.

Quay, H. C. (1986b). A critical analysis of DSM-III as a taxonomy of psychopathology in childhood and adolescence. In T. Millon & G. L. Klerman (Eds.), *Contemporary directions in psychopathology* (pp. 151–165). New York: Guilford Press.

Quinsey, V. L., & Marshall, W. L. (1983). Procedures for reducing inappropriate sexual arousal: An evaluation review. In J. G. Greer & I. R. Stuart (Eds.), *The sexual aggressor: Current perspectives on treatment* (pp. 267–289). New York: Van Nostrand Reinhold Co.

Rabiner, C. J., Wegner, J. T., & Kane, J. M. (1986). Outcome study of first-episode psychosis, I. Relapse rates after 1 year. *American Journal of Psychiatry, 143,* 1155–1158.

Rabkin, J. G., & Struening, E. L. (1976). Life events, stress, and illness. *Science,194,* 1013–1194.

Rachman, S. J. (1974). Primary obsessional slowness. *Behaviour Research and Therapy, 11,* 463–471.

Rachman, S. J. (1978). *Fear and courage.* San Francisco: Freeman.

Rachman, S. J. (1983). Obstacles to the successful treatment of obsessions. In E. B. Foa & P. M. G. Emmelkamp (Eds.), *Failures in behavior therapy* (pp. 35–57). New York: Wiley.

Rachman, S. J. (1984). The experimental analysis of agoraphobia. *Behaviour Research and Therapy, 22,* 631–640.

Rachman, S. J., & Hodgson, R. (1974). Synchrony and desynchrony in fear and avoidance. *Behaviour Research and Therapy, 12,* 311–318.

Rachman, S. J., & Hodgson, R. J. (1980). *Obsessions and compulsions.* Englewood Cliffs, NJ: Prentice-Hall.

Rachman, S. J., & Wilson, G. T. (1980). *The effects of psychological therapy* (2nd ed.). New York: Pergamon Press.

Rapoport, J. L. (1983) The use of drugs: Trends in research. In M. Rutter (Ed.), *Developmental neuropsychiatry* (pp. 385–403). New York: Guilford Press.

Rapoport, J. L. (1988). The neurobiology of obsessive-compulsive disorder. *Journal of the American Medical Association, 260,* 2888–2890.

Raps, C. S., Peterson, C., Reinhard, K. E., & Abramson, L. Y. (1982). Attributional style among depressed patients. *Journal of Abnormal Psychology, 91,* 102–108.

Ratner, S. C. (1967). Comparative aspects of hypnosis. In J. Gordon (Ed.), *Handbook of clinical and experimental neurosis.* New York: Macmillan.

Ray, O. S. (1972). *Drugs, society and human behavior.* St. Louis: C. V. Mosby.

Rechtschaffen, A., & Kales, A. (Eds.) (1968) *A manual of standard terminology, techniques and scoring system for sleep stages of human subjects.* Bethesda: HEW Neurological Information Network.

Redmond, D. E., Jr., (1985). Neurochemical basis for anxiety and anxiety disorders: Evidence from drugs which decrease human fear or anxiety. In A. H Tuma & J. Maser (Eds.), *Anxiety and the anxiety disorders* (pp. 533–555). Hillsdale, NJ: Laurence Erlbaum.

Reed, T. E. (1985). Ethnic differences in alcohol use, abuse, and sensitivity. A review with genetic interpretation. *Social Biology, 32,* 195–209.

Regier, D. A., & Burke, J. D., Jr., (1985). Epidemiology. In H. I. Kaplan & B. J. Sadock (Eds.), *Comprehensive Textbook of Psychiatry/IV* (4th edition), Vol. 1 (pp. 295–312). Baltimore: Williams & Wilkins.

Reich, W. (1933/1949). *Character analysis* (3rd ed.). New York: Farrar, Straus and Giroux.

Reinisch, J. M. (1981). Prenatal exposure to synthetic progestins increases potential for aggression in humans. *Science, 211,* 1171–1173.

Reisberg, B. (Ed.) (1983). *Alzheimer's disease.* New York: The Free Press.

Reisenzein, R. (1983). The Schachter theory of emotion: Two decades later. *Psychological Bulletin, 94,* 239–264.

Reitan, R. M., & Davison, L. A. (Eds.) (1974). *Clinical neuropsychology: Current status and applications.* Washington, DC: V. H. Winston & Sons.

Rescorla, R. A. (1988). Pavlovian conditioning: It's not what you think it is. *American Psychologist, 43,* 151–160.

Reveley, A. M., Reveley, M. A., Clifford, C. A., & Murray, R. M. (1982, March 6). Cerebral ventricular size in twins discordant for schizophrenia. *Lancet,* 540–541.

Reveley, A. M., Reveley, M. A., & Murray, R. M. (1983, August 27). Enlargement of cerebral ventricles in schizophrenics is confined to those without known genetic predispositions. *Lancet,* 525.

Reynolds, C. F., III & Kupfer, D. J. (1987). Sleep research in affective illness: State of the art circa 1987. *Sleep, 10,* 199–205.

Richardson, S., & Tolis, G. (1984). Gonadal dysfunction in anorexia nervosa. In N. S. Shah & A. G. Donald (Eds.), *Psychoneuroendocrine dysfunction.* New York: Plenum.

Rickels, K. (1981). Benzodiazepines: Use and misuse. In D. F. Klein & J. Rabkin (Eds.), *Anxiety: New research and changing concepts* (pp. 1–24). New York: Raven.

Riley, K. C. (1984). Unraveling hysteria: A neuropsychological investigation of Briquet syndrome. Unpublished Doctoral Dissertation, University of Texas at Austin, 1984.

Rimland, B. (1964). *Infantile autism.* New York: Meredity Publishing Co.

Rimland, B. (1978). Savant capabilities of autistic children and their cognitive implications. In G. Serban (Ed.), *Cognitive defects in the development of mental illness* (pp. 43–65). New York: Brunner/Mazel.

Ritvo, E. R., Freeman, B. J.,Mason-Brothers, A., Mo, A., & Ritvo, A. M. (1985). Concordance for the syndrome of autism in 40 pairs of afflicted twins. *American Journal of Psychiatry, 142,* 74–77.

Rivinus, T. M., Biederman, J., Herzog, D. B., Kemper, K. et al. (1984). Anorexia nervosa and affective disorders: A controlled family history study. *American Journal of Psychiatry, 141,* 1414–1418.

Roberts, J. A. F. (1952). The genetics of mental deficiency. *Eugenics Review, 44,* 71–83.

Roberts, L. (1988). Study raises estimate of Vietnam war stress. *Science, 241,* 788.

Robertson, H. A., Martin, I. L., & Candy, J. M. (1978) Differences in benzodiazepine receptor binding in Maudsley reactive and Maudsley non-reactive rats. *European Journal of Pharmacology, 50,* 455–457.

Robins, E. (1981). *The final months: Study of the lives of 134 persons who committed suicide.* New York: Oxford University Press.

Robins, E., & Guze, S. B. (1970). Establishment of diagnostic validity in psychiatric illness: Its application to schizophrenia. *American Journal of Psychiatry, 126,* 983–987.

Robins, L. N. (1966). *Deviant children grown up.* Baltimore: Williams & Wilkins.

Robins, L. N. (1978). Aetiological implications in studies of childhood histories relating to antisocial personality. In R. D. Hare, & D. Schalling (Eds.), *Psychopathic behaviour: Approaches to research* (pp. 256–271). Chichester, England: Wiley & Sons.

Robins, L. N., Helzer, J. E., & Davis, D. H. (1975). Narcotic use in Southeast Asia and afterward. *Archives of General Psychiatry, 32,* 955–961.

Robins, L. N., Helzer, J. E., Weissman, M. M., Orvaschel, H., Gruenberg, E., Burke, J. D. Jr., & Regier, D. A. (1984). Lifetime prevalence of specific psychiatric disorders in three sites. *Archives of General Psychiatry, 41,* 949–958.

Robinson, R. G., Boston, J. D., Starkstein, S. E., & Price, T. R. (1988) Comparison of mania and depression after brain injury: Causal factors. *American Journal of Psychiatry, 145,* 172–178.

Rodnick, E., & Shakow, D. (1940). Set in the schizophrenic as measured by composite reaction time index. *American Journal of Psychiatry, 90,* 214–255.

Rogers, R. (1987). APA's position on the insanity defense: Empiricism versus emotionalism. *American Psychologist, 42,* 840–848.

Rokeach, M. (1964). *The three Christs of Ypsilanti.* New York: Vintage.

Rose, R. J., Reed, T., Bogle, T. (1987). Asymmetry of *a-b* ridge count and behavioral discordance of monozygotic twins. *Behavior Genetics, 17* 125–140.

Rosenbaum, G., Shore, D. L., & Chapin, K. (1988). Attention deficit in schizophrenia and schizotypy: Marker versus symptom variables. *Journal of Abnormal Psychology, 97,* 41–47.

Rosenhan, D. L. (1973). On being sane in insane place. *Science, 179,* 250–258.

Rosenthal, D. (1963). *The Genain Quadruplets.* New York: Basic Books.

Rosenthal, D. (1970). *Genetic theory and abnormal behavior.* New York: McGraw-Hill.

Rosenthal, D., Wender, P. H., Kety, S. S., Schulsinger, F., Welner, J., & Ostergaard, L. (1968). Schizophrenics' offspring reared in adoptive homes. In D. Rosenthal & S. S. Kety (Eds.), *The transmission of schizophrenia* (pp. 377–391). Oxford: Pergamon.

Ross, D. M., & Ross, S. A. (1976). *Hyperactivity: Research, theory and action.* New York: Wiley.

Ross, E. D., & Rush, A. J. (1981). Diagnosis and neuroanatomical correlates of depression in brain-damaged patients. *Archives of General Psychiatry, 38,* 1344–1354.

Ross, T. A. (1937). The common neuroses. Baltimore: Wood.

Roth, M. (1986). The association of clinical and neurological findings and its bearing on the classification and aetiology of Alzheimer's disease. *British Medical Bulletin, 42,* 42–50.

Rottenberg, H., Waring, A., & Rubin, E. (1981). Tolerance and cross-tolerance in chronic alcoholics: Reduced membrane binding of ethanol and other drugs. *Science, 213,* 583–585.

Rounsaville, B. J., Weissman, M. M., Kleber, H., & Wilber, C. (1982). Heterogeneity of psychiatric diagnosis in treated opiate addicts. *Archives of General Psychiatry, 39,* 161–166.

Roy, A. *Hysteria* (1982). Chichester, England: Wiley.

Roy, A. (1985). Early parental separation and adult depression. *Archives of General Psychiatry, 42,* 987–991.

Royce, J. R., & Covington, M. (1960). Genetic differences in the avoidance conditioning of mice. *Journal of Comparative and Physiological Psychology, 53,* 197–200.

Rozin, P. (1976). The psychological approach to human memory. In M. R. Rosenzweig & E. L. Bennett (Eds.), *Neural mechanisms of learning and memory* (pp. 3–46). Cambridge, Massachusetts: MIT Press.

Rubinow, D. R., Roy-Byrne, P., Hoban, M. C., Gold, P. W., & Post, R. M. (1984). Prospective assessment of menstrually related mood disorders. *American Journal of Psychiatry, 141,* 684–686.

Rudel, R. G. (1980). Learning disability: Diagnosis by exclusion and discrepancy. *Journal of the American Academy of Child Psychiatry, 19,* 547–569.

Rush, J. A., Erman, M. K., Giles, D. E., Schlesser, M. A., Carpenter, G., Nishendu, V., & Roffwarg, H. P. (1986). Polysomnographic findings in recently drug-free and clinically remitted depressed patients. *Archives of General Psychiatry, 43,* 878–884.

Russell, D. E. H. (1983). The incidence and prevalence of intrafamilial and extrafamilial sexual abuse of female children. *Child Abuse and Neglect, 7,* 133–146.

Russell, G. F. M., Szumkler, G. I., Dare, C., & Eisler, I. (1987). An evaluation of family therapy in anorexia nervosa and bulimia nervosa. *Archives of General Psychiatry, 44,* 1047–1056.

Rutter, D. R. (1979). The reconstruction of schizophrenic speech. *British Journal of Psychiatry, 134,* 356–359.

Rutter, M. (1972). Relationships between child and adult psychiatric disorders. *Acta Psychiatrica Scandinavica, 48,* 3–21.

Rutter, M. (1981). Psychological sequelae of brain damage in children. *American Journal of Psychiatry, 138,* 1533–1544.

Rutter, M. (1982). Cognitive deficits in the pathogenesis of autism. *Journal of Child Psychology and Psychiatry, 24,* 513–531.

Rutter, M., & Garmezy, N. (1983). Developmental psychopathology. In E. M. Hetherington (Ed.), *Socialization, personality, and social development* (pp. 775–911). New York: John Wiley & Sons.

Saccuzzo, D. P., & Braff, D. L. (1981). Early information processing deficit in schizophrenia: New findings using schizophrenic subgroups and manic control subjects. *Archives of General Psychiatry, 38,* 175–179.

Saccuzzo, D. P., & Schubert, D. L. (1981). Backward masking as a measure of slow processing in schizophrenia spectrum disorders. *Journals of Abnormal Psychology, 90,* 305–312.

Sachar, E. J. (1981). Psychobiology of affective disorders. In E. R. Kandel & J. H. Schwartz (Eds.), *Principles of neural science* (pp. 611–619). New York: Elsevier/North Holland.

Sackheim, H. A., Nordlie, N. W., & Gur, R. C. (1979). A model of hysterical and hypnotic blindness: Cognition, motivation, and awareness. *Journal of Abnormal Psychology, 88,* 474–489.

Sacks, O. (1974). *Awakenings.* New York: Vintage Books.

Sacks, O. (1985). *The man who mistook his wife for a hat.* New York: Summit Books.

Saghir, M. T., & Robins, E. (1973). *Male and female homosexuality: A comprehensive investigation.* Baltimore: Williams & Wilkins.

Sainsbury, P. (1968). Suicide and depression. In A. Coppen & A. Walk (Eds.), *Recent developments in affective disorders: A symposium* (pp. 1–13). London: Royal Medico-Psychological Association.

Salkovskis, P. M., & Harrison, J. (1984). Abnormal and normal obsessions—A replication. *Behaviour Research and Therapy, 22,* 549–552.

Sarason, I. G. (1972). *Abnormal psychology: The problem of maladaptive behavior.* New York: Appleton-Century-Croft.

Sarbin, T. R. (1981). On self-deception. In T. A. Sebeok & R. Rosenthal (Eds.). *The Clever Hans phenomenon: Communication with horses, whales, apes, and people* (pp. 200–235). New York: New York Academy of Sciences.

Sartorius, N., Shapiro, R., & Jablensky, A. (1974). The international pilot study of schizophrenia. *Schizophrenia Bulletin, 1,* 21–35.

Satterfield, J. H., Hoppe, C. M., & Schell, A. M. (1982). A prospective study of delinquency in 110 adolescent boys with attention deficit disorder and 88 normal adolescent boys. *American Journal of Psychiatry, 139,* 795–798.

Satterfield, J. H., Satterfield, B. T., & Schell, A. M. (1987). Therapeutic interventions to prevent delinquency in hyperactive boys. *Journal American Academy of Child and Adolescent Psychiatry, 26,* 56–64.

Schact, T., & Nathan, P. E. (1977). But is it good for the psychologists?: Appraisal and status of DSM-III. *American Psychologist, 32,* 1017–1025.

Schacter, S. (1982). Recidivism and self-cure of smoking and obesity. *American Psychologist, 37,* 436–444.

Schafer, R. (1948). *The clinical application of psychological tests: Diagnostic summaries and case studies* (Menninger Foundation monograph series No. 6). New York: International Universities Press.

Schafer, R. (1954). *Psychoanalytic interpretation in Rorschach testing.* New York: Grune & Stratton.

Schallert, T. (1983). Sensorimotor impairment and recovery of function in brain-damaged rats: Reappearance of symptoms during old age. *Behavioral Neuroscience, 97,* 159–164.

Schalling, D. (1978). Psychopathy-related personality variables and the psychophysiology of socialization. In R. D. Hare & D. Schalling (Eds.), *Psychopathic behaviour: Approaches to research* (pp. 85–106). Chichester, England: Wiley & Sons.

Schatzman, M. (1973). Paranoia or persecution: The case of Schreber. *History of Childhood Quarterly, 1,* 62–88.

Schellenberg, G. D., Bird, T. D., Wijsman, E. M., et al. (1988). Absence of linkage of chromosomal 21q21 markers to familial Alzheimer's disease. *Science, 241,* 1507–1510.

Schenk, L., & Bear, D. (1981). Multiple personality and related dissociative phenomena in patients with temporal lobe epilepsy. *American Journal of Psychiatry, 138,* 1311–1316.

Schmauk, F. J. (1970). Punishment, arousal, and avoidance learning in sociopaths. *Journal of Abnormal Psychology, 76,* 325–335.

Schoeneman, T. J. (1977). The role of mental illness in the European witch hunts of sixteenth and seventeenth centuries: An assessment. *Journal of the History of the Behavioral Sciences, 13,* 337–351.

Schofield, W., & Balian, L. (1959). A comparative study of personal histories of schizophrenic and nonpsychiatric patients. *Journal of Abnormal and Social Psychology, 59,* 216–225.

Schomer, D. L. (1983). Partial epilepsy. *The New England Journal of Medicine, 309,* 536–539.

Schonfeld, I. S., Shaffer, D., O'Connor, P., & Portnoy, S. (1988). Conduct disorder and cognitive functioning: Testing three causal hypotheses. *Child Development, 59,* 993–1007.

Schou, M. (1988). Lithium treatment of manic-depressive illness: Past, present, and perspectives. *Journal of the American Medical Association, 259,* 1834–1836.

Schreiber, F. (1973). *Sybil.* Chicago: Henry Regnery. (Reprints of Warner Paperback Library, New York, 1974).

Schuckit, M. A. (1985a). Ethanol-induced changes in body sway in men at high alcoholism risk. *Archives of General Psychiatry, 42,* 375–379.

Schuckit, M. A. (1985b). A one-year follow-up of men alcoholics given disulfiram. *Journal of Studies on Alcohol, 46,* 191–195.

Schulsinger, F. (1972). Psychopathy: Heredity and environment. *International Journal of Mental Health, 1,* 190–206.

Schulsinger, F., Kety, S. S., Rosenthal, D., & Wender, P. H. (1979). A family study of suicide. In M. Schou & E. Stromgren (Eds.), *Origin, prevention and treatment of affective disorders* (pp. 277–287). London: Academic Press.

Schuster, C. R., Renault, P. F., & Blaine, J. (1979). An analysis of the relationship of psychopathology to non-medical drug use. In R. W. Pickens & L. L. Heston (Eds.), *Psychiatric factors in drug abuse* (pp. 1–19). New York: Grune & Stratton.

Schwartz, R. H., & Wirtz, P. (1988). Suicide attempts by high school students. *American Journal of Psychiatry, 145,* 537.

Scott, J. P. (1968). *Early experience and the organization of behavior.* Belmont, CA: Wadsworth.

Scoville, W. B., & Milner, B. (1957). Loss of recent memory after bilateral hippocampal lesions. *Journal of Neurology, Neurosurgery, and Psychiatry, 20,* 11–21.

Searles, J. S. (1985). A methodological and empirical critique of psychotherapy outcome meta-analysis. *Behaviour Research and Therapy, 23,* 453–463.

Searles, J. S. (1988). The role of genetics in the pathogenesis of alcoholism. *Journal of Abnormal Psychology, 97,* 153–167.

Seidman, L. J. (1983). Schizophrenia and brain dysfunction: An integration of recent neurodiagnostic findings. *Psychological Bulletin, 94,* 195–238.

Seif, M. N., & Atkins, A. L. (1979). Some defensive and cognitive aspects of phobias. *Journal of Abnormal Psychology, 88,* 42–51.

Selfe, L. (1977). *Nadia: A case of extraordinary drawing ability in an autistic child.* New York: Academic Press.

Seligman, M. E. P. (1970). On the generality of the laws of learning. *Psychological Review, 77,* 406–418.

Seligman, M. E. P. (1975). *Helplessness: On depression, development, and death.* San Francisco: Freeman.

Selye, H. (1976). *Stress in health and disease.* Reading, MA: Butterworth.

Shader, R. I., Scharfman, E. L., & Dreyfuss, D. A. (1986). A biological model for selected personality disorders. In A. M. Cooper, A. J. Frances, & M. H. Sacks (Eds.), *Psychiatry Volume 1: The personality disorders and neuroses* (pp. 41–51). Philadelphia: Lippincott.

Shah, A., & Frith, U. (1983). An islet of ability in autistic children: A research note. *Journal of Child Psychology and Psychiatry, 24,* 613–620.

Shakow, D. (1977). Segmental set: The adaptive process in schizophrenia. *American Psychologist, 32,* 129–139.

Shalev, A., & Munitz, H. (1986). Conversion without hysteria: A case report and review of the literature. *British Journal of Psychiatry, 148,* 198–203.

Shapiro, S., Skinner, E. A., Kessler, L. G., Van Korff, M., German, P. S. et al. (1984). Utilization of health and mental health services. *Archives of General Psychiatry, 41,* 971–978.

Shapiro, D. A., & Shapiro, D. (1982). Meta-analysis of comparative outcome studies: A replication and refinement. *Psychological Bulletin, 92,* 581–604.

Sheard, M. H. (1980, April). The biological effects of lithium. *Trends in Neuroscience,* 85–86.

Sheehan, D. V. (1982, September). Current perspectives in its treatment of panic and phobic disorders. *Drug Therapy,* 179–193.

Shepher, D. (1971). Mate selection among second generation kibbutz adolescents and adults. Incest avoidance and negative imprinting. *Archives of Sexual Behavior, 1,* 293–307.

Sherrington, R., Brynjolfsson, J., Petursson, H., Potter, M., Dudleston, K. et al. (1988). Location of a susceptibility locus for schizophrenia on chromosome 5. *Nature, 336,* 164–167.

Sherwood, G. G., & Gray, J. E. (1974). Two "classic" behavior modification patients: A decade later. *Canadian Journal of Behavioral Science, 6,* 420–427.

Shields, J. (1982). Genetical studies of hysterical disorders. In A. Roy (Ed.), *Hysteria* (pp. 41–56). Chichester, England: Wiley.

Shimkunas, A. M. (1972). Demand for intimate self-disclosure and pathological verbalizations in schizophrenia. *Journal of Abnormal Psychology, 80,* 197–205.

Shneidman, E. (1972). Classifications of suicidal phenomena. In B. Q. Hafen & E. J. Faux (Eds.), *Self destructive behavior: A national crisis* (pp. 10–22). Minneapolis: Burgess.

Shneidman, E. (1985). *Definition of suicide.* New York: Wiley-Interscience.

Siegel, C., Waldo, M., Mizner, G., Adler, L. E., & Freedman, R. (1984). Deficits in sensory gating in schizophrenic patients and their relatives: Evidence obtained with auditory evoked responses. *Archives of General Psychiatry, 41,* 607–612.

Sigvardsson, S., von Knorring, A-L., Bohman, M., & Cloninger, C. R. (1984). An adoption study of somatoform disorders I. The relationship of somaticization to psychiatric disability. *Archives of General Psychiatry, 41,* 853–859.

Silverman, J. (1964). Scanning-control mechanism and "cognitive filtering" in paranoid and nonparanoid schizophrenia. *Journal of Consulting Psychology, 28,* 385–393.

Silver, J. (1967). Variations in cognitive control and psychophysiological defense in the schizophrenias. *Psychosomatic Medicine, 24,* 225–251.

Simons, A., Garfield, S. L., & Murphy, G. E. (1984). The process of change in cognitive therapy and pharmacotherapy for depression. *Archives of General Psychiatry, 41,* 45–51.

Simons, A. D., Murphy, G. E., Levine, J. L., & Wetzel, R. D. (1986). Cognitive therapy and pharmacotherapy for depression. *Archives of General Psychiatry, 43,* 43–48.

Simons, R. F., MacMillan, F. W., III, & Ireland, F. B. (1982). Reaction-time crossover in preselected schizotypic subjects. *Journal of Abnormal Psychology, 91,* 414–419.

Singer, M. T., & Wynne, L. C. (1965). Thought disorder and family relations of schizophrenics: IV. Results and implications. *Archives of General Psychiatry, 12,* 201–212.

Sirois, F. (1982). Epidemic hysteria. In A. Roy (Ed.), *Hysteria* (pp. 101–115). Chichester, England: Wiley.

Sitaram, N., Nurnberger, J. I., Jr., Gershon, E. S., & Gillin, J. C. (1982). Cholinergic regulation of mood and REM sleep: Potential model and marker of vulnerability to affective disorder. *American Journal of Psychiatry, 139,* 571–576.

Sizemore, C. C., & Pittillo, E. (1977). *I'm Eve.* New York: Jove/HBC.

Skinner, B. F. (1938). *The behavior of organisms: An experimental analysis.* Englewood Cliffs, NJ: Prentice-Hall.

Skinner, H. A. (1981). Toward the integration of classification theory and methods. *Journal of Abnormal Psychology, 90,* 68–87.

Skodol, A. E., Rosnick, L., Kellman, D., Oldham, J. M., & Hyler, S. E. (1988). Validating structured DSM-III-R personality disorder assessments with longitudinal data. *American Journal of Psychiatry, 145,* 1297–1299.

Slater, E. (1961). The thirty-fifth Maudsley lectures: 'Hysteria 311.' *Journal of Mental Science, 107,* 359–381.

Slater, E. (1982). What is hysteria. In A. Roy (Ed.), *Hysteria* (pp. 37–40). Chichester, England: Wiley.

Slater, E., & Cowie, V. (1971). *The genetics of mental disorders.* London: Oxford University Press.

Slater, E., & Glithero, E. (1965). A follow-up of patients diagnosed as suffering from "hysteria." *Journal of Psychosomatic Research, 9*, 9–13.

Slovenko, R. (1980). Law and psychiatry. In H. I. Kaplan, A. M. Freedman, & B. J. Sadock (Eds.), *Comprehensive textbook of psychiatry/III* (3rd ed.), (Vol. 3) (pp. 3043–3090). Baltimore: Williams & Wilkins.

Smith, D. W. (1970). *Recognizable patterns of human malformation*. Philadelphia: W. B. Saunders.

Smith, M. L., Glass, G. V., & Miller, T. I. (1980). *The benefits of psychotherapy*. Baltimore: Johns Hopkins University Press.

Snyder, M. L., Smoller, B., Strenta, A., & Frankel, A. (1981). A comparison of egotism, negativity, and learned helplessness as explanations of poor performance after unsolvable problems. *Journal of Personality and Social Psychology, 40*, 24–30.

Snyder, S. H. (1978). The opiate receptor and morphine-like peptides in the brain. *American Journal of Psychiatry, 135*, 645.

Snyder, S. H. (1980). *Biological aspects of mental disorder*. New York: Oxford University Press.

Snyder, S. H. (1984). Drug and neurotransmitter receptors in the brain. *Science, 224*, 22–31.

Sobell, M. B., & Sobell, L. C. (1984). The aftermath of heresy: A response to Pendery *et al*'s (1981) critique of "Individualized Behavior Therapy for Alcoholics." *Behaviour Research and Therapy, 22*, 413–440.

Solanto, M. V. (1984). Neuropharmacological basis of stimulant drug action in attention deficit disorder with hyperactivity: A review and synthesis. *Psychological Bulletin, 95*, 387–409.

Solomon, R. L. (1980). The opponent-process theory of acquired motivation: The costs of pleasures and the benefits of pain. *American Psychologist, 39*, 691–712.

Solomon, R. L., & Corbit, J. D. (1974). An opponent-process theory of motivation. I. Temporal dynamics of affect. *Psychological Review, 81*, 119–145.

Solovay, M. R., Shenton, M. E., Gasperetti, C., Coleman, M., Kestnbaum, E., & Holzman, P. S. (1986). Scoring manual for the thought disorder index. *Schizophrenia Bulletin, 12*, 483–496.

Sommer, R., & Whitney, G. (1961). The chain of chronicity. *American Journal of Psychiatry, 118*, 111–117.

Sommerschield, H., & Reyher, J. (1973). Posthypnotic conflict, repression, and psychopathology. *Journal of Abnormal Psychology, 82*, 278–290.

Spanos, N. P. (1978). Witchcraft in histories of psychiatry: A critical analysis and alternative conceptualization. *Psychological Bulletin, 85*, 417–439.

Spanos, N. P., Weekes, J. R., Menary, E., & Bertrand, L. D. (1986). Hypnotic interview and age regression procedures in the elicitation of multiple personality symptoms: a simulation study. *Psychiatry, 49*, 298–311.

Spiegel, D., Hunt, T., & Dondershine, H. E. (1988). Dissociation and hypnotizability in posttraumatic stress disorder. *American Journal of Psychiatry, 145*, 301–305.

Spiegel, R., & Aebi, H. J. (1983). *Psychopharmacology: An introduction*. New York: Wiley & Sons.

Spitz, R. A. (1945). Hospitalism: An inquiry into the genesis of psychiatric conditions in early childhood. *Psychoanalytic Study of the Child, 1*, 53–74.

Spitzer, R. L. (1975). On pseudoscience in science, logic in remission, and psychiatric diagnosis: A critique of Rosenhan's "On being sane in insane places." *Journal of Abnormal Psychology, 84*, 442–452.

Spitzer, R. L., & Fleiss, J. L. (1974). A re-analysis of the reliability of psychiatric diagnosis. *British Journal of Psychiatry, 125,* 341–347.

Spitzer, R. L., Skodol, A. E., Gibbon, M., & Williams, J. B. W. (Eds.) (1981). *DSM-III case book*. Washington, DC: American Psychiatric Association.

Spitzer, R. L., Skodol, A. E., Gibbon, M., & Williams, J. B. W. (1983). *Psychopathology: A Casebook*. New York: McGraw-Hill.

Squire, L. R. (1982). The neuropsychology of human memory. *Annual Review of Neuroscience, 5,* 241–273.

Squires, K. C., Chippendale, T. J., Wrege, K. S., Goodin, D. S., & Starr, A. (1980). Electrophysiological assessment of mental function in aging and dementia. In L. W. Poon (Ed.), *Aging in the 1980s* (pp. 125–134). Washington, DC: American Psychological Association.

St. George-Hyslop, P. H., Tanzi, R. E., Polinsky, R. J., Haines, J. L., Nee, L., et al. (1987). The genetic defect causing familial Alzheimer's disease maps on chromosome 21. *Science, 235,* 885–890.

Stampfl, T. G., & Levis, D. J. (1967). Essentials of implosive therapy: A learning-theory based psychodynamic behavioral therapy. *Journal of Abnormal Psychology, 72,* 496–503.

Starkman, M. N. (1988). Phenomenology and family history of affective disorder in Cushing's disease. *American Journal of Psychiatry, 145,* 390–391.

Steinbrueck, S. M., Maxwell, S. E., & Howard, G. S. (1983). A meta-analysis of psychotherapy and drug therapy in the treatment of unipolar depression with adults. *Journal of Consulting and Clinical Psychology, 51,* 856–863.

Stekel, W. (1924). *Peculiarities of behavior, Vol 1*. New York: Boni & Liveright.

Steketee, G., & Foa, E. B. (1985). Behavioral treatment of obsessive-compulsive disorder. In D. Barlow (Ed.), *Clinical handbook of psychological disorders: A step-by-step treatment manual* (pp. 69–144). New York: Guilford Press.

Steketee, G., Foa, E. B., & Grayson, J. B. (1982). Recent advances in the behavioral treatment of obsessive-compulsives. *Archives of General Psychiatry, 39,* 1365–1371.

Stephens, J. H. (1978). Long-term prognosis and follow-up schizophrenia. *Schizophrenia Bulletin, 4,* 25–47.

Stern, C. R. (1984). The etiology of multiple personalities. In B. G. Braun (Ed.), *Symposium on multiple personality*. *The Psychiatric Clinics of North America, 7,* 149–159.

Stern, S. L., Dixon, K. N., Nemzer, E., Lake, M. D., Sansone, R. A et al. (1984). Affective disorder in the families of women with normal weight bulimia. *American Journal of Psychiatry, 141,* 1224–1227.

Stoil, M. J. (1987/88). The case of the missing gene: Hereditary protection against alcoholism. *Alcohol Health & Research World, 12,* 130–136.

Stoller, R. J. (1980). Gender identity disorders. In H. I. Kaplan, A. M. Freedman, & B. J. Sadock (Eds.), *Comprehensive textbook of psychiatry/III* (3rd ed.), *Vol. 2* (pp. 1695–1705). Baltimore: Williams & Wilkins.

Stoller, R. J. (1982). Transvestism in women. *Archives of Sexual Behavior, 11,* 99–115.

Stone, M. H. (1980). *The borderline syndromes: Constitution, personality, and adaptation*. New York: McGraw-Hill.

Stone, M. H. (1988). Toward a psychobiological theory of borderline personality disorder: Is irritability the red thread that runs through borderline conditions? *Dissociation, 1,* 2–15.

Strachan, A. M. (1986). Family intervention for the rehabilitation of schizophrenia: Toward protection and coping. *Schizophrenia Bulletin, 12,* 678–698.

Striegel-Moore, R. H., Silberstein, L. R., & Rodin, J. (1986). Toward an understanding of risk factors in bulimia. *American Psychologist, 41,* 246–263.

Strub, R. L., & Black, F. W. (1977). *The mental status examination in neurology.* Philadelphia: F. A. Davis.

Strupp, H. H. (1978). Psychotherapy research and practice: An overview. In S. L. Garfield & A. E. Bergin (Eds.), *Handbook of psychotherapy and behavior change* (pp. 3–22). New York: Wiley.

Strupp, H. H., Hadley, S. W., & Gomes-Schwartz, B. (1977). *Psychotherapy for better or worse.* New York: Jason Aronson, Inc.

Sullivan, H. S. (1954). *The psychiatric interview.* New York: Norton.

Summers, W. K., Maovski, L. V., Marsh, G. M., Tachiki, K., & Kling, A. (1986). Oral tetrahydroaminoacridine in long-term treatment of senile dementia, Alzheimer type. *The New England Journal of Medicine, 315,* 1241–1245.

Suomi, S. J., & Harlow, H. F. (1977). Production and alleviation of depressive behaviors in monkeys. In J. D. Maser & M. E. P. Seligman (Eds.), *Psychopathology: Experimental models* (pp. 131–173). San Francisco: W. H. Freeman.

Suomi, S. J., Kraemer, G. W., Baysinger, C. M., & DeLizio, R. D. (1981). Inherited and experiential factors associated with individual differences in anxious behavior displayed by Rhesus monkeys. In D. F. Klein & J. Rabkin (Eds.), *Anxiety: New research and changing concepts* (pp. 179–199). New York: Raven.

Susman, V. L., & Katz, J. L. (1988). Weaning and depression: Another postpartum complication. *American Journal of Psychiatry, 145,* 498–501.

Sussman, N., & Hyler, S. E. (1980). Factitious disorders. In H. I. Kaplan, A. M. Freedman, & B. J. Sadock (Eds.), *Comprehensive textbook of psychiatry/III* (3rd ed.) *Vol. 2* (pp. 2002–2014). Baltimore: Williams & Wilkins.

Sutcliffe, J. P., & Jones, J. (1962). Personal identity, multiple personality, and hypnosis. *International Journal of Clinical and Experimental Hypnosis, 10,* 231–269.

Sutherland, G. R. (1983). The fragile X chromosome. In G. H. Bourne & J. F. Danielli (Eds.), *International review of cytology* (Vol. 81) (pp. 107–143). New York: Academic Press.

Sutker, P. B., & Allain, A. N. Jr. (1987). Cognitive abstraction, shifting, and control: Clinical sample comparisons of psychopaths and nonpsychopaths. *Journal of Abnormal Psychology, 96,* 73–75.

Swanson, J. M., & Kinsbourne, M. (1979). State-dependent learning and retrieval: Methodological cautions and theoretical considerations. In J. F. Kihlstrom & F. J. Evans (Eds.), *Functional disorders of memory* (pp. 275–299). Hillsdale, NJ: Lawrence Erlbaum.

Swedo, W. E., Rapoport, J. L., Leonard, H., Lenane, M., & Cheslow, D. (1989). Obsessive-compulsive disorders in children and adolescents. *Archives of General Psychiatry, 46,* 335–341.

Sweeney, P. D., Anderson, K., & Bailey, S. (1986). Attributional style in depression: A meta-analytic review. *Journal of Personality and Social Psychology, 50,* 974–991.

Symons, D. (1979). *The evolution of human sexuality,* New York: Oxford University Press.

Szasz, T. S. (1970). *Ideology and insanity.* Garden City, NY: Doubleday & Co.

Tarter, R. E., McBride, H., Buonpane, N., & Schneider, D. U. (1977). Differentiation of alcoholics: Childhood history of minimal brain dysfunction, family history, and drinking pattern. *Archives of General Psychiatry, 34,* 761–768.

Taylor, C. B., Bandura, A., Ewart, C. K., Miller, N. H., & DeBusk, R. F. (1985). Exercise testing to enhance wives' confidence in their husbands' cardiac capabilities soon after clinically uncomplicated acute myocardial infarction. *American Journal of Cardiology, 55,* 635–638.

Taylor, D. (1984). Psychoanalytic contributions to the understanding of psychiatric illness. In P. McGuffin, M. F. Shanks, & R. J. Hodgson (Eds.), *The scientific principles of psychopathology* (pp. 623–676). London: Grune & Stratton.

Taylor, E. A. (1986). Childhood hyperactivity. *British Journal of Psychiatry, 149,* 562–573.

Taylor, M. A., Greenspan, B., & Abrams, R. (1979). Lateralized neuropsychological dysfunction in affective disorder and schizophrenia. *American Journal of Psychiatry, 136,* 1031–1034.

Taylor, W. S., & Martin, M. F. (1944). Multiple personality. *Journal of Abnormal and Social Psychology, 39,* 281–300.

Tearnan, B. H., Telch, M. J., & Keefe, P. (1984). Etiology and onset of agoraphobia: A critical review. *Comprehensive Psychiatry, 25,* 51–62.

Teasdale, T. W., Owen, D. B. (1984). Heredity and familial environment in intelligence and educational level—A sibling study. *Nature, 309,* 620–622.

Telch, M. J. (1988). Combined pharmacological and psychological treatments for panic sufferers. In S. Rachman & J. D. Maser (Eds.), *Panic: Psychological perspectives* (pp. 167–187). Hillsdale, NJ: Lawrence Erlbaum.

Telch, M. J. (1989). Role of cognitive appraisal in panic-related avoidance. *Behavior Research and Therapy.*

Telch, M. J., Agras, W. S., Taylor, C. B., Roth, W. T., & Gallen, C. C. (1985). Combined pharmacological and behavioral treatment for agoraphobia. *Behaviour Research and Therapy, 23,* 325–335.

Telch, M. J., Brouillard, M., Telch, C. F., Agras, W. S., & Taylor, C. B. (1989). Role of cognitive appraisal in panic-related avoidance. *Journal of Abnormal Psychology.*

Telch, M. J., Lucas, J. A., & Nelson, P. (1989). Nonclinical panic in college students : An investigation of prevalence and symptomatology. *Journal of Abnormal Psychology, 98,* 300–306.

Tellegen, A., Lykken, D. T., Bouchard, T. J., Wilcox, K. J., Rich, S., & Segal, N. L. (1988). Personality similarity in twins reared apart and together. *Journal of Personality and Social Psychology, 54,* 1031–1039.

Tennant, C. (1988). Parental loss in childhood: Its effect in adult life. *Archives of General Psychiatry, 45,* 1045–1050.

Tennant, C., Smith, A., Bebbington, P., & Hurry, J. (1981). Parental loss in childhood: Relationship to adult psychiatric impairment and contact with psychiatric services. *Archives of General Psychiatry, 38,* 309–314.

Terr, L. C. (1983). Chowchilla revisited: The effect of psychic trauma four years after a school bus kidnapping. *American Journal of Psychiatry, 140,* 1543–1550.

Ter-Pogossian, M. M., Raschle, M. E., & Sobel, B. E. (1980, October). Positron-emission tomography. *Scientific American, 176.*

Teuber, H. L. (1975). Recovery of function after brain injury in man. In *Outcome of severe damage to the nervous system,* Ciba Foundation Symposium 34. Amsterdam: Elsevier North-Holland.

Thigpen, C. H., & Cleckley, H. (1954). A case of multiple personality. *Journal of Abnormal and Social Psychology, 49,* 135–151.

Thigpen, C. H., & Cleckley, H. M. (1957). *The 3 Faces of Eve.* New York: Popular Library.

Thomas, A., Chess, S., & Birch, H. G. (1968). *Temperament and behavior disorders in children.* New York: New York University Press.

Thompson, R. F. (1986). The neurobiology of learning and memory. *Science, 233,* 941–947.

Thornhill, R., & Thornhill, N. W. (1983). Human rape: An evolutionary analysis. *Ethology and Sociobiology, 4,* 115–173.

Thorpe, G. L., & Burns, L. E. (1983). *The agoraphobic syndrome: Behavioral approaches to evaluation and treatment.* Chichester, England: Wiley.

Tienari, P., Sorri, A., Lahti, I., Naarala, M., Wahlberg, K.-E., Ronkko, T., Pohjola, J., & Moring, J. (1985). The Finnish adoptive family study of schizophrenia. *Yale Journal of Biology and Medicine, 58,* 227–237.

Tomlinson, B. E., Blessed, G., & Roth, M. (1968). Observations on the brains of non-demented old people. *Journal of Neurological Science, 7,* 331–356.

Torgersen, S. (1979). The nature and origin of common phobic fears. *British Journal of Psychiatry, 134,* 343–351.

Torgerson, S. (1983). Genetic factors in anxiety disorders. *Archives of General Psychiatry, 40,* 1085–1089.

Tourian, A. Y., & Sudbury, J. B. (1978). Phenylketonuria. In J. B. Stanbury, J. B. Wyngaarden, & D. S. Fredrickson (Eds.), *The metabolic basis of inherited disease* (pp. 240–255). New York: McGraw-Hill.

Tracy, F., Donnelly, H., Morgenbesser, L., & MacDonald, D. (1983). Program evaluation: Recidivism research involving sex offenders. In J. G. Greer & I. R Stuart (Eds.), *The sexual aggressor: Current perspectives on treatment* (pp. 198–213). New York: Van Nostrand Reinhold Co.

Trautner, R. J., Cummings, J. L., Read, S. L., & Benson, D. F. (1988). Idiopathic basal ganglia calcification and organic mood disorder. *American Journal of Psychiatry, 145,* 350–353.

Treiser, S. L., Cascio, C. S., Donohue, T. L., Thoa, N. B., Jacobowitz, D. M., & Kellar, K. J. (1981). Lithium increases serotonin release and decreases serotonin receptors in the hippocampus. *Science, 213,* 1529–1531.

Trimble, M. R. (1981). *Post-traumatic neurosis.* Chichester, England: Wiley.

Trower, P., & Turland, D. (1984). Social phobia. In S. M. Turner (Ed.), *Behavioral theories and treatment of anxiety* (pp. 321–365). New York: Plenum.

Tsuang, M. T., Dempsey, G. M., & Rauscher, F. (1976). A study of "atypical schizophrenia:" Comparison with schizophrenia and affective disorder by sex, age of admission, precipitant, outcome, and family history. *Archives of General Psychiatry, 33,* 1157–1160.

Tsuang, M. T., Lyons, M. J., & Faraone, S. V. (1987). Problems of diagnosis in family studies. *Journal of Psychiatric Research, 21,* 391–399.

Turner, R. J., & Wagonfeld, M. O. (1967). Occupational mobility and schizophrenia: An assessment of the social causation and social selection hypotheses. *American Sociological Review, 32,* 104–113.

Turner, S. M., Beidel, D. C., & Nathan, R. S. (1985). Biological factors in obsessive-compulsive disorders. *Psychological Bulletin, 97,* 430–450.

Tutko, T. A., & Spence, J. T. (1962). The performance of process and reactive schizophrenics and brain injured subjects on a conceptual task. *Journal of Abnormal Psychology, 65,* 387–394.

Tyler, P. A. (1984). Homosexual behavior in animals. In K. Howells (Ed.), *The psychology of sexual diversity* (pp. 42–62). Oxford: Basil Blackwell.

Vaillant, G. E. (1975). Sociopathy as a human process: A viewpoint. *Archives of General Psychiatry, 32,* 178–183.

Vaillant, G. E. (1978). The distinction between prognosis and diagnosis in schizophrenia: A discussion of Manfred Bleuler's paper. In L. C. Wynne, R. L. Cromwell, & S. Matthysse (Eds.), *The nature of schizophrenia: New approaches to research and treatment* (pp. 637–640). New York: Wiley.

Vaillant, G. E. (1983a). *The natural history of alcoholism.* Cambridge, MA: Harvard University Press.

Vaillant, G. E. (1983b). Natural history of male alcoholism V: Is alcoholism the cart or the horse to sociopathy? *British Journal of Addiction, 78,* 317–326.

Vaillant, G. E. (1984). The disadvantages of DSM-III outweigh its advantages. *American Journal of Psychiatry, 141,* 542–545.

Vaillant, G. E., Gale, L., & Milofsky, E. S. (1982). Natural history of male alcoholism II. The relationship between different diagnostic dimensions. *Journal of Studies on Alcohol, 43,* 216–232.

Vaillant, G. E., & Milofsky, E. S. (1982a). The etiology of alcoholism: A prospective viewpoint. *American Psychologist, 37,* 494–503.

Vaillant, G. E., & Milofsky, E. S. (1982b). Natural history of male alcoholism IV. Paths to recovery, *Archives of General Psychiatry, 39,* 127–133.

Vaillant, G. E., & Perry, J. C. (1980). Personality disorders. In H. I. Kaplan, A. M. Freedman, & B. J. Sadock (Eds.), *Comprehensive textbook of psychiatry/III* (3rd ed.) *Vol. 2* (pp. 1562–1590). Baltimore: Williams & Wilkins.

Valenstein, E. S. (1973). *Brain control: A critical examination of brain stimulation and psychosurgery.* New York: Wiley.

Valenstein, E. S. (Ed.) (1980). *The psychosurgery debate: Scientific, legal, and ethical perspectives.* San Francisco: Freeman.

Valzelli, L. (1981). *Psychobiology of aggression and violence.* New York: Raven Press.

Vaughn, C. C., & Leff, J. P. (1976). The influence of family and social factors on the course of psychiatric illness: A comparison of schizophrenic and depressed neurotic patients. *British Journal of Psychiatry, 129,* 125–137.

Veith, I. (1965). *Hysteria: The history of a disease.* Chicago: University of Chicago Press.

Vischi, T. R. (1984). Overview of mental health services cost issues. In Z. Taintor, P. Widen, & S. A. Barrett (Eds.), *Cost considerations in mental health treatment: Settings, modalities, and providers* (pp. 5–9). Washington, DC: U.S. Government Printing Office.

Vogel, F., & Motulsky, A. G. (1979, 1986). *Human genetics: Problems and approaches.* New York: Springer Verlag.

Vogel, G. W., Vogel, F., McAbee, R. S., & Thurmond, A. J. (1980). Improvement of depression by REM sleep deprivation. *Archives of General Psychiatry, 37,* 247–253.

Volpe, J. J., & Hill, A. (1983). Current concepts of intraventricular hemorrhage and its sequelae. In M. Wolraich & D. K. Routh (Eds.), *Advances in developmental and behavioral pediatrics (Vol. 4)* (pp. 205–234). Greenwich, CT: JAI Press Inc.

Von Zerssen, D. (1982). Personality affective disorders. In E. S. Paykel (Ed.), *Handbook of affective disorders* (pp. 212–228). New York: Guilford Press.

Wachtel, P. L. (1973). Psychodynamics, behavior therapy, and the implacable experimenter: An inquiry into the consistency of personality. *Journal of Abnormal Psychology, 82,* 324–334.

Waldrop, M. F., & Halverson, C. F. (1971). Minor physical anomalies and hyperactive behavior in young children. In J. Hellmuth (Ed.), *Exceptional infant: Studies in abnormalities,* (Vol. 2) (pp. 343–380). New York: Brunner/Mazel.

Walker, E. (1981). Attentional and neuromotor functions of schizophrenics, schizoaffectives, and patients with other affective disorders. *Archives of General Psychiatry, 38,* 1355–1358.

Walker, J. I., & Brodie, H. K. H. (1980). Paranoid disorders. In H. I. Kaplan, A. M. Freedman, & B. J. Sadock (Eds.), *Comprehensive textbook of psychiatry/III* (3rd Edition), *Vol. 2*(pp. 1288–1300). Baltimore: Williams & Wilkins.

Warburton, D. (1987). Chromosomal causes of fetal death. *Clinical Obstetrics and Gynecology, 30,* 268–277.

Ward, C. H., Beck, A. T., Mendelson, M., Mock, J. E., & Erbaugh, J. K. (1962). The psychiatric nomenclature: Reasons for diagnostic disagreement. *Archives of General Psychiatry, 7,* 198–205.

Ward, I. L. (1984). The prenatal stress syndrome: Current status. *Psychoneuroendocrinology, 9,* 3–11.

Warner, R. (1978). The diagnosis of antisocial and hysterical personality disorders. *Journal of Nervous and Mental Disease, 166,* 839–845.

Watson, J., & Rayner, R. (1920). Conditioned emotional reaction. *Journal of Experimental Psychology, 3,* 1–22.

Watson, J. D., & Crick, F. H. (1953). Molecular structure of nucleic acids: A structure for deoxyribonucleic acids. *Nature, 171,* 737–738.

Watt, N. F., Anthony, E. J., Wynne, L. C., & Rolf, J. E. (Eds.) (1984). *Children at risk for schizophrenia: A longitudinal perspective.* Cambridge: Cambridge University Press.

Watt, N. F., Fryer, J. H., Lewine, R. R. J., & Pentky, R. A. (1979). Toward longitudinal conceptions of psychiatric disorder. In B. A. Maher (Ed.), *Progress in experimental personality research* (pp. 199–283). New York: Academic Press.

Watt, N. F., Grubb, T. W., & Erlenmeyer-Kimling, L. (1982). Social, emotional, and intellectual behavior at school among children at high risk for schizophrenia. *Journal of Consulting and Clinical Psychology, 50,* 171–181.

Watt, N. F., & Lubensky, A. W. (1976). Childhood roots of schizophrenia. *Journal of Consulting and Clinical Psychology, 44,* 363–375.

Wehr, T. A., Sack, D. A., & Rosenthal, N. E. (1987). Seasonal affective disorder with summer depression and winter hypomania. *American Journal of Psychiatry, 144,* 1602–1603.

Weinberger, D. R., & Berman, K. F. (1988). Speculation on the meaning of cerebral metabolic hypofrontality in schizophrenia. *Schizophrenia Bulletin, 14,* 157–168.

Weiner, D. B. (1979). The apprenticeship of Philippe Pinel: A new document, "Observations of citizen Pussin on the insane." *American Journal of Psychiatry, 136,* 1128–1134.

Weiner, I. B. (1982). *Child and adolescent psychopathology.* New York: Wiley.

Weiner, R. D. (1984). Does electroconvulsive therapy cause brain damage? *The Behavioral and Brain Sciences, 7,* 1–53.

Weintraub, M. I. (1983). *Hysterical conversion reactions: A clinical guide to diagnosis and treatment.* New York: SP Medical and Scientific Books.

Weintraub, S., & Mesulam, M.-M. (1987). Right cerebral dominance in spatial attention: Further evidence based on ipsilateral neglect. *Archives of Neurology, 44,* 621–625.

Weiskrantz, L. (1980). Varieties of residual experience. *Quarterly Journal of Experimental Psychology, 32,* 365–385.

Weiss, G. (1983). Long-term outcome: Findings, concepts, and practical issues. In M. Rutter (Ed.), *Developmental neuropsychiatry* (pp. 422–436). New York: Guilford Press.

Weiss, J. M. (1977). Psychological and behavioral influences on gastrointestinal lesions in animal models. In J. D. Maser & M. E. P. Seligman (Eds.), *Psychopathology: Experimental models* (pp. 232–269). San Francisco: Freeman.

Weiss, J. M., Glazer, H. I., Pohorecky, L. A., Bailey, W. H., & Schneider, L. H. (1979). Coping behavior and stress-induced behavioral depression: Studies of the role of brain catecholamines. In R. A. Depue (Ed.), *The psychobiology of the depressive disorders. Implications for the effects of stress* (pp. 125–160). New York: Academic Press.

Weissman, M. M., Wickramaratne, P., Merikangas, K. R., Leckman, J. F., Prusoff, B. A., Caruso, K. A., Kidd, K. K., & Gammon, G. D. (1984). Onset of major depression in early childhood: Increased familial loading and specificity. *Archives of General Psychiatry, 41,* 1136–1143.

Wells, C. E. (1978). Chronic brain disease: An overview. *American Journal of Psychiatry, 135,* 1–12.

Wender, P. H., Kety, S. S., Rosenthal, D., Schulsinger, F., Ortmann, J., & Lunde, I. (1986). Psychiatric disorders in the biological and adopted individuals with affective disorders. *Archives of General Psychiatry, 43,* 923–929.

Wender, P. H., Reimherr, F. W., & Wood, D. R. (1981). Attention deficit disorder (minimal brain dysfunction) in adults. *Archives of General Psychiatry, 38,* 449–454.

Wender, P. H., Rosenthal, D., Kety, S. S., Schulsinger, F., & Welner, J. (1974). Crossfostering: A research strategy for clarifying the role of genetic and experiential factors in the etiology of schizophrenia. *Archives of General Psychiatry, 30,* 121–128.

Wender, P. H., Rosenthal, D., Kety, S. S., Schulsinger, F., & Welner, J. (1973). Social class and psychopathology in adoptees: A natural experimental method for separating the roles of genetic and experimental factors. *Archives of General Psychiatry, 23,* 318–325.

Wertz, R. T., Weiss, D. G., Aten, J. L., Brookshire, R. H., Garcia-Bunuel, L. et al. (1986). Comparison of clinic, home, and deferred language treatment for aphasia. *Archives of Neurology, 43,* 653–658.

West, D. J., & Farrington, D. P. (1973). *Who becomes delinquent?* London: Heinemann.

West, D. J., & Farrington, D. P. (1977). *The delinquent way of life.* London: Heinemann.

Westmoreland, B. F. (1980). Organic mental disorders associated with epilepsy. In H. I. Kaplan, A. M. Freedman, & B. J. Sadock (Eds.), *Comprehensive textbook of psychiatry/III* (3rd ed.), (Vol. 2) (pp. 1469–1482). Baltimore: Williams & Wilkins.

Whitman, F. (1980). The pre-homosexual male child in three societies: The United States, Guatemala, Brazil. *Archives of Sexual Behavior, 9,* 87–99.

White, F. J., & Wang, R. Y. (1983). Differential effects of classical and atypical antipsychotic drugs on A9 and A10 dopamine neurons. *Science, 221,* 1054–1057.

White, R. W. (1963). Ego and reality in psychoanalytic theory: A proposal regarding independent ego energies. *Psychological Issues, Monograph No. 11, 3,* 1–202.

Wickelgren, W. A. (1979). Chunking and consolidation: A theoretical synthesis of semantic networks, configuring in conditioning, S-R versus cognitive learning, normal forgetting, the amnesic syndrome, and the hippocampal arousal system. *Psychological Review, 86,* 44–60.

Widiger, T. A., & Frances, A. (1985). The DSM-III personality disorders. *Archives of General Psychiatry, 42,* 615–623.

Widiger, T. A., & Frances, A. (1987). Interview and inventories for the measurement of personality disorders. *Clinical Psychology Review, 7,* 49–75.

Widom, C. S. (1977). A methodology for studying noninstitutionalized psychopaths. *Journal of Consulting and Clinical Psychology, 45,* 674–683.

Widom, C. S. (1978). A methodology for studying non-institutionalized psychopaths. In R. D. Hare & D. Schalling (Eds.), *Psychopathic behaviour: Approaches to research* (pp. 71–84). Chichester, England: Wiley & Sons.

Wikler, A. (1980). *Opioid dependence.* New York: Plenum Press.

Willerman, L. (1973). Activity level and hyperactivity in twins. *Child Development, 44,* 288–293.

Willerman, L. (1979). *The psychology of individual and group differences.* San Francisco: Freeman.

Willerman, L., Loehlin, J. C., & Horn, J. M. (in preparation). An adoption study of parent-child resemblance on the MMPI—A preliminary report, 1989.

Williams, R. S., Hauser, J. L., Purpura, D. P., DeLong, G. R., & Swisher, C. N. (1980). Neuropathologic studies in four retarded persons with autistic behavior. *Archives of Neurology, 37,* 749–753.

Wilsnack, S. C., & Wilsnack, R. W. (1979). Sex roles and adolescent drinking. In H. T. Blane & M. E. Chafetz (Eds.), *Youth, alcohol, and social policy* (pp. 183–224). New York: Plenum Press.

Wilson, G. T. (1984). Behavior therapy. In R. J. Corsini (Ed.), *Current psychotherapies* (pp. 239–278). Itasca, IL: F. E. Peacock Publishers, Inc.

Wilson, L., & Kihlstrom, J. F. (1986). Subjective and categorical organization of recall during posthypnotic amnesia. *Journal of Abnormal Psychology, 95,* 264–273.

Wing, J. K., Cooper, J. E., & Sartorius, N. (1974). *The description and classification of psychiatric symptoms: An instruction manual for the PSE and Catego system.* London: Cambridge University Press.

Winkelstein, W., Lyman, D. M., Padian, N., Grant, R., Samuel, G., et al. (1987). Sexual practices and the risk of infection by the human immunodeficiency virus. The San Francisco Men's Health Study. *Journal of the American Medical Association, 257,* 321–325.

Winnicott, D. W. (1965). *The maturational process and the facilitating environment.* New York: International Universities Press.

Winokur, G. (1977). Delusional disorder (paranoia). *Comprehensive Psychiatry, 18, 511–521.*

Winokur, G. (1979). General discussion, Part II. In J. E. Barrett, R. M. Rose, & G. L. Klerman (Eds.), *Stress and mental disorder* (pp. 145–150). New York: Raven Press.

Winokur, G. (1985). Family psychopathology in delusional disorder. *Comprehensive Psychiatry, 26,* 241–248.

Wise, R. A. (1988). The neurobiology of craving: Implications for the understanding and treatment of addictions. *Journal of Abnormal Psychology, 97,* 118–132.

Wishnie, H. A. (1975). Inpatient therapy with borderline patients. In J. E. Mack (Ed.), *Borderline states in psychiatry* (pp. 41–62). New York: Grune & Stratton.

Witkin, H. A., Mednick, S. A., Schulsinger, F. et al. (1977). Criminality, aggression and intelligence among XYY and XXY men (pp. 165–187). In S. A. Mednick & K. O. Christiansen (Eds.), *Biosocial bases of criminal behavior*. New York: Gardner Press.

Wolff, P. H. (1972). Ethnic differences in alcohol sensitivity. *Science, 175,* 449–450.

Wolff, P. H. (1973). Vasomotor sensitivity to alcohol in diverse mongoloid populations. *American Journal of Human Genetics, 25,* 193–199.

Wolff, P. H., Gunnoe, C., & Cohen, C. (1985). Neuromotor maturation and psychological performance: A developmental study. *Developmental Medicine and Child Neurology, 27,* 344–354.

Wolfgang, M. E., Figlio, R. M., & Sellin, T. (1972). *Delinquency in a birth cohort*. Chicago: University of Chicago Press.

Wolkin, A., Angrist, B., Wolf, A., Brodie, J. D., Wolkin, B., Jaeger, J., Cancro, R., & Rotrosen, J. (1988). Low frontal glucose utilization in chronic schizophrenia: A replication study. *American Journal of Psychiatry, 145,* 251–253.

Wolpe, J. (1958). *Psychotherapy by reciprocal inhibition*. Stanford: Stanford University Press.

Wolpe, J. (1982). *The practice of behavior therapy* (3rd ed.) New York: Pergamon Press.

Wong, D. F., Wagner, H. N., Tune, L. F., Dannals, R. F., Pearlson, G. D., Links, J. M., Tamminga, C. A., Bronssole, E. P., et al. (1986). Positron emission tomography reveals elevated D_2 dopamine receptors in drug-naive schizophrenics. *Science, 234,* 1558–1563.

Wooden, K. (1980). Case history of Charles Manson. In W. Aiken, & H. LaFollette (Eds.), *Whose child? Children's rights, parental authority, and state power* (pp. 44–54). Totowa, NJ: Littlefield, Adams & Co.

World Health Organization (1979). *Schizophrenia: An international follow-up study*. Chichester, England: Wiley.

Wurtman, R. J. (1983, May 21). Behavioral effects of nutrients. *Lancet I,* 1145–1147.

Wurtman, R. J. (1985, January). Alzheimer's disease. *Scientific American, 252,* 62–74.

Wurtman, R. J., & Wurtman, J. J. (1989, January). Carbohydrates and depression. *Scientific American, 260,* 68–75.

Yablonsky, L. (1965). *The tunnel back: Synanon*. New York: Macmillan.

Yakovlev, P. I., & Lecours, A. (1967). The myelogenetic cycles of regional maturation of the brain. In A. Minkowski (Ed.), *Regional development of the brain in early life* (pp. 3–65). Oxford: Blackwell Scientific Publications.

Yarnell, H. (1940). Fire-setting in children. *American Journal of Orthopsychiatry, 10,* 272–286.

Yeudall, L. T., Fromm-Auch, D., & Davies, P. (1982). Neuropsychological impairment of persistent delinquency. *Journal of Nervous and Mental Disease, 170,* 257–265.

Yochelson, S., & Samenow, S. E. (1976). *The criminal personality. Vol. I: A profile for change*. New York: Jason Aronson.

Zajonc, R. B. (1980). Feeling and thinking: Preferences need no inferences. *American Psychologist, 35,* 151–175.

Zeigarnik, B. V. (1965). *The pathology of thinking*. New York: Consultants Bureau.

Ziegler, F. J., Imboden, J. B., & Meyer, E. (1960). Contemporary conversion reactions: clinical study. *American Journal of Psychiatry, 116,* 901–910.

Zigler, E. (1984). A developmental theory on mental retardation. In B. Blatt & R. J. Morris (Eds.), *Perspectives on special education: Personal orientations* (pp. 173–209). Glenview, IL: Scott, Foresman.

Zilbergeld, B. (1983). *The shrinking of America: Myths of psychological change.* Boston: Little, Brown.

Zilbergeld, B., & Evans, M. (1980, August). The inadequacy of Masters and Johnson. *Psychology Today, 29–43.*

Zilboorg, G., & Henry, G. W. (1941). *A history of medical psychiatry,* New York: Norton.

Zis, A. P., & Goodwin, F. K. (1982). The amine hypothesis. In E. S. Paykel (Ed.), *Handbook of affective disorders* (pp. 175–190). New York: Guilford Press.

Zohar, J., Mueller, E. A., Insel, T. R., Zohar-Kadouch, R. C., & Murphy, D. L. (1987). Serotonergic responsivity in obsessive-compulsive disorder: Comparison of patients with healthy controls. *Archives of General Psychiatry, 44,* 946–951.

Zubenko, G. S., Huff, J., Beyer, J., Auerbach, J., & Teply, I. (1988). Familial risk of dementia associated with a biologic subtype of Alzheimer's disease. *Archives of General Psychiatry, 45,* 889–893.

Zuger, B. (1984). Early effeminate behavior in boys: Outcome and significance for homosexuality. *Journal of Nervous and Mental Disease, 172,* 90–97.

Addendum to Bibliography

Dische, S. et al. (1983). Childhood nocturnal enuresis: Factors associated with outcome of treatment with an enuresis alarm. *Developmental Medicine & Child Neurology, 25,* 67-80.

Frith, C. D., & Done, D. J. (1988). Towards a neuropsychology of schizophrenia. *British Journal of Psychiatry, 153,* 437-443.

Fuller, R. K. et al. (1986). Disulfiram treatment of alcoholism. *Journal of the American Medical Association, 256,* 1449-1455.

Gazzaniga, M. S., & LeDoux, J. E. (1978). *The integrated mind.* New York: Plenum.

Guillemin, R., & Burgus, R. (1976). The hormones of the hypothalamus. In *Readings from Scientific American, Progress in psychobiology.* San Francisco: Freeman. Pp. 134-141.

Harach, J. L. (1982). The dopamine hypothesis. An overview of studies with schizophrenic patients. *Schizophrenia Bulletin, 8,* 438-469.

Harpur, T. J., Hare, R. D., & Hakstian, A. R. (1989). Two-factor conceptualization of psychopathy: Construct validity and assessment implications. *Psychological Assessment, 1,* 6-17.

Hunt, J. McV. (1941). The effects of infant feeding-frustration upon adult hoarding in the albino rat. *Journal of Abnormal Psychology, 36,* 338-360.

Lewy, A. J., Sack, R. L. Miller, L. S., & Hoban, T. M. (1987). Antidepressant medication and circadian phase-shifting effects of light. *Science, 235,* 352-354.

Lewy, A. J., Wehr, T. A. Goodwin, F. K., Newsome, D. A., & Markey, S. P. (1980). Light suppresses melatonin secretion in humans. *Science, 210,* 1267-1269.

Liversedge, L. A., & Sylvester, J. D. (1955). Writer's cramp and conditioning therapy. *Bulletin of the British Psychological Society, 26,* 19 (Abstract).

Lothstein, L. M. (1983). *Female to male transsexualism: Historical, clinical and theoretical issues.* London: Routledge.

McNally, R. J. (1987). Preparedness and phobias: A review. *Psychological Bulletin, 101,* 283-303.

Stiles, W. B., Shapiro, D. A., & Elliot, R. (1986). Are all psychotherapies equivalent? *American Psychologist, 41,* 165-180.

Trimble, B. K., & Baird, P. A., (1978). Maternal age and Down's syndrome. *American Journal of Medical Genetics, 2,* 1-5.

Van Kamen, D. P., Bunney, W. E., Jr., Docherty, J. P., Marder, S. R., Ebert, M. H. et al. (1982). *d*-Amphetamine-induced heterogeneous changes in psychotic behavior in schizophrenia. *American Journal of Psychiatry, 139,* 991-997.

Weinberger, D. R. Berman, K. F., & Zec, R. F. (1986). Physiological dysfunction of dorsolateral prefrontal cortex in schizophrenia. I. Regional cerebral blood flow evidence. *Archives of General Psychiatry, 43,* 114-124.

Whitlock, F. A. (1967). The aetiology of hysteria. *Acta Psychiatrica Scandanavica, 43,* 144-162.

Name Index

Subject Index